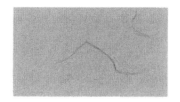

PSYCHOTHERAPY WITH SUICIDAL PEOPLE

PSYCHOTHERAPY WITH SUICIDAL PEOPLE
A Person-centred Approach

Antoon A. Leenaars

John Wiley & Sons, Ltd

Other Wiley Editorial Offices

John Wiley & Sons Inc., 111 River Street, Hoboken, NJ 07030, USA

Jossey-Bass, 989 Market Street, San Francisco, CA 94103-1741, USA

Wiley-VCH Verlag GmbH, Boschstr. 12, D-69469 Weinheim, Germany

John Wiley & Sons Australia Ltd, 33 Park Road, Milton, Queensland 4064, Australia

John Wiley & Sons (Asia) Pte Ltd, 2 Clementi Loop #02-01, Jin Xing Distripark, Singapore 129809

John Wiley & Sons Canada Ltd, 22 Worcester Road, Etobicoke, Ontario, Canada M9W 1L1

Wiley also publishes its books in a variety of electronic formats. Some content that appears
in print may not be available in electronic books.

Library of Congress Cataloging-in-Publication Data

Leenaars, Antoon A.
   Psychotherapy with suicidal people : a person-centred approach /
Antoon A. Leenaars.
      p.   cm.
Includes bibliographical references and index.
   ISBN 0-470-86341-2 (cloth : alk. paper) – ISBN 0-470-86342-0 (paper : alk. paper)
   1. Suicidal behavior.   2. Client-centered psychotherapy.   I. Title.

RC569.L44   2003
616.85′84450651–dc21

                                        2003014216

British Library Cataloguing in Publication Data

A catalogue record for this book is available from the British Library

ISBN 0-470-86341-2 (hbk)
ISBN 0-470-86342-0 (pbk)

Typeset in 10/12pt Palatino by TechBooks, New Delhi, India

This book is printed on acid-free paper responsibly manufactured from sustainable forestry
in which at least two trees are planted for each one used for paper production.

To my beloved grandmother, Cornelia van Hooijdonk
(nee. Huubrects, 5th August 1883 to 15th December 1956),
who was my first mentor on life.

CONTENTS

ABOUT THE AUTHOR

Dr Leenaars is a registered psychologist in private practice in Windsor, Canada, and is a member of the Department of Public Health Sciences at the Karolinska Institutet, Sweden, and was a member of the Department of Clinical and Health Psychology at the University of Leiden, The Netherlands. He was the first Past President of the Canadian Association for Suicide Prevention (CASP), and is a past President of the American Association of Suicidology (AAS), the only non-American to date.

He has collaborated with 100 colleagues in over 20 nations, and has published over 100 professional articles or chapters on violence, trauma, suicide, homicide, genocide, and related topics. He has published 10 previous books, and is Editor-in-Chief of *Archives of Suicide Research*, the official journal of the International Academy for Suicide Research. Dr Leenaars is a recipient of the International Association for Suicide Prevention's Stengel Award, CASP's Research Award, and AAS's Shneidman Award, for outstanding contribution in research in suicidology. He is recognized for his international efforts in suicide prevention, and has served as an expert witness in legal cases dealing with wrongful death, suicide, and homicide.

PREFACE

It is 5 December 2000 and I am in the Hotel De Doelen, room 3—an apartment in the loft—overlooking the Rapenburg Canal in Leiden, beginning to write this book. De Doelen is a 1600s patrician mansion. Leiden is The Netherlands' oldest academic city, the home of the historic University that bears the city's name. One can wish no better place to write a book.

This book is about unique people—some suicidal and some that died by suicide. The book follows the direction of Henry (Harry) Murray: "Never denigrate a fellow human being in fewer than 2000 words." The main problem facing this book is the one that is the classical issue of psychiatry/psychology itself: the mind–body problem or the admissibility of introspective qualitative accounts as opposed to objective quantitative reports. This debate resonates to Windelband's (1904) division of two possible approaches to knowledge; that is, between the nomothetic and the idiographic. The nomothetic approach deals with generalizations, using tabular, statistical, arithmetic, demographic, quantitative methods, whereas the idiographic approach involves the intense study of individual(s) (particulars). The latter typically involves the use of qualitative methods, via clinical case study, history, biography, and so on (although at times, as studies of suicide notes show, quantitative methods can also be used). In the study of each unique individual, personal documents are frequently used; for example, treatment notes, medical reports, diaries, autobiographies, third-party interviews and, if I may, suicide notes. The nomothetic approach is well engrained in suicidology, psychology, psychiatry, and science in general. Keeping in mind that a preface represents a compromise for an author between the press for greater inclusion and the need to restrict oneself to a representative introduction, the idiographic approach may need some further explication.

Gordon Allport (1942, 1962) outlined a classical statement on the advantages of the idiographic approach. Allport (1962) began with the fact that psychology is "committed to increasing man's understanding of man", both the general and the particular. This is true whether one is a psychiatrist, psychologist, social worker, medical doctor, psychiatric nurse, crisis counsellor, minister, Elder, or whatever. We are deeply interested in the individual personality—and how to treat that person. Over a century ago, John Stuart Mill proposed that we make distinctions about the general and the particular in science. He showed that both the general and the unique are critical for science's development. Mill, Freud, Allport, have all argued that for the study of human events one needs both the general and the individual. Allport's classical argument is as follows:

> Suppose we take John, a lad of 12 years, and suppose his family background is poor; his father was a criminal; his mother rejected him; his neighbourhood is marginal. Suppose that 70 percent of the boys having a similar background become criminals. Does this mean that John himself has a 70 percent chance of delinquency?
>   Allport answers: Not at all. John is a unique being.
>
> (Allport, 1962, p. 411)

Allport noted that the real issue, whether utilizing the idiographic approach or the nomothetic approach, involves methods that are rich, flexible, and precise, that "do justice to the fascinating individuality" of each individual. This fascinating individuality is humankind's complexity and this is as true for suicide as for any other behaviour. Suicide is complex—more complex than most of us imagine. It is a multidimensional malaise, with both conscious and unconscious elements. That is why I began this book with some introductory chapters on suicide and its complexity to suggest a frame—like a nautical chart for a voyage—to understand the suicidal person better. In that regard, Karl Menninger has provided us with an important dictum that is worth remembering: "The patient is always right." It is our task in psychotherapy to find out "how he/she is right".

A criticism in the field today is that the qualitative study of our clinical cases is open to different interpretations and, thus, open to a myriad of applications (Leenaars et al., 2002b). Runyan (1982a), for example, has noted that "it is claimed that Freud's case studies suffer from the critical flaw of being open to many interpretations". Of course, it is a truism that the studies of most people's lives are open to any number of theoretical templates. Some—for example, Gergen (1977)—have gone as far as to claim that the events of people's lives allow the investigator freedom to simply support his or her formulations. One can say whatever one wishes about the patient, the treatment, the death, and so on. This misuse is possible, not only in a case study but, I would add, in any type of research. Statistics too, in quantitative studies of effective intervention, can be manipulated by one's formulations as, for example, the gun control debate in the field illustrates. Among others, Runyan (1982a) has suggested that to avoid such misuse, one must "critically evaluate alternative explanations and interpretations". This multiple perspective approach has been one of the richest contributions in the field (Leenaars, 1988a), and gives the main coordinates for this book—and should be for our clinical practice. Indeed, being open to all views constitutes the very richness of human reason. Ultimately, of course, from this phenomenological view, as humans, we can only make formulations about events (Husserl, 1973), whether a suicide, suicidal behaviour or, as Kuhn (1962) showed, even science.

On one more issue, some (such as B.F. Skinner) argue that theory should not play any role in psychotherapy. This view holds that treatment (as the argument also goes in research) should be atheoretical. However, as has been discussed for millennia (e.g., Heraclitus, Plato, Freud, Durkheim, Shneidman, Farberow), theory, explicit and implicit, plays some role in research and in developing implications and applications for response from these studies (Leenaars et al., 1997). A frequent problem is that the theory is simply not stated. The clinician is then left to wonder what the information, whether from quantitative research or qualitative case study, means for him/her as he/she is found with a suicidal person in a howling storm. Yet, it is only with theory, as William James suggested at the end of the 1800s, that we can sort out experience. This book is one attempt to sort out the suicidal mess, and Leiden is the perfect setting in which to do so. I hope that the voyage has some utility in the treatment of suicidal people and I welcome all research, quantitative and qualitative, on what I write. I espouse an empirically based intervention.

The *a priori* assumption in this book: The reader already knows something about psychotherapy, counselling, crisis intervention, and so on. No one book can teach a person to be a therapist; it requires an education and experience. Thus, this book assumes a therapist's orientation, whether cognitive-behavioural, psychodynamic, relational, problem-centred, psychoanalytic, whatever. It does not teach a therapy; rather, it charts the howling seas of anguish to address the archetypal rage in the suicidal person. It offers an empirically supported definition, with applications across age, gender, historical time, and so on, as well as countries (few explanations of suicide exist globally). This understanding of suicide provides, by inference, the implications and applications for response in this book. Psychotherapy follows understanding the unique person—Sylvia, Scott, Jeff, Vincent, and any suicidal person that you will meet in the fight to stay alive (Eros over Thanatos).

These views should not be seen as coming from a non-researcher. One of my identities is as a researcher; for example, I am an inaugural member of the International Academy for Suicide Research (IASR), and am the Editor-in-Chief of their journal, *Archives of Suicide Research* (ASR). Indeed, the use of case studies (the idiographic approach, qualitative research: Leenaars, 2002) does not mean that John Stuart Mill's set of basic rules for science have to be abandoned. In his *System of Logic*, Mill (1984) reported a set of Canons for inductively establishing causality. These are the Methods of Difference, of Agreement and Difference, of Residues, and of Concomitant Variation. In my own study of suicide notes, for example, Mill's Method of Difference does not need to be abandoned, as the comparison between genuine and simulated suicide notes illustrates. John Stuart Mill has handed many of us a career.

* * *

The decision to write this book was finally made on 4 September 2000, when I was at the De Doelen with my close friend, Harvard psychiatrist, John T. Maltsberger—he prefers room 13, the grand Dutch style bedroom in the hotel, with an authentic turn-of-the-century 1800 Delft tile fireplace. He, suicidologist Edwin Shneidman, and fellow researcher David Lester (the most prolific writer in the field), urged this project on me. David Lester, John T. Maltsberger, Konrad Michel (head of the Switzerland-based Aeschi group on psychotherapy with suicidal people), and Edwin Shneidman were kind enough to consult with me here and there on the text. David Lester read the entire text, making numerous suggestions for improvement.

I have often corresponded with these colleagues and others—to name any is to miss too many—on the topic of suicide and its application to psychotherapy. The content of this book reflects their knowledge, and I am grateful to each of them.

Since my early studies in suicide, Dr Shneidman (I call him Ed) has been pivotal to my thinking (Leenaars, 1993a, 1999a). Shneidman taught: "We ought to know what we are treating." He believes that we will treat mental health problems, for example, suicide, more effectively only when we develop "clear and distinct" understanding of the suicidal person—each suicidal person. This book is an attempt to meet that challenge. His insights, in fact, are found throughout this volume, but of course, the words and conclusions are my own.

I recently asked Dr Shneidman what I should tell the readers of this book about psychotherapy; he offered the following (see *Newslink*, **27**, p. 7, for details):

> Suicide is about a person . . . a person wanting to stop pain, what I call psychache.
> Psychotherapy tries to mollify the pain. It is an anodyne. In a sense, suicide prevention tries to mollify the whole person.
> What works in psychotherapy is a view held by Sigmund Freud, William James, Erwin Stengel [*and I would add, Edwin Shneidman*], not Pavlov, Skinner or any reductionistic view. [*Ed strongly believes this point!*]
> Our treatment, psychotherapy, whatever, should address the person's story, not the demographic, nosological categories or this or that fact. It is not what the clinician knows. It is the clinician's understanding of the person's story, each individual's own story. It says, "Please tell me who you are . . . what hurts?"
> Not, "Please fill out this form . . . and give me samples of your body fluids."

Shneidman, said, however, "the practical" disadvantage of this approach is that it requires more than a few moments per patient. Suicide prevention is not an efficiency operation; it is a human exchange.

The relationship is the *sine qua non* of psychotherapy with suicidal people. There is no question: *attachment* is critical. This conclusion is based on evidence-based practice (Task Force on Empirically Supported Therapy Relationships, 2001). Our relationship in psychotherapy should be what Martin Buber (1970) called, I/Thou, not I/It. There is a definite need for a therapeutic alliance (or rapport). To put it simply: What works is quality care. This is as true in the therapy room as in the operating room. "Psychotherapy", Shneidman said, "is concerned with what kind of person that individual is."

Effective psychotherapy should be person-centred—or, if you prefer, patient-centred. Person-centred or patient-centred psychotherapy is derived from the focus on the individual—the individual in his/her entirety; i.e., biological, psychological, sociological, and so on. This is why it is also sometimes called multicomponent or multimodal psychotherapy. This simply means that it is not only psychotherapy alone—cognitive, interpersonal, whatever—that is most useful, but it may be even more effective in some cases in combination with medication—and removing the gun from the house may be even more effective. Of course, if you have read any of my papers, you will note that it is implied that my perspective includes a cognitive one (with deep thanks to Aaron T. Beck). To conclude, my approach, as you will read, is best called person-centred.

The one additional suicidologist that I do need to mention is Susanne Wenckstern (you'll find numerous references to her as co-author in my publications). Her efforts have been essential, not only as a fellow scientist and clinician, but as my wife. She served, in fact, not only as a consultant to this book, but as my personal secretary to the project. My children, Lindsey, Heather, and Kristen, since I wrote my first book, *Suicide Notes* (wherein I wrote, "despite the occasional, 'No dada, Me!'") have once more allowed me to study—and have now even served as secretaries to this book. Lindsey—who now studies psychology—went over the references twice. Sherry Purdie, as she has done faithfully for three decades, typed many of the first drafts. William Bakker, the owner of De Doelen, and his staff, have made Dutch hospitality matchless. They allowed me to have a place with a sign "Niet Storen" ("Do not Disturb"). I visited and wrote this book on a number of subsequent visits to the De Doelen, spending about 20% of my weekends in Europe in the last years, writing. I thank all the people who have fostered the development of this book.

A book is obviously written for the reader, you, and, as a final opening remark, there is one apology: There are no universal formulations in this book on how to respond to highly lethal people. When the subject matter is psychotherapy with suicidal people, we can be no more accurate than the available ways of responding, our subject matter, permits. The yearning for universal treatment laws, understandably, exists. Yet, as Drs Freud, Lester, Maltsberger, Michel, Shneidman, and Wenckstern advise, the search for a singular universal response is a chimera. There is no cookbook! As for any health clinician, say a cardiologist, the outline for psychotherapy as found in a book is not that simple in the trenches, whether in the therapy room or operating room. You—the psychiatrist, psychologist, Samaritan, social worker, counsellor, nurse, and so on—must constantly learn. I hope that this book assists, as there is no escape from the following fact: Suicidal people can be treated effectively.

Leiden, 2003

ACKNOWLEDGEMENTS

First and foremost, I need to make explicit my debt to Dr Edwin Shneidman. Not only is his education central to my suicidological career, but also he provided kind permission to reprint, present, and discuss his publications, consultations, and so on. Further, he permitted—in fact, encouraged—the reader to copy and/or use his ideas. The same is true of my ideas in this volume, including the TGSP (Chapter 6).

Specifically, because of the standards in permission, Dr Shneidman provided permission to reprint a number of published matter and material that he reproduced over and over in his own publications. This includes, but is not limited to, the following: The Facts and Myths of Suicide, The Commonalities of Suicide, The Needs of Suicidal People, The Psychological Distress Questionnaire, and parts of the following publication: Shneidman, E. (1997). The psychological autopsy. In L. Gottschalk et al., *Guide to the Investigation and Reporting of Drug Abuse Deaths* (pp. 79–210). Washington, DC: USDHEW, US Government Printing Office (by permission of E. Shneidman).

The objective of the International Academy for Suicide Research (IASR) is the promotion of high standards of research and scholarship in the field of suicidal behaviour. It fosters communication and cooperation. I am honoured to have chaired IASR's task force for future study of suicide. The task force findings resulted in a report and the task force encouraged its dissemination; thus, parts of the report are reproduced here with permission and encouragement, specifically: Leenaars, A., De Leo, D., Diekstra, R., Goldney, R., Kelleher, M., Lester, D. and Nordstrom, P. (1997). Consultations for research in suicidology. *Archives of Suicide Research*, 3, 139–151. (By permission of A. Leenaars, Chair of task force and Editor-in-Chief of *Archives of Suicide Research*.)

One further acknowledgement is needed. Once more, I had the honour of chairing an international group in the field, the International Working Group on Ethical and Legal Issues in Suicidology. The working group also included: C. Cantor, J. Connolly, M. EchoHawk, D. Gailiene, Z. He, N. Kokorina, D. Lester, A. Lopatin, M. Rodriguez, L. Schlebusch, Y. Takahashi, and L. Vijayakumar, and produced a number of reports (see details in Chapter 21). Yet, the task force also produced a full report, that was never published, but is presented here in Chapter 21, Ethical and Legal Issues. One view on ethics would be myopic in our global world. The wider perspective allows us to better understand not only the ethical and legal issues in the field, but also suicide. It allows us to say more than "in the Western world".

Grateful acknowledgement is also made for the inclusion in this volume of some of my papers that have been revised, modified, updated, edited, or otherwise. The book is, in fact, based on three decades of study in the field, and these are some of the key publications that were used to establish an empirically, peer-review-based practice for this book:

Leenaars, A. (1991). Suicide notes and their implications for intervention, *Crisis, 12*, 1–20. (By permission of Hogrefe & Huber Publishers, Gottingen, Germany.)

Leenaars, A. (1992). Suicide notes, communication, and ideation. In R. Maris, A. Berman, J. Maltsberger & R. Yufit (Eds), *Assessment and prediction of suicide* (pp. 337–361). New York: Guilford Press. (By permission of Guilford Publications, New York, USA.)

Leenaars, A. (1994). Crisis intervention with highly lethal suicidal people. *Death Studies,* **18**, 341–359. (Reproduced by permission of Taylor & Francis, Inc., Philadelphia, USA, http://www.routledge-ny.com.)

Leenaars, A. (1994). Justin: A case discussion of a suicide attempt in a four year old boy. In A. Leenaars & D. Lester (Eds), *Suicide and the unconscious* (pp. 139–174). Northvale, NJ: Jason Aronson Inc. (By permission of Jason Aronson, Inc., Northvale, NJ, USA.)

Leenaars, A. (1996). Suicide: A multidimensional malaise. (The Presidential Address.) *Suicide and Life-Threatening Behavior,* **26**, 221–236. (By permission of Antoon Leenaars and Guilford Publications, New York, USA.)

Leenaars, A. (1997). Rick: A suicide of a young adult. *Suicide and Life-Threatening Behavior,* **27**, 15–27. (By permission of Guilford Publications, New York, USA.)

Leenaars, A. (2001). Controlling the environment to prevent suicide. In D. Wasserman (Ed.). *Suicide: An unnecessary death* (pp. 259–263). London: Martin Dunitz. (By permission of Martin Dunitz, London, UK.)

Leenaars, A. & Wenckstern, S. (1998). Sylvia Plath: A protocol analysis of her last poems. *Death Studies,* **22**, 615–635. (Reproduced by permission of Taylor & Francis, Inc., Philadelphia, USA, http://www.routledge-ny.com.)

Part I

UNDERSTANDING

Suppose we take Jeff, a lad of 18 years, and suppose his family background is marked with depression; he is isolated; his pain is unbearable; and he sees no escape from his malaise, but suicide. Suppose that 70% of such young adults, having a similar background, become suicidal. Does that mean that Jeff himself has a 70% chance of killing himself? Echoing Allport, Murray, and Shneidman, the answer is—not at all. Jeff is a unique being.

We must do justice to the fascinating individuality of each person. This fascinating individuality of each person is humankind's complexity and this is as true for suicide as for any behaviour. Suicide is complex. It is a multidimensional malaise, with both conscious and unconscious elements. This is the reason why I begin this section with a few chapters to allow one to understand suicide perhaps a little better; not only suicide in general (the 70%), but suicide in the individual (the Jeffs).

Shneidman taught that: "We ought to know what we are treating." He believes that we will treat such problems as suicide more effectively only when we develop "clear and distinct" understanding of suicide. Indeed, he believes that, in the study of large issues like suicide, there is a natural progression from conceptualization to understanding and then to application and practice. This part serves somewhat like a prolegomenon to our topic: psychotherapy with a suicidal person. It consists of four chapters: an overview of suicide; a definition of suicide as a multidimensional malaise, based on the empirical study of the person's own last narrative, the suicide note; a study of the conscious and unconscious processes in suicide; and an explication to cognition, communication and suicide notes—from the story to the mind. The latter chapter is critical because it highlights how the narrative aspects of human life, in their "sameness", show the prominent or common psychological threads that allow *a* person to jump into the suicidal abyss.

Chapter 1

SUICIDE

Death is difficult to understand. Death is mysterious. It is almost universally feared and remains forever elusive. This is especially so with suicide. Almost all of us are bewildered, confused, and even overwhelmed when confronted with suicide. Yet, for some it is a final solution. Perplexing for most, it is actively sought by a few. Paradoxically, these few same people are probably the least aware of the essence of reasons for doing so. Understanding suicide, and death, is a complex endeavour for all.

DEFINITION OF SUICIDE

Briefly defined, suicide is the human act of self-inflicted, self-intentioned cessation (Shneidman, 1973). Suicide is not a disease (although there are many who think so); it is not a biological anomaly (although biological factors may play a role in some suicides); it is not an immorality (although it has often been treated as such); and it is not a crime in most countries around the world (although it was so for centuries).

It is unlikely that any one view or theory will ever define or explain phenomena as varied and as complicated as acts of human self-destruction. Our own initial definition is fraught with complexities and difficulties.

The history of our key word provides only initial assistance. "Suicide", in fact, is a relatively recent word. According to *The Oxford English Dictionary*, the word was used in 1651 by Walter Charleton when he said: "To vindicate one's self from ... inevitable Calamity, by Sui-cide is not ... a Crime." However, the exact date of its first use is open to some question. Some claim that it was first used by Sir Thomas Browne in his book, *Religio Medici*, published in 1642. Edward Philips, in his 1662 edition of his dictionary, *A New World of Words*, claimed to have invented the word. The word "suicide" does not appear in Robert Burton's *Anatomy of Melancholy* (1652 edition), nor in Samuel Johnson's *Dictionary* (1755). Before the introduction of the word, other terms, of course, were used to describe "the act"— among them self-destruction, self-killing, self-murder, and self-slaughter. Burton's phrases for suicide include "to make way with themselves" and "they offer violence to themselves". The classical (and current) German term is in keeping with this tradition—Selbstmord, or self-murder. Other countries around the world have their own words and definitions.

In the present scene, two major efforts to define the term are provided by teams of experts—the first American, and the second international: Rosenberg, Davidson, Smith, Berman, Garter, Gay, Moore-Lewis, Mills, Murray, O'Carroll, and Jobes (1988); and Leenaars, De Leo, Diekstra, Goldney, Kelleher, Lester, and Nordstrom (1997). An extensive quote of the latter group will be presented in Chapter 5. An excellent scholarly discussion of the problem of definition was offered by Douglas (1967), who outlined the fundamental dimensions of meanings that are required in the formal definition of suicide, which include aspects of initiation, willing, motivation, and knowledge. The international team (Leenaars et al., 1997) suggests that one must consider issues beyond clear definition, e.g., circumstances, medical lethality, intent. As you will read, clear definition is needed before assessment and treatment.

Suicide may today be defined differently depending on the purpose of the definition—medical, legal, administrative, etc. In the United States and Canada (and most of the countries reporting to the World Health Organization), suicide is defined (by a medical examiner or coroner) as one of the four possible modes of death. An acronym for the four modes of death is NASH: natural, accidental, suicidal, and homicidal. This fourfold classification of all deaths also has its problems. Its major deficiency is that it treats the human being in a Cartesian fashion, namely as a biological machine, rather than appropriately treating him or her as a motivated biopsychosocial organism. That is, it obscures the individual's intentions in relation to his or her own cessation and, further, completely neglects the contemporary concepts of psychodynamic psychology regarding intention, including unconscious motivation.

There is no universally accepted definition of suicide today. In fact, there never was one. Indeed, there are numerous definitions. Varah (1978) has collated a variety of definitions, and here is a sampling:

> Erwin Ringel (Austria): Suicide is the intentional tendency to take one's own life.
>
> Charles Bagg (United Kingdom): Suicide is the intentional act of taking one's life either as a result of mental illness (these illnesses frequently though not always causing distress to the individual carrying out the act) or as a result of various motivations which are not necessarily part of any designated mental illness but which outweigh the instinct to continue to live.
>
> Walter Hurst (New Zealand): The decision to commit suicide is more often prompted by a desire to stop living than by a wish to die. Suicide is a determined alternative to facing a problem that seems to be too big to handle alone.
>
> Sarah Dastoor (India):
>   I vengeful, killer, hate—inspired—so I die
>   I guilty, sinner, trapped—escaping life
>   I hoping rebirth, forgiveness divine—live again
>
> Tadeusz Kielanowski (Poland): Suicide is the most tragic decision of a man who found nobody to hold out a hand to him.

Soubrier (1993, p. 33), in his review of this topic, concluded: "A major issue in suicidology is the following: Do we have a common definition of suicide?"

The topic of definition of suicide was the focus of an entire book by Shneidman (1985). His book, *Definition of Suicide*, can be seen as a necessary step to a more effective understanding and treatment of suicide. It argued that we desperately need a clarification of the definitions of suicide—definitions that can be applied to needful persons—and he defined suicide as:

> Currently in the Western world, suicide is a conscious act of self-induced annihilation, best understood as a multidimensional malaise in a needful individual who defines an issue for which the suicide is perceived as the best solution. (Shneidman, 1985, p. 203)

This definition should not be seen as the final word, but will be used here as a *mnemonic* for understanding the event.

EPIDEMIOLOGY OF SUICIDE

It is generally believed that many actual suicides fail to be certified as suicides. Be that as it may, most suicidologists (e.g., O'Carroll, 1989) agree that official statistics on suicide can validly be used and, furthermore, Sainsbury and Barraclough (1968) have shown that cross-national comparisons can be not only validly but reliably made. Suicide rates vary from country to country (Lester, 1992). Table 1.1 shows suicide rates in 12 countries/regions of the world based primarily on the data from the World Health Organization (WHO, yearly; see www.who.int), obtained from Dr David Lester (personal communication, 12 February 2002).

The 12 nations/cultures are: Australia, Ireland, Turtle Island, Lithuania, China, Russia, United States, Cuba, South Africa, Japan, India and the Netherlands. These are the home countries of the individuals who comprise the International Working Group on Ethical and Legal Issues in Suicidology (see Chapter 21). They give us a sample of the rates of suicide around the world.

Table 1.1 Suicide rates for 12 nations/cultures

	1901	1950	1970	1980	1985	1990	1995
Australia	11.9	9.3	12.4	11.0	11.5	12.9	12.0
Ireland	2.9	2.6	1.8	6.3	7.8	9.5	11.3
Turtle Island	—	—	—	—	—	59.5[a]	—
Lithuania	—	—	—	—	34.1	26.1	44.0
China[b]	—	—	—	—	—	28.7[c]	—
Netherlands	5.8	5.5	8.1	10.1	11.3	9.7	10.1
USA	—	11.3	11.6	11.9	12.3	12.4	11.9
Cuba	—	—	11.9	—	—	—	20.3
South Africa[d]	—	—	—	—	—	17.2	—
Japan	17.7	19.6	19.2	17.7	19.4	16.4	17.2
India	—	—	9.1	6.3	7.1	8.9	9.7
Russia	—	—	—	34.6	31.2	26.5	41.5

[a] Rate based on one Inuit community. Abbey et al. (1993).
[b] WHO rates are only on a 10% sample—and separated rural/urban—so no single rate is available.
[c] Phillips and Liu (1996) 1990–1994 (cited in Lester, 1997).
[d] Rates never calculated for blacks. Schlebusch (personal communication) provided an estimated 1990 rate.

The WHO data start in 1901. The data are now published online at www.who.int and not in books. Fewer countries have data online. The WHO does not report data for distinct cultural groups; thus, there are no comprehensive data for the Native people of Turtle Island (now called North America). The rates in some aboriginal communities on Turtle Island are unbelievably high (Leenaars et al., 1999a). Within the context of very low rates historically, Abbey et al. (1993), have reported rates of 59.5 to 74.3 per 100 000 in one group, the Inuit in the Arctic. The young males are the highest risk group; for example, Wotton (1985), reported a rate as high as 295 per 100 000 for 15- to 25-year-olds in one community. This is epidemic.

Data from India are available, but not easily accessible and not well known; the India data reported here are from Lester et al. (1999). South Africa reports only crude numbers, but not for blacks. In the past, sometimes South Africa counted Asians and coloureds in addition to whites, but it is unclear why they did so, making the South African rates from the WHO probably unreliable and invalid. Lourens Schlebusch (personal communication, 27 March 2002), provided the following comment, with the cautionary note about "the only suicide rates": "Some of the studies show that in 1990 the overall suicide rate was 17.2 per 100 000, which is slightly higher than the WHO's reported world average of 16 per 100 000." More recent efforts are underway in South Africa to develop more accurate mortality statistics (Schlebusch & Bosch, 2000). China also lacks data; the rates reported by the WHO are based on only 10% of the sample. Phillips and Liu (1996, cited in Lester, 1997), provide an estimate for 1990–1994; this is the best estimate available. Other nations, for example, Lithuania and Russia, only have more recent data. Still others, for example, Cuba has provided only sporadic data. With all these caveats, Table 1.1 presents the data available from 1901, 1950, 1970, 1980, 1985, 1990, 1995. It is the best snapshot that we can get on the epidemiology (with thanks to David Lester, my forever-statistical consultant and friend).

Not only do national statistics vary but substantial variations in suicide for sub-groups also occur in these nations (e.g., age, gender, ethnicity). Age is an especially important demographic variable as children and adolescents also commit suicide. Although suicide is rare in children under 12, it occurs with greater frequency than most people imagine (we shall meet such a 4-year-old in this volume), and suicide is also an alarming problem in adolescents in many parts of the world, especially for older boys. The tragedy of adolescent suicide is especially poignant because the life expectancy of these youths is greatest in terms of both interval of years and the diversity of experiences that should await them (a few such cases will be presented later). Nonetheless, it is young adults (i.e., 18–25) and the elderly (i.e., above 55 or 60) who are most at risk. In the United States, it is the elderly who are at highest risk, again especially the males (who will also be found in this book). However, that trend is not always true in other nations. In many nations, for example, the rate of suicide for young adults is as high, if not higher, than for the elderly in some countries. In females, the highest rate occurs in middle adulthood, often the 40s. (In China, females have a higher rate than males (Phillips & Liu, 1996).)

Although space here does not allow for more detailed discussion of the epidemiology, the reader is referred to reviews (e.g., Lester, 1992) on the topic.

HISTORY OF SUICIDE

The modern era of the study of suicide—at least in the Western world—began around the turn of the twentieth century, with two main threads of investigation, the sociological and psychological, associated primarily with the names of Emile Durkheim (1858–1917) and Sigmund Freud (1856–1939), respectively. Much earlier, during the classical Greek era, suicide was viewed in very specific ways, but almost always negatively. Pythagoras of Samos (around 530 BC), who introduced the theory of number to understand man and the universe ("Number is all things and all things are number"), proposed that suicide would upset the spiritual mathematics of all things. All was measurable by number, and to exit by suicide might result in an imbalance, unlike other deaths that were in harmony with all things. Plato's position (428–348 BC), best expressed in the *Phaedo* in his quotation from Socrates, is as follows:

> Cebes, I believe . . . that the gods are our keepers, and we men are one of their possessions. Don't you think so?
>   Yes, I do, said Cebes.
>   Then take your own case. If one of your possessions were to destroy itself without intimation from you that you wanted it to die, wouldn't you be angry with it and punish it, if you had any means of doing so?
>   Certainly.
>   So if you look at it in this way I suppose it is not unreasonable to say that we must not put an end to ourselves . . .

There are, however, provisions for exceptions. The above quotation continues:

> . . . until God sends some compulsion like the one which we are facing now.

The compulsion, of course, was the condemnation by the Athenian court of Socrates for "corrupting the minds of the young and of believing in deities of his own invention instead of the gods recognised by the state" (*Apology*). Socrates then drank poison, hemlock.

Although Plato allowed for exceptions, he echoed Pythagoras; suicide was wrong and against the state. He writes in *The Laws*:

> But what of him . . . whose violence frustrates the decree of Destiny by self-slaughter though no sentence of the state required this of him, no stress of cruel and inevitable calamity has driven him to the act, and he has been involved in no desperate and intolerable disgrace, the man who thus gives unrighteous sentence against himself from mere poltroonery and unmanly cowardice? Well, in such a case, what further rites must be observed, in the way of purification and ceremonies of burial, it is for Heaven to say; the next of kin should consult the official canonists as well as the laws on the subject, and act according to their direction. But the graves of such as perish thus must, in the first place, be solitary . . . further they must be buried ignominiously in waste and nameless spots . . . and the tomb shall be marked by neither headstone nor name.

Aristotle (384–322 BC), Plato's most famous but rebellious student, also espoused the view that suicide was against the State and, therefore, wrong. Man was answerable to the State and thus liable for wrongdoing and was to be punished for wrongful acts. Suicide is one such act. In book 3 of the *Nicomachean Ethics*, Aristotle noted that:

> ... to die to escape from poverty or love or anything painful is not the mark of a brave man, but rather of a coward; for it is softness to fly from what is troublesome, and such a man endures death not because it is noble but to fly from evil.

Suicide is categorically seen as unjust. The suicide is "the worst man". In the only other reference on suicide, Aristotle is explicit; in book 5 of the *Ethics* he writes:

> ... one class of just acts are those acts in accordance with any virtue which are prescribed by the law; e.g., the law does not expressly permit suicide, and what it does not expressly permit it forbids. Again, when a man in violation of the law harms another (otherwise than in retaliation) voluntarily, he acts unjustly, and a voluntary agent is one who knows both the person he is affecting by his action and the instrument he is using; and he who through anger voluntarily stabs himself does this contrary to the right rule of life, and this the law does not allow; therefore he is acting unjustly. But towards whom? Surely towards the state, not towards himself. For he suffers voluntarily, but no one is voluntarily treated unjustly. This is also the reason why the state punishes; a certain loss of civil rights attaches to the man who destroys himself, on the ground that he's treating the state unjustly.

Epicurus (341–270 BC), another well-known Greek philosopher, was also opposed to suicide. He stated, "... the many at one moment shun death as the greatest of all evils, and another yearn for it as a respite from the evils of life."

In classical Rome, in the centuries just before the Christian era, life was held rather cheap and suicide was viewed either neutrally or, by some, positively. The Roman Stoic, Seneca (4 BC–65 AD), in one of his famous "Letters to Lucilius" wrote,

> Living is not as long as he can ... He will always think of life in terms of quality not quantity ... Dying early or late is of no relevance, dying well or ill is ... even if it is true that while there is life there is hope, life is not to be bought at any cost.

Zeno (around 490 BC), a Greek and the founder of Stoic philosophy, hanged himself after putting his toe out of joint in a fall at age 98. The history of Rome is filled with such incidences, where life was given up for seemingly trivial reasons. Seneca went as far as to call self-murder a "great freedom". Seneca's wish: "Death lies near at hand." Seneca killed himself (by opening his veins). The emperor Nero, had ordered his death because Seneca was accused of plotting against him; and Seneca's death became glorified and respected with great reverence at that time (Van Hooff, 1990). The history of Rome's civilization itself was, indeed, inimical; the life-style in Rome truncated that civilization's very existence, and this can be summed up in Zeno's most famous appeal for suicide:

> To sum up, remember the door is open. Be not a greater coward than the children, but do as they do. When things do not please them, they say, "I will not play anymore." So when things seem to you to reach that point, just say "I will not play anymore" and so depart, instead of staying to make moan.

The Old Testament does not directly forbid suicide, but in Jewish law suicide is wrong. Life had value. In the Old Testament one finds only six cases of suicide: Abimelech, Samson, Saul, Saul's armour-bearer, Ahithapel, and Zimni. The New

Testament, like the Old, did not directly forbid suicide. During the early Christian years, in fact, there was excessive martyrdom and tendency towards suicide, resulting in considerable concern on the part of the Church Fathers. Suicide by these early martyrs was seen as redemption and thus, to stop the suicides, the Fathers began increasingly to associate sin and suicide. In the fourth century, suicide was categorically rejected by St Augustine (354–430). Suicide was considered a sin because it precluded the possibility of repentance and because it violated the Sixth Commandment, "Thou shalt not kill." Suicide was a greater sin than any other sin. One might wish to avoid suicide, more than any other sin. This view was elaborated by St Thomas Aquinas (1225–1274) who emphasized that suicide was not only unnatural and antisocial, but also a mortal sin in that it usurped God's power over man's life and death (echoing the views of Aristotle, but now suicide is not against the State, but against God, the Church). By 693, the Church, at the Council of Toledo, proclaimed that individuals who attempted suicide were to be excommunicated. The notion of suicide as sin took firm hold and for hundreds of years played an important part in Western man's view of self-destruction. Only during the Renaissance and the Reformation did a different view emerge, although, as Farberow (1972) has documented, the Church remained powerful and opposed to suicide among the lower classes into the twentieth century, although it was not the only view. "In the Western world" philosophy was presenting different perspectives.

The writers and philosophers from the 1500s began to change the views on suicide. William Shakespeare (1564–1616), for example, has provided us with an excellent array of insights. Minois (1999), in his review of the history of suicide in Western culture, underscores that Shakespeare illustrates how "dramatically" the attitudes had changed by this time. Shakespeare wrote a number of tragedies, with 52 suicides occurring in his plays (Minois, 1999). Shakespeare was a superb suicidologist. Who can forget one of the most famous passages ever written on the topic? William Shakespeare's *Hamlet*, act 3, scene 1:

> To be or not to be: that is the question.
> Whether 'tis nobler in the mind to suffer
> The slings and arrows of outrageous fortune,
> Or to take arms against a sea of troubles,
> And by opposing end them. To die; to sleep;
> No more; and by a sleep to say we end
> The heart-ache and the thousand natural shocks
> That flesh is heir to, 'tis a consummation
> Devoutly to be wish'd. To die, to sleep; . . .

There were many philosophers during the Renaissance ages that argued the opposition to suicide. René Descartes (1596–1650) is a good example. Yet, at the same time, the complexity on the topic increased. The French philosopher, Jean-Jacques Rousseau (1712–1778), attempted to free the suicide from evil. He emphasized the natural state of the human being, i.e., innocence. Rousseau transferred sin from the individual to society, making the person and people generally good (and innocent) and asserting that it is society that makes them bad. Suicide is caused by society; the individual is not to blame for his/her death. The disputation as to the locus of blame—whether in man or in society—is a major theme that dominates the history of thought about suicide subsequently. David Hume (1711–1776) was one of the first major Western philosophers to discuss suicide apart from the concept of sin. In his essay, "On Suicide", intentionally published by him a year after his death, he refutes the view of suicide as a crime by arguing that suicide is not a transgression of our duties to God, to our fellow citizens, or to ourselves. Suicide is a right. He asserts that

> ... prudence and courage should engage us to rid ourselves at once of existence when it becomes a burden.... If it be no crime in me to divert the Nile or Danube from its course, were I able to effect such purposes, where then is the crime in turning a few ounces of blood from their natural channel?

This is based on his view: "The life of a man is of no greater importance to the universe than that of an oyster." He even touches on the topic of survivorship, suggesting that one does not harm one's family, neighbours with suicide. Suicide is simply a right.

Whereas Hume tried to decriminalise suicide and make it our right, others, including Immanuel Kant (1724–1804), wrote that human life was sacred and should be preserved, in an antistoic sense, at any cost. There was an abundance of different views by the 1700s, the period of the Enlightenment. Johann Wolfgang von Goethe (1749–1832), in his novel *The Sorrows of Young Werther*, presents, for example, the opposite view to Kant's (see Chapter 2). Life does not need to be preserved. There is a right to death. Werther killed himself in the face of unbearable emotional pain. The book is a story of Werther's intoxication—"complete possession", "flood of emotions", in which "everything around about ceased to exist", "the purest joy of life", "Heaven"—with Lotte, who is betrothed to and marries another. Werther killed himself with the pistol Lotte's father had given him.

Werther had a strong impact in Europe; Goethe himself became known only as "the author of Werther". Even the clothes Werther wore became fashionable. A contagious suicide effect (sometimes called the Werther effect) seemed to occur, a concern that preoccupies many suicidologists to this day (although archival research by Thorson and Öberg (2003) has questioned the existence of the Werther effect after the publication of Goethe's book). As an important aside, it should be noted that Goethe himself battled against his own emotional difficulties, for example, working on Faust for 60 years until he had completed it.

During more recent times, other main threads of suicidal study evolved. Existentialism, for example, has brought suicide into sharp focus, best exemplified in Albert Camus's *The Myth of Sisyphus* (1955). In the opening lines, he wrote:

> There is but one truly serious philosophical problem, and that is suicide. Judging whether life is or is not worth living amounts to answering the fundamental question of philosophy. All the rest and whether or not the world has three dimensions, whether the mind has nine or twelve categories—comes afterwards.

Yet, the answer to Camus's question may not be obvious. What he meant by the philosophical problem is somewhat like the following: "If life has no meaning, life is not worth living; life is meaningless; therefore, one ought to kill oneself." Camus himself, however, opposed suicide. He stated, in fact, that even if life is meaningless, suicide is not just. Camus disagreed with the first premise; he argued that meaninglessness, whether painful or otherwise, does not suggest that life be not worth living. He saw the argument as faulty reasoning. (I will return to the "On 'Therefore'" in the suicidal mind in Chapter 12.) Camus, thus, opposes suicide, although his quote on suicide may well be the most famous of the last century, albeit often misunderstood. Every veteran and aspiring suicidologist knows the quote.

The two giants in the field of suicidal theorizing at the turn of the twentieth century were Durkheim and Freud. Durkheim in *Suicide* (1951) focused on society's inimical effects on the individual, while Freud, eschewing the notions of either sin or crime, gave suicide back to man, but put the locus of action in man's unconscious. Since around 1900, a host of psychological theories, aside from those of Freud, have focused on the individual; for example, those of Alfred Adler, Ludwig Binswanger, Aaron T. Beck, Carl G. Jung, Karl Menninger, George Kelly, David Lester, Henry A. Murray, Edwin Shneidman, Harry Stack Sullivan, and Gregory Zilboorg, to name a few (Leenaars, 1988a). Indeed, our view of the history of suicide shows not only a constant development in defining suicide, but also that suicide is open to various constructions (as we will learn in Chapter 2).

CONTEMPORARY DEVELOPMENTS IN SUICIDOLOGY

In *The Oxford English Dictionary*, the arbiter of the English language, we read:

Suicidology (F suicide sb^2 + ology). The study of suicide and its prevention. Hence suicido-logist.

[1929: W.A. Bongar in *Psychiatrisch-Juridisch Gelshap*. . . . "De wetenschap selfmoord, de suicidologie (cursivering van mij) zou men haar kunnen noemen, is ruim een eeuw oud" (p. 3).]

1964: E.S. Shneidman in *Contemporary Psychology*, lx, 371–372. I thank Louis Dublin, Grand Old Man in Suicidology, for this book because in it he has given us all new clues to suicide.

1967: *Bulletin of Suicidology*, July 7/2. The 10-point programme outlined is a mutual enterprise whose successful development depends on the active interest, support and activities of suicidologists. 1969—1976—.

The "fulcrum moment", as Edwin Shneidman himself called it, of contemporary suicidology occurred several minutes after he discovered several hundred suicide notes in a coroner's vault in 1949 in Los Angeles. At that moment he had a glimmering that the vast potential value of the notes could be immeasurably increased if he did not read them, but rather compared them blindly, in a controlled experiment, with simulated suicide notes, elicited from matched non-suicidal persons. John Stuart Mill's Method of Difference came to Shneidman's side and contemporary suicidology, the seeds for the study of contemporary suicidal phenomena, were sown.

Maris (1993) has outlined the evolution of suicidology since that critical event. As one reads Maris's paper, one becomes aware of suicidology's vastness today. Suicidology is a multidisciplinary enterprise. It is the study of psychological, biological, cultural, sociological, interpersonal, intrapsychic, logical, conscious and unconscious and philosophical elements in the suicidal event. Shneidman, and most suicidologists agree, has always insisted that suicidology is not reducible to any one of its domains.

Maris (1993) provides a long list of subdisciplines, including psychology, medicine, psychiatry, sociology, anthropology, epidemiology, criminology, nursing, biology, philosophy, religion, education, literature, etc., all of which make contributions to suicidology. As Maris (1993) notes, that list "could be extended or refined almost indefinitely".

From the embryonic beginnings in the vault, suicidology has become an expanded discipline. It involves survivorship. It involves crisis work on telephone hotlines. It involves research in laboratories and in natural field settings. It involves associations such as the American Association for Suicidology, the Canadian Association for Suicide Prevention, and the International Association for Suicide Prevention. It involves a research group, the International Academy of Suicide Research; an academy dedicated to enhancing the research in the field. It involves training and practice. Thus suicidology today not only includes the study of suicide but also its prevention, including psychotherapy.

SUICIDE FACTS AND MYTHS

The lore about suicide contains a large number of interesting and esoteric items. People in general are not only perplexed and bewildered by self-destructive behaviour, but they also believe a number of misconceptions of suicide. Here are some common fables and facts about suicide, formulated by Shneidman around 1952 and incorporated into a number of publications (e.g., Shneidman & Mandelkorn, 1967):

1. Fable: *People who talk about suicide don't commit suicide.*
   Fact: Of any 10 persons who kill themselves, 8 have given definite warnings of their suicidal intentions.

2. Fable: *Suicide happens without warning.*
   Fact: Studies reveal that the suicidal person gives many clues and warnings regarding suicidal intentions.

3. Fable: *Suicidal people are fully intent on dying.*
   Fact: Most suicidal people are undecided about living or dying, and they "gamble with death", leaving it to others to save them. Almost no one commits suicide without letting others know how they are feeling.

4. Fable: *Once a person is suicidal he or she is suicidal forever.*
   Fact: Individuals who wish to kill themselves are suicidal only for a limited period of time.

5. Fable: *Improvement following a suicidal crisis means that the suicidal risk is over.*
   Fact: Most suicides occur within about three months following the beginning of "improvement", when the individual has the energy to put his or her morbid thoughts and feelings into effect.

6. Fable: *Suicide strikes much more often among the rich—or, conversely, it occurs most exclusively among the poor.*
   Fact: Suicide is neither the rich person's disease nor the poor person's curse. Suicide is very "democratic" and is represented proportionately among all levels of society.

7. Fable: *Suicide is inherited.*
   Fact: Suicide is not inherited. It is an individual pattern.

8. Fable: *All suicidal individuals are mentally ill, and suicide always is the act of a psychotic person.*
   Fact: Studies of hundreds of genuine suicide notes indicate that although the suicidal person is extremely unhappy, he or she is not necessarily mentally ill.

There is also the misconception that we talk about "myths" as if we know what people believe. Studies by McIntosh et al. (1983) and Leenaars et al. (1988) addressed this topic. Their findings support the belief that people's knowledge regarding some facts of the above are quite high and generally well above what was anticipated from the previous anecdotal literature. People with direct experience of suicide seem to know more (Durocher et al., 1989). On the other hand, older people seem to fare the poorest in their knowledge (Leenaars et al., 1991). Yet, the series of studies also raised some questions, for example, "is 'suicide is inherited' always a fable?" As we will learn, this is a legitimate question, somewhat different from the views held in the 1950s (see also Chapter 19).

ATTEMPTED SUICIDE

A previous attempt is one of the best clues to future attempts (Beck et al., 1979). However, not all previous attempters go on to attempt again [or kill themselves; about 15% do so versus 1.5% for the general population (Lester, 1992; Leenaars & Lester, 1994)]. Although it is obvious that one has to "attempt" suicide in order to commit it, it is equally clear that the event of "attempting suicide" does not always have death (cessation) as its objective. It is acknowledged that often the goal of "attempted suicide" (such as cutting oneself or ingesting harmful substances) is to change one's life (or to change the behaviour of the "significant others" around one) rather than to end it. On some rare occasions death is actually intended and only luckily avoided. However, I wish to stress, as have others (e.g., Stengel, 1964), that it is useful to think of the "attempter"—now often referred to as the parasuicide—and the "completer" as two sets of overlapping populations: (1) a group of those who attempt suicide, a few of whom go on to commit it, and (2) a group of those who commit suicide, many of whom previously attempted it. A great deal has to do with *perturbation* and *lethality* associated with the event.

Perturbation refers to how upset (disturbed, agitated, sane–insane) the individual is—rated as low–medium–high (or alternatively on a 1 to 9 scale)—and may be measured by various means (e.g., self-reports, biological markers, psychological tests, observations). Lethality is roughly synonymous with the "deathfulness" of the act and is an important dimension in understanding any potentially suicidal individual. Lethality can be rated as low–moderate–high (or alternatively on a 1 to 9 scale). An example for measuring lethality is the following assessment item, derived from Shneidman (1967): "During the last 24 hours, I felt the chances of my actually killing myself (committing suicide and ending my life) were: absent, very low, low–medium, fifty-fifty, high–medium, very high, extra high (came very close to actually killing myself)." A critical distinction in suicide is that lethality—not perturbation—kills. All sorts of people are highly perturbed but are not suicidal. The ratio between suicide attempts and completions is about 4:1 to about 10:1—one committed suicide for every 4–10 attempts; however, in young people, some reports have the ratio at 50:1, or even 100:1. The ratio, in fact, appears to vary significantly between nations and across risk groups, sex, age, and so on.

The "attempter" (along with individuals who engage in self-assaultive and self-mutilative behaviour) and the "completer" share some commonalities; however, they are, by and large, operationally quite different. There is a third group, the "contemplators", whose numbers are so vast that it is difficult to begin to highlight their commonalities, which are again quite different (we will meet both attempters and contemplators in this volume). Shneidman (1985) has presented the differences between suicide and attempted suicide. He suggests, for example, that whereas the common stimulus in suicide is unendurable psychological pain, in attempted suicide it is intense, potentially endurable, psychological pain. As another example, whereas the common purpose in suicide is to seek a solution to an overbearing problem, in attempted suicide it is to reduce tension and to evoke a response. However, there are also similarities, although the content of such characteristics may be quite different. Shneidman (1985) provided the following examples: the common stressor in both is frustrated needs; and the common consistency in both is with lifelong adjustment patterns.

A study—a rare opportunity to actually compare attempters and completers—actually found that there might be more similarities than differences (Leenaars et al., 1992). Archival research—a comparison of suicide notes written by individuals who killed themselves and notes, sometimes called *parasuicide notes*, by individuals who made highly lethal attempts—found only a few differences (see Chapter 2). Attempters see their act as a style of life, being too weak to cope with life's ever-present difficulties, and lacking in social integration. Suicide attempts may become a way of life. The empirical observations on this topic are sparse and Smith and Maris (1986) have called for extensive research in this area.

Suicide attempts have many meanings and, whatever the level of lethality, ought to be taken seriously. A person who attempts suicide may not necessarily mean that he/she wants to die but that the situation was so intense that he/she had to communicate the pain. Words like "manipulation" or "blackmail" or "attention" add only a pejorative emotional tone, revealing our own attitudes and fears.

PARTIAL DEATH AND SUBSTITUTES FOR SUICIDE

Freud (1974a), Shneidman (1963), Murray (1967), and others have speculated that beyond intentional suicides, there is a vast array of subintentional inimical be-haviours. The very life-style of some individuals seems to truncate and demean their life so that they are as good as dead. In 1901, Freud stated:

> It is well known that in the severe cases of psychoneurosis instances of self injury are occasionally found as symptoms and that in such cases suicide can never be ruled out as a possible outcome of the physical conflict... many apparently accidental injuries that happen to such patients are really instances of self-injury. (pp. 178–179)

Freud further notes that such self-destruction is not rare. Often alcoholism, drug addiction, mismanagement of physical disease, auto accidents, and masochistic behaviour can be seen in this light. Farberow (1980) has edited a book on "the many faces of suicide". Therein, he asks a number of relevant questions. For example:

- Why did a person stop taking insulin when he knew he had to take it regularly to stay well, or even to stay alive?
- Why did a person, knowing what drugs can do to you, get hooked?
- Why did a person drive so fast on the curving mountain roads when he had known for the last three months how bad his brakes were?

There may be no intent to kill oneself, but the person is "as good as dead". Karl Menninger, the chief theorist on the concept of partial death, in *Man Against Himself* (1938), writes of (1) *chronic* suicide—including asceticism, martyrdom, neurotic in-validism, alcohol addiction, antisocial behaviour, and psychosis; (2) *focal* suicide—focusing on a limited part of the body—including self-mutilation, multiple surgery, purposive accidents, impotence, and frigidity; and (3) *organic* suicide—focusing on the psychological factors in organic disease, especially the self-punishing aggres-sive and erotic components. Freud (1974a) has speculated that there is, in fact, a suicidal thread (or death instinct) in all of us.

A related concept is of "subintentioned death" (Shneidman, 1963). This concept as-serts that there are many deaths that are neither clearly suicidal nor clearly acciden-tal or natural, but deaths in which the decedent played some covert or unconscious role in "permitting" his or her death to occur, either "accidentally" or by "inviting" homicide, or by unconsciously disregarding what could be a life-extending medical regimen, and thus dying sooner than "necessary". Freud (1974a) speculated:

> Anyone who believes in the occurrence of half-intentional self-injury—if I may use a clumsy expression—will be prepared also to assume that in addition to consciously intentional suicide there is such a thing as half-intentional self-destruction (self-destruction with an unconscious intention), capable of making skilful use of a threat of life and of disguising it as a chance mishap. (pp. 180–181)

PSYCHOLOGICAL THEORIES OF SUICIDE

The modern era of the psychological study of suicide began around the turn of the twentieth century with the investigations of Sigmund Freud (1974a, 1974b, 1974c,

1974g, 1974h, 1974i, 1974j, 1974k, 1974l, 1974n). Freud's clinical research suggested to him that the root cause of suicide, within a developmental context, was the experience of loss or rejection of a significant, highly cathected object (i.e., a person). In 1920, Freud further developed what he termed a "deeper interpretation" of what leads someone to kill himself after such a loss or rejection. He stated:

> Probably no one finds the mental energy to kill himself unless, in the first place, in doing so he is at the same time killing an object with whom he has identified himself and, in the second place, is turning against himself a death wish which had been directed against someone else. (Freud, 1974i, p. 162)

Freud—eschewing the two popular notions about suicide at the turn of the twentieth century—sin and crime—placed the focus of blame on the person; specifically, in the person's unconscious. Since around 1900, there have been a host of psychological theories besides Freud's that have attempted to define suicide. Indeed, a—if not the—major advance in the psychology of suicide in the last century was the development of various models beyond Freud's that have attempted to understand this complicated human act, the most noteworthy of which has been Edwin Shneidman.

Suicide is open to various psychological constructions. In his famous experiment on volume where the experimenter pours fluid from a short, fat beaker into a tall, thin one, Piaget (1970) has demonstrated that the young child will say there is more fluid in either the first or second beaker. The child is centred on only one dimension to the exclusion of others. Later in human development, the child can take into account both dimensions simultaneously and use multiple perspective on the same event. To be decentred in general is to be able to take an abstract view of things, rather than to be influenced totally by the characteristics of concrete particulars ("stimulus bound"). To view suicide only from Freud's original view is perhaps to be too concrete and stimulus bound. To introject only Freud's or any other specific view may be seen as acting like the young preconservative child, i.e., centred. Although Freud provided a sound basis in the very early years of suicidology, what we have discovered thus far about suicide is that it may best be defined from multiple perspectives: not being concrete but also not being overinclusive. In this sense, it may be wise to follow Kelly's (1955) dictate of constructive alternativism:

> We take the stand that there are always some alternative constructions available to choose among in dealing with the world. No one needs to paint himself into a corner; no one needs to be completely hemmed in by circumstances; no one needs to be the victim of his biography. (p. 15)

Here, I have decided to present four points of view: psychoanalytic (Freud); cognitive-behavioural (Beck); social learning (Lester); and multidimensional (Shneidman). I hope in some way to clarify the central issue—understanding why human beings commit suicide. Let me begin with a few remarks by Shneidman on the topic of theory in general.

Shneidman (1985) suggests that a psychological theory regarding suicide should begin with the question, "What are the interesting common psychological dimensions of committed suicide?", not "What kind of people commit suicide?". This question, according to Shneidman, is critical; for they (the common dimensions) are what suicide is. Not necessarily the universal, but certainly the most frequent or common characteristics provide us with a meaningful conceptualization regarding suicide.

Most frequently, non-professionals identify external causes (e.g., ill health, being left by a lover, losing one's fortune, etc.) as what is common in suicide. A recent downhill course (e.g., drop in income, sudden acute alcoholism, a change in work, and divorce or separation) can, indeed, be identified in suicide. However, although there are always situational aspects in every suicidal act, these are only the precipitating events. Suicide is more complex. Suicide is a multidetermined event. How can we understand these psychological complexities?

Suicide is a multidimensional malaise. It is an intrapsychic drama on an interpersonal stage. From this psychological view (Leenaars, 1988a, 1989a, 1989b, 1994) we will define suicide with the key ideas of the four suicidal theories mentioned above: Psychoanalytic (Sigmund Freud), Cognitive-Behavioural (Aaron T. Beck), Social Learning (David Lester), and Multidimensional (Edwin Shneidman).

The four perspectives will be presented in the form of protocol sentences or what might be construed to be aphorisms. Protocol sentences are testable hypotheses, and in that sense they are like aphorisms. An aphorism is a short statement stating a truth. It is a principle expressed tersely in a few telling words. A major difference between protocol sentences and aphorisms is that the latter tend to be general. Although protocol sentences may be general, they must be testable (although some form of specificity is implied for the sentence to be testable). One must be able to determine the truth or falsity of the statement. Aphorisms, if they are true, should also be subject to the possibility of verification (falsifiability). The protocol procedure was first introduced by Carnap (1959) and applied in my own research in suicide for over three decades. Protocol sentences (or aphorisms) are one means of defining an event. It is obvious, as Shneidman (1984) noted, that one way to discuss suicide is to do so aphoristically.

Psychoanalytic

As I have already mentioned, Sigmund Freud first formulated the psychoanalytic perspective early in the twentieth century. Other noteworthy suicidologists in this tradition are Karl Menninger, Henry A. Murray, and Gregory Zilboorg. Here are some protocol sentences (or aphorisms) derived from Freud's work.

1. Suicide is motivated by unconscious intentions. Even if the person communicates that he or she has consciously planned suicide, the focus of the action is in the unconscious.
2. The root cause of suicide is the experience of loss and rejection of a significant highly cathected object (i.e., a person)—the person, in fact, is singly preoccupied with this loss/rejection.
3. The suicidal person feels quite ambivalent. He/she is both affectionate and hostile towards a lost/rejecting person.

4. The suicidal person is, in some direct or indirect fashion, identifying with a rejecting or lost person. Attachment, based upon an important emotional tie, is the meaning of identification.
5. The suicidal person exhibits an overly regressive attachment—"narcissistic identification"—with the object. He/she behaves as if he/she were reacting to another person.
6. The suicidal person is angry at the object although the feelings and/or ideas of vengefulness and aggression are directed towards him/herself.
7. The suicidal person turns back upon him/herself murderous wishes/ impulses/needs that had been directed against the object.
8. Suicide is a fulfilment of punishment; i.e., self-punishment.
9. The suicidal person experiences a sense of guilt or self-criticism. The person develops prohibitions of extraordinary harshness and severity towards him/herself.
10. The suicidal person's organization of experiences is impaired. He/she is no longer capable of any coherent synthesis of his/her experience.

Cognitive-Behavioural

The cognitive-behavioural perspective is most widely associated with Aaron T. Beck and his colleagues (1963, 1967, 1971, 1975a, 1975b, 1976, 1978, 1979a, 1979b). George Kelly, Albert Ellis, and Don Meichenbaum are also associated with this view. The following 10 protocol sentences are deduced from Beck's writings:

1. Suicide is associated with depression. The critical link between depression and suicidal intent is hopelessness.
2. Hopelessness, defined operationally in terms of negative expectations, appears to be the critical factor in the suicide. The suicidal person views suicide as the only possible solution to his/her desperate and hopelessly unsolvable problem (situation).
3. The suicidal person views the future as negative, often unrealistically. He/she anticipates more suffering, more hardship, more frustration, more deprivation, etc.
4. The suicidal person's view of him/herself is negative, often unrealistically. He/she views him/herself as incurable, incompetent, and helpless, often with self-criticism, self-blame, and reproaches against the self (with expressions of guilt and regret) accompanying this low self-evaluation.
5. The suicidal person views him/herself as deprived, often unrealistically. Thoughts of being alone, unwanted, unloved, and perhaps materially deprived are possible examples of such deprivation.
6. Although the suicidal person's thoughts (interpretations) are arbitrary, he/she considers no alternative, accepting the validity (accuracy) of the cognitions.
7. The suicidal person's thoughts, which are often automatic and involuntary, are characterized by a number of possible errors, some so gross as to constitute distortion; e.g., preservation, overgeneralization, magnification/minimization, inexact labelling, selective abstraction, negative bias.

8. The suicidal person's affective reaction is proportional to the labelling of the traumatic situation, regardless of the actual intensity of the event.
9. Irrespective of whether the affect is sadness, anger, anxiety, or euphoria, the more intense the affect the greater the perceived plausibility of the associated cognitions.
10. The suicidal person, being hopeless and not wanting to tolerate the pain (suffering), desires to escape. Death is thought of as more desirable than life.

Social Learning

The social learning view has been summarized by Lester (1987): Albert Bandura and psychologists in the classical (Pavlov) and operant (Skinner) traditions are the best-known theorists in this view. The 10 aphorisms of this paradigm are as follows:

1. Suicide is a learned behaviour. Childhood experiences and forces in the environment shape the suicidal person and precipitate the act.
2. Child-rearing practices are critical, especially the child's experiences of punishment. Specifically, the suicidal person has learned to inhibit the expression of aggression outward and simultaneously learned to turn it inward upon him/herself.
3. The suicide can be predicted based on the basic laws of learning. Suicide is shaped behaviour—the behaviour was and is reinforced in his/her environment.
4. The suicidal person's thoughts provide the stimuli; suicide (response) is imagined. Cognitions (such as self-praise) can be reinforcers for the act.
5. The suicidal person's expectancies play a critical role in the suicide—he/she expects reinforcement (reward) by the act.
6. Depression, especially the cognitive components, is strongly associated with the suicide. Depression goes far towards explaining suicide. For example, depression may be caused by a lack of reinforcement, learned helplessness, and/or rewarded.
7. Suicide can be a manipulative act. Others reinforce this.
8. Suicide is not eliminated by means of punishment.
9. The suicidal person is non-socialized. He/she has not been sufficiently socialized into traditional culture. The suicidal person has failed to learn the normal cultural values, especially towards life and death.
10. The suicide can be reinforced by a number of environmental factors, for example, subcultural norms, suggestions on television, gender preferences for specific methods, suicide in significant others (modelling), a network of family and friends, cultural patterns.

Multidimensional

The psychologist who has consistently argued for a multidimensional view is Shneidman (1967, 1973, 1980, 1981a, 1982a, 1985, 1991, 1993—see Leenaars, 1999a). Here is a brief summary, utilizing our previous procedure, of his work:

1. The suicidal person is in unbearable psychological pain. The person is focused almost entirely on this unbearable emotion (pain), and especially one specific (an arbitrarily selected) way to escape from it.
2. The suicidal person experienced a situation that is traumatic (e.g., poor health, rejection the spouse, being married to a non-supportive spouse). What is implied is that some needs are unfulfilled, thwarted, or frustrated.
3. For the suicidal person, the idea of cessation (death, stopping, or eternal sleep) provides the solution. It permits him/her to resolve the unbearable state of self-destructiveness, disturbance, and isolation.
4. By the suicide, the person wishes to end all conscious experience. The goal of suicide is cessation of consciousness and the person behaves in order to achieve this end.
5. The suicidal person is in a state of heightened disturbance (perturbation), e.g., he/she feels boxed in, rejected, harassed, unsuccessful, and especially hopeless and helpless.
6. The suicidal person's internal attitude is ambivalence. The suicidal person experiences complications, concomitant contradictory feelings, attitudes and/or thrusts (not only towards him/herself and other people but towards the act itself).
7. The suicidal person's cognitive state is constriction (tunnel vision, a narrowing of the mind's eye). He/she is figuratively intoxicated or drugged by his/her overpowering emotions and constricted logic and perception.
8. The suicidal person needs or wishes to egress. He/she wants to leave (the scene), to exit, to get out, to get away, to be gone, not to be around, to be "elsewhere"... not to be.
9. There is a serial pattern to the suicide. The suicidal person exhibits patterns of behaviour that diminish or truncate his/her life, which subtract from its length or reduce its scope.
10. The person's suicide has unconscious psychodynamic implications.

Summary

To summarize, suicide is best understood as a multidimensional human malaise. What we have discovered so far is that suicide can be defined differently from various psychological points of view. I do not mean to suggest that all these views are mutually exclusive or equally accurate or helpful for psychotherapy—we do not have to follow the cognitive processes of the suicidal person. Nor do I believe that my protocol (aphorism) method is the only way to outline a point of view; indeed, it may well lose some of the complexity in the theories themselves. It is, however, one way to understand the event.

The real importance of protocol sentences is that they must be verifiable. In that regard, what aphorisms of Freud or Beck or Lester or Shneidman are true? What are empirical? Suicidology's future endeavour, in general, will be the need to develop some form of empirical verification of the various constructions of the event. Research will be an important aspect of such efforts. I do not mean to suggest only the controlled experiment. But, following Allport (1942) and Maslow (1966), we must be open-minded, utilizing both ideographic and nomothetic approaches. Suicide is plagued by the difficulty of obtaining data (Maris, 1981). In my own research, I have utilized suicide notes as my database. Despite their limitations (Leenaars, 1988a), suicide notes have been historically useful in describing the suicide since the individual is at the final throes of the life vs death decision. Other documents as well as statistics, third-party interviews, and the study of non-fatal suicide attempters have a place in understanding suicidal phenomena—if the data are put in the context of broad theoretical formulations about suicide and personality functioning in general.

Although misuse of psychological theory(ies) is possible (e.g., finding support only for one's view and, thus, acting like the suicidal person him/herself), theoretical formulations have an important place in the use of personal documents (e.g., suicide notes) and in any form of research. Research must be embedded in theory. To avoid our constriction, I would argue that we must critically evaluate alternative explanations and interpretations. We must no longer look at suicide from Freud's perspective alone but from Beck's, Lester's, Shneidman's, and so on. Indeed, a comprehensive model will be presented in Chapter 2.

Theory, explicit and implicit, plays some role in research whether solving a specific problem, testing an existing theory, developing new theories, or expanding existing theories. The problem is that frequently the theory is not articulated. Regrettably, much of the research on suicide is atheoretical. Equally regrettable, often remediators have no stated conceptualization or, more accurately, the conceptualization is characterized, if I can use Beck's descriptions, by a number of cognitive errors, some so gross as to constitute distortion; e.g., perseveration, overgeneralization, magnification/minimization, inexact labelling, selective abstraction, bias. One is simply too centred. I do not mean to suggest that my view solves the problem, but I hope to have clarified the issue—psychologically, suicide is best understood from different points of view, especially if that theory is to be useful in intervention.

An understanding of suicide can be used to assist us in preventing the event. Psychotherapy must follow empirically verified definition. When understanding is centred and not based on any sound empiricism, remediation (i.e., prevention, intervention, and postvention) is likely to be ineffective. Hopefully, the definition of suicide derived from the four points of view will be a beginning to assist a needful individual in some way in therapy.

As a final comment, I do not mean to suggest that psychology alone has a role in defining suicide. It is not sufficient to define the entire event. It would, in fact, seem most accurate to define suicide as an event with biological (including biochemical, neuropsychological), sociocultural, interpersonal, philosophical/existential, psychological, and other aspects. All empirical definitions may assist us in psychotherapy with suicidal people.

Of course suicide is more than I have so far isolated. The common thread, however, in all the views so far presented is that there is a consistency to all suicides, namely with lifelong adjustment patterns (Shneidman, 1985). Suicide has a history.

THEORETICAL/CLINICAL OBSERVATIONS

This section consists of six parts, all focused on clarifying suicide: biological roots, brain dysfunctions, physical disabilities and illness, depression, specific precipitating events, and the family system.

Biological Roots

"No brain, no mind" is one of Henry Murray's reminders to his student Edwin Shneidman (Shneidman, 2001). Yet, of late—if I am allowed a difference between Dr Shneidman and myself—he has overly forgotten this teaching; he calls himself a radical mentalist (personal communication, November 2001). Dr Shneidman's (2001) current belief is somewhat akin to Descartes' (1972). Descartes is best known for his statement, "Cogito ergo sum". This is radical mentalism. Dr Shneidman's position is "Cogito ergo suicide". My own view is akin to his 1985 position in *Definition of Suicide*, in which he states his principles (see his Chapter V, "A formal definition, with explication"). He writes that, "...suicide is a multifaceted event and that biological, cultural, sociological, interpersonal, intrapsychic, logical, conscious and unconscious, and philosophical elements are present, in various degrees, in each suicidal event" (p. 202). When I discussed the topic in November 2001 at Ed's home, he stated that he was wrong then. His current position is best stated in his book, *The Suicidal Mind* (1996)—see also his letter in the *New England Journal of Medicine* (Shneidman, 1992). In 2001, Shneidman stated his current position thus: "I do not think that the key answers about suicide are to be found in the brain; I think that the key action is in the mind" (p. 74). I think that he was right in 1985. Descartes led us astray, so did Shneidman. If I am allowed one disagreement with Dr Shneidman, it would be this: Shneidman led us astray. (I think, if I dare, that Henry Murray would agree with me.) I believe that the suicidal mind is the suicidal brain and the suicidal brain is the suicidal mind. To understand suicide, we need to understand these roots of suicide and much more. Utilizing only one of these views is too reductionistic. The key answers are to be found in the brain and the mind—and elsewhere.

Stoff and Mann's (1997) edited volume begins to outline the current understanding of the neurobiology of suicide. Their book is an essential read for any aspiring psychotherapist.

On a critical note, however, one could see Stoff and Mann's view to be equally too reductionistic. Suicide is no more or less the suicidal brain, than the suicidal mind. Stoff and Mann write:

> ...efforts aimed at identifying the potentially suicidal individual using demographic, social developmental and psychological factors offer too weak a prediction to be of substantial clinical utility. It is believed that the biological perspective, which has grown out of the expanding research on the biological basis of mood disorders, is a predominant approach to suicide research. It can assist in the investigation of risk factors that predispose a person to suicidal behavior and that increase understanding of etiology, treatment, and ultimately, prevention. (p. 1)

Utilizing only this view will lead us as much astray as Shneidman. Once more, we need all perspectives. Suicide is complex, more complex than most people are aware. It is not only the suicidal brain. It is not only the suicidal mind. All avenues are legitimate ways to understand and prevent suicide. Psychotherapy, in fact, is only one way to intervene; the one focused on in this book.

The classical study in suicidology of the biological roots was by Asberg et al. (1976). They identified 5-H1 AA in cerebrospinal fluid as a biochemical marker in some suicides. This study marked the beginning of empirical biological suicidology. Yet, although the Asberg study is now over 25 years old, there is relatively little secure knowledge regarding the neurobiology of suicide today (Hawton & van Heeringen, 2000). Despite a recent flood of information regarding biological correlates of suicide, much of it lacks scientific rigour, but less so than a few decades ago (Motto & Reus, 1991; Rifai et al., 1992). Lester (1992), in a review of this area, suggested that the "research has been quite poor" (p. 27). Sample sizes are small. Confounding variables, e.g., postmortem delay, have added to the confusion. Depression or other psychiatric disorders have rarely been controlled. Studies of biological correlates across the life-span (Motto & Reus, 1991), as well as specific groups—e.g., the elderly (Rifai et al., 1992)—have concluded that biological conjectures about the common precipitants of suicide, are, in fact, premature—of course, the same can be said about the psychological study, sociological, and so on. Indeed, the science has led us to some important roots in suicide (Stoff & Mann, 1997).

Despite the state of the art, suicide must be seen as a biological event (and much more). Possible markers, isolated to date, include urinary 17-hydroxycorticosteroids (17-OHCS), cortisol in plasma and cerebrospinal fluid, cerebrospinal fluid 5-hydroxyindoleacetic acid, tritiated imiprimine binding, 3-methoxy-4-hydroxyphenylglycol and homovanillic acid, urinary norepinephrine/epinephrine ratio; and thyroid-stimulating hormone response to thyrotropin-releasing hormone. Slaby (1992), in his comment about this field, and others (e.g., Maltsberger, 2002) are optimistic about our biological understanding of suicide, especially in the relation of suicide to affective disorders (e.g., manic-depressive disorder) and their neurobiological correlates, resulting in direct implications for medication (see Chapter 19). At least, in some suicides, biological correlates are strikingly relevant (we will comment about this topic in more detail later, see Chapter 19).

Brain Dysfunction and Learning Disabilities

The importance of brain dysfunction in children and its relation to learning disabilities is well documented. The relation of brain dysfunction and socio-emotional problems in people is, however, a more neglected topic in the literature. Not only does a learning disability render a person at risk for socio-emotional problems including suicide, but there are also particular subtypes of learning disabilities and these different subtypes may result in different levels of risk. Rourke and Fisk (1981) have documented that different patterns of cerebral dysfunction and their resulting learning disability(ies) render a person at risk for different types of socio-emotional disturbances. They report three major subgroups. The first group has a right brain dysfunction, and such people are prone to learning problems with non-verbal, visual information. They may show the following socio-emotional problems: not paying attention to visual objects including other people; rarely expressing emotions appropriately in their facial expressions; having a voice that can be expressionless; being very talkative; talking to self; having flow problems in their speech; and being awkward socially. The second group has a left brain dysfunction, and such people are prone to learning problems with verbal information. They may show the following socio-emotional problems: rarely initiating conversations; having problems paying attention, for example, in conversation; being brief and often concrete in their remarks; often stating "I don't know" to questions; and some are very impulsive, not thinking before they act. The third group has both left and right brain dysfunction and exhibit a conglomerate of symptoms.

Other more specific cerebral deficits render people at risk for other specific problems such as planning, sequencing social events, and so on. Attention deficit/hyperactivity disorder (ADHD), in all its subtypes, is an example. Although further empirical studies need to be conducted in the neuropsychology of suicides, these observations clearly warrant attention. Indeed, Rourke et al. (1989) have shown that one possible adolescent and adult outcome of childhood central processing deficiencies is suicidal behaviour as well as other socio-emotional problems. They have suggested that it is especially the first pattern associated with right brain dysfunction that predisposes those afflicted to adolescent and adult suicide risk. The brain is so critical in risk.

Physical Disabilities and Illness

I would be remiss if I did not at least note the importance of physical problems in suicidal behaviour in some people (Barraclough, 1986; Stenger & Stenger, 2000). Physical illness interacts with an individual's emotional functioning; indeed, some illnesses directly affect one's emotions. Empirical study regarding illness and suicide is urgently needed; currently research suggests that some physical illnesses are associated with suicidal behaviour, including anorexia, bulimia, diabetes, epilepsy, traumatic brain injury, and muscular dystrophy (Barraclough, 1986). Some individuals with physical disabilities who are at risk are those with limb amputations or spinal injuries resulting in quadriplegia. Individuals with terminal illness such as AIDS appear also to be at high risk (Fryer, 1986; Marzuk, 1989). However, it is important to realize that not all such people are suicidal and that research is needed to substantiate these views.

Depression

It was once believed that all suicidal people were depressed, but this is a myth. The fact is that not all suicidal people are depressed, and that not all depressed people are suicidal. Depression and suicide are not equivalent. Yet, Lester (1992) has noted that depression distinguishes many suicidal people from non-suicidal groups. Depression can be noted in mood and behaviour (ranging from feeling dejected and hesitancy in social contacts, to isolation and serious disturbance of appetite and sleep), verbal expression (ranging from talks about being disappointed, excluded, blamed, etc., to talk of suicide, being killed, abandoned, helpless), and fantasy (ranging from feeling disappointed, excluded, mistreated, etc., to suicide, mutilation, loss of a significant person) (Pfeffer, 1986). Behaviours such as excessive aggressiveness, change in work performance, and expressions of somatic complaints or loss of energy, have all been associated with depression. However, not all depression is overt, especially in youth. Some children and especially teenagers (and some adults) exhibit what has been termed masked depression (see Chapter 9 for details). They dissemble. Anorexia, promiscuity and drug abuse, for example, have been associated with depression. It is important to remember, however, that depression does not equal suicide in a simple one to one fashion. Most suicides experience unbearable pain, but not necessarily depression (Shneidman, 1985). The unbearable emotion might be hostility, anxiety, despair, shame, guilt, dependency, hopelessness, or helplessness. What is critical is that the emotion—pain—is unbearable. Unendurable psychological pain is the common stimulus in suicide (Shneidman, 1985), not depression alone (see Chapters 2 and 19 for further details).

Specific Environmental Precipitating Events

A current popular formulation regarding suicide is that suicide is simply due to an external event; for example, a rejection, the influence of the music of a pop singer, whatever. Although precipitating events (e.g., deprivation of love, sexual abuse, being bullied, death of parent, divorce, a rejection) do occur in the suicides of people, this may be less frequent in children. We are here reminded of a clinical example, which is quite similar to one reported by Menninger (1938): A 16-year-old was found dead in a car, having died of carbon monoxide poisoning. People were perplexed, "Why did this young person from an upper-middle-class family kill himself?" The parents found out that his girlfriend rejected him on the day of his suicide. That was the reason: when a young man gets rejected and is so in love, he may kill himself. A few friends and his teachers knew that he had been having problems in school. That was the reason. A few others knew that his father was an alcoholic and abusive. That was the reason. His physician knew that he had been adopted and had been recently upset about that. She knew the real reason. And others knew. . . .

Shneidman (1985) has noted that the common consistency in suicide is not the precipitating event, but life-long coping patterns (see Chapter 2 for details). One can see continuity despite developmental changes. People who kill themselves experience a steady toll of threat, stress, failure, challenge, and loss that gradually undermines their adjustment process. Suicide has a history.

This view does not mean to suggest that an environmental stimulus is not critical; it may in fact, be, to use a popular metaphor, the straw that breaks the camel's back. One event needs special mentioning, bullying—or, if you will, abuse. We all remember the bully on our own schoolyards (although they are also in the workplace, or home, or anywhere). The bully, according to *The Oxford English Dictionary*—the

OED—is: "A person who uses strength or power to coerce or intimidate weaker persons." Bullies persecute, intimidate, oppress. Dickens's Mr Bumble is a good example: "a big mean guy" according to my 11-year-old daughter, Kristen. But, as Charles Dickens wrote in *Oliver Twist* (1966 edition, p. 287), "Mr. Bumble . . . had a decided propensity for bullying . . . and, consequently, was (it is needless to say) a coward."

This goes beyond an environmental stimulus in some suicidal people. In a landmark case in Vancouver, Canada, on 26 March 2002, the court found a 16-year-old female bully guilty for uttering a series of physical threats (e.g., "You're fucking dead"). The victim, Dawn-Marie Wesley, a 14-year-old girl, had killed herself on 10 November 2000. She named the bullies in her suicide note (which she concluded with the prototypical, "I love you all so much"). Of course, the suicide was more complex, but in the suicidal equation of Dawn-Marie, Provincial Court Judge Jill Rounthwarte stated, "threatening conduct . . . caused Dawn to fear for her safety, a fear that was entirely reasonable in all of the circumstances". Of course, this implies that environmental control (e.g., zero tolerance in the schools) may be an important avenue to prevent the needless death of other Dawn-Maries (see Chapter 19).

There are, of course, many threats, stresses, and so on. One further stimulus that has frequently been identified as a possible precipitating event, especially in young people, and is worth mentioning here, is the death of a parent (Pfeffer, 1986). Indeed, when the death occurs by suicide, everyone in the family may be at risk. There are survivor pains.

This discussion also raises the issues of the contagion (copycat) effect. Some years ago in Japan, an 18-year-old pop idol, Yukiko Okada, after a fight with her lover, leaped to her death from the building that housed her recording company in Tokyo. In the 17 days following her suicide, the suicide toll reached 33 young people. Philips (1986) is often credited with documenting the fact that such cluster suicides do occur in teenagers and young adults, even more than in adults. Suicide clusters have, in fact, been reported in Japan, North America and across the world. Brenner (1988) has, however, shown that a contagion effect may not exist in the very young, for example, in boys (5–14 years old). Aside from clustering, the impact of suggestion is also seen in the effect of media reporting of suicide. Most recently, it has been noted that there may be particular characteristics of those "contagion" suicides (Brent, 1992; Martin, 1998). This is an area for further study (Lester, 1992).

Family Background

A review of the literature (e.g., Berman & Jobes, 1991; Corder & Haizlip, 1984; Corder et al., 1974; Leenaars, 1988b; Leenaars & Wenckstern, 1991; Maris, 1985; Pfeffer, 1986; Richman, 1993; Toolan, 1981; Seiden, 1984) suggests that the family system and its functioning is a central factor associated with suicide and suicidal behaviour in children, adolescents, and even older people, although by no means do all families show these characteristics—some, none at all. Nevertheless, a few common observations of families will be provided, followed by a few specific additional observations for teenagers:

1. There is, at times, a lack of generational boundaries in suicidal families. There is an insufficient separation of the parent from his/her family of origin. For example, grandparents may take over the parenting role.
2. The family system is often inflexible. Any change is seen as a threat to the survival of the family. Denial, secretiveness, dissembling and especially a lack of communication characterize the family's interactions, even in the suicides of the elderly. One 8-year-old boy reported to me, "If I try to kill myself, maybe my dad will listen." Additionally in teenagers, such families have strong discipline patterns and limit setting that bind the individual in his/her identity development, which is critical at this time of a person's life. Parents may interfere in the romantic relationships of their children, even in late adolescence.
3. At times, there is a symbiotic parent–child relationship. A parent, usually the mother, is too attached to the youth. Not only is such a relation disturbing, but the parent also does not provide the emotional protection and support that a parent usually provides intuitively to a youth as he/she grows. Sometimes the parent treats the child as an "adult". One such teenager tried to break this bond by attempting to kill herself in her mother's prized car, while another—a straight A student—intentionally obtained a B, resulting in a parent–child conflict and a suicide attempt by the youth. Additionally, it has been noted repeatedly in children that if such a parent dies, the child may commit suicide to be magically reunited with that same parent.
4. Long-term disorganization (malfunctioning) has been noted in these families; for example, mother's or father's absence, divorce, alcoholism, or mental illness. In teenage girls there is a very high rate of incest, compared with the general population. Even in the suicides of adults, and even more so the elderly, these types of disorganization have been observed. One such 74-year-old female tried to kill herself, stating in a note that she had not seen her children for 20 years.

In addition, three differentiating observations about the families of suicidal teenagers have been made. First, adolescents in such families often feel a lack of control over their environment, stemming from rigid family rules or symbiotic relationships. Second, adolescence is a time of stress and turmoil. It is not, as some believe, a time of simple joy and peace. Often, parents do not allow any conflict, turmoil, and development to occur. Third, recent family disorganization—for example, recent moves, unemployment in the home, physical or mental illness, parental conflict—has been noted in the family.

Berman (1986), by way of critique of some of this literature, has argued that much of the research is not scientifically controlled. For example, the research has not compared suicidal youth and their families with other troubled or non-troubled youth and their families. More recent reviews (Hawton & van Heeringen, 2000) offer no new research-based insights. Are the familial/interpersonal factors identified due to psychopathology, and not suicide risk *per se*? What are the familial risk factors? Are there protective factors? The conclusions offered above about the families of some suicidal people should be considered only tentative pending further study.

BEHAVIOURAL CLUES

In understanding suicide, we need to be aware of behaviours that are potentially predictive of suicide. However, there is no single definitive predictive behaviour. The two concepts that have already been discussed, and may be helpful here, are lethality and perturbation. The clues below are applicable to all age groups although the mode of expression may differ depending on age and numerous other factors.

Previous Attempts

Although it is obvious that one has to "attempt" suicide in order to commit it, it is equally clear that the event of "attempting suicide" need not have death as its objective. As noted earlier, it is useful to think of overlapping populations: (a) a group of those who attempt suicide, and a few of whom go on to commit it, and (b) a group of those who commit suicide, and a few who previously attempted it. A previous attempt is a good clue to future attempts, especially if no assistance is obtained after the first attempt. However, not all previous attempters make another attempt (or kill themselves). All too frequently such behaviour is not taken seriously. I recall an 11-year-old (very depressed) girl who cut her wrists at school and the principal's response was merely, "She is just trying to get attention." What an extreme way to get attention! The girl was moderately lethal and highly perturbed, requiring considerable intervention.

Verbal Statements

As with behaviour, the attitude towards individuals making verbal threats is too frequently negative. Statements are seen as "just for attention". This attitude results in ignoring the behaviour of a person who is genuinely perturbed and potentially suicidal. The important question is, "Why use this way of getting attention when there are so many other constructive ways?"

Examples of verbal warnings are: "I'm going to kill myself" or "I want to die", both being very direct. Other more indirect examples are: "I am going to see my (deceased) wife" or "I know that I'll die at an early age".

Cognitive Clues

The single most frequent state of mind of the suicidal person is constriction (Hughes & Neimeyer, 1990). There is a tunnel vision; a narrowing of the mind's eye. There is a narrowing of the range of perception or opinions or options that occur to the mind. Frequently, the person uses words like "only", "always", "never", and "forever". For example: "No one will ever love me. Only mom loved me"; "John was the only one who loved me"; "My boss will always be that way"; and "Either I'll kill my husband or myself". A 40-year-old bank manager, who had recently been fired from his job, expressed the constriction as follows: "Either I get my job back or I'll kill myself."

Emotional Clues

The person who is suicidal is often highly perturbed; he or she is disturbed, anxious, perhaps agitated. Depression, as already noted, is frequently evident. Suicidal people may feel boxed in, rejected, harassed, and unsuccessful. Some frequent feelings reported by patients are anger, anxiety, emptiness, loneliness, loss, and sadness. A common emotional state in most suicidal people is hopelessness or helplessness. Some statements may signal hopelessness: "Nothing will change. It will always be this way." Whereas helplessness may be verbalized as: "There is nothing I can do. There is nothing my children can do to make a difference."

Sudden Behavioural Changes

Changes in behaviour are also suspect. Those who may be at risk are the outgoing individual who suddenly becomes withdrawn and isolated and the normally reserved individual who starts being outgoing and seeking thrills. Such changes are of particular concern when a precipitating painful event is apparent. Changed performance in school or work, such as sudden failure, may be an important clue. Making final arrangements, such as giving away a record collection, a favourite watch, or other possessions, may be ominous and often not responded to by the receiver; the receiver is simply too pleased to get the "gift". A sudden preoccupation with death, such as reading and talking about death, may be a clue. Nonetheless, constructive discussion of this topic such as a class project for a university student may be helpful for the individual and his/her classmates.

Life-Threatening Behaviour

I recall that a 9-year-old boy who killed himself had previously been seen leaning out of an open window in his apartment, and, at another time, playing with a gun. I know of a 24-year-old male who died in a single car accident on an isolated road after having had several similar accidents following rejections by his girlfriend. I know of a 70-year-old female who died from drug mismanagement, despite the nurse in her residence controlling her medication. Self-destruction is not rare. Often alcoholism, drug addiction, mismanagement of medical treatment, and automobile accidents can be seen in this light, as previously discussed.

Suicide Notes

Like previous attempts and verbal statements, suicide notes are important clues; however, they are often read but not listened to by the reader. Notes are very rarely written by children, but are somewhat more frequent among adolescents. About 18–37% of adults leave notes (samples have varied greatly).

Because the topic of notes warrants a book by itself (Leenaars, 1988a), let me here state only that if one wants to understand the event, there is no better source than the words of the suicide, words that he/she wrote minutes before death (we will use such documentation throughout this book to illustrate not only a way to understand the events, but also individual suicidal people). A sample of notes will be presented in Chapter 7.

GENDER

The basic sex difference in suicide is that males kill themselves more than females [although this is not evident in China (Pritchard, 1996)]. In contrast, females attempt suicide more often than males, and this sex difference has been found in almost all nations (Lester, 1988a, 1992). The male–female difference in suicide has, in fact, remained fairly stable, even in other eras. The generally accepted male–female ratio of completed suicides is 3–4 males to 1 female, but there is great variation around the world.

Explanations in the literature (Leenaars, 1988c, 1988d) have varied. Females use different and less lethal methods (drugs vs shooting). Individuals with severe psychiatric disorders have higher rates of suicide and men are more likely to be diagnosed with such disorders. There are alternative social expectations for men and women in trauma that make males act more catastrophically. Yet, Shneidman (1985) has argued that genotypic similarities may be more prevalent than differences. Indeed, my own research (Leenaars, 1988c, 1988d) on suicide notes of males and females confirms this (see Chapter 2). Pain is pain. Frustrated needs are frustrated needs. Constriction is constriction. Perhaps there are phenotypic differences (e.g., method, diagnostic label) in suicide but not genotypic ones across sex? Could the high rates of completed suicide in males be more influenced by gender roles than by psychological factors? As Greenglass (1982, p. 256) noted:

> Since the beginning of recorded history, being male or female has been one of the most significant characteristics of a person. Sex and gender not only determine the kinds of experiences people have, but they also significantly influence the way people perceive and act toward each other. Moreover, socio-cultural expectations have been integrated into elaborate gender-role systems, which have an enormous impact on all areas of psychological and social functioning.

Tomlinson-Keasey and colleagues (1986), in their study of gifted female suicides, came to the same conclusion as my study of notes. They found that the markers (e.g., mental dysfunction, a history of problems) of suicide were the same in both sexes. Others (e.g., Canetto, 1994) have cited such factors as socio-economic disadvantage, unemployment, hostile relationships and a history of suicidal behaviour among friends and family as relevant to the suicides of women. Such factors have also been observed in the suicides of men (Lester, 1988a, 1992; Tomlinson-Keasey et al., 1986). The area is, however, plagued by stereotypes (Canetto, 1994). For example, the division of women's suicides as irrational and men's as rational is not supported in the data (Leenaars, 1988c, 1988d), and reflections on this topic are most relevant (Lester, 1988a). Equally, maybe one should ask, especially for its implication for treatment: "Why are women *not* killing themselves?"

A LIFE-SPAN PERSPECTIVE OF SUICIDE

There are various ways in which life's—including the suicidal person's—time-lines can be conceptualized. Though suicide is in many ways the same across the entire life-span, understanding suicide from a developmental perspective is productive (Leenaars, 1991a). My comments here are a brief summary of the area; there is no intent to be exhaustive.

Maris (1991) has provided a developmental perspective of suicide. He states that "The suicidal act is a process, a convergence of many factors over time...suicide is not one thing and is not the simple product of an acute crisis." He argues that the person's history (or "career" as he terms it) is always relevant to that person's self-destruction. Yet, Shneidman (1991) has argued that although it may be useful to group suicides under "adolescent or adult, or middle age or old", there is only suicide: "There is only human suicide and all of it is to be understood in terms of the same principles."

An American, as an example, dies by his/her own hand, on average, every 17 minutes. However, this differs depending on the time-line/age (as well as other major demographic factors; sex, gender, race/ethnicity, and so on). The rate of suicide varies depending on developmental age. Lester (1991a) looked at international trends across the life-span and illustrated, as we noted earlier, that there are different rates of suicide for different ages in different countries.

Developmental ages (or time-lines) have their unique—despite common— psychological issues. In line with the epidemiological findings that there are different rates of completed suicide across the life-span—and such rates differ from country to country—research and clinical findings, indeed, show that there may well be unique psychological issues at different ages for the suicidal person.

Although the "trunk" of suicide (referring back to Shneidman's definition—see page 5) may be the same, there appear to be differences in such psychological issues as "I love you"; "This is me"; "I am caving-in"; "I want to be gone"; "I am weakened"; "This is the only thing I can do". These differences may be more quantitative, however, than presence or absence. Richman (1991, 1993) shows us that suicide in the elderly, for example, is not to be understood primarily or even solely as a result of being old. As in other age groups, suicide in the elderly is multifaceted: sociological, biological, and cultural correlates may vary with age (Leenaars, 1991a).

Stack (1991), for example, presented the social correlates of suicide by age. Stack states that "correlates of suicidal behavior that vary by age include the position of the age group in society's institutional structure: the economy, religion, and family".

He shows us that there are different correlates depending on age such as the high divorce rates for young adults, the disproportional investment in motherhood by middle-aged females, and physical illness in the elderly. Stack (1991) has also shown that the impact of the media on the rate of suicide is different for different ages and that it is especially the adolescents that are affected by the media and subsequent acts of violence, including suicide.

Thus, understanding the time-lines in the suicidal process has a pivotal place in the study of the suicidal person. Much greater attention by clinicians and researchers alike is needed.

CULTURAL VARIATION

Suicide is complex; and culture is one important aspect of the complexity. Much of our understanding, including Shneidman's definition, has, however, a Western orientation. Shneidman (1985) stated that his proposed definition is applicable *only to the Western world* and notes that this caution needs to be given "so that cross-cultural comparisons do not make the error of assuming that a suicide is a suicide" (p. 203). To be effective in intervention, cultural diversity in the suicidal event must be understood.

It is probable that the individual, family, or community outside of the Western hemisphere does not share our commonly held views of suicide (e.g., as portrayed in the media). Here I will illustrate this view with examples from a few cultures to highlight our myopia, and return to this topic in detail in Chapter 21, with the assistance of the International Working Group on Ethical and Legal Issues in Suicidology.

In Japan, according to Iga (1993), for example, suicide, though not welcomed, has traditionally been accepted. Japan has never prohibited suicide and attempted suicide, except in the early eighteenth century. Suicide is seen as a personal problem in Japan (Iga, 1993; Takahashi, 1993). To understand suicide in Japan, Iga writes, one must especially understand Japanese views of death. These views are based on the idea of *mujo*, the sense of eternal change. Death is welcomed by many Japanese as an emancipation as, for example, illustrated in medieval times when many priests and their followers drowned themselves in the ocean, believing that they were going to *Saiho Jodo*, "Buddha Land". Death allowed one to identify with one's ancestor, and to have a continuing life (Shneidman's "*post-self*"). Suicide was no exception.

Aboriginal (or indigenous) people in North America (i.e., Turtle Island) have, as another example, their own diverse frameworks on death and suicide (Connors, 1995; Leenaars et al., 1999a). Historically, the loss of the traditional holistic view and the process of "acculturation"—a genocide—to the majority culture and its devastating impact are embedded in the trauma of the high rate of suicide in these people. This is true about many aboriginal people around the world, such as the Aborigines in Australia (Leenaars et al., 1999a). Although I cannot begin to address the complexity here, perhaps a look at the past in one group, the Northern

Cheyenne, may assist heuristically. Barter and Weist (1970) have extensively investigated patterns of suicide in the Northern Cheyenne people in Montana, US. They report that, contrary to the belief that suicide was rare in the early history of the Northern Cheyenne, they found documentation of 25 suicide deaths between 1830 and 1884. Suicide warriors, however, who were generally, though not always, young men who vowed to die in battle, committed the majority of these deaths. Barter and Weist (1970) noted:

> If a certain young man wished . . . he could make a vow that in the next battle, when the enemy began to close in, he would drive a pin into the ground and tie himself to it. This meant that he would take a stand there and not retreat, fighting until the enemy was driven back or he was killed . . . A man who vowed to take such a stand was called a suicide warrior and it was a great thing to die fighting in this way.

This self-sought "glorious" death afforded the suicide high prestige, with corresponding increased self-esteem—which, from our view, must appear to be a denial of death. As a similar example, Crazy Horse, the well-known Lakota Chief, always stated as he went into battle, "Today is a good day to die." The suicide pattern shifted dramatically, however, during the reservation period (1884–1949) and again during the contemporary reservation period (1950–1969) reflecting, according to Barter and Weist, cultural changes in the Northern Cheyenne. This epidemic of suicide occurred among many indigenous people around the world, but not all. Much seems to be associated with whether or not they were subjected to genocide (Leenaars et al., 1999a). Furthermore, the example of the suicide warrior as a cultural variation on the meaning of suicide illustrates that cultures are not static, but are ever-changing entities. We need to bear in mind that, even if one achieves some familiarity and comfort in working with people of a certain ethnic group or culture, that culture is constantly evolving and changing.

A subtle but important difference must be raised in the discussion about accepted suicide in cultures so far. Durkheim (1951) referred to such exceptions as "altruistic suicide". There are, in fact, examples of altruistic suicide, not only in Japan and among Aboriginal people around the world, but in almost all cultures, from antiquity to the present. Examples can be found among many peoples, from the Christian martyrs into the eighteenth century, to the practice of self-immolation not only in India, but Vietnam, Korea, and many regions of the world, to the now so-called suicide terrorist—or suicide bomber in the media—in the Middle East. There have always been exceptions throughout regions and ages.

Durkheim further explicated that some suicides are not only seen as a right but as a duty. "Society", states Durkheim, "compel(s) some of its members to kill themselves" (p. 220). Socrates was an example. Some altruistic suicides are obligatory, some are optional, and some are acute—those committed by martyrs or heroes. In all these examples, martyrdom is a motivation, whether it is to extol a religious belief, or to have honour in battle, or to pay homage to some other ideal. For some people, these exceptions give them the right to suicide—yet others see such acts as primitive and violent rationalizations. The deaths at the World Trade Center on 11 September 2001 sadly portray one of the most recent examples. How do we understand such suicides? Durkheim also questioned their motives:

All these cases have for their root the same state of altruism which is equally the cause of what might be called heroic suicide. Shall they alone be placed among the ranks of suicides and only those excluded whose motive is particularly pure? But first, according to what standard will the division be made? When does a motive cease to be sufficiently praiseworthy for the act it determines to be called suicide? (p. 240)

Durkheim's questions lead to others: Are there rights to suicide? And what are the implications of such suicidal people for the psychotherapist? How do we respond to such a person—a martyr, a suicidal person, etc.? These questions have implications for our response—more so in some cultures than in others. How would one treat Socrates or Crazy Horse?

Other cultures have different meanings, as we will see later. Even within North America, there is a richness and great diversity of peoples, e.g., aboriginal peoples, Afro-Americans, Inuit people, French Canadians, and so on. It is erroneous to assume that there is *one* commonly held definition or understanding of suicide (or death more generally). Suicide needs to be understood within a heuristic framework of the dominant culture/society, while appreciating and being sensitive to its specific understandings. This is true around the world and has direct implications and applications to treatment.

Simply put, suicide has different meanings for different people; and this is true for our suicidal patients. Culture is an especially powerful vehicle for meaning, and interventionists must be aware of these differences. To be insensitive to this issue in understanding suicide will likely result not only in problems in knowledge but also difficulties, even suicidogenic ones, in suicide prevention among different cultural groups.

SUICIDE PREVENTION

The classical approach to the prevention of mental health problems and public health problems is that of Caplan (1964) who distinguished the concept of primary, secondary, and tertiary *prevention*. The more commonly used concepts for these three modes of prevention are *prevention*, *intervention*, and *postvention*, respectively. All have a place in preventing suicide.

- *Prevention* relates to the principle of good mental hygiene in general. It consists of strategies to ameliorate the conditions that lead to suicide. "To do"—*venire*—something before the dire event occurs. Primary prevention is best accomplished through education. Such education, given the complexity of suicide, is enormously complicated, and is almost tantamount to preventing human misery.
- *Intervention* relates to the treatment and care of a suicidal crisis or suicidal problem. Also termed secondary prevention, it involves doing something during the event. A great deal has been learned about how to intervene—in crisis intervention and psychotherapy—with suicidal people. Obviously, suicide is not solely a medical problem and many persons can serve as life-saving agents. Nonetheless, professionally trained people—psychologists, psychiatrists, social workers, and psychiatric nurses—continue to play the primary roles in intervention.

- *Postvention*—a term introduced by Shneidman in 1971—refers to those things done after the dire event has occurred. Postvention deals with the traumatic after-effects in the survivors of a person who has committed—or attempted—suicide. It involves offering psychological services to the bereaved survivors. It includes working with all survivors who are in need—children, parents, teachers, friends, and so on.

To address these approaches in more detail warrants a separate volume for each topic; our focus here will be on intervention—primarily risk assessment and psychotherapy. I would like to digress, however, and add a few special comments on suicide prevention in schools (Leenaars & Wenckstern, 1990), probably because I have long advocated that the schools will be critical in preventing youth suicide (Leenaars, 1985). The response to suicide has to be complex in our communities and with our young people; the tragedy of Columbine High School in the United States of America in 1999 attests to this fact. Schools, for example, as suggested by the US Secretary's Task Force on Youth Suicide (1989) and the US Surgeon General, Satcher (1998), offer an excellent opportunity of reaching a large number of young people. Staff in schools, in fact, must act as "reasonably prudent persons". The decision of the US Ninth Circuit Court of Appeals in *Kelson* vs *The City of Springfield*, 1985, supports this view. In that case, the parents of a 14-year-old boy sued the school for negligence, complaining that the school had a duty to provide training in suicide prevention and that the school had failed to do so. The case was admissible to court because the court—though settlement was finally made out of court—held that a person might bring action against a school for non-prudent behaviour.

Although prevention efforts should be part of a comprehensive prevention–intervention–postvention plan, it is generally agreed that the most cost-efficient and potentially constructive avenue in public health problems is prevention (primary prevention). Prevention demands great patience and long-term commitment of resources and should not be confused with the intervention that suicidal people need. Prevention is for education, not intervening with lethal people. Suicidal young people need more than education; they often need psychotherapy.

We should critically reflect about our programmes. The prevention of (teenager) suicide must be part of a comprehensive programme that addresses all aspects of the prevention–intervention–postvention model.

RATIONAL SUICIDE, ASSISTED SUICIDE AND EUTHANASIA

In August 1991, Derek Humphry's book *Final Exit* reached the bestseller list for advice books in the *New York Times*. To date, this book has sold more copies than any other book on suicide. The book highlights a topic that all those working with suicidal people must face. Derek Humphry and the Hemlock Society (and similar people/groups world wide; see Chapter 21) do not advocate suicide *per se*. The society believes that suicide and assisted suicide, carried out in the face of terminal illness causing unbearable suffering, should be ethically and legally acceptable. Old age, in and of itself, is stated by the Hemlock Society *not* to be a cause for suicide.

But, whether we like it or not, terminal illness in some people is sufficient cause. The views about the right to die are, however, not uniform. Dr Kevorkian ("Dr Death"), for example, disassociates himself from the Hemlock Society (and other right-to-die groups) (Humphry, 1993). Kevorkian believes we should, without further debate, provide assisted suicide to those who request such a procedure (Kevorkian, 1988).

People in different countries have different views on the topic (Battin, 1993), and an array of distinct perspectives by an international group will be presented at the end of this volume. In the Netherlands, for example, euthanasia for the terminally ill was legalized on 1 April 2002; the first nation to do so in the world. The law will guarantee protection from prosecution for the physician who performs euthanasia, provided a set of guidelines (the "carefulness requirements") are met.

Suicide by the terminally ill, and perhaps even the non-terminally ill, requires understanding: Is it rational? What are the possible alternatives? Is it legitimate to withhold or withdraw life support? Can a case be made for euthanasia? Should we condone or approve assisted suicide? Euthanasia refers to the practice, after treatment has failed, of allowing the person to die with physician assistance. Assisted suicide is different; it refers to the practice of providing the means by which the person can end his/her own life, but is not physician assisted (see Chapter 21 for details). The above are all relevant questions for the psychotherapist working with suicidal people—especially those who are terminally ill.

On the issue of "rational" suicide, Diekstra (1992) has suggested that the word "rational" should be eliminated from our discussion on this topic. "Rational" is a construction. He asks, "When is any behavior just 'rational' or not?" It is a misleading term.

Obviously old age is not a reason for suicide. Many elderly people, including those that are terminally ill, are suicidal if their pain has become unbearable. Recovery, however, from the suicidal state is possible. Whether such pain ends in recovery or death depends partly on the relationship of the older person to family and to us, the psychotherapists. Rapport or therapeutic alliance is so critical, even in these cases. The decision to kill oneself is a process. It calls into question one's history, especially one's attachments, including those who are terminally ill. It is often an evaluation that one's past, present and future relationships offer some hope, something bearable that stops the exit. Attachments are so crucial: They often alleviate the unbearable pain.

Richman (1991) believes that the above ideas are critical to the topic at hand and argues against the right to die. He and others state that suicide, including suicide by the terminally ill, is never based only on being ill. Sigmund Freud is a dramatic example, because his work in mental health is so influential. Freud killed himself (with his physician's assistance). Was it, as he stated, because of his terminal illness? Or was it because he had been severely depressed at the time? He had been overwhelmed by World War II and had notable problems in his adjustment after moving to England. Was Freud's suicide due only to his terminal illness? Does Freud's suicide differ in its essence from other suicides? Humphry would say yes; Richman would say no. There are other questions—for example, was Freud's death a suicide? Would it be more appropriate to call it self-determined death or free death or voluntary death? These and other questions will be critical for the psychotherapist. When are suicide, assisted suicide, and euthanasia acceptable and when not? Are they ever?

Let me offer a story: I remember once witnessing the after effects of a suicide of an elderly male, age 84. His wife had died 3 months earlier; he had cancer; his car was in the shop; he had no family; and he chose to jump 22 stories to his death. That was tragic. What was even more tragic for me was watching the people in his building, a senior citizen apartment house with no social services, next to my office building. I remember seeing an older woman on the fifth floor look and look, as did others, at the body for one and a half hours. What services had the man needed? Would psychotherapy have been an alternative? Could someone have helped him with his crisis? And what about the other people? Is it humane to allow these senior people to be forced to witness such a death? Was the man terminally ill and, if so, would euthanasia (by a family doctor) or assisted suicide be more humane? And even if he was terminally ill, could we, as therapists, have helped to ease his pain? Could his death have been prevented?

The importance of the discussions on euthanasia and assisted suicide is that it raises questions that psychotherapists must reflect upon (see Chapter 21). Are we, for example, willing to provide the treatment, psychotherapy or otherwise, that elderly people need? Are we willing to support hospice care for those who are dying? Are politicians and the public willing to provide the money for the services that elderly people need? Or that terminally ill people need? There are many questions regarding euthanasia and assisted suicide. The issue of the right to die must be discussed by society in general, and psychotherapists in particular, well beyond the realm of suicidology. It will probably be a critical issue for psychotherapists in the twenty-first century.

THE TEN BEST BOOKS

What are the 10 top books in suicidology? I was once asked this question and it seems appropriate to answer it here, to provide an aspiring or veteran psychotherapist with a sort of "who's who" in the field. The ten classics—and this is subjective—are: E. Durkheim (1951), *Suicide*; P. Friedman (Ed.) (1967), *On Suicide* (a discussion of the Vienna Psychoanalytic Society); S. Freud (1974g), *Mourning and Melancholia*; K. Menninger (1938), *Man Against Himself*; A. Henry and J. Short (1954), *Suicide and Homicide*; E. Shneidman and N. Farberow (Eds) (1957), *Clues to Suicide*; C. Cain (Ed.) (1972), *Survivors of Suicide*; C. Varah (Ed.) (1985), *The Samaritans*; E. Shneidman (1985), *Definition of Suicide*; and K. Hawton and K. van Heeringen (eds) (2000), *The International Handbook of Suicide and Attempted Suicide* (although E. Stengel (1994), *Suicide and Attempted Suicide* and N. Kreitman (1977), *Parasuicide* are notable classics on attempted suicide). If I could add one, I would add a biological text, but it is unclear which one. The obvious names are M. Asberg, J. Mann, P. Nordstorm, H. Van Praag, A. Roy, and L. Traskman-Bendz. Shneidman (2000) and Maltsberger (2002) have suggested that the authoritative volume is D. Stoff and J. Mann (1977), *The Neurobiology of Suicide: From the Bench to the Clinic*. Thus, I will accept this edited volume to be included in the Ten Best Books for now. I write "for now" because the advances in biological sciences have been exponential (Maltsberger, 2002; Stahl, 2000). This is the test of a growing science.

CONCLUDING REMARKS

The present chapter is a prologue to the understanding of suicide. Suicide is a multifaceted event. Understanding such an event is a complex endeavour; yet not to do so, as a psychotherapist, may well be suicidogenic. Some things can be learned. There is much left to learn. The need to intervene with suicidal people prompts us, even necessitates us, to understand the nature of suicide. In this volume, I will share the knowledge I have gained while working with suicidal people. Therapists need to know what they are treating.

Chapter 2

SUICIDE: A MULTIDIMENSIONAL MALAISE

No one really knows why human beings commit suicide. One of the questions asked most frequently about suicide is: "Why do people kill themselves?" or, more specifically, "Why did that individual commit suicide?" People are perplexed, bewildered, confused, and even overwhelmed when they are confronted with suicide. Indeed, the very person who takes his/her own life may be, at the moment of decision, the least aware of the essence of the reasons for doing so. Understanding suicide, like understanding any complicated human act, is a complex endeavour, involving knowledge and insight drawn from many points of view. This is true for all people working in suicidology. My goal here is to provide a point of view on the questions, based on my studies of suicide over the years. My hope is that the perspective will be useful whether one is answering the crisis line, counselling the acute suicidal patient, surviving a loved one's suicide or, with the current task, especially providing psychotherapy with suicidal patients.

Most frequently, as we have learned, people identify external causes (e.g., ill health, being abandoned by a lover, losing one's income) as the reason the person killed him/herself. This view is too simplistic, although often the suicidal person holds that perspective. This is not to suggest that a recent traumatic event (e.g., drop in income, a change in work, a divorce, a grade of F) cannot be identified in many suicides. However, although there are always situational aspects in every suicidal act, they form only one aspect of the complexity.

Suicide is a multidimensional malaise (Shneidman, 1985). There are biological, psychological, intrapsychic, logical, conscious and unconscious, interpersonal, sociological, cultural, and philosophical/existential elements in the suicidal event, to name a few. It thus seems reasonable that we would be perplexed and bewildered about answering the question "Why?".

Any element of the malaise is a legitimate avenue to understanding suicide. Studies of serotonin have a place, as have studies of the effect of gun control, as have studies of cultural diversity. In fact, I oppose any reductionistic model in understanding suicide. Much of current thought about suicide is, from my view, too mechanistic. Suicide is a multifaceted event and is open to study by multiple disciplines, and herein I offer a psychological/psychiatric perspective by a suicidologist. Let me here, in fact, state that I agree with Shneidman (1985) that the psychological dimensions of suicide are the "trunk" of suicide. Shneidman (1985), using an arboreal image, wrote:

> An individual's biochemical states, for instance, are the roots. An individual's method of suicide, the contents of the suicide note, the calculated effects on the survivors and so on, are the branching limbs, the flawed fruit, and the camouflaging leaves. But the psychological component, the problem solving choice, the best solution of the perceived problem, is the main "trunk". (pp. 202–203)

From a psychological point of view, I would like to offer a few observations on the question "Why?". Of course, one should understand that these ideas are not exhaustive. They are ideas gleaned from significant suicidologists in our psychological history that have some empirical support. Specifically, the clinicians are: A. Adler, L. Binswanger, S. Freud, C.G. Jung, K.A. Menninger, G. Kelly, H.A. Murray, E.S. Shneidman, H.S. Sullivan and G. Zilboorg.

As a crucial final point of introduction, there are, of course, views that theory should not play a role in understanding suicide. Suicidology should only be tabular and statistical. However, I believe that theory, explicit and implicit, plays a key role in understanding any behaviour (and for the clinician, it is essential). Theory is the foundation in science (Kuhn, 1962). Newton, Einstein and all great scientists are great because they were theorists. It is only through theory that we will sort out the "mess of experience" (Wm James). In fact, it can be argued that "sciences have achieved their deepest and most far-reaching insights by descending below the level of familiar empirical phenomena" (Hempel, 1966, p. 77). Theory may well be in the eye of the beholder (Kuhn, 1962), but it is pivotal in scientific understanding whether one is a researcher, crisis worker or clinician. There is nothing as useful as good theory. I would go even further: I believe that we can only have our understanding (theory) of the patient. People must make formulations about things to understand them (Husserl, 1973). Thus, it would be wise to borrow the ideas of our leading theorists, as we began to see in Chapter 1, to answer the question, "Why?".

SUICIDE NOTES

How can we answer our initial questions? How do we look at suicide? Our answers, whether theoretical or not, should be based on logical and empirical fact (Ayer, 1959). Shneidman and Farberow (1957a), Maris (1981) and others have suggested the following alternatives at scientifically answering these questions: statistics, third-party interviews, the study of non-fatal suicide attempters and documents (including personal documents). All of these have their limitations. Statistics reflect by themselves only numbers and are, at best, only a representation of the true figures. A third-party interview, sometimes called a psychological autopsy, can only provide a point of view, which is not the suicide's view. Non-fatal attempters may be different from completers. Documents may provide, to use the words of Maris (1981), only a snapshot of an event that requires a full-length movie. But sometimes they provide a vignette of sufficient length so that some essential essences of the entire movie can be reasonably inferred. Indeed, all the alternatives have their limitations and strengths.

Of course, there is the problem of obtaining any of these data: statistics, interviews, reports by attempters and personal documents. The database for potential explanations of suicide is conspicuously absent. Maris (1981) points out that this is because "most researchers have been trapped by either the Scylla of official or 'vital' statistics or the Charybdis of individual case histories".

A related (if not embedded) problem is the one that is the ubiquitous issue of psychology itself: the mind–body problem; or, the admissibility of introspective accounts as opposed to objective reports. This resonates to Windelband's (1904) division of two possible approaches to knowledge between the nomothetic and the idiographic. The tabular, statistical, arithmetic, demographic, nomothetic approach deals with generalizations, whereas the idiographic approach involves the intense study of individuals—the clinical methods, history, biography. In this latter approach personal documents are frequently utilized—personal documents such as letters, logs, memoirs, diaries, autobiographies, suicide notes. Let us, before addressing the topic at hand, explore the views on the idiographic approach in more detail; the other—the nomothetic approach—is well engrained in psychology and science in general.

Allport (1942) has provided us with a classic statement on the advantages of the idiographic approach, noting that personal documents have a significant place in psychological research. Shneidman (1980), in *Voices of Death* (a book about letters, diaries, notes and other personal documents relating to death), has stated that such "documents contain special revelations of the human mind and that there is much one can learn from them". Although Allport (1942) cites some shortcomings in the use of personal documents in psychological science—unrepresentativeness of sample, self-deception, blindness to motives, errors of memory—he makes a clear case for the use of personal documents, citing the following: learning about the person, advancing both nomothetic and idiographic research, and aiding in the aims of science—understanding, prediction, and control. As an interesting footnote to his trailblazing work (Shneidman, 1980), Allport wrote about diaries, memoirs, logs, letters, autobiographies, but it did not occur to his capacious mind to think of perhaps the most personal document of all: suicide notes.

As an association, I recall being introduced to Beck's work, *Cognitive Therapy and the Emotional Disorders* (Beck, 1976), as a graduate student. I remember reading and re-reading this book. What struck me at that time was Beck's ability to provide an aspiring clinician with the actual protocols of patients that we meet in our offices. I learned how the patient's "pain" is embodied in his/her language and how we can use these protocols to understand him/her from the cognitive view. Even if one does not adhere to Beck's view, his perspective has provided many of us with a sound clinical view of people's cognitions/protocols. Using extensive personal documents (Allport, 1942), Beck and associates have developed our understanding of people through their own words.

My study of suicide is equally not defensive about the use or pleading for the occasional admissibility of personal documents, whether the person's own words, narratives or otherwise. On the contrary, it emphasizes their special virtues and their special power in doing the main business of psychology—the intensive study of the person.

Furthermore, the use of personal documents (or narratives) does not mean that the essential method of science—i.e., Mill's method of difference—has to be abandoned, as the comparison between genuine and simulated suicide notes clearly illustrates. I believe that personal documents provide a unique place in human science where maximum relevance can be mated with acceptable precision. There are not many marriages like that in psychology, to generate intervention strategies.

Suicide notes are the ultrapersonal documents. They are the unsolicited productions of the suicidal person, usually written minutes before the suicidal death. They are an invaluable starting point for comprehending the suicidal act and for understanding the special features of the people who actually commit suicide and what they share in common with the rest of us who have only been drawn to imagine it. Suicide notes are a way through the looking glass to suicide, although, unlike Alice, we will not find "beautiful things" there, but unbearable pain.

Early research (e.g., de Boismont, 1856; Wolff, 1931) on suicide notes largely utilized an anecdotal approach that incorporated descriptive information. Subsequent methods of study have primarily included classification analysis and content analysis. Only a very few studies, however, have utilized a theoretical–conceptual analysis, despite the assertion in the first formal study of suicide notes (Shneidman & Farberow, 1957a) and in ongoing discussion (Diamond et al., 1995) that such an approach offers much promise. Over 25 years ago I addressed this lack by applying a logical, empirical analysis to suicide notes. The method permits a theoretical analysis of suicide notes, augments the effectiveness of controls, and allows us to develop some theoretical insight into the vexing problem of suicide. It is this mode of analysis that we propose to follow here in this book to provide a theory to understand, and by implication, intervene with the suicidal patient.

The method has previously been described in detail (Leenaars, 1988a; Leenaars & Balance, 1984a). Essentially, it treats the notes as an archival source. This source is subjected to the scrutiny of control hypotheses, following an *ex post facto* research design (Kerlinger, 1964). The major problem with the current type of research is the lack of control over extraneous variables and the large number of potentially important antecedent variables, and thus there is the danger of misinterpreting relationships. Kerlinger (1964) suggested that these problems can be largely overcome by explicitly formulating not just a single hypothesis, but several "control" hypotheses as well. This would call for suicide notes to be recast in different theoretical contexts (hypotheses, theories, models) for which lines of evidence of each of these positions can then be pursued in the data. Carnap's logical and empirical procedures (1959) can be utilized for such investigations. To date, the theories of 10 suicidologists—Adler, Binswanger, Freud, Jung, Menninger, Kelly, Murray, Shneidman, Sullivan and Zilboorg—have been investigated. Carnap's positivistic procedure (1959) calls for the translating of theoretical formulations into observable (specific) protocol sentences in order to test the formulations. For example, a core aspect of the theories of the 10 suicidologists is that the stimulus for suicide is unbearable pain; thus, a protocol sentence under this rubric would be as follows: "Suicide has adjustive value and is functional because it stops painful tension and provides relief from intolerable psychological pain." The protocol sentences express the meaning of a given theory as they are matched empirically, by independent judges, with the actual data. Next, one introduces the method of induction from the available verified protocol for the discovery of general insights and to allow further theory building to occur.

To summarize from a series of empirical studies (e.g., age, sex, method used) of the theories of the 10 suicidologists, a number of theoretical propositions (or protocol sentences) have been identified to be observable in various samples of notes, the actual words of a suicidal person (much like our patient's in the psychotherapy room). Shneidman and Farberow (1957a) had introduced the technique of studying genuine suicide notes by comparing them, in a blind study, with simulated suicide notes. These later notes can be elicited from non-suicidal people, based on John Stuart Mill's method of difference. These differences are assumed to be actually absent in the non-suicidal person, allowing us to know not only the narratives of suicidal people, but also how they differ from those who have only been drawn to imagine being suicidal. The initial study (Leenaars, 1988a, 1989a) isolated 100 protocol sentences—10 from each of the 10 theorists. These were reduced to 35 sentences; 23 protocol sentences were found that highly predicted (described) the content of suicide notes (i.e., one standard deviation above the mean of observations) and 17 protocol sentences that significantly discriminated genuine suicide notes from simulated notes (i.e., control data) (see Chapter 7). Five sentences were found to be both predictive and descriptive, resulting in the final 35 empirically verified sentences.

Specifically, a study was undertaken of 60 suicide notes (Leenaars, 1989a), representing suicides from across the adult life-span, representing both sexes. A cluster analysis (Varaclus procedure, oblique principal component; SAS, 1985) was undertaken to reduce the 35 protocol sentences, both highly predictive and discriminative, to a meaningful empirical schema. Our analysis produced a classification of eight discrete clusters (when an eigenvalue of 1.00 was used as the criterion). This number of clusters accounted for 56% of the variance. The eight clusters identified by a word or short phrase were as follows: I, Unbearable Psychological Pain; II, Interpersonal Relations; III, Rejection–Aggression; IV, Inability to Adjust; V, Indirect Expressions; VI, Identification–Egression; VII, Ego; and VIII, Cognitive Constriction. Subsequently, from a series of studies, a meta-frame to organise the clusters into intrapsychic and interpersonal elements was proposed (Leenaars, 1988a, 1989a, 1989b, 1995). Suicide can be theoretically understood from the proposed theory (templates, constructs, or frames) to be outlined next in detail, but first allow me one final philosophical point on theory.

Theory gives us patterns or templates (that is one of the reasons why the subtitle of my book, *Suicide Notes*, is *Predictive clues and patterns*). Plato called it, forms; Plotnius, a seal; Jung, archetypes; Murray, "unity thema"; and Shneidman, commonalities. A philosophical question for millennia has been: How can we have patterns, templates, seals, commonalities, or whatever we call "it"? Or to restate the question from a clinical view: If Jennifer and Jeff are suicidal, how are they really the same ... or, scientifically stated, alike and different? What is her/his suicidal nature? Are there predictive clues or patterns and, if so, what are they and what are their implications and applications for psychotherapy (or any treatment)? Without the "sameness", there can be no seals or patterns or templates for understanding, prediction and control. We need to know, not necessarily the universal, but, at least, what is most common, the same—despite the ever-flowing buzzing of life (James, 1890), i.e., flux, change, difference, and so on.

A THEORY OF SUICIDE

Theory must begin with definition. Thus, to begin, let me offer once more, as a mnemonic, the formal definition of suicide by Shneidman (1985, p. 203):

> Currently in the Western world, suicide is a conscious act of self-induced annihilation, best understood as a multidimensional malaise in a needful individual who defines an issue for which suicide is perceived as the best solution.

Suicide is not simply a psychopathological entity in the DSM-IV (American Psychiatric Association, 1994). I do not agree, as I noted earlier, with those who point to an external stress as the cause of suicide. I also do not agree that it is only pain. I tend to place the emphasis on the multideterminant nature of suicide. Suicide is *intrapsychic*. It is stress and pain, but not simply the stress or even the pain, but the person's inability to cope with the event or pain. The issue of any schema about human personality, i.e., personology (Murray, 1938), is one that makes an individual an individual. It should be the study of the whole organism, not only the stress or pain. People do not simply commit suicide because of pain, but because the pain is unbearable; they are mentally constricted; they have a mental/emotional disorder; they cannot cope, and so on.

However, from a psychological view, suicide is not only intrapsychic, it is also *interpersonal* (or, stated differently, it is both an inner and outer phenomenology). The suicidal individual is not only depressed, mentally constricted and so on, but he or she is also cut off from loved ones, ideals and/or even the community. The suicidal person is estranged. People live in a world (a society). Individuals are interwoven; the suicidal person, painfully so. I disagree with those who point to only some intrapsychic aspects such as anger turned inward or primitive narcissism to explain suicide. Suicide occurs in a person *and* between people (or some other ideal; e.g., health). This is not a Cartesian dichotomy; it is rather a dynamic interactional system. Yet, the intrapsychic world is figural. Suicide occurs as a solution in a mind. The mentalistic processes are the foreground (such as the pain, depression). This is an important difference. It is in the inner world in which a person makes the decision to jump, shoot, etc. It is here that he or she decides, "This is the best solution." To put it simply: No drama, no stage. It is the intersection between the two phenomenologies that is essential to understand in suicide. It is, for example, not simply unemployment on the stage, but how the person's drama unfolds on this very personal, individual stage. Metaphorically speaking, suicide is an intrapsychic drama on an interpersonal stage.

Two concepts, as I noted in Chapter 1, that have been found to be essential and helpful in understanding the malaise are lethality and perturbation (Shneidman, 1973, 1980, 1985, 1993). Lethality refers to the probability of a person killing him/herself, and on quantification scales ranges from low to moderate to high. It is a psychological state of mind. Perturbation refers to subjective distress (disturbed, agitated, sane–insane), and can also be rated from low to moderate to high. Both concepts are needed to frame the following theory. It is important to note that one can be perturbed and not suicidal. Lethality kills, not perturbation.

To begin: Suicide can be clinically understood from at least the following templates or patterns (Leenaars, 1988a, 1989a, 1989b, 1995):

Intrapsychic

I Unbearable Psychological Pain
The common stimulus in suicide is unendurable psychological pain (Shneidman, 1985, 1993). The enemy of life is pain. The suicidal person is in a heightened state of perturbation, an intense mental anguish. What the author, William Styron (1990), called "The howling tempest of the brain." It is the pain of feeling pain. Although, as Menninger (1938) noted, other motives (elements, wishes) are evident, the person primarily wants to flee from pain experienced in a trauma, a catastrophe. The fear is that the trauma, the crisis, is bottomless—an eternal suffering. The person may feel any number of emotions such as boxed in, rejected, deprived, forlorn, distressed, and especially hopeless and helpless. It is the emotion of impotence, the feeling of being hopeless–helpless that is so painful for many suicidal people. The situation is unbearable and the person desperately wants a way out of it. The suicide, as Murray (1967) noted, is functional because it abolishes painful tension for the individual. It provides escape from intolerable suffering.

II Cognitive Constriction
The common cognitive state in suicide is mental constriction (Shneidman, 1985). Constriction (i.e., rigidity in thinking, narrowing of focus, tunnel vision, concreteness, etc.) is the major component of the cognitive state in suicide. The person is figuratively "intoxicated" or "drugged" by the constriction; the intoxication can be seen in emotions, logic, and perception. The suicidal person exhibits at the moment before his/her death only permutations and combinations of a trauma (e.g., business failure, political scandal, poor health, and rejection by spouse). The suicidal mind is in a special state of relatively fixed purpose and of relative constriction. In the face of the painful trauma, a possible solution became *the* solution. This constriction is one of the most dangerous aspects of the suicidal mind.

III Indirect Expressions
Ambivalence, complications, redirected aggression, unconscious implications, and related indirect expressions (or phenomena) are often evident in suicide. The suicidal person is ambivalent. There are complications, concomitant contradictory feelings, attitudes and/or thrusts, often towards a person and even towards life.

Not only is it love and hate but it may also be a conflict between survival and unbearable pain. The person experiences humility, submission, devotion, subordination, flagellation, and sometimes even masochism. Yet, there is much more. What the person is conscious of is only a fragment of the suicidal mind (Freud, 1974g). There are more reasons to the act than the suicidal person is consciously aware of when making the final decision (Freud, 1974g; Freud, 1974h; Leenaars, 1988a, 1993b). The driving force may well be unconscious processes.

IV   Inability to Adjust

People with all types of problems, pains, etc., are at risk for suicide. Psychological autopsy studies suggest that as many as 90% of people who kill themselves have some symptoms of psychopathology and/or problems in adjustment (Hawton & van Heeringen, 2000; Wasserman, 2001). Up to 60% appear to be related to mood disorders (although likely lower in teenagers). Although the majority of suicides may, thus, fit best into mood nosological classifications (e.g., depressive disorders, manic-depressive disorders), other emotional/mental disorders have been identified. For example, anxiety disorders, schizophrenic disorders (especially paranoid type), panic disorders, borderline disorders, antisocial disorders, have been related to suicides (Sullivan, 1962, 1964; Leenaars, 1988a). Anxiety may well be an equally important pain, next to depression (Fawcett, 1997). Schizophrenics have a very high rate (about 5%—not the often cited 10%) (Palmer & Bostwick, 2002). Yet, there are other disorders not specified that may result in risk. From the autopsy data, it is learned that as many as 10% may have no disorder identifiable in DSM-IV (or some other classification scheme). The person may simply be so paralysed by pain that life, a future, etc., are colourless and unattractive.

Depression in its varieties is, thus, the most frequent disorder (and full discussion would require a separate text); however, it must be understood by any clinician that not all suicidal people are depressed, and that not all depressed people are suicidal. It is often cited that 15% of people who develop depression ultimately kill themselves. Bostwick (2000) has, however, clearly demonstrated in a meta-analysis of the research that this is a myth. It may well, in fact, be as low as 2%. Most important, it is essential to remember that suicidal people experience unbearable pain, not always depression, and even if they do experience depression, the critical stimulus is the "unbearable" nature of the depression (as in some other mood). Suicidal people see themselves as being in unendurable pain and unable to adjust. Their state of mind is, however, incompatible with accurate discernment of what is going on. Having the belief that they are too weak to overcome difficulties, such people reject everything except death—they do not survive life's difficulties.

V   Ego

The ego with its enormous complexity (Murray, 1938) is an essential factor in the suicidal scenario. The OED defines ego as "the part of the mind that reacts to reality and has a sense of individuality". Ego strength is a protective factor against suicide. The biological perspective has equally argued this conclusion; van Praag (1997) has, for example, clearly documented a biological aspect to suicidal people: increased susceptibility to stressors, labile anxiety and aggression regulation. Suicidal people frequently exhibit a relative weakness in their capacity to develop constructive tendencies and to overcome their personal difficulties (Zilboorg, 1936). The person's ego has likely been weakened by a steady toll of traumatic life events (e.g., loss, rejection, abuse, failure). This implies that a history of traumatic disruptions—*pain*—placed the person at risk for suicide; it is probable that it mentally and/or emotionally handicapped the person's ability to develop mechanisms (or ego functions) to cope. There is, to put it in one simple word, *vulnerability*. There is a lack of resilience. A weakened ego correlates positively with suicide risk.

Interpersonal

VI *Interpersonal Relations*
The suicidal person has problems in establishing or maintaining relationships (object relations). There frequently is a disturbed, unbearable interpersonal situation. A calamity has prevailed. A positive development in those same disturbed relationships may have been seen as the only possible way to go on living, but such development was seen as not forthcoming. The person's psychological needs are frustrated. Suicide appears to be related to an unsatisfied or frustrated attachment need, although other needs, often more intrapsychic, may be equally evident, e.g., achievement, autonomy, dominance, honour. Suicide is committed because of thwarted or unfulfilled needs—needs that are often frustrated interpersonally.

The possible needs that are frustrated or blocked are expansive. Here is a partial list of needs, adopted from Henry A. Murray's *Explorations in Personality* (1938):

- *Abasement*. To submit passively to external force; accept injury, criticism, punishment; to surrender; become resigned to fate; blame or belittle self.
- *Achievement*. To accomplish something difficult; master, manipulate, organize physical objects, human beings or ideas; to overcome; to excel oneself.
- *Affiliation*. To enjoyably cooperate or reciprocate with an allied other; to please and win affection; to adhere or remain loyal to a friend or group.
- *Aggression*. To overcome opposition forcefully; to fight; to attack or injure another; to oppose forcefully or punish other.
- *Autonomy*. To get free, shake off restraint; break out of social confinement; avoid or quit activities of domineering authorities; be independent and free.
- *Counteraction*. To make up for failure by restriving; overcome weakness or repress fear; to maintain self-respect and pride on a high level; overcome.
- *Defendence*. To defend or vindicate the self against assault, criticism, blame; conceal or justify a misdeed, failure, or humiliation.
- *Deference*. To admire and support a superior; praise, honour or eulogize; yield eagerly to influence of another; emulate an exemplar.
- *Dominance*. To control other humans; influence or direct others by command, suggestion or persuasion; or to dissuade, restrain, or prohibit others.
- *Exhibition*. To make an impression; be seen and heard; to excite, amaze, fascinate, entertain, shock, intrigue, amuse, or entice others.
- *Harmavoidance*. To avoid pain, physical injury, illness, and death; escape from a dangerous situation; to take precautionary measures.

- *Infavoidance.* To avoid humiliation; avoid or quit conditions that lead to scorn, derision, indifference, or embarrassment.
- *Inviolacy.* To protect the self; remain separate; maintain distance; to resist others' intrusion on one's own psychological space; remain isolated.
- *Nurturance.* To gratify the needs of another person, especially one who is weaker; to feed, help, support, console, protect, comfort; to nurture.
- *Order.* To put things or ideas in order; to achieve arrangement, balance, organization, tidiness and precision among things and ideas.
- *Play.* To act for "fun". To enjoy relaxation of stress; to laugh and make jokes; to seek pleasurable activities for their own sake.
- *Rejection.* To exclude, abandon, expel, separate oneself or remain indifferent to a negatively seen person; to snub or jilt another.
- *Sentience.* To seek and enjoy sensuous experience; to give an important place to creature comforts and satisfaction of the senses—taste, touch.
- *Succorance.* To have one's needs gratified by the sympathetic aid of another; be supported, sustained, guided, consoled, taken care of, protected.
- *Understanding.* To ask questions; be interested in theory; speculate, analyse, generalize; to want to know the answers.

VII   *Rejection–Aggression*

The rejection–aggression hypothesis was first documented by Stekel in the famous 1910 meeting of the Psychoanalytic Society in Freud's home in Vienna (Friedman, 1967). Adler, Jung, Freud, Sullivan, and Zilboorg have all expounded variations of this hypothesis. Loss is central to suicide; it is, in fact, often a rejection that is experienced as an abandonment. It is an unbearable narcissistic injury. This injury is part of a traumatic event that leads to pain and, in some, self-directed aggression. In the first controlled study of suicide notes, Shneidman and Farberow (1957a) reported, for example, that hate directed towards others and self-blame are both evident in notes. The suicidal person is deeply ambivalent and, within the context of this ambivalence, suicide may become the turning back upon oneself of murderous impulses (wishes, needs) that had previously been directed against a traumatic event, most frequently someone who had rejected that individual. Biological research in the field has demonstrated a neurobiological link between aggression and suicide. Despite a minimizing of this fact by some (e.g., Shneidman, 1985), aggression, whether other or self-directed, has for example an association to serotonin dysfunction (Asberg et al., 1976). Freud's hypothesis appears to have a biological basis within the biopsychosocial view of suicide. Aggression is, in fact, a common emotional state in suicide. Suicide may be veiled aggression—it may be murder in the 180th degree (Shneidman, 1985).

VIII   *Identification–Egression*

Freud (1974g, 1974i, 1974j) hypothesized that intense identification with a lost or rejecting person or, as Zilboorg (1936) showed, with any lost ideal (e.g., health, youth, employment, freedom), is crucial in understanding the suicidal person. Identification is defined as an attachment (bond) based upon an important emotional tie with another person (object) (Freud, 1974i) or any ideal. If this emotional need is not met, the suicidal person experiences a deep pain (discomfort). There is an intense desperation and the person wants to egress, i.e., to escape. Something must be done to stop the anguish. The suicidal person wants to leave, to exit, to get out, to get away, to be gone, to be elsewhere . . . not to be . . . to be dead. Suicide becomes the only solution and the person plunges into the abyss.

Summary

In concluding, the theory outlined is only one point of view. Yet, the elements, I believe, have utility in understanding suicide. Indeed, to begin to address the question, "Why do people kill themselves?" or, more specifically, "Why did that individual commit suicide?", we need a psychology of suicide. We must answer the question, "What are the important common psychological dimensions of suicide?"—rather than, "What kind of people commit suicide?" The question is critical, for these common dimensions (or "sameness") are what suicide is. Not necessarily the universal, but certainly the most frequent or common characteristics provide us with a meaningful conceptualization of suicide. The history of suicidology (psychiatry, psychology, sociology, and so on) gives us the ideas, concepts, formulations, and so on, and science gives us the observable "valid" ones. This is the best of all possible psychologies, an empirically supported one. The theory outlined is an attempt to do that. There are few such theories in suicidology. It provides an answer to the question posed; it presents some common elements to answer, why Jeff killed himself.

These elements, common to suicide, furthermore highlight that suicide is not only due to external "stress" or pain or even unattachment. The common consistency in suicide is, in fact, with lifelong adjustment patterns (Shneidman, 1985). Suicidal people have experienced a steady toll of life events; i.e., threat, stress, failure, loss and challenge—or, in one word, pain—that has undermined their ability to cope. Suicide has a history.

Our lives, suicidal or not, are elliptical (Shneidman, 1985). This concept is not new; Heraclitus of Ephesus (circa 500 BC) held the view (Freeman, 1971). Friedrich Nietzsche called it the eternal return of the same (Nietzsche, 1966). It is the question of "sameness". T.S. Eliot (1944) wrote:

> We shall not cease from exploration
> And the end of all our exploring
> Will be to arrive where we started
> And know the place for the first time

The "sense of sameness is the very keel or backbone of our thinking" (James, 1890). This is from the point of view of a mind, of course. "Sameness" allows us to be a little wiser. An unbroken flow of life—events, traumas, and so on—would result in endless and often disabling problems in life and thus in the therapy room. All would be in flux. All would be a buzz. Sameness is identity, whether good or bad, whether life-enhancing or suicidal-inducing. Sameness allows us to know psychological (theoretical) laws, whether idiographic or nomothetic. It allows us to understand suicide and suicidal behaviour in that person and people. A philosophical question—and most relevant to the clinical question at hand—is: "Does anything remain the same in the flow of life?" To use Hegel's answer, there is identity in diversity. Plato first attributes the theory of a universal or common in the flux to Heraclitus, at least. There is "sameness".

The practical application in the therapy room is the following: Our patients' stories are always the same; this is as true about suicide as about anything else in people's lives. Life follows a non-Euclidean geometry defined so that all lines converge. Nature—at least some of it—also follows the rule. Koestler's comets, for example, move in very elongated ellipses. The suicidal history is elliptical—the eternal return of the same, even though there is change. Life is always in flux and equidistant to the constant. The constants are templates ("sameness").

Hopefully, the synthesis presented will provide a useful clinical perspective for many in suicidology on "Why people kill themselves?" and, as we will see, on "How do we intervene with suicidal people?".

SOME OBSERVATIONS

Theory should be empirically observable. This is the place of research in science. Thus, I would like to turn to research, examining the theory in terms of scientific evidence: age (with special reference to adolescents), sex, method, attempters, cross-culture, and cross-time.

Age

Shneidman and Farberow (1957a), in the first empirical studies of suicide, indicated that psychological aspects of suicide vary with age. However, too few studies have examined the obvious clinical critical element; for example, very few studies on suicide notes have examined this variable. The research (Darbonne, 1969a; Leenaars & Balance, 1984b, 1984c; Lester & Hummel, 1980; Lester & Reeve, 1982; Tuckman et al., 1959), however, consistently supported Shneidman and Farberow's (1957a) claim. Despite great similarities, there are differences in suicide across the life-span.

A problem with the studies of suicide and age is that various researchers have divided their age samples differently, resulting in some difficulties in direct comparison among studies. Leenaars (1988a), in the hope of bringing some clarity to the area, proposed a schema that was not only based on extensive research on adult development (Colarusso & Nemiroff, 1981; Kimmel, 1974) but also on Erikson's theoretical model on the stages of such development (Erikson, 1963, 1968), with the understanding that overlap between these groups, as well as even more varied classification within these groups, is possible. It is critical, however, to understand that, from a developmental view, age is not a mere demographic variable; it is a genotypic view. The groups, with Erikson's characteristics and proposed age range (with the proviso that no developmental age can be strictly reduced to chronological age) are as follows:

1. Adolescence (Erikson's stage, identity vs identity confusion; chronological age, 12 to 18)

2. Young Adulthood (Erikson's stage, intimacy vs isolation; chronological age, 18 to 25).
3. Middle Adulthood (Erikson's stage, generativity vs stagnation; chronological age, 25 to 55).
4. Late Adulthood (Erikson's stage, integrity vs despair; chronological age, 55 and over).

Leenaars (1989b, 1991b) studied 60 suicide notes, representing the specific adult age ranges and found that there were more similarities than differences on the psychological dimensions across the adult life-span. However, differences were noted. About the intrapsychic drama, we learned that people in young and middle adulthood are more indirect and ambivalent in their suicide (Indirect Expression). Or the converse, people in late adulthood are more direct, showing less redirected aggression, complications, and unconscious implications. Older adults are perhaps less confused about their suicide, having a stronger ongoing wish to die.

Young adults appear to be less able to cope with life's demands (Inability to Adjust). Young adults, compared to other adults, appear to be more diagnosable, if one wishes to use such labels, with a mental disorder. Young adults more frequently consider themselves too weak to function effectively, being unable to survive life's difficulties.

Young adults also appear to exhibit more often a weakened ego (Ego). More than people in middle and late adulthood, young adults exhibit a relative weakness in their capacity to develop constructive tendencies (e.g., love and work) and to overcome personal difficulties. This is, of course, closely associated to the high incidence of Inability to Adjust in this group. Young adults more often lack ego strength.

The interpersonal stage differs also in some ways. We learned that Interpersonal Relations are more often critical in young adulthood although it is pivotal to remember that "object relations" are common in all suicides. Yet, as Erikson (1963, 1968) noted, intimacy versus isolation is the major conflict for young adults. Often, suicidal young people feel a sense of total rejection. More often than other adults, young adults describe in their notes disturbed, unbearable interpersonal situations (although the relationship is often to a person, it may be to another ideal).

Related to the relationship aspect is the fact that young adults also exhibit more aspects of Identification–Egression than do people in late adulthood, but not middle adulthood. Intensive identification (or bond) with a lost or rejecting person or any ideal (e.g., youth, sanity, employment) is critical in understanding suicide, especially in young adults. The loss precipitates an ego regression in which everything, including the self, is repudiated and the person gives up on life.

We can, thus, tentatively conclude that the proposed theory is applicable across the adult life-span. These are the commonalities or similarities. The specific difference, however, may reflect age-specific stressors or concerns that may be important in understanding suicide. Specific differences across the adult life-span, of course, are an issue of more or less, not of presence or absence (Leenaars, 1988a).

Age: Adolescents

The adult studies beget some main questions in suicide prevention, especially because considerable attention has been given to suicide in youth world wide. First, what are the psychological factors that explain suicide in adolescents? Second, are suicide notes and, by implication, suicide different or similar across the life-span? To answer these questions, let me provide some background on suicide in teenagers.

Suicide is a major cause of death in the young (Berman & Jobes, 1991; Bertolote, 1993). This event is truly tragic because life expectancy for adolescents is the greatest in terms of both the interval of years lost and the diversity of experience that should await them (Leenaars, 1991a). Official suicide statistics, which have been proved to be underestimates (e.g., Jobes et al., 1987), nevertheless show that up to 20% of all male deaths and 28% of female deaths among adolescents in the industrialized world are caused by suicide. Among adolescents, suicide ranks among the first three causes of death. These shocking descriptive statistics are truly alarming, calling for greater research efforts.

Despite increasing research efforts (see King, 1997; Lester, 1992), the psychological factors for suicide in this age group remain largely unexplored. There is a growing body of empirically based knowledge; but, like much of suicidology, these studies are atheoretical (Leenaars et al., 1997) and provide limited insight into the suicidal mind of a young person. There are, in fact, very few studies that are able to give an insight into the reasons why young persons decide to end their lives (King, 1997). In addition, as we have learned, the opportunities that are available for potential explanations, given the very nature of the act, are limited (Maris, 1981).

Given all the limitations of data collection methods, the data, as we have learned, that are most neglected are the documents or narratives (e.g., suicide notes) from the adolescents themselves who died by suicide. To date, there are only three studies in the literature on the writings of adolescents (Leenaars et al., 2001b; McBride & Siegel, 1997; Posner et al., 1989). The study by Posner and his colleagues provides a descriptive analysis of teenager suicide notes; and McBride and Siegel, following a hypothesis by Rourke et al. (1989), noted evidence of pathognomonic signs for learning disabilities in the writings of adolescents.

The main reason for the lack is obtaining notes from adolescents—and this is related to a main question on the topic, namely how representative note-writers are to the general population, with reports ranging from 18 to 37% of suicides leaving notes (Leenaars, 1988a; O'Connor et al., 1999). Further, previous studies do not report the incidence of notes in subpopulations, e.g., adolescents. For example, the largest sample archived is 721 notes from 1945 to 1954, obtained by Shneidman and Farberow (1957a) from the Los Angeles Coroner's Office. Most of these notes are not marked with demographic characteristics. Out of a sample so marked, only 2% were from adolescents. A subsequent descriptive analysis of the sample of 1983–1984 notes from the Los Angeles County Coroner's Office, out of 127 notes, only 4 notes (3.2%) met the age range of adolescents. Leenaars and colleagues (2001b) presented a comprehensive theoretical study of the suicide notes of teenagers, derived from a large sample of over 2000 notes.

Leenaars and colleagues (2001b) studied 80 suicide notes, representing the adolescent and adult age ranges. As predicted by developmental theory (Erikson, 1963, 1968; Leenaars, 1991a), and as abundant studies show, there are psychological aspects that may be distinctly age-specific (again, a statement of more or less).

An important finding of the study is that the eight-fold theoretical clusters derived from the literature in suicidology may be as applicable to adolescents as to adults. Thus, previous results (e.g., Leenaars, 1988a, 1989a, 1989b, 1996) on the adult life-span can be tentatively applied to teenagers. The results allow us to speculate in favour of the conclusion that there may be similarities or commonalities ("sameness") in suicidal behaviour across the life-span (based on interpretations of suicide note protocols); of course, our sample does not include children, a group with increasingly noted suicide risks (Orbach, 1988; Pfeffer, 1986). Importantly, there are differences in the age groups, supporting our previous conclusions about differences across the life-span, depending on age.

We can, thus, tentatively conclude that the proposed theoretical formulation to understand why adolescents kill themselves may well be applicable to adults in some ways. These are commonalities or similarities. The specific differences, however, may reflect age-specific processes or (risk) factors that may be important in understanding suicide in adolescents. As a cautionary note, we do not wish to imply that our study has identified the causal links to suicide in teenagers, only some common and maybe differentiating factors or characteristics of the adolescents' suicidal mind (as we had previously discovered with adults). These characteristics may well be associated to heightened risk.

Based on the results, the teenagers appear to score higher than adults on Cognitive Constriction, Indirect Expressions, Rejection–Aggression and Identification–Egression. Given the attention to youth suicide, I will discuss these findings in more detail—and later address the other developmental groups as they arise. On the intrapsychic level of analysis, it appears that suicidal adolescents, at the moments before their death, may be highly cognitively constricted. They are singly preoccupied with one trauma (e.g., rejection of girl/boyfriend, conflict with a parent, being bullied), offering only variations of this one circumstance in their last narrative. Their death is probably highly correlated to their tunnel vision, funnelled through words like "always", "no one", "all", and "never". They choose death out of an overwhelmingly constricted mind.

Intrapsychically, they may be equally quite confused and contradictory in their mind. They may be ambivalent, often expressing love–hate towards the same person (one writes, "I hate you mom ... All my love, your daughter"). Yet, there are probably many more reasons for the act than those consciously recognized by the teenager. Not only is the mind constricted, but it is likely to be a confused, complicated mind. There appear to be many unconscious processes in their decision. They not only define the problem narrowly, but also the solution.

At an interpersonal level, the teenager often notes life's circumstances or situations, notably a loss, failure, and abandonment. The loss of the girl/boyfriend, for example, may well be an overwhelming and unbearable narcissistic injury. The ambivalent adolescent reacts with anger and vengefulness towards the traumatic event, frequently a rejecting person. He/she wants to kill and hopes that his/her suicide will have an evil impact on the survivor(s) as, for example, one teenager concluded his note, "P.S. Happy Father's Day".

Finally, also at an interpersonal level, the adolescents may be deeply attached (identification) with the lost person, or other ideal (e.g., straight A's), often at a symbiotic level. It is likely that they are unwilling or unable to accept the injury and want to egress. The teenager kills him/herself to escape.

From Erikson's developmental perspective (1963, 1968), adolescence is seen as the time for identity (ego) development with its complexity (e.g., individuality, sameness and continuity, wholeness and synthesis, social solidarity). It is a difficult transition and can be strongly affected by overidentification (to the point of total loss of self) with specific people or ideals (e.g., straight A's). The symbiosis may often be to a girl/boyfriend (or other peer), which is clearly reflected in the teenager's suicide note. Cognitively, often in adolescence, there appears to be a lack in the ability to abstract, being quite prone to fixation on one event or circumstance, as often noted in our suicide group. One frequently sees a flood of confusion in the teenager's conscious cognitive processes, although equally, unconscious processes may occur. As Frager and Fadiman (1984) note about the adolescent stage in the life cycle: "Although many aspects of the search for senses of identity are conscious, unconscious motivation may also play a major role. At this stage, feelings of acute vulnerability may alternate with great expectations of success" (p. 156).

The suicidal teenager's mind may not only be lacking in abstraction; it may be confused and limited. Suicidal teens are likely to be quite vulnerable, although this is often true of teenagers. Suicidal teenagers especially feel unable to cope with life's demands. Identity "is accrued confidence that the inner sameness and continuity, prepared in the past are matched by the sameness and continuity of one's meaning from others" (Erikson, 1963, pp. 261–262). In the suicidal teenager, all meaning may be lost; he/she is likely to be so overwhelmed with, for example, loss or failure. It is probably a deep injury, resulting in great confusion about his/her identity, i.e., a lack of certainty about who one is, without, for example, the boy/girlfriend. They are not a separate and distinct entity (identity diffusion). The loss of the overattachment (overidentification) to the object probably results in unbearable pain and the need to escape. As Erikson (1968) noted, "in the social jungle of human existence there is no feeling of being alive without a sense of identity" (p. 130). In the suicidal teenager, in fact, it may well be that death is chosen reactively because there is no "I" without the girl/boyfriend, straight A's or whatever.

In summary, we can tentatively conclude that our theoretical factors may be critical in adolescent suicide. Of course, all the factors or characteristics in the study were noted in some teenagers. Equally, we did not study many other factors, which may be relevant to self-chosen death. Suicide in teenagers, as in all ages, is complex and multidetermined, and our findings need to be placed in a broader context and perspectives of suicide (and developmental psychology in general) (Leenaars, 1991a; King, 1997). There are no obvious singular reasons why teenagers kill themselves.

Our results about adolescents offer a preliminary integration of existing theory about suicide across the life-span and provide a step towards model building of the unique features of suicide in teenagers, based on their own narratives. While there appear to be commonalities in suicides, there may well be differences. The person's age, such as adolescence, is quite relevant in understanding the event. Indeed, I believe, as a developmentalist, that a life-span developmental perspective is vital in understanding the teenagers' suicide, but also that we need to situate the suicidal event in the proper biopsychosociocultural, temporal, and individual dynamic context (King, 1997; Leenaars, 1991a; Michel & Valach, 1997). Such an integrated perspective may have utility in future predictive studies and, most important, in prevention and intervention with suicidal teenagers.

Our main conclusion about adolescent suicide is in support of the theory that it may be useful to look at the psychological aspects, both intrapsychic and interpersonal, from a life-span developmental perspective, although underlying commonalities may equally be meaningful (Shneidman, 1991). As predicted by developmental theory (Erikson, 1963, 1968; Leenaars, 1991a), and as the study shows, there may be aspects that are highly related to age-specific processes. Not only is this true for adolescents, but it is especially true for young adults. Young adults appear to exhibit significantly different patterns than other adults and teenagers, consistent with previous research (Leenaars, 1989a, 1989b). In the study by Leenaars et al. (2001b), young adults' pattern seems to be especially influenced by intrapsychic constructs of Unbearable Psychological Pain, Inability to Adjust, and Ego, again suggesting that young adult suicides may have a high relation to the crystallization of mental disorders in this age group. Obviously, each suicide must still be understood with awareness that some of the distinctiveness between suicides may well be a reflection of developmental age, as well as other aspects of the diversity among individuals. This is as true for teenagers as for adults.

In summary, our main conclusion about age is in support of the theory that there may be more similarities in suicide than differences. It may be useful to look at the core psychological aspects, both intrapsychic and interpersonal, from a life-span developmental perspective, but the underlying commonalities appear equally meaningful (Shneidman, 1991). Indeed, greater psychological commonalities than differences are to be expected in all suicidal events, by virtue of their human quality (Shneidman, 1991). Yet, as predicted by developmental theory (Erikson, 1963, 1968; Leenaars, 1991a), and as the studies show, there may be aspects that are distinctly age specific. By implication, each suicidal patient must still be understood with awareness that some of the distinctiveness between suicides may well be a reflection of developmental age—or other aspects of diversity in individuals.

Sex

Are women's suicides psychologically different from those of men? That is an important question, especially since the basic sex difference in suicide is that males kill themselves more than females (Canetto & Lester, 1995), except in China. Men kill themselves about three times more often than females (Diekstra, 1996; Gulbinat, 1996; Lester, 1992).

Gender differences in research on suicide have been, until recently, a neglected topic. Although not the primary focus of the research, early researchers (Cohen & Fiedler, 1974; Lester & Reeve, 1982) reported the following type of sex differences: males appear to be more direct and more negative; females exhibit a greater concern for others; males express fewer negative emotions; and females are more disorganized. However, those early studies can be questioned, being mainly anecdotal. Their suggestion, for example, that women are more disorganized and disturbed is not based on a clear and precise methodology.

Within the context of the growing literature on gender psychology in general, Leenaars (1988a, 1988c, 1988d), examining 40 suicide notes that were matched for age and sex, reported no sex differences on the intrapsychic and interpersonal aspects discussed earlier. There appear to be no sex differences on such issues as "I love you", "I'm in unbearable pain", "I'm hopeless and helpless", "I cannot cope", and "This is the only way out for me".

Tomlinson-Keasey et al. (1986) presented a converging view that there may be more similarities than differences in core psychological aspects across the sexes in their prospective investigation of suicide among gifted women. In 1970, Shneidman (1971) investigated the lives of five male suicides. These men had been subjects in the famous Terman longitudinal study of gifted individuals and Shneidman isolated a number of markers (e.g., conspicuous instability; depression; problems in relationships, especially early ones) that predicted the suicides. Tomlinson-Keasey et al. (1986) used the same markers in eight women who committed suicide in the Terman subjects and concluded that Shneidman's markers were applicable for both men and women. These results support the view that there may be significant similarities across sex, and suggested that the outlined theory can be applied to both women and men; this is not to say that there are no differences, but only that, from a clinical perspective, we can use the same basic constructs to understand the suicidal person. We also wish to state that much greater study is needed, for example, "Why do women exhibit three times better well-being than men?".

Method of Suicide

People appear to have a preferred method of suicide (Lester & Murrell, 1980). In fact, modern theories of the impact of restricting availability of methods for suicide (e.g., gun control in Canada [Lester & Leenaars, 1993]) are based upon the assumption that most people will not switch from their preferred method of suicide should it be unavailable during a suicidal crisis (Clarke & Lester, 1989). People in general, furthermore, perceive different methods (e.g., guns vs pills) differently and believe that individuals who use different methods are psychologically different (Lester, 1988b). Yet, it must be asked: Do the psychological characteristics of the suicidal individual make a difference in the method chosen for suicide?

Leenaars (1990) examined a sample of 42 suicide notes from which the method of suicide was known. The methods were classified, utilizing a scheme presented by Lester (1983) as active (firearms, hanging, and stabbing) or passive (drugs and poisons). The notes were matched for age and sex. No differences were reported, converging with previous studies in the area of suicide notes (Leenaars & Lester, 1988–89; Lester, 1971, 1983). The negative findings can be made more noteworthy if one observes that previous research, investigating the psychological characteristics of the suicidal person with data other than suicide notes, has also only found negative results (Lester, 1970a, 1970b, 1971; Lukianowicz, 1974; Noreik, 1975). Of course, there is the old problem here (and in other aspects of this issue) of "accepting the null hypothesis in science", although from a clinical view we cannot wait to respond. (We will also rediscuss the topic on modes of environmental control to prevent suicide in Chapter 19.)

Attempters

As noted in Chapter 1, although it is obvious that one has to "attempt" suicide in order to commit it, it is equally clear that "attempting suicide" does not always have death (cessation) as its objective. "Completing suicide", in contrast, typically, despite ambivalence, does have death as its objective. I believe, as have others (e.g., Stengel, 1964), that it is useful to think of the "attempter"—sometimes referred to as a type of parasuicide (see Chapter 5 for details)—and the "completer", as two overlapping populations: (1) a group of those who attempt suicide, a few of whom go on to commit it and (2) a group of those who commit suicide, many of whom have previously attempted it. The question, thus, can be raised: Are these two groups psychologically the same and/or different? Shneidman (1985) has concluded "that suicide and parasuicide are, by and large, operationally quite different" (p. 214). Research on suicidal individuals has, however, revealed only a number of differences between attempted suicides and completed suicides (e.g., Davis, 1967; Shneidman & Farberow, 1961; Wilkins, 1967). Much greater research is, thus, needed on this topic.

Attempted suicide is much more common than completed suicide. It has been identified that about 3.5 to 4 attempts occur for each completed suicide (Shneidman & Farberow, 1961; Schmidtke, 1997). Yet, because many gestures at attempted suicide result in such little damage that the attempts do not get counted by official agencies, it has been estimated that there are probably 8 to 10 suicide attempts for every completed suicide. It would be pertinent to point out here that scholars are divided on the merits of studying attempted suicides. The prevailing view has long been that because attempters and completers are two different, though overlapping populations, little can be learned about completed suicides by studying attempted suicides in isolation (Lester, 1970c). However, the availability of individuals who attempted suicide for completing questionnaires and participating in interviews has led to their use as "substitute" subjects (Neuringer, 1962). Lester and colleagues (1975), furthermore, have suggested that dividing a group of suicidal subjects by the seriousness of their suicidal intent would permit identification of features that might increase (or decrease) linearly with increasing suicidal intent—a point also made by Leenaars et al. (1997; see Chapter 5).

There is a need for studies of suicide that compare attempters with completers (Smith & Maris, 1986). Are there commonalities? Are there differences? As noted earlier, there have actually been very few studies to answer these questions. Thus, we need to ask: Is our theory of suicide only applicable to completers, or can we also apply it to attempters—all, some or most? These are critical questions for prevention, and by implication, psychotherapy. One avenue for such investigations is to compare the notes written by both groups, something generally neglected to date in the literature, except for the publication by Leenaars et al. (1992), and I will here report the findings of this sole study. As an important aside, I wish to follow my earlier suggestion (Leenaars, 1988a) that, by definition, only the notes written by completers should be called suicide notes. Attempters may write similar letters but it would be wrong to call them suicide notes. Some people call such letters parasuicide notes; yet, I am uncertain whether this is the best term (see Chapter 5).

It has been estimated that about 18 to 37% of completers leave a note. Notes of attempters are rarer. Only about 2% of attempters leave a note, although it is impossible to be conclusive here because most such documents are destroyed, hidden, etc., by the writer and/or his/her family. We simply do not have a conclusive answer to these questions. Let us now turn to the findings of the study by Leenaars et al. (1992).

The purpose of the study by Leenaars and his colleagues was to investigate suicide notes and parasuicide notes for the presence of the eight clusters (and the individual protocol sentences) that had been discussed earlier. The methods were the same.

The sample of parasuicide notes consisted of 18 letters written by individuals who attempted suicide. The notes of the attempters were obtained through the cooperation of a police department in a southwestern American town. There were regrettably no formal estimates of lethality of the attempts (see Chapter 5). This was not possible because police protocol would not allow for such a procedure, though the use of a lethality estimate would have been more desirable. Who were these attempters? Were they people of high lethality or low or moderate lethality? We know that the attempts were lethal enough to result in police involvement and the need for medical attention. Generally, based on consultation where possible, it is our impression that the attempts were of moderate to high lethality (e.g., Smith et al., 1984; see Chapter 5).

Each parasuicide note was matched for age (±2 years) and sex with a suicide note written by an individual who killed him/herself. These notes were obtained from my archives. All notes were written by individuals in adulthood (i.e., 18 and above), with an age range from 18 to 70 for the parasuicide notes and from 19 to 72 for the suicide notes.

The comparison on the eight clusters produced no significant differences. The suicide notes and parasuicide notes did not differ on the eight psychological characteristics. Only one specific protocol difference (item 13 under Inability to Adjust; see Chapter 6) was found between the notes. The protocol item, namely that the individual considers him/herself too weak to overcome his/her personal difficulties and therefore rejects everything to cope with the difficulties of life, was rated as more often true of parasuicide notes ($\chi^2(1, N = 36) = 5.0$, $p < 0.05$). It would appear—at least tentatively—that perhaps attempters relatively more often see themselves as unable to adjust to life's difficulties, although they are not diagnosed as having a mental disorder more frequently. Yet, from a statistical point of view, the sole finding could be one of chance. Even this observation would need replication.

The lone result is very limited, especially given the belief that attempters are different from completers. On the other hand, maybe the psychological characteristics of suicide identified in this book are as applicable to highly lethal attempters as they are to completers. There are, indeed, significant commonalities between attempters and completers (Shneidman, 1985). Perhaps those identified here are indeed some of those similarities, and thus, have an application for psychotherapy. It is likely, in fact, that there is a continuum of suicidal behaviour, not merely a dichotomy of attempters and completers.

In their study, Leenaars and colleagues (1992) also reviewed the literature comparing completers and attempters (Davis, 1967; Lester & Wright, 1973; Wilkins, 1967). This literature was reviewed and protocol sentences were derived from this review. This literature also allowed for prediction of direction between our groups in the hypotheses (Greenwald, 1975), a way to address the relevance of negative findings. Some 20 protocol sentences, both whether more common in completers or attempters, were identified and these were compared in the suicide and parasuicide notes.

The comparison on the 20 protocol sentences produced only a few additional significant findings.

Parasuicide notes expressed greater evidence that the attempt was a life-style ($\chi^2(1, N = 44) = 4.83$, $p < 0.05$). Opposite to the prediction, it was also noted that attempters in their notes more often suggested a lack of social integration ($\chi^2(1, N = 44) = 4.36$, $p < 0.05$).

Suicide notes and parasuicide notes may differ; yet, they may be more similar than different. Completers and attempters (at least those studied), based on their notes, appear not to differ in such characteristics as pain, aggression, cognitive constriction, hopelessness, psychopathology, and relationships.

Suicide attempts evoke response in others. Indeed, the act may well be undertaken with a general disregard for a beloved person, spouse, society, etc., to evoke a response in them. The act, for the attempter, may become a way to cope, not to die. It is noteworthy that only a few attempters actually commit suicide; yet, having made an attempt is a good predictor of self-harming behaviour in the future. If our speculations are correct, when do these self-harming individuals become mortality statistics? When does their self-harming life-style become impetus enough to add to a complex equation to wish to die? Echoing others (e.g., Shneidman, 1985), we urgently need to do research on suicide–parasuicide comparisons to answer these possibly life-saving questions.

Our findings have clinical implications. Maybe we can treat the attempters as we should have the completers. Maybe completers let us know what and how to do psychotherapy with suicide attempters and all suicidal people. Our theory, at least, appears to be as applicable to attempters as to completers. Maybe these completers have told us what to treat. Maybe their stories do provide an avenue to rescue.

Cross-Culture

Much of our understanding of suicide may be culture specific. Shneidman's (1985) definition, as discussed in Chapter 1, has a Western orientation ("In the Western world"). Thus, caution is needed in the field. Shneidman (1985) noted that when making "cross-cultural comparisons, do not make the error of assuming that a suicide is a suicide" (p. 203).

Studies of suicide in different cultures and nations, for example, the Japanese-American (Iga, 1993) and Japan (Takahashi, 1993), show that our Western theories of suicide may not be shared. Suicide has different meanings for different people. Culture is an especially powerful vehicle for meaning. Insensitivity to this fact will likely result in problems in our understanding of "Why?". Despite this fact, extensive international research is only about a decade old, especially spurred on by the World Health Organization (WHO) and international associations such as the International Academy for Suicide Research (IASR) and the International Association for Suicide Prevention (IASP).

There are only a few studies, for example, on suicide notes from different countries. Leenaars (1992a), noting that Canada has a higher rate of suicide than the United States (Leenaars & Lester, 1992), examined 56 suicide notes from Canada and the United States, and matched the writers for age and sex (this was the first cross-cultural study of suicide notes). None of the intrapsychic or interpersonal aspects differed. Leenaars et al. (1994a) examined 70 suicide notes from Germany and the United States, matching the writers for age and sex. None of the variables reached significance. Subsequently, studies from Northern Ireland (O'Connor & Leenaars, 2003), Hungary (Leenaars et al., 1998b), Russia (Leenaars et al., 2002c), and Australia (Leenaars et al., 2003) supported this observation. Primarily, differences observed were within the interpersonal realm, but rarely. Maybe culture affects these aspects more than issues of pain, mental blindness, and so on. Interpersonal or social characteristics, or the context, may be most relevant to explain differences. But not intrapsychic ones. Cultures differ!

Suicide notes, and by implication, the psychological dimension of suicide, may be similar in Canada, Germany, Hungary, the United States, and so on. It is probable that pain is pain, rejection is rejection, an egression is an egression, and so on in people from various cultures, although their mode of expression may differ. Yet, there are questions about how different the United States, Canada, and Germany are compared to cultural differences with Japan and South Africa. What about India (Leenaars et al., in progress)? It appears, yes. Methodologically, there are limitations to the studies to date in universal application. Further cross-cultural study will be essential as, with the twenty-first century, we move into a global world. It is important not only for progress in suicidology but for effective treatment, that research findings in one nation be replicated in other nations.

On a fulcrum note, it may still be cautiously assumed that the multidimensional theory is applicable to other cultures. There is some cross-cultural reliability; this is rare in suicidology. Broad theoretical comparisons may bring out similarities, but we should continue to isolate the factors responsible for differences among individuals. We simply do not know whether the suicide of the Japanese is the same or different from the American or whether the suicide of the Inuk in Canada's Arctic is the same or different from other Canadians. Suicidology must answer these questions in this decade.

Cross-Time

An historical review of suicide will show that people's conceptions about suicide have changed over time. Plato's position in *The Phaedo* is different, for example, from David Hume's in "On suicide" and, for further comparison, is different from Albert Camus's in *The Myth of Sisyphus*. Rarely, however, has it been asked whether the psychological aspects are different or similar during different time periods. Has suicide changed, and with it the implications? Leenaars (1988a), in a study of suicide notes, has reported on the question, "Are suicides psychologically different today than in the past?" More specifically, I asked, "Has suicide changed or remained constant specifically between 1945–1954 and 1983–1984?"

Sixty-six notes, matched for age and sex, written in 1945–1954 and in 1983–1984, were examined. These two samples allowed us to investigate the question about the general nature of suicide over the 40-year period, a period of considerable turmoil in history, from World War II through Vietnam. The results suggested that the psychological aspects of suicide are generally ubiquitous across time—at least for these 40 years in the United States. Thus, the theory appears to be as applicable to the forties as to the eighties. Maybe these are commonalities or similarities. Maybe there are greater psychological commonalities than differences in suicide. Generally, I believe that our findings regarding suicide are as applicable today as they were 40 years ago.

AN IDIOGRAPHIC SUMMARY

Our attempt to address the question "Why do people kill themselves?" has, I hope, brought us closer to an answer. We now see that suicide, indeed, can be best understood as a multidimensional malaise. It is constituted, at least, by intrapsychic aspects (unbearable pain, cognitive constriction, indirect expressions, inability to adjust, ego) and interpersonal aspects (interpersonal relations, rejection–aggression, identification–egression). Suicide has adjustive value for the individual, not survival value (Murray, 1967). It is perceived, consciously and unconsciously, as the best solution to a problem. My main conclusion is in support of Shneidman (1985) that there are more psychological commonalities than differences despite noted differences in developmental age. These observations are tentatively true across sex, culture, time, and method chosen for suicide (and maybe other factors in our suicidal patients). Yet, a good theory in suicidology must also have sound clinical utility. Next, I will briefly address the applicability of my schema by examining the application of the theory to a historical note, with much more detailed studies throughout this volume. Indeed, this book is about case studies.

To recapitulate: Studies in 1945–1954 and in 1983–1984 indicated that suicide has generally been the same across this short time span. We can raise the question of whether notes from very much earlier times would be the same or different; for example, Thomas (1980) presented an idiographic (unique) study of an ancient Egyptian suicide note, written about 4000 years ago. Thomas suggested that the note communicated (among other factors) the following: a painful situation that may have been more fantasy than reality; an inability to adjust, related to a deeply depressed emotional state; a cognitive state that was constricted if not delusional (e.g., "no one loved him", "the world is only full of sin"); and a perception that all, even his own soul, had forsaken him. Suicide was seen as "sweetness" and "joy" for this Egyptian. It was a welcome escape. Thomas, indeed, reflected on the stability of the man's personality. The man who committed suicide wrote:

> Death is before me today, As a man longs to see his house. When he has spent years in captivity.

There are a number of other historical suicide notes worthy of an archival dig. Johann W. Goethe (1749–1832), in his novel *The Sorrows of Young Werther*, presents a simulated—not genuine—suicide note. Werther, as we noted in Chapter 1, killed himself in the face of his unbearable anguish. It is a story of a traumatic painful event—the unrequited love of Lotte. It is a story of Werther's intoxication—"flood of emotions", "everything around about ceased to exist"—with Lotte who is betrothed and marries another. The book itself is written as if it were the personal documents—letters, the diary—of Werther. *The* final document, a suicide note, reads as follows:

> Everything is so calm around me and my soul is so calm. I thank thee, Lord who gives these last moments. This warmth, this strength!
>
> I step to the window, my dearest, and see, and still see through the stormy, fleeting clouds some stars in the eternal heavens. No, you will not fall! The Eternal Father carries you near his heart, and me. I see the stars of the shaft of the Dipper, the loveliest of all the constellations. When I left you at night and passed your gate, it was in front of me.
>
> With what intoxication have I so often looked at it, raised up my hands to it as a symbol, and made it a sacred token of my bliss! And even now—oh Lotte, what is there that does not remind of you? Are you not about me always? And have I not, like a child, greedily seized every trifle which you, dear saint had touched!
>
> Beloved silhouette! I return it to you, Lotte, and ask that you take good care of it. I have bestowed a thousand, thousand kisses on it, waved a thousand greetings to it whenever I went out and returned home.
>
> I left a note for your father entreating him to protect my body. In the church yard there are two linden trees, in a far corner, next to the field, there I wish to rest. He can and will do this for his friend. Do ask him too. I will not ask pious Christians to allow their bodies to lie next to that of a poor, unhappy man. Oh I wished you would bury me by the wayside, or in a lonely valley, that priest and Levite might cross themselves as they pass the stone which marked the spot, and the Samaritan may shed a tear.

There Lotte! I do not shudder to take the cold, dreadful cup from which I am to drink the ecstasy of death! You have given it to me, and I do not fear. All, all the desires and hopes of my life are fulfilled. So cold, so stiff to knock at the iron gate of death.

That I might have been granted the happiness to die for you, Lotte, to sacrifice myself for you! I would die gladly, I would die cheerfully, if I could restore the peace and happiness of your life. But alas! It was granted to but a few noble souls to shed their blood for those they loved, and by their deaths to kindle for them a new life enhanced a hundredfold.

I want to be buried in these clothes, Lotte. You have touched and sanctified them. I have also asked your father to carry out this request. My soul hovers over the coffin. Let them not search through my pockets. This rose-coloured ribbon which you wore on your bosom the first time I met you surrounded by your children—oh! Kiss them a thousand times and tell them the fate of their unhappy friend. The darlings! how they swarm around me. Oh! how I attached myself to you, how I could not keep away from you from the first moment! Let this ribbon be buried with me. You gave it to me on my birthday! How eagerly I accepted all this! Alas! I did not think the way would lead to this!—Be calm! I beg you, be calm!

They [the pistols] are loaded—The clock strikes twelve! So be it then!—Lotte! Lotte! Farewell! Farewell![1]

How can we understand Werther's suicide? Using the theory outlined in this chapter, we can observe within the context of Werther's life, as described by Goethe, the following unity thema:

Intrapsychic

I Unbearable Psychological Pain

Young Werther was, according to his own communication, in what he perceived to be a traumatic situation, the unrequited love of Lotte. He was experiencing unendurable psychological pain. In the note, Werther wrote about only one thing: his love for Lotte ... yet, other motives appear evident. Werther was perturbed, experiencing feelings of pitiful forlornness, deprivation, distress, and grief. He felt boxed in ... and especially hopeless (Lotte was the only one) and helpless (there is nothing I can do ... nothing anyone can do). Suicide had a functional value—it provided relief from intolerable suffering.

II Cognitive Constriction

Werther's suicide note was about only one thing, a trauma—his love for Lotte. Werther's emotional state was overpowering; his own word was "intoxication". His thoughts were constricted on his loss. He provided only permutations and combinations of this grief provoking content in the note. Lotte was "heaven" and "the purest joy of life".

III Indirect Expressions

Themes of submission and devotion, subordination and masochism were evident. The only happiness was to die for Lotte, to sacrifice (punish) himself for Lotte to "restore the peace and happiness of your life". Death was the only solution ... yet,

---

[1] Translated from German by Susanne Wenckstern.

much more than the written words described Werther's life; Unconscious psycho-dynamic implications are evident in his last letter, calling for even deeper interpretation of *The Sorrows of Young Werther*.

IV   *Inability to Adjust*

At the end, Werther needed to adapt but he was paralysed. His life was colourless and all had become wholly unattractive.

V   *Ego*

The pain alone did not account for Werther's suicide; Goethe describes Werther's ego as a critical aspect in the suicide. Unresolved problems, obstacles, etc., were evident in Werther. He wanted to sacrifice himself (self-punishment). The suicide was accomplished due to a relative weakness in his capacity for developing constructive tendencies—*Thanatos overcame Eros*.

Interpersonal

VI   *Interpersonal Relations*

Werther's interpersonal relations were disturbed. The relation to Lotte was disturbing (to him, Lotte, her husband and her family). His attachment to Lotte was painfully (too) intimate and, given Lotte's own affection for him and a deep ambivalence, was simultaneously stimulated and inhibited. Werther's need for attachment was frustrated. The relation had been doomed to failure from the beginning since Lotte had been betrothed to another before they met. Other needs (Murray, 1938) identified in the text are abasement, autonomy, dominance, exhibition, and order.

VII   *Rejection–Aggression*

In the end, Werther was singly preoccupied with the loss and rejection. He believed that Lotte was the only possible way to go on living. He was weakened and narcissistic. Werther, in fact, was described in the book as a narcissistic person.

VIII   *Identification–Egression*

Werther's identification (attachment) with a rejecting and lost person (Lotte) was deep and painful. He was unwilling to accept these painful emotions which made it possible for him to accept death willingly. He wanted to egress—to be gone. His only ideal (or solution) was beyond life, "the ecstasy of death". Like so many suicides, Werther fantasized that all would be well in the next life; he and Lotte would be reunited forever.

Analysis of Werther's Note

The actual protocol sentences from Chapter 6 that were verified in Werther's note are as follows: Unbearable Psychological Pain, 1, 2, 3, 6; Cognitive Constriction, 7, 8, 9; Indirect Expressions, 11, 12; Inability to Adjust, 15; Ego, 16, 17, 18; Interpersonal Relations, 21, 23, 24; Rejection–Aggression, 26, 27; Identification–Egression; 33, 34, 35. (The reader may wish to attempt his/her own rating; see Chapter 6.)

Thus, it can be concluded that the theory is applicable to the case of Werther, a case that is over 200 years old. At the very least, I can conclude that Goethe and I agree about "Why people kill themselves". Maybe there are significant commonalities or forms or "sameness" in "Why?" that theoretical suicidologists have been articulating for centuries.

CONCLUDING REMARKS

People in general have considerable difficulty appreciating significant characteristics of suicidal individuals. Most fortunately, a host of suicidologists have given us a rich history of theory for understanding suicide. These suicidologists point out that in life people—and Sylvia or Vincent—are somehow at once both the same and in flux. I have learned that the suicidal history is elliptical and thus understandable, predictable, and controllable. I will go even a little further—although it may be seen as arrogance—that this fact of suicidal nature is sound clinical wisdom. We owe our ancestors in suicidology a great deal. Their theories provide the foundations for our field and our aspirations for rescue. These building blocks define the event. In fact, according to Shneidman (1985), even further clearer theory building will be the most important direction for progress in the field.

The main conclusion from my studies is that there may be more commonalities ("sameness") in suicide than differences. There are core dynamics across time and maybe even across culture. By virtue of our human quality, whether male or female, greater similarities than differences are to be expected in all suicidal events (Shneidman, 1991). Maybe there are forms, seals, archetypes, unity thema, commonalities, or whatever we wish to call it. Yet, although there are probably commonalities across the life-span, there may be intrapsychic and interpersonal aspects that are distinctly specific, especially in terms of developmental age. Despite clear and distinct commonalities, each individual must still be, however, understood idiosyncratically with awareness of developmental age, sex, culture, (historical) time, and so on.

We need to continue to develop models (Goffman, 1974; Kuhn, 1962) to understand suicide—and the suicide of that individual, whether Susan or Peter. We need models that can be researched and, most importantly, can be made useful and life saving. This is true for clinicians, researchers, community based individuals, clergy, Elders, survivors—all who work at suicide prevention. It is also true for psychotherapists who are bent on changing the life-long adjustment patterns of the suicidal person, not only to help to rescue the patient today, but to assist for the future. We hope to change the deadly "sameness". The goal is simple: to help the suicidal person to cope with life.

Chapter 3

UNCONSCIOUS PROCESSES

Suicide is a *conscious* act. It is a conscious act of self-induced annihilation. This is not to say that there are no vital unconscious elements in the total scenario. In other words:

> ... it is meant to indicate that, by definition, suicide can occur only when an individual has some conscious mediation or, better, some conscious intention to stop his or her own life. There is always an element of some awareness and conscious intentionality in suicide. (Shneidman, 1985, p. 204)

On the other hand, the driving force may well be *unconscious process*. By definition, one must be conscious of the act to kill oneself, but the conscious aspect of the human mind is only one part of the act. The unconscious is a vast domain and I believe a key to our understanding.

THE UNCONSCIOUS

Consciousness (including the precise moment at which I decide to kill myself) is composed of only what I am aware of at that moment. Consciousness is, indeed, important in understanding a complicated human act like suicide. Yet, there is much more. We have long known that, beyond the conscious ones, there are many thoughts and feelings connected with what we do.

The unconscious is probably one of Sigmund Freud's most important concepts (Ellenberger, 1970; Fenichel, 1954; Heidbreder, 1933). Its appeal is probably that one can explain a variety of phenomena from dreams to slips of the tongue to the writing of suicide notes. One can show that these are phenomena related to and emanating from the unconscious mind.

Freud first began to postulate the unconscious from his work with his patients while studying with Breuer in the 1880s. Freud was most interested in symptoms due to hysteria such as functional blindness and glove anaesthesia. One of Breuer's patients, Anna O., had been especially significant to Freud. She was a young woman whose hysterical symptoms had developed out of a childhood experience. For Freud, "I do not want to feel any painful sensation is the first and final motive of defence" (Fenichel, 1954, p. 161). Symptoms—and I would add suicide—can be seen as a defence (or a solution) to pain. In treatment, Anna O. became aware of the root of her anguish. Breuer's and Freud's interpretation was that an original experience had aroused pain that had been prevented from expressing itself in a normal fashion. Rather, the pain became expressed in a symptom. The symptom, thus, was neither physical nor conscious in origin.

Freud postulated that for many of his patients' symptoms—expressions of pain—there were no physical determinants and no conscious reasons. The person, for example, suffering from hysterical blindness had not decided to be blind. Freud's patient could describe essential details about the blindness; yet, was unaware of critical aspects.

Thus, Freud (1974e) wrote:

> The assumption of the existence of something mental that is unconscious is necessary and legitimate. It is necessary because the data of consciousness have a very large number of gaps in them; both in healthy and in sick people, psychological acts often occur which can be explained only by presupposing other acts, of which nevertheless, consciousness is afforded no evidence. At any given moment consciousness includes only a small content, so that the greater part of what we call conscious knowledge must be for very considerable periods of time, in a state of latency, that is to say, of being psychically unconscious. The assumption of an unconscious, is moreover, a perfectly legitimate one inasmuch as postulating it, we are not departing a single step from our customary and generally accepted mode of thinking. (p. 166)

What one knows about one's behaviour provides only a fragmentary aspect of the total personality. This is not to say that it is insignificant, only that it is not the driving force behind behaviour. The unconscious is the driving force. The unconscious is active, dynamic, and personal. In a sense, Freud here anthropomorphizes all of mental life. He describes the unconscious as if it were distinctly personal, as personal as the people we meet in everyday life.

Within psychology, there is a resurgence of interest in the unconscious, even among the more cognitive views (see Bowers & Meichenbaum, 1984; Kral & Johnson, 1996). Indeed, we do not have to forgo the concept because Freud postulated it. Epstein (1994), for example, suggested that there is cognition outside of awareness that "automatically, effortlessly, and intuitively organises experience and directs behavior" (p. 710). The concept of the unconscious is, indeed, well accepted, well beyond the original dynamic view—and is essential to understand suicide (Leenaars & Lester, 1996). Kral and Johnson offer self-deception (i.e., "motivated nonawareness of conflicting beliefs or selves" (p. 71)) as one example of unconscious cognitive processes, a dissembling that one can see in subsequent cases, such as Rick. Empirical work, even with autonomic (sympathetic) arousal, supports the existence of the concept of the unconscious. Psychologists, even the empirical ones, now acknowledge the need for the concept to explain a wide array of behavior—this is true for suicide.

Thus, in order to understand human acts including suicide, one must introduce the unconscious. Suicidology would be overly barren without it. Suicidologists can learn much about suicide with a perspective focused on the unconscious processes.

A SERENDIPITOUS FINDING

A series of studies spanning the last four decades (e.g., Leenaars, 1979, 1985, 1986, 1987, 1988a, 1988b, 1988c, 1989a, 1989b, 1990; Leenaars & Balance, 1981, 1984a, 1984b, 1984c; Leenaars et al., 1985, 2001b) introduced an empirical approach to suicide notes, which presented a method for the theoretical analysis of suicide notes. To date, as outlined in Chapter 2, the theories of 10 suicidologists have been investigated (Leenaars, 1988a); specifically, studies of Adler, Binswanger, Freud, Jung, Menninger, Kelly, Murray, Shneidman, Sullivan, and Zilboorg have been undertaken. A specific series of studies (Leenaars, 1987; Leenaars et al., 1985) on Shneidman's formulations of suicide revealed that important unconscious processes were present in over half of the suicide notes studied, regardless of age and sex. It was also found that unconscious processes were significantly more frequently observed in genuine suicide notes than in simulated suicide notes (Leenaars, 1986). The specific protocol sentence or classification derived from Shneidman's work (1980, 1981a, 1985) was: "In the suicide note, the person's communication appears to have unconscious psychodynamic implications." Very few variables to date have been observed to be so critical in suicide notes, and thus, by implication, suicide.

It is most pertinent that independent clinical judges had made these observations with substantial interjudge reliability. It was also shown that the judges were able to obtain an overall average (presence or absence) score–rescore agreement significantly greater than chance. Thus, some aspects of reliability have been documented about the scoring of unconscious processes in suicide notes.

A serendipitous observation was found when a cluster analysis was undertaken (Leenaars, 1986, 1987). The unconscious forces were grouped with a set of protocol sentences labelled *relations*. Specifically, the protocol sentence was grouped with a dyadic event, a calamitous relationship, the withdrawal of a key significant other person, expressions of love and hate towards a person, an ambivalent attitude towards a person, perceiving another person as dooming one to death, and feeling hopeless and helpless about establishing meaningful relations. It appeared that the unconscious processes were most associated with these relational aspects of suicide, whether with a person or some other ideal (e.g., freedom, health).

Regrettably, however, when the judges were asked what the unconscious process might be and how they reached their conclusion, no agreement was reached. One judge cited concepts and decision rules based on psychoanalytic defence mechanisms, whereas the other cited concepts and rules that were generally derived from Shneidman's work. Of course, theorists themselves tend to disagree generally about such concepts. Freud cited intense identification with a lost or rejecting object *and* aggression turned inward as the critical variables. Shneidman would cite intense (unbearable) psychological pain, with accompanying constriction, hopelessness, push for egression, etc.—probably sparked underneath by dramatically frustrated psychological needs that are critical in the individual's make-up. Other suicidologists, for example, Beck, Menninger, Lester, Zilboorg, etc., cite other notions. It is hence understandable that individuals would respond in different ways to these exceedingly complex issues.

Concepts such as "unconscious" are not as readily observed as manifest content. This, of course, was true in the case of Anna O. Further procedures were needed, such as providing more structured classification or operational definitions about the nature of the latent (i.e., unconscious) content and decision rules or guidelines for assigning a vote to the classification.

A STUDY: AN INTRODUCTION

Dreams have often been subjected to latent analysis. Since both dreams and suicide notes can be seen as a response, as it were, to the blank card of the Thematic Apperception Test, both are amenable to the rules of thematic interpretation in general. The primary difficulty in conducting research on latent concepts is that observation and interpretation tend to be subjective (Kerlinger, 1964). After all, unconscious processes cannot be assessed directly (Freud, 1974e), but only analysed from the distorted manifest content. Freud (1974h) proposed that wishes, needs, motivations, etc. that are related to psychological conflict or pain are frequently repressed into the unconscious and, subsequently, expressed in dreams and, although the mental processes are different in some ways, (Freud, 1974a, 1974h), in every day life (e.g., verbal expressions, writings). These expressions are, however, *distorted* and thus the unconscious forces (latent content) cannot be assessed directly (Freud, 1974e). However, they can be assessed *indirectly* from the distortions in the verbalizations, associations, etc. (Freud, 1974f).

Based on Freud's perspective, Foulkes (1978) attempted to develop *objective* general principles to describe the types of distortions that commonly occur in the manifest content of dreams; these principles can be equally applied to suicide notes and other thematic material. Foulkes's Scoring System for Latent Structure (1978) is an objective and explicit system. He proposed that unconscious forces be presented in linguistic form in psychologically meaningful units, namely subject–verb–object relationships. Table 3.1 presents a summary of Foulkes's scoring classifications. As an analysis technique, Foulkes's Scoring System is unique and innovative because it attempts to establish a reasonable and orderly set of rules for the analysis of latent content.

Foulkes's scoring system for the interpretation of the latent content in these personal documents was used in a study of suicide notes (Leenaars & McLister, 1989; McLister & Leenaars, 1988; McLister, 1985) to examine genuine suicide notes and simulated suicide notes (as control data). Based on previous research it was predicted that unconscious forces would be present in the statements of the genuine suicide notes more frequently than in the simulated notes, i.e., more distortions would be identified in genuine notes according to established operational definitions.

A Study: The Method

Two independent raters, with graduate training in psychology, served as the judges. The judges were blind to the purpose of the study. As suggested by Leenaars (1986)

Table 3.1 Foulkes's scoring classifications

Classifications	Examples
Interactive Verbs	
Moving Towards	loving, wanting, needing, accepting, liking, helping
Moving From	withdrawing, disconnecting, disenfranchising, detaching from
Moving Against	being aggressive towards, rejecting, dominating, controlling, exploiting
Creating	discovering, nurturing, inventing
Associating Verbs	
With	associated with
Equivalence	being identical to
Means	acting as the means/medium
Nouns	
Father	father, older man
Mother	mother, older woman
Parent	scored when sex of parent is unknown
Sibling	brother, sister
Spouse	spouse, peer of opposite sex in long-term relationship
Peer Male	males of approximately same age
Peer Female	females of approximately same age
Children	males/females of younger age
Ego	self
Symbolic	animals, material objects, thoughts

Author's note: This table is based on material from the work of David Foulkes and is used here with Dr Foulkes's permission.

and recommended by Foulkes (1978), judges received considerable instructions in the scoring system and were trained on a large sample of suicide notes ($N = 63$). The judges' scoring agreement reached at least 90% on all classifications before initiating the study.

The judges were then asked to score the 33 genuine and 33 simulated suicide notes in Shneidman and Farberow (1957a). Shneidman and Farberow had randomly obtained (with the cooperation of the Los Angeles County Coroner's office) the 33 genuine notes from a sample of 721 suicide notes and had subsequently obtained the 33 simulated notes from independent, non-suicidal individuals who were matched by sex, age, and occupation. The judges were unaware of the use of simulated notes as control data.

As recommended by Foulkes (1978), the judges scored the suicide notes independently and, subsequently, met to reconcile their scoring to minimize deviation from the scoring rules. The reconciled scores were employed in the data analysis.

The judges read Foulkes's (1978) description of the rules for the Scoring System for Latent Structure. Every sentence in a note is scored on the basis of explicit rules—not intuition, theoretical tenets, etc.—with relationships as the conceptual unit of analysis. Every sentence is scored for subject (noun), verb (Interactive or Associative) and object (noun). The rules are briefly summarized below.

Verbs are scored as either Interactive or Associative (see Table 3.1). Interactive statements are scored for subject–verb–object relationships, using the verb categories of

Moving Toward, Moving From, Moving Against, and Creating. Associative statements are scored when nouns are linked by relationships defined as With, Equivalence, and Means. Interactive verbs can be modified. Modifications that enhance the intensity of the relationship are scored "+" and those that diminish the intensity of the relationships are scored "−".

Foulkes lists the various noun categories (see Table 3.1). Self is scored as Ego. Nouns are scored using the categories; for example, persons of the same generation as the Ego are scored as Sibling, Spouse, Peer Male, or Peer Female depending on their sex and relationship to Ego. Nouns can be modified. Nouns described in terms that are positive or enhance their adequacy are scored "+" and nouns described in terms that are negative or diminish their adequacy are scored "−".

The decision rules for scoring Ego are described by Foulkes (1978). Every interactive statement is considered to be a self-statement, so either the subject or the object must be scored as Ego. Ego may be the subject or the object in a statement, but may not be both. Thus, the scoring system requires that the writer of the note "is located in, at least, one pole of every scored interactive relationship" (Foulkes, 1978, p. 208). This assumption is based on Freud's statement that "Dreams are completely egotistical". A similar assumption has been made about other expressions of a person (Freud, 1974f) and can be readily applied to suicide notes. Ego is either stated directly in a note or can be inserted into the context by being represented in a note in several ways and/or times through *identification* with extraneous persons (and/or other objects). Other things being equal, since the suicidal person is the author of the note, he/she is the subject of each sentence. The principle is called active voice; i.e., the subject is Ego [although this can be "modified by 'identification' rules which align Ego with persons of like age and sex" (Foulkes, 1978, p. 210)]. If the object of the sentence is clearly the writer, the object is scored as Ego. Ego can be scored only once in each sentence, even in sentences like "I hate myself". The latter reflexive type sentences are scored as modifying Ego (as in our case, Negative or "−") but do not constitute interactive statements. When neither the subject nor the object is explicitly described as Ego in a note, decision rules are applied to infer Ego. The primary identifications are by active-voice, by sex, and by age. More complex rules are also provided when statements describe, for example, third persons and symbolic interactions. All interactive statements that cannot be scored directly from the text, but call for decision rules to be applied, constitute one type of distortion.

Foulkes also explains that, in certain circumstances, associative statements lead to a transformation of interactive statements, following Freud's dictum that associations or contextual data are given a priority if available. Nouns in interactive statements can be replaced (transformed) with nouns that have been linked to them in associative statements. For example, if, in a note, the person writes "I hate x" and "x goes with spouse" then, one can conclude that "I hate spouse". Associative sentences are exempt from the rule that Ego must be scored in each sentence; i.e., third-person sentences can occur, following Freud's resolution that associations, etc., are not always ego-cathected (or significant). The example above illustrates the exemption. When associative statements result in transformations of interactive statements, it implies that a distortion has occurred (although different from distortions related solely to interactive statements). Thus, two types of distortions are scored in the system: one related to associative transformations and the other to cases in which interactive statements cannot be scored directly from the text.

The scoring rules are only summarized here and are described in detail by Foulkes (1978).

A Study: The Results

Following Foulkes's rules of analysis (1978), the results indicated that genuine and simulated suicide notes did not differ in distortions related to associative transformations. In the interactive statement only 7.87% of the genuine notes and 5.42% of the simulated notes contained such transformations. This finding is probably related to the fact that free associations cannot be obtained for suicide notes as they can for dreams, and that this type of distortion is generally dependent on associations. Subsequent references to distortions refer to cases in which interactive statements could *not* be scored directly from the text. It was here that a significant finding was observed: genuine suicide notes contained significantly more distortions than the simulated notes.

Of the genuine suicide notes, 21 contained distortions—almost two-thirds of the notes—and distortions were associated with 25.2% of the interactive statements. Of the simulated suicide notes, 12 contained distortions—about one-third of the notes—and distortions were associated with 11.82% of the interactive statements. A large proportion of the distortions in both the genuine (86.40%) and simulated (80.77%) notes involved the employment of the decision rules to determine whether the Ego should be scored in the position of subject or object of an interactive relationship between two third persons or between a third person and an object.

No differences were found in the frequency with which each interactive verb (Moving Towards, Moving From, and Moving Against) was noted in genuine and simulated notes. Moving Towards was scored most frequently; Moving Towards accounted for 67.45% of the interactive statements in the genuine notes.

As specified in the scoring rules, Ego was scored as the subject or object in 100% of the interactive statements. Spouse was the next most frequently employed noun; relationship between Ego and Spouse accounted for 57.22% of the interactive statements in the genuine notes. Analysis indicated that only Father and Spouse were significantly more often scored in genuine notes. Spouse was employed in 32 genuine notes (although this, in part, is probably reflective of the fact that the notes in Shneidman and Farberow (1957a) were written only by married individuals).

A Study: Conclusions

The procedures outlined, thus appeared to have been useful in research on the unconscious processes in suicide notes and would very likely be so with other clinical material, like the patient's narrative, which is thematic in nature. Even if one does not accept the psychoanalytic assumptions given, one is still confronted with the fact that blind-to-the-hypotheses judges scored latent content (i.e., distortions) more frequently in genuine notes than in simulated ones. Although further validity studies are warranted with Foulkes's system, the procedures in this study subjected the investigation of unconscious psychodynamic forces in suicide notes to the first reported, structured, objective analysis in the literature. The fact that both studies— one with clinical judgements and the other with operational definitions—report similar findings and that Foulkes's system can be applied to dream reports, suicide notes and possibly other thematic material begin to add some support to the idea that the distortions as operationally defined may well measure what they purport to measure.

SPECULATIONS ON THE UNCONSCIOUS

An obvious concern is the following: Are we, indeed, measuring what we are purporting to be measuring? It may well be, as some would argue, that we are simply measuring the confusion associated with the mental state that precedes suicide. The suicidal person may simply be unaware ("unconscious") of aspects of the information processing. However, such a perspective is in contrast to Freud (1974f) when he suggested that *distortions* (as well as displacements, bizarreness, etc.) measure the *dynamic unconscious*. The focus in this view—implied in Foulkes's system—is on repressed unconscious processes (e.g., wishes, needs). As Eagle (1987) has noted, this is an issue of markedly different theoretical tenets; i.e., different conceptions of the unconscious. The ideas in this chapter are largely based on a number of tenets of dynamic or psychoanalytic psychology. It accepts the distinction between manifest and latent. It accepts that latent implications (i.e., unconscious processes) are important in understanding a suicidal person. It accepts that there are procedures to infer the latent implications from the manifest content in suicide notes. For example, it implies that distortions are symptomatic of unconscious forces. In contrast, the more simple behavioural view would be one that accepts that the person is *only* unaware ("unconscious") of processes that influence the behaviour that would occur when the suicidal person decides to end his/her life due to mental constriction, unbearable pain, hopelessness–helplessness, etc. This is in sharp contrast to some of the more comprehensive cognitive-behavioural views. I do not mean to suggest that cognitive processes do not occur; rather, I believe that both cognitive and dynamic and other processes [e.g., biological (especially in mood disorders), socio-cultural, philosophical] occur in an individual who defines an issue for which suicide is perceived as the best solution. My point is that it is possible to understand suicide from a perspective of unconscious forces. Further analysis with thoughts and observations of various diverse theorists on latent content are needed although a critical shortcoming of such investigations, as in all studies of completed suicide, will be the availability of adequate data (e.g., associations) (Maris, 1981). If we, for example, could put the suicide notes in the context of the authors' lives, we could make greater use of associations and more to understand the event.

In the study reported above, the results support the observation that genuine suicide notes contain more unconscious implications than simulated notes. The second, more formal, study substantiated the finding of an earlier one by utilizing

an objective scoring system. Significantly more distortions in the interactive statements of individuals who wrote genuine suicide notes than matched individuals
who wrote simulated suicide notes were found. Distortions are reflections of latent
content (Freud, 1974f; Foulkes, 1978). Genuine suicide notes more often called for
decision rules to be applied about the latent meaning in the interactive statements.
A large proportion (86.4%) of the distortions involved deciding whether the Ego
should be scored in the position of object or subject of an interactive relationship
between two third persons or between a third person and an object. One possible
interpretation of these findings is that the manifest content of a suicide note may
not be identical with all of the writer's wishes, needs, etc. By analysing the latent
content, we may be able to uncover some of these underlying forces. For example,
it may be assumed, from my perspective, that attachments are very important in
suicide, although I would add that "attachment" is extremely complicated.

Suicide is often interpersonal in nature (Freud, 1974i). I have suggested that *unconscious* processes are related to this interpersonal aspect of suicide (Leenaars, 1986).
Freud (1974i) speculated on the latent interpretation of what leads someone to kill
oneself, in the following:

> Probably no one finds the mental energy required to kill himself unless, in the first
> place, in doing so he is at the same time killing an object with whom he had identified
> himself and, in the second place, is turning against himself a death wish which had
> been directed against someone else. (p. 162)

The person had developed a strong identification with a person (or, as Zilboorg
(1936) has shown, some other ideal). Attachment, based upon an important emotional tie with another person, is for Freud (1974j) the meaning of identification;
not only does the person (or other ideal) exist outside, it becomes introjected into
one's own personality. The attachment is deep within one's unconscious. As Litman (1967) noted, our "ego is made up in large part of identifications" (p. 333).
These identifications are especially associated with our earliest attachments (e.g.,
parents) and significant people (e.g., spouse, child). With loss, rejection, etc., the
energy (libido) in this attachment is withdrawn, but the person continues to exhibit
an overly painful attachment. As Fenichel (1954) noted, "the loss is so complete that
there is no hope of regaining it. One is hopeless . . . and helpless" (p. 400). Freud
had articulated the importance in attachment in his analysis of Anna O. and Dora,
a patient who had been suicidal. In both it was the relation to father that was so
painful and critical in their development. The loss does not need, I believe, to be
actual. It may be fantasized like the attachment itself. It is the attachment substantiated by our research that is the basic unconscious process, not the death wish.
Although aggressive wishes, whether inward or outward, occur in some suicides,
it is primarily identification that is a key in most suicides. Suicide is more an outcome of frustrated attachment needs (wishes) than of aggressive wishes. The loss
of the attachment, often experienced as abandonment, at both the more obvious
manifest level and the deeper latent level fuels the pain that becomes unbearable:
No love, no life.

The dynamics in suicide, I believe, are thus related to a key significant other person
and other people (e.g., father, mother)—although other ideals may be the object for

the attachment. Further, the need in these relations is often one of moving towards (attention, approval, gratitude, affection, love, sex, etc.) rather than moving against or moving away. According to Horney (1950), from whom Foulkes developed his schema for interactive verbs, such a person evaluates his/her life according to how much one "is liked, needed, wanted, or accepted". This type of person is self-effacing and has a continual wish (or need) for attachment—"attention, approval, gratitude, affection, love, sex". To be loved is to be safe. This type of person will sacrifice all to be loved. Horney wrote:

> While curtailed in any pursuit on his own behalf, he is not only free to do things for others but, according to his *inner dictates*, should be the ultimate helpfulness, generosity, considerateness, understanding, sympathy, love, and sacrifice. In fact, love and sacrifice in his mind are closely intertwined: he should sacrifice everything for love—love is sacrifice. (Horney, 1950, p. 220; my emphasis)

Although other needs may be present, it is the need for attachment, within a historical context, that is central in most suicide.

Freud himself had associated suicide and love; indeed, his only overt suicide threats, years before his suicide, occurred during his engagement to his wife-to-be, Martha Bernays (Litman, 1967). According to Jones (1953–1957), Freud had decided to commit suicide if he lost Martha. In a letter to Martha, Freud wrote:

> I have long since resolved on a decision, the thought of which is in no way painful, in the event of my losing you. That we should lose each other by parting is quite out of the question. You would have to become a different person, and of myself, I am quite sure. You have no idea how fond I am of you, and hope I shall never have to show it. (Jones, 1953–1957, p. 132)

Freud was quite attached to Martha and, as his history revealed, other ideals, i.e., health.

It is equally noteworthy that Karl Menninger, when asked (Jacobs & Brown, 1989) if he would change any aspect of his triad of motives in suicide—to kill, to be killed, to die—he stated: "I think there is one more unconscious motive to add to the triad. I think some love gets into suicide motivation" (p. 484).

It is likely that a group of suicidal individuals are, in fact, quite pathological in their love. In his analysis of Freud's speculation on suicide, Litman (1967, p. 340) wrote:

> ... Freud often referred to certain dangerous ways of loving, in which the ego is "overwhelmed" by the object. Typically, the psychic representations of the self and other are fused and the other is experienced as essential for survival.

We term such attachments "symbiotic" and it is likely that "symbiotic love is a potential precursor of suicide" (Litman, 1967, p. 340). Some suicide notes, but not all, exhibit such unhealthy love—we will meet such people later in the case presentations. For many suicidal people, it is simply the loss that they cannot bear. The loss is so complete that there is no hope of living. The pain is unbearable.

Suicide occurs in a needful individual.

> It is difficult to conceptualise an individual committing suicide apart from that individual seeking to satisfy certain inner felt needs... there can never be a needless

suicide...it focally involves the attempt to fulfil some urgently felt psychological needs. Operationally, these heightened unmet needs make up, in a large part, what the suicidal person feels (and *reports*). (Shneidman, 1985, pp. 208–209; my italics)

If we let the unconscious speak in the suicidal person's own report, the suicide note, we learn: The suicidal person is not so much withdrawing, detaching from, disconnecting, disenfranchising nor being aggressive towards, rejecting, dominating, controlling, exploiting but loving, needing, wanting, liking, accepting. In the suicidal person, love and sacrifice are closely intertwined. A person sacrifices everything for love...love may well be a driving force in suicide.

A CASE ILLUSTRATION

By way of concluding this chapter, I would like to present an analysis of the suicide notes of Natalie, a case that Shneidman (1980) and I (2002) have discussed in detail.

Natalie, a 39-year-old woman, killed herself. What is instructional about this case in suicidology is that in addition to her suicide notes, there exist over 100 separate documents. They include the following: early school records, teachers' notes to her parents, physicians' reports, school evaluations, college records, several psychological tests, numerous questionnaires that she had completed, dozens of letters and miscellaneous personal documents. These personal documents and other records provide us with the associations that are lacking in suicide notes. They allow us to get a clearer glimpse of her life, including her conscious and unconscious mind. Shneidman (1980) has presented a full account of the case.

Let me begin with Natalie's five suicide notes, cited verbatim.

1. To her adult friend:

   Rosalyn—Get Eastern Steel Co.—Tell them and they will find Bob right away. Papa is at his business. Betty is at the Smiths—Would you ask Helene to keep her until her Daddy comes—so she won't know until he comes for her. You have been so good—I love you—Please keep in touch with Betty—Natalie.

2. To her eldest daughter:

   Betty, go over to Rosalyn's right away—Get in touch with Papa.

3. To her ex-husband, from whom she was recently divorced:

   Bob—I'm making all kinds of mistakes with our girls—They have to have a leader and everyday the job seems more enormous—You couldn't have been a better Daddy to Nancy and they do love you—Nancy misses you so and she doesn't know what's the matter—I know you've built a whole new life for yourself but make room for the girls and keep them with you—Take them where you go—It's only for just a few years—Betty is almost ready to stand on her own two feet—But Nancy needs you desperately. Nancy needs help—She really thinks you didn't love her—and she's got to be made to do her part for her own self-respect—Nancy hasn't been hurt much yet—but ah! the future if they keep on the way I've been going lately—Barbara sounds warm and friendly and relaxed and I pray to God she will understand just a little and be good to my girls—They need two happy people—not a sick mixed-up mother—There will be a little money to help with extras—It had better go that way than for more pills and more doctor bills—I wish to God it had been different but be happy—but please—stay by your girls—And just one thing—be kind to Papa—He's done everything he could to try to help me—He loves the girls dearly and it's right that they should see him often—Natalie

Bob—this afternoon Betty and Nancy had such a horrible fight it scares me. Do you suppose Gladys and Orville would take Betty for this school year? She should be away from Nancy for a little while—in a calm atmosphere.

4. To her stepfather:

Papa—no one could have been more kind or generous than you have been to me—I know you couldn't understand this—and forgive me—The lawyer had copy of my will—Everything equal—the few personal things I have of value—the bracelet to Nancy and my wedding ring to Betty—But I would like Betty to have Nana's diamond—have them appraised and give Betty and Nancy each half of the diamonds in the band. Please have somebody come in and clean—Have Bob take the girls away immediately—I don't want them to have to stay around—You're so good Papa dear——

5. To her two children:

My dearest ones—You two have been the most wonderful things in my life—Try to forgive me for what I've done—your father would be so much better for you. It will be harder for you for awhile—but so much easier in the long run—I'm getting you all mixed up—Respect and love are almost the same—Remember that—and the most important thing is to respect yourself—The only way you can do that is by doing your share and learning to stand on your own two feet—Betty, try to remember the happy times—and be good to Nancy. Promise me you will look after your sister's welfare—I love you very much—but I can't face what the future will bring.

To analyse the latent meaning of Natalie's suicide, let me now return to one of Natalie's notes. Table 3.2 presents a note scored by Foulkes's system.

From the analysis, we learn: Natalie was deeply attached to her father. The distortions in her notes relate to her father. Natalie was aware of some vital aspects of her act, as her notes show, but probably not all. It is possible that the original attachment had aroused unbearable pain that could not be expressed. A driving force, I believe, to Natalie's death was her need for attachment to her father.

Given my focus on interpersonal relations, it is clearly evident from the documents related to Natalie's life that her relationships were disturbing. She had experienced considerable loss and rejection in her attachments, not only from her ex-husband but also (and deeper) from her father. The identification had great similarity in its development, I suspect, as in Anna O. and Dora. In a letter about her troubled life, Natalie said this about her father: "I adored my father from afar. Our occasional meetings were unsatisfactory—my father is a very brilliant man—however, he has little use for me—he lives 20 minutes away but has been in our home only once for a few minutes in the past two years." Elsewhere she wrote: "I adored my father from afar. Our occasional meetings were very unpleasant but it was a very shallow relationship." Natalie clearly identifies with her father in these words; she is and wants to be attached to him. Her relationship with her father, as with her ex-husband, was, however, under a constant strain—her wishes, needs, etc., were unsatisfied and frustrated.

Table 3.2 An illustration of a suicide note scored by Foulkes' system

Text	Scoring	Distortion
Bob—I'm making all kinds of mistakes with our girls -	Ego (+) moving against (+) children [Ego with (+) children] Spouse with (+) children] -	
They have to have a leader and everyday the job seems more enormous -	(−) Ego (−) creating (+) children [(−) Ego creating (+) children ((−) means (+) children]	
You couldn't have been a better Daddy to Nancy and they do love you— -	[(+) Spouse with child] Ego (+) moving towards spouse	(+) Children to ego
Nancy misses you so and she doesn't know what's the matter	(−) Ego (+) moving towards spouse	Child to ego
I know you've built a whole new life for yourself	Spouse (−) creating (+) ego	Life to ego
but make room for the girls -	Spouse moving towards (+) ego	(+) Children to ego
and keep them with you— Take them where you go— It's only for just a few years—Betty is almost ready to stand on her own two feet—	[Spouse (+) with (+) children] [Spouse (−) with (+) children] (−) Ego moving from spouse	 Child to ego
But Nancy needs you desperately	(+) Ego (−) moving towards spouse	Child to ego
Nancy needs help [from you] -	Spouse (−) moving towards ego [Spouse (−) moving towards ego (child ((−) means child)]	Child to ego
She really thinks you didn't love her and she's got to be made to do her part for her own self-respect	Spouse (−) moving towards (−) ego	Child to ego
Nancy hasn't been hurt much yet—	Ego (−) moving against child	
but ah! the future if they keep on the way I've been going lately—	Ego (−) moving against child	
Barbara sounds warm and friendly and relaxed and I pray to God	Ego moving towards father	God to father
she will understand [me] just a little	[(+) peer female (−) with ego]	
and be good to my girls— -	Peer female moving towards (−) ego Ego moving towards (+) spouse (+) Children moving towards	(+) Children to ego

Table 3.2   (*continued*)

Text	Scoring	Distortion
They need two happy people—	(+) ego	Peer female to ego
not a sick mixed-up mother—	(+) Children (−) moving towards (−) ego	
- -		
	[Money (+, − with extras]	
There will be a little money	[Money with (+) child]	
to help with the extras	[Extras with (+) child]	
It had better go that way		
than for more pills	[Money (−) with (+) pill]	
and more doctor bills.	[Money (−) with (−) father]	
I wish to God	Ego moving towards father	God to father
It had been different but be		
happy—but please—stay by		
your girls	[Spouse with (+) children]	
And just one thing—be		
kind to Papa—	Ego moving towards father	Spouse to ego
- -		Father-in-law to father
He's done everything		Father-in-law to
he could to try to help		father
me—	Father (+, −) moving towards ego	Father-in-law to father
- -	Father (+) moving towards ego	(+) Children to
He loves the girls dearly		ego
		Father-in-law to father
and it's right		
that they should see him	Ego (+) moving towards father	(+) Children to
often—		ego
- -		
Natalie		Father-in-law to father

Natalie's personal documents are filled with overpowering pain. She was frantic. Pitiful forlornness, deprivation, distress, and grief were all evident in her "emotional intoxication". Feelings (and ideas) of vengefulness and aggression towards herself appear to be evident—especially submission. Her note to her husband is manifestly a painful *mea culpa*. She took all the blame. She punished herself. She was passive, fearing aggression and violence. All of the feelings are expressed overtly in her final letters. It is easy to detect the anger towards her ex-husband and her father. She also exhibited love, concern, etc., towards others (her stepfather, her children).

Our latent analysis would suggest that a primary attachment—love—of Natalie's be towards her father. She so desperately needed to be loved by him and to love him. Her notes and other documents are marked by ambivalence—love and hate. At the end, Natalie was boxed in, passive, rejected, and especially helpless and hopeless; yet, it is affection, approval, love, etc., that are so central in her notes. She needed to move towards people. For example, she writes, "I pray to God" which, if one accepts the premises in this chapter, translates to "I move towards my father". As another example, she writes, "He's done everything he could to try to help me", which means "My father—albeit both positive and negative—moves towards me". There are a number of such expressions in her notes. The unbearable pain is associated with, I suspect, unconscious processes of identification with her ex-husband and (at a deeper level) her father.

All this discussion about Natalie's father does not imply that her mother was not an important attachment. I merely wish to emphasize the loss/rejection—the pain—in her moving towards father. Indeed, love for/love from mother was always central to Natalie's life. Natalie's mother died at age 67. (This is presumably why there is no reference to her in Natalie's notes.) Natalie was then 36—at a period in her life when her anguish began to be increasingly overpowering. She wrote at that time, "I love her more than anyone else on earth". Elsewhere, she described her attachment to her mother as "my perfect relationship with my mother". Natalie's attachment to her mother cannot be overstated. She once wrote about her mother: "My mother was overly generous towards me and wanted to make up for my not having a father." One can only wonder what the loss of this "perfect" attachment meant to Natalie both consciously and unconsciously. Natalie herself died a few years later at age 39.

By way of a suicidological footnote, it is worth noting that around this time her favourite book was Karl Menninger's *Man Against Himself*.

As can be gleaned from Natalie's notes, she was not only figuratively overcome by her pain but also by her perception and ideas. Her notes are full of permutations and combinations of grief-provoking content (despite the ever-present thrust of ambivalence). She believed that her life was hard, futile. She was occupied with the following: "I can't face what the future brings." She said that she was "making all kinds of mistakes". She clearly believed, with flawless logic from her perspective, that once she was dead it would be "so much easier" for her children, her ex-husband, herself—everybody. She almost stated the following prototypical sentences in the documents: "Everyone will be much better off when I'm dead. Everything will be much better when I'm dead." She would sacrifice everything for love.

Natalie's suicide, from my perspective, is much less logical than she believed. Here, for example, is some of Shneidman's analysis of the content in her notes in relation to cognition (1980):

> Natalie's suicide note to her children is filled with contradictions and inconsistencies. (We remember that when she was tested as a child, the psychologist called her extremely logical.) In the suicide note, the implicit logical arguments flow back and forth, between assertion and counterassertion, never with any resolution. Here are some examples: She says, in effect, you will stay with your father, you should love your father, I know that you cannot love your father but at least you must respect him. She then almost free-associates to the word "respect" and argues, rather lamely, that love and respect are almost the same anyway, and in case that argument is not persuasive (which it is not), then one should, at least, respect one's self. The logic wanders; yet for Natalie, the logic made sense: It is her argument about *her* father.

Another sad example: She says to her children, You must stand on your own two feet, but she also implies that the point of her removing herself from their lives is so that they can be reunited with their father—as, probably, she unconsciously yearns to be reunited with her father.

To tell one's children in a suicide note to remember the happy times certainly has some contradictory element in it, on the very face of it. I love you so much, she says, but the end result of her actions is to make them orphans. She adds, I can't face what the future will bring, but she then takes her life largely because of the haunting, inescapable past. And finally, there is her statement, "I'm getting you all mixed up", which obviously betokens the confusion not in their minds but in her own. (pp. 66–67)

One wonders about what the unconscious is expressing here.

One can conclude that Natalie was emotionally perturbed; Natalie's notes (and her history) attest to the fact that she had difficulties developing constructive and loving attachments. She had suffered defeat, which, at the time of her death, she felt she could not overcome. The active withdrawal by key significant others—notably at an unconscious level, the desertion of her father and probably the death of her mother—plunged Natalie into despair, grief, hopelessness, and helplessness. She was not able to go on; she described herself as "a sick mixed-up mother". Indeed, her notes suggest that she was figuratively "drugged" by overpowering emotions and constricted perceptions. Her history was full of these "mixed-up" states, which one of her doctors described as "neurotic tendencies". From Freud's perspective these symptoms had developed out of childhood experiences. Life, in fact, she said, "seems so enormous".

When Natalie was in her mid-thirties, a medical doctor had noted that she was on "the verge of a nervous breakdown". Natalie went to see a therapist. About this treatment, Natalie wrote, "my tension symptoms are so chronic and severe that they must have their origin in my childhood". Regrettably the therapist's notes are unavailable. Did Natalie gain some insight into the rejection by her father? The attachment to her mother? Her husband failed to support her in her treatment, seeing Natalie's problem as exaggerated and therapy as "plain silly".

She was often strikingly ambivalent about treatment. At one time, she wrote:

I feel now that a psychologist is the last thing in the world I need to see. Now I am just capable of furnishing (earning) part of our monthly needs and being a wise mother to my girls.

She saw herself as hopeless and helpless, not knowing "the rudiments of daily living". Life was painful, noting that "the slightest response is a strain".

We know, as noted in the police report at her death, that she was seeing a psychologist three times weekly. One can conclude that at some time her pain in her conscious *and* unconscious mind became *unbearable*. Suicide became the only solution.

In the end, Natalie appeared to have been so preoccupied with her trauma that she was unaware of how to adjust and she chose cessation. We would here follow Shneidman's belief that: Each individual tends to die as he or she has lived, especially as he or she has previously reacted in periods of threat, stress, failure, challenge, shock and loss. Her history, as shown through the looking glass of her suicide notes, was so important in her conscious choice of death. Yet, it is likely that her unconscious dynamics—to be loved, to love—were major determinants of her suicide.

CONCLUDING REMARKS

Suicide is complex, more complicated than the suicidal person's conscious mind had been or can ever be aware. Deep is the pain; love even deeper than agony. Deep are identifications. Attachments to people may well be the deepest and, as we will learn, critical if we are to intervene with suicidal people effectively.

Chapter 4

COGNITION, COMMUNICATION, AND SUICIDE NOTES

To be seriously concerned with understanding suicide leads one to a most challenging task, the prediction of suicide. The problem of predicting those who will eventually kill themselves is one that has plagued suicidology since the very origin of these efforts. Traditional sources on suicide prediction include non-fatal suicide attempters, general statistics, third-party (survivor) interviews. Each of these sources has brought clinicians closer to predicting the event. Yet there is, at least, one other source that, I believe, can be rewarding in our quest, namely the person's own words (Allport, 1942).

Although there is considerable controversy surrounding the usefulness of personal words or documents and other introspective communication (Runyan, 1982a, 1982b; Windelband, 1904), Allport (1942) notes that personal documents have a significant place in social science. Allport made a clear case for their use citing the following: learning about the person (such as his/her ideation), advancing nomothetic and idiographic understanding, and aiding in the aims of science in general—understanding, prediction, and control. These are the very aims of sound assessment, and prediction of suicide, and its intervention.

Perhaps the most personal document of all is the *suicide note*. It is the unsolicited communication of a suicidal person, usually written minutes before the suicidal death. It is, as we have seen, an invaluable starting point for comprehending the suicidal act, for predicting such events, and for developing an action plan for psychotherapy.

COGNITION, COMMUNICATION, AND NOTES

Suicide notes are without question a communication—a written communication (Hayakawa, 1957). Often the note is a final communication, a last desperate act of saying something to someone. To understand the communication, we must see the relation of the note to ideation, ideation—that may well often be hidden from direct observation.

The problem of the relation between communication (including the written one such as a note) and ideation (or cognition) is a historical one. Some, such as Muller

(1887), suggested that the two are simply identical. A few, such as Berkeley (Bolton, 1972), see no relation at all. There have been a host of schools (e.g., association psychology, Gestalt psychology, Wurzburg) that have expanded on the relation, all with different points of view. Not without controversy, today the relation between communication and cognition is seen as existing, but as complex (e.g., Bolton, 1972; Piaget, 1970, 1972; Vygotsky, 1962). The relation is seen not merely as an association or as static, but rather as dynamic. To present a comprehensive discussion of such a relationship is well beyond the scope of this chapter; let it suffice to say that the relation is not a thing but a process.

Cognition or ideation is for oneself, whereas communication is usually for others (Vygotsky, 1962). This difference in function reflects real differences in process. Often our thoughts are more abstract than our specific words. Judgements need to be made regarding whether a specific written or oral communication is a reflection of a thought. Yet, we have to study words, talk, notes, diaries, etc., to infer ideation. We typically communicate in words although as Furth (1966) has shown, thinking is possible without language (as for example, in the deaf). We cannot directly study a person's ideation. We infer, given the relation of cognition to words.

In line with this volume, it is important to note that ideation is engendered by our needs, pain, interests, etc. The relation, as we have said, between word and thought is dynamic. Vygotsky (1962) stated that, "The relation between thought and word is a living process." Freud (1979a, 1974h) proposed that needs, wishes, etc., although often repressed in the unconscious, are expressed in dreams and everyday life; e.g., verbal expressions, writings. Freud (1974f) further suggested that conscious and unconscious ideation can be assessed in communication (see Chapter 3). As Vygotsky noted on the dynamic relation, "A word is a microcosm of human consciousness." This is the main tenet of the thematic tradition, which is espoused here.

It is my belief that this is why the study of the suicidal person's own words and notes has been so fruitful. Suicide notes are windows to the mind of the deceased. In the same way, other communication (such as recorded talk, diaries) of a suicidal person offers us a living process to his/her cognition.

CONSIDERATIONS PRELIMINARY TO PREDICTION

Interpretation of clinical material usually includes or implies prediction of the patient's future behaviour as well as a description of his/her present ideation. One can go so far as to say that prediction from clinical material such as communications, notes, diaries, etc., is one of the primary purposes of interpretation (understanding) in a clinical setting. The interpretation, "The patient is suicidal", is certainly a prediction that the patient is in danger of attempting and/or completing suicide. How does one make such a prediction? To answer this question prediction should not be seen as separate from understanding.

During the last century, applied psychology has been involved with the use of tests to study intelligence, memory, anxiety, depression, etc. One of the major movements has been the projective one. Henry Murray (1943), following the earlier pioneer Herman Rorschach, saw the projective procedures as "useful in any comprehensive study of personality". These procedures are based on the premise that people, when they speak or write, "draw on the fund of their experiences and express their sentiments and needs, whether conscious or unconscious". Murray's description of how the process operates was, in part, derived from Freud's description of defensive operation but Murray stressed that the process was natural and defensiveness may or may not play a role (Exner, 1986). As simply put by John Exner, "any stimulus situation that is not structured to elicit a specific class of response, as are arithmetic tests, true–false inventories, and the like, may evoke the projective process" (1986, p. 16). Murray's *Thematic Apperception Test* (TAT) is a prime example within this tradition. Through an error in printing, one of the cards in the TAT (card 16) is blank; it was retained, however, in the TAT itself. Elsewhere, I (Leenaars, 1988a) have argued that a suicide note can be seen, as it were, as a response to this blank card of the TAT. The suicide note (and the suicidal person's communication in general) can, thus, be seen in a similar fashion as the communications in thematic tests (e.g., TAT, CAT, MAPS). They are windows to a person's cognition/ideation and can be analysed for "thematic meaningfulness" (Shneidman, 1949, 1951).

It is likely that a layperson—with some beginner's luck, and without the benefit of any constructs or templates to understand suicide—may make valid and important interpretations. However, no true clinician would engage in such action, especially in terms of predicting life and death. Pertinent and sound understanding is needed in suicide prediction. What is required, from my view, is a theoretical context of suicide and personality functioning in general to understand the communication and, by implication, the ideation of a potential suicidal individual and its potential implications for predictions. The templates (or patterns or frames) proposed here are ones that not only provide such a view but also have, at least, some *empirical support*. As a word of caution, Murray (1943) has noted that some interpretations may "do more harm than good, since the apparent plausibility of clever interpretations creates convictions which merely serve to confirm the interpreter in the error of his ways" (p. 6).

REVIEW OF THE LITERATURE

One, if not *the*, reason why it is so difficult to predict suicide is that we usually deal with the end result. In other mental health areas, we are not faced with this obstacle. For example, if we wish to predict a learning disability, we can make some interpretations, check them, try again, etc. In suicide, obviously, we cannot. As Joseph Zubin (1974) argued, given this situation, "unravelling the causes after the fact is well-nigh impossible" but, if I may add, possible. We are, however, restricted *at this time* by a fact noted by James Diggory (1974): "The belief that suicidal behaviours are predictable can be valid only as a belief *in principle*, not *in fact*" (p. 59).

Over the last five decades or so, despite these and similar critical observations, a large number of attempts at constructing tests for suicide prediction and related phenomena have been made. Probably one of the best tests is Shneidman's simple measure (1973) or, more accurately, question: "During the last 24 hours, I felt the chance of my actually killing myself (committing suicide and ending my life) was: absent, low, fifty–fifty, high, very high (came very close to actually killing myself)." Clinical experience has shown that many patients can predict their own suicide potential (and are often relieved to find someone willing to talk about their own ominous prediction).

Aaron Beck and his colleagues (e.g., 1967, 1974a, 1974b, 1974c, 1975a, 1975b, 1979a) are probably most noteworthy in their endeavours to construct scales for prediction related to suicide. Their tests include: the Beck Depression Scale, the Hopelessness Scale, the Suicidal Intent Scale, and the Scale for Suicide Ideation. The research on these scales (including very critical reviews and research) is too vast to be discussed here. A large number of other possible scales have been presented to assess and predict suicide and a few, as we will see later, are very useful.

Instruments of prediction equally call for reflection. Motto (1985) has provided us with some important insights into problems about prediction, which are worthy of review here. He cites the following: a suitable criterion measure (predictive validity); the degree to which the scale agrees with other measures (concurrent validity); applicability of the scale to various populations; the willingness of clinicians, crisis workers, physicians, etc., to use a scale that is not consistent with their own intuition; and the use of a rater who knows what the scale measures (criterion contamination). There is, at least, one additional concern that is fundamental to prediction and the development of a test, namely the base rate problem or the frequency of a given condition in a population to which the test is applied (Meehl & Rosen, 1955). These are challenges ahead of us in our efforts to predict and, if I may add, control suicide.

SUICIDE NOTES

Suicide notes are the ultra-personal documents (Leenaars, 1988a; Shneidman, 1980). They are the unsolicited productions of the suicidal person, usually written minutes before the suicidal death. They are an invaluable starting point for comprehending the suicidal act and for understanding the special features about people who actually commit suicide and what they share in common with the rest of us who have only been drawn to imagine it (Leenaars, 1988a, Leenaars & Balance, 1984a; Shneidman 1980, 1985; Shneidman & Farberow, 1957a).

It should be noted at the beginning, however, that the study of suicide notes has a number of limitations. Only about 12 (maybe 18) to 37% of suicides leave notes (Leenaars, 1988a; Shneidman & Farberow, 1957a; O'Connor et al., 1999). Thus, the conclusion about the psychology of suicide (and the implication for intervention) may contain some bias. However, since the first systematic study of suicide notes, few differences have been reported between individuals who left notes and those who did not.

Erwin Stengel (1964) noted:

> Whether the writers of suicide notes differ in their attitudes from those who leave no notes behind it is impossible to say. Possibly, they differ from the majority only in being good correspondents. At any rate, the results of the analysis of suicide notes are in keeping with the observation . . . common to most suicidal acts. (pp. 44–45)

Sampling differences exist, given the nature of some suicides. Fishbain et al. (1984) reported that suicide-pact victims more frequently leave a note. Fishbain et al. (1987) noted that subintentional suicides (e.g., Russian roulette deaths) were significantly less likely to leave a note. Researchers have reported differences in various aspects of samples. Michel (1988) reported that young people are more likely to leave a suicide note, whereas Posner et al. (1989) found no such higher rate. Samples vary: indeed, some studies report that males leave more notes, while others report the same for females, the young, the old, and so on. Leenaars and Lester (1988–89) have pointed out that caution is in order when inferring conclusions from small samples, although the clinician must respond even in a case of one.

Early research (e.g., Wolff, 1931) on suicide notes largely utilized an anecdotal approach that incorporated descriptive information. Subsequent methods of study have primarily included classification analysis and content analysis. Currently, there are well over 100 published articles on suicide notes; an extensive review with an annotated bibliography has been presented elsewhere (Leenaars, 1988a). Some of this research is very relevant in showing the predictive power of communication and notes. Shneidman and Farberow's early studies (1957a, 1957b; Farberow & Shneidman, 1957) allowed us to conclude that suicidal individuals are prone to fallacies in their cognitive processes; that the wish to kill, the wish to be killed, and the wish to die were evident; and that the suicidal person departs with hate and self-blame. Subsequent studies have isolated the following clinically relevant factors in notes: psychic tension (Wagner, 1960); depression (Capstick, 1960); mental confusion (Spiegel & Neuringer, 1963); unfulfillable desires, high perturbation, intolerable inner tension, unrealistic expectations of others, personal devaluation, and feelings of worthlessness (Bjerg, 1967); hostility (Tuckman & Ziegler, 1968); positive affect, e.g., "love" (Ogilvie et al., 1969); heightened dependency needs, problems in maintaining relationships, and veiled aggression (Darbonne, 1969b); the act as justified and the need to be forgiven for it (Jacobs, 1971); involvement with fantasy (Lester, 1971); unable to distinguish the subjective from the objective, oversimplification, thinking that everything is obvious, rigid, fatalistic, projection, and unable to distinguish feelings and the outside world (Tripodes, 1976); constriction (Henken, 1976); ambivalence (i.e., simultaneous presence of love and hate), shame and disgrace (Shneidman, 1980); idiosyncrasies in ideation (Shneidman, 1981b); cognitive impairment in positive evaluation (Schwilbe & Rader, 1982); specific people, places and things are negated while generalized others are seen as more positive (Edelman & Renshaw, 1982); a fatalistic attitude (Peck, 1983); and ambivalent attachment to a person (Posner et al., 1989).

Only a very few of the above studies on suicide notes have utilized a theoretical–conceptual analysis despite the belief, since the first formal study of suicide notes, that such contributions offer a rich potential (Shneidman & Farberow, 1957a). In a series of studies spanning over 25 years, the author introduced a logical, empirical approach to suicide notes and from these studies we have learned that the cognitions, communications, and notes of the suicidal person are highly associated with the following: unbearable psychological pain, cognitive constriction, indirect expressions, inability to adjust, ego, interpersonal relations, rejection–aggression, and identification–egression.

Research on the communication and notes has indicated general applicability to most suicides. Yet, is it applicable to others who make attempts or only think about the event? As outlined in detail in Chapter 2, research (Leenaars et al., 1992) indicates that there may well be few differences between suicide notes and *parasuicide notes* of highly lethal individuals. Parasuicide notes are communications written by individuals who attempted to kill themselves (or engaged in some other form of parasuicidal behaviour including cognition).

Leenaars et al.'s research (1992) is most pertinent here because it suggests that the protocols, outlined earlier, have applicability to suicide and attempted suicide. In the archival study—a comparison of suicide notes written by individuals who killed themselves and notes by individuals who attempted suicide—Leenaars et al. (1992) undertook the comparison of the eight patterns (and individual protocol sentences) as possible predictors of the communications of completers and attempters. The attempters were of moderate to high lethality. No difference on the eight clusters was found; only one protocol difference was noted, namely that attempters see themselves more often as too weak to cope with life's difficulties, although their notes were not more frequently judged to be indicative of pathology. Although there are differences between attempters and completers (see Leenaars, et al., 1992; Shneidman, 1985), it may well be that the psychological characteristics (or "unity thema") outlined here are as applicable to attempters as to completers. It is likely that there is a continuum of suicidal behaviour, not merely a dichotomy of attempters and completers. If so, the suicidal profile identified earlier may be clinically useful in not only understanding suicide but also parasuicidal behaviour. The profile may well, thus, be clinically useful in assessing and predicting suicide and suicide attempters. This line of reasoning would suggest that the profile outlined may be useful in understanding not only notes, but other suicidal communication, and, by implication, ideation.

THEMATIC GUIDE FOR SUICIDE PREDICTION

From research, the Thematic Guide for Suicide Prediction (TGSP) has been developed (Leenaars, 1988a, 1992b) and will be presented in Chapter 6. The structure of the TGSP is, thus, based on decades of research on suicide notes, recognizing suicide as a human malaise with considerable psychological variability. Independent research on suicide notes (O'Connor et al., 1999) and biographical studies of suicides (Lester, 1994) have supported not only the utility of the approach, but also its clinical utility. The TGSP is a 35-item measure that can be applied to an individual's communication, whether written or spoken, following the long tradition of thematic measurement. It provides an inferential guide to suicidal ideation. The guide consists of eight separate subscales with predictive and differentiating items: *unbearable psychological pain*; *cognitive constriction*; *indirect expressions*; *inability to adjust*; *ego*; *interpersonal relations*; *rejection-aggression*; and *identification-egression*. It is *critical* to understand that the TGSP is not a test like the TAT, MAPS, etc., but how one analyses/interprets the actual protocols. It is a guide or outline for assessment or evaluation of the spoken or written words of an individual. It allows one to assess and qualitatively predict a person's suicidal ideation, following the premise that prediction is based on understanding. It provides the templates, much like the views on interpretation presented on the TAT in Shneidman's book, *Thematic Test Analysis*. The TGSP is presented in Chapter 6 with specific instructions (derived from the research and clinical studies), identifying data, and so on.

Our research experience, outlined in detail elsewhere (Leenaars, 1988a), with independent judges has raised a number of potential but obvious concerns with clinicians using the scales:

1. The TGSP can probably only be used by professionally trained clinicians. Attempts in research to utilize, for example, undergraduate psychology students produced very unreliable results, suggesting the problem of clinical prediction.
2. Clinicians can be, following Exner (1986), overincorporaters or underincorporaters. The former are slow, excessive, overly perfectionistic; the latter are *very* quick, resulting in poor ratings and excessive blunders.
3. Motivational issues may affect judgements.

We have also noted that the more frequently a patient's protocols are matched (or verified) with the items of the TGSP, the more ominous is the predictive value of those items. It should be remembered that some items have a differentiating value despite infrequent occurrence. It is the richness of the words, communication and notes that provide the clues to understanding the person. As one uses the guide with a patient (whether via written or oral communication), an infrequently observed item on the TGSP may well be important in understanding that individual.

One possible critical response to the TGSP is the following: It appears to generate numbers, but it is not clear what these numbers tell us about suicide prediction. Such a comment, I believe, is based largely on a statistical approach to prediction. This is the quantitative approach, and a simplistic one at that. This is only one avenue in assessment and in its rigid form is discrepant from the qualitative movement. The use of only the statistical view is a *cognitively simple* (as George Kelly used the term) construal. I believe that to understand suicide we need the statistical approach, the qualitative approach, and much more (see Leenaars et al., 2002b).

As a reminder, the TGSP should not be used alone. It must not be used in a vacuum. Rather, it should be utilized within a context of clinical judgement that includes other tests, observations, etc. There is no such thing as *the* test.

CONCLUDING REMARKS

Not without controversy, suicide notes and other personal communications—such as the words of our patients in our therapy rooms—are a microcosm of human cognition. They are an invaluable starting point not only for understanding what Melville called the "damp, drizzly November of my soul" but also for assessing, predicting and intervening with suicidal people. Indeed, in my school of thought, understanding and prediction are intertwined. We must understand what we wish to rescue.

It is probable that no protocol of any person (including a suicide note) will provide all of the communication needed to assess and predict suicide. Such communication and, by implication, cognition, will have to be placed in the context of that person's life. It is likely that a number of tests, interviews, scales, etc., will be needed to understand such a complex human behaviour as suicide. No one test or guide will give the answer. There is not *the* bump on the head that will tell us if a patient is suicidal or not, even less the size telling us how suicidal that person is. The TGSP is only one tool. Furthermore, all understanding ultimately depends on the skill of the clinician. In that sense, suicide risk prediction is a task like many others that a sound clinician faces—the problem of understanding a number of evaluations about the same person. We will now turn to this key aspect of successful psychotherapy with suicidal patients.

Part II

SUICIDE RISK ASSESSMENT

The concept of assessment is preferential to that of diagnosis. I do not wish to imply that I am only critical of the DSM (or ICD) approach to suicide, only that a diagnostic approach alone would be suicidogenic. There is no one diagnosis of "Suicide Disorder". The DSM approach is insufficient for suicide risk assessment. There is no "one bump on a person's head". Equally, the search for a singular test or question to predict *the* bump is a chimera, a conceptual fabrication. Such a search is at a pre-understanding stage of cognition (maybe somewhat akin to what Piaget calls a "concrete operational stage"). It would be an overly constricted suicidological mind (much like the suicidal mind). To quote Henry Murray, "Never denigrate a fellow human being in fewer than 2000 words." I follow Murray's and Shneidman's lead in their interest in assessment. My own, Thematic Guide for Suicide Prediction (TGSP), is in this tradition.

The six chapters in Part II reflect my interest in the assessment process. The first three offer a schema to understand the suicidal mind, the suicidal brain. After a review of the field—which concludes that few tests are sufficiently useful or empirical—a theory of suicide is provided. Without theory, the psychologist, psychiatrist, social worker, psychiatric nurse, and so on, are only left to wonder what the person's stories mean. These three chapters offer an empirically supported definition— Shneidman has always argued that defining suicide should be our main effort in suicidology—with application across age, gender, culture, method used, historical time, and so on. In these chapters, the reader will find an overview of prediction and assessment, a guide to understand the suicidal person's narrative, and a practice section to allow one to reliably hear the suicidal cry, whether found in suicide notes, poems, or therapeutic protocols. The real value of these chapters is the homework assignments in this part. It invites the reader to listen to the suicidal story, then to understand it with some common, empirically validated characteristics, to prepare for effective intervention. This part is homework for the reader. It provides the lessons to be done at home by the practising or aspiring suicidologist. It is the work to understand the suicidal patient—there is no substitute.

The chapters in this part allow one to assess the narrative aspects of a suicidal life, in their "sameness" or commonalities. The common are the "threads" of behaviour that run through the life history. There are threads, the consistencies in every case, both certain common characteristics of suicide and, certain features of that individual's life. Suicidal people in our psychotherapy rooms have, in general, enormous consistencies—but they are also unique.

Allport, Murray, and Shneidman have explicitly supported the intense personal study of suicidal lives. Our study, as in all psychotherapeutic situations, is interested in each unique Jeff (or Bill, or Mary). One is not limited here by actual clinical cases, but can also study artistic works, writings, and poems. Sylvia Plath and Vincent van Gogh are two such examples; both show us more of the suicidal mind (and the suicidal brain). Likewise, on a day-to-day basis, we are interested in each unique patient. Our practical question is: How do we assess that individual's suicide risk? Who is this (suicidal) person?

Part II concludes with three chapters, all offering intensive idiographic study of individuals and allowing one to evaluate one's homework. Reliability has utility in both the laboratory and the therapy room. The chapters are: a protocol analysis of Sylvia Plath's last poems; a psychological autopsy of a suicidal patient, who killed himself while in psychotherapy (highlighting the suicidal marker of dissembling); and an example of a psychological autopsy carried out in an adversarial setting, the courtroom. The last chapter equally examines some issues in a related deliberate violence, homicide.

Chapter 5

CLINICAL EVALUATION OF SUICIDE RISK

No one really knows how to assess suicide risk perfectly. One of the questions most frequently asked about suicide risk is: "How do you predict suicide risk?", or, more specifically, "How do you assess and/or predict each unique individual's suicide risk?". Indeed, suicide risk assessment may well be the most complex clinical task that psychiatrists, psychologists, and other mental health professionals face. If we are to confront this complexity, we will see that assessment and prediction are interwoven with understanding.

As we learned earlier, one reason, if not *the* reason, why it is so difficult to predict suicide is that we usually deal only with the end result. With other mental health issues, we are not faced with this obstacle. For example, if we wish to predict schizophrenia, we can make some hypotheses, investigate them, refine them, and so forth. In suicide, obviously, we cannot do this. The search for *the* test or *the* clue or . . . of predicting a behaviour as complex as suicide is a wishful fancy. There is no *one* test. There is no *one* clue.

Clinicians wishing to understand and predict any behaviour have long ago abandoned the notion of using one criterion. To use just one test is, in fact, to regress to the days of phrenology, when it was believed that if we could find the right bump on a person's head we would know his/her personality, IQ, level of depression, etc.— and, I assume, his/her suicidal tendencies. Even the earliest use of standardized procedures in mental health (e.g., Galton's questionnaire methods, Cattell's mental tests, Binet's test) was criticized as needing to address this problem (Anastasi, 1982). In response to the recognition of such simplification, clinicians developed a wide-ranging approach (e.g., interviews, tests, observations, third-person consultations, use of personal documents) and acknowledged the need to use their clinical judgement to understand the observations. I believe that if we are to predict suicide we must adopt such a comprehensive approach, or we will be forever searching for the "bump" that will tell all.

PREDICTION VERSUS ASSESSMENT

In the 1960s and 1970s, there was a focus on the prediction of suicide, and suicidologists believed that it would eventually be possible to predict which individuals out of a population would ultimately complete suicide (Beck et al., 1974a). However, it was soon realized that the statistical rarity of suicide and the imperfection of the prediction instruments led to an enormously large number of false positives—so many, in fact, that the prediction instruments were of little use to clinicians or to those planning suicide prevention services (Lester, 1974).

In the 1980s and 1990s, the focus shifted to assessment (Maris et al., 1992); that is, rather than predicting the future occurrence of suicide in people, the intent was to assess potentially suicidal people in a more general sense, taking into account all their life experiences and psychological characteristics that are relevant to future suicidal behaviour. Indeed, it is my belief that prediction and assessment are mutual processes and that any separation is artificial. They are not separate categories.

Assessment requires clear definition. *What* is *it* that we are assessing? One value of the DSM, despite its limitations, is that it teaches you to think in concise, standardized definitions of terms. This, as we learned from Shneidman (1985) is, however, complex. Despite the complexity, there have been some attempts. Recently, I had the opportunity to chair a task force of the International Academy for Suicide Research (IASR) on that very topic (although the complete report extends beyond the topic—the focus is on future direction for study in suicide). I will here, with permission, quote what was stated about definitions (the complete text was published in *Archives of Suicide Research*, 1997, vol. 3, pp. 139–151). I cannot write it any better than on that occasion:

> A. *Definitions.* Suicide today is defined differently depending on the purpose of the definition—medical, legal, administrative, etc. In most countries reporting to the World Health Organization (WHO), suicide is defined as one of four possible modes of death. An acronym for the four modes of death is NASH: natural, accidental, suicidal, and homicidal. This fourfold classification of all deaths has its problems. Its major deficiency is that it treats the human being in a Cartesian fashion. It obscures the individual motivations, intentions and much more, never mind the degree of these characteristics.
>
> Yet, it is essential that matters relating to suicide be operationally defined in order to facilitate comparisons and to measure efficacy of interventions both intranationally and internationally. Even if we simply divided suicide into (a) suicide and (b) non-fatal suicidal behaviour (or simply, suicidal behaviour), obscurity would occur. Non-fatal suicidal behaviour would encompass suicidal ideas and suicidal acts; yet here issues of nomenclature are rife.
>
> Clustering of suicidal ideation amongst suicidal behaviour has and may continue to create confusions. Ideas are separate from actions, which is equivalent to saying that ideation *per se* does not imply any consequent behaviour. Obviously, defining in a simple, clinically sounding way non-fatal suicidal behaviour (or just suicidal behaviour) is a much more complicated issue.
>
> Suicidal ideas, for example, may themselves be divided into those signifying that life is not worth living and those signifying that death is preferable. The hierarchy of ideas is further extended by active consideration of methods including the where, the when, the how, and the consequences. There is a further step in the hierarchy if the methods and attendant circumstances are both practical and accessible. Such a hierarchical model of suicidal ideas should not presuppose that the individual

moves up or down the hierarchy in a linear manner but the clear definition of where his/her ideas rest on such a continuum would clarify comparisons. To begin such clarification, a major international project is needed to clearly define terms, concepts, etc.

Efforts to begin to address these issues have promised hope; yet, to date, there is no accepted nomenclature. The word "parasuicide" is a good example. Parasuicide, first introduced by Kreitman, Philip, Greer and Bagley (1969), is typically defined (see Kerkhof, Schmidtke, Bille-Brahe, De Leo & Lonnqvist, 1994) as:

> An act with non-fatal outcome, in which an individual deliberately initiates a non-habitual behaviour that, without intervention from others, will cause self-harm, or deliberately ingests a substance in excess of the prescribed or generally recognized therapeutic dosage, and which is aimed at the realising change which the subject desired via the actual or expected physical consequences.

The definition includes numerous self-harm acts including suicide attempts. Yet, the words, parasuicide and suicide attempt lack specificity. What are we referring to by the terms? For example, in parasuicide as defined, a person who fortuitously survives an attempt by a shotgun is clustered with a person who mismanages his/her prescription pills. Even at the front lines of suicide prevention, these events mean different things. Simply defining something does not make it useful. According to the majority of the authors of this paper, parasuicide, in fact, has not helped in our steps forward and we recommend dropping the use of the word.

The minority report, however, sees a value in the term "parasuicide", both at an individual level and an international one. First, words imply meaning. Consider the term, attempted suicide; if we call a certain behaviour an attempted suicide; then, we imply an attempt to bring about a fatal outcome—but then hastily add we truly mean that always or most of the time not. Then we are already in a terminological mess. Second, terms have social and emotional meaning; for example, if we say that an adolescent girl, who after a quarrel with a boyfriend swallows a limited number of benzodiazepines of low lethal potentiality, made an attempted suicide; then attached to the label are far-reaching consequences (Diekstra & van der Loo, 1978). The term of attempted suicide, according to this minority view, is more a prescription than a description (Diekstra, 1997). Parasuicide is offered as a more objective term, concluding that it is in no way a matter of indifference what term is used. Clinicians, policymakers, etc., are affected by the words. The terms, in fact, that we use in the field and disseminate have important individual, social and political implications.

The term "parasuicide" may also be useful at an international level in cross-cultural studies (to avoid confusion in determination of suicidal intention). This is one of the key values seen of the term, "parasuicide" by the investigators in the WHO/EURO Multicentre Study on Parasuicide. It allowed various countries in Europe to study non-fatal suicide acts without addressing the various meanings that different cultures apply to such behaviour. The problem, however, with a term like parasuicide is that it encompasses such a broad range of behaviours that it may easily become a non-discriminative and therefore non-significant category itself.

To begin to address these issues and to develop a basic nomenclature, we propose some basics, which are consistent with other independent endeavours (Rosenberg, Davidson, & Smith, 1988). At the very minimum, the following should be considered: defining suicidal acts, definition of circumstances, definition of medical lethality and definition of intent. These aspects will be addressed briefly below.

B. *Defining suicidal acts.* Suicidal acts should be operationally defined. Such definitions must include clear-cut descriptions of methods and medical lethality. The WHO now gives a list of methods, which should form the basis of future comparisons. Assessment of lethality includes not only methods but also attendant circumstances.

Before such assessments are made, it is therefore necessary to operationalize the circumstances.

C. *Definition of circumstances.* Such definition must include whether the person was alone at the time and, secondly, whether he was likely to remain alone until the methods had had, or had ceased to have an effect. If in the presence of others or likely to be discovered by others a judgement would have to be made as to whether these others would prevent the act, allow the process to continue without intervention or facilitate the process.

D. *Definition of medical lethality.* After method and attendant circumstances have been defined, then gradation of medical lethality is allowed. Medical lethality refers to the degree that a method causes or is sufficient to cause death. The assumption is that acts of high lethality are failed suicides and acts of low lethality have other personal or social meanings. Suicidal behaviour is taken to exclude other high-risk behaviours, e.g., cliff climbing, car speeding and alcohol and substance misuse.

E. *Definition of intent.* There should be a distinction between medical lethality and suicidal intent. Intent is defined as to have suicide or deliberate self-killing as one's purpose. Intent includes issues such as "definition of circumstance". Evidence of intent to die rather than knowledge that death will follow should be the basis for the definition. It may well be that how intent is handled is the most important aspect of the definitions. Formal suicide intent scales may be of assistance; however, a recent review of such scales for specific use with adolescence (with application across the lifespan) by the National Institute of Mental Health (NIMH) of the United States concluded that *few, if any, are useful* (Garrison, Lewinsohn, Marsteller, Langhinrichsen, & Lann, 1991). Yet, the NIMH group did isolate two intent scales that had sound empirical support. They are as follows: (1) Beck Suicide Intent Scale (BSIB) (Beck, Beck, & Kovacs, 1975; Steer & Beck, 1988), and (2) Lethality of Suicide Attempt Rating Scale (LSARS) (Smith, Conroy, & Ehler, 1984).

All this is not meant to suggest that other scales may not be useful, only that there are abundant reliability and validity issues in measuring intent.

There are different and further ideas on definition. Rosenberg and his colleagues (1988) have provided an excellent operational criterion to define intent in a standardized fashion, that has not only clinical, but also forensic implications. These research ideas give us an empirical basis for aiding us in preventing suicide. Yet, as a clinician, in psychotherapy, I must constantly strive to be cognitively complex in the definition of intent (Kelly, 1955). One cannot be constricted.

LETHALITY AND PERTURBATION

In assessing suicide risk in people, we need to be aware of behaviours that are potentially predictive of suicide. However, there is no such definitive behaviour. Suicide is a multidimensional malaise (Leenaars, 1988a; Shneidman, 1980, 1985). Two concepts—introduced earlier, but so essential in clinical prediction that I repeat myself here—that have been found to be essential and helpful in understanding the malaise are *lethality* and *perturbation* (Shneidman, 1973, 1980, 1985, 1993). Lethality refers to the probability of a person killing him/herself, and on quantification scales ranges from low to moderate to high. It is a psychological state of mind. Perturbation refers to subjective distress (disturbed, agitated, sane–insane, decomposed), and can also be rated from low to moderate to high. Both have to be evaluated. It is important to note that one can be perturbed and not suicidal. Lethality kills, not perturbation. Perturbation is often relatively easy to evaluate; lethality is not. A professional probably best assesses lethality *with* experience in the area of suicidology. The concepts of lethality and perturbation are, thus, critical in one's professional assessment and prediction.

TESTS TO PREDICT SUICIDE

Numerous attempts at constructing tests for suicide prediction and related phenomena have been made, but have mostly met with failure. In response to awareness of the inherent difficulties in predicting suicide, the National Institute of Mental Health (NIMH) of the United States organized a think tank in the assessment of suicidal behaviour (Lewinsohn et al., 1989). They reviewed all available assessment instruments used to study suicidal behaviour. Their conclusion was: *Few, if any, are useful*. The NIMH group found numerous problems in the instruments; for example, ambiguity of the purpose of the instrument, insufficient attention to validity, the lack of discrimination between suicide risk and other forms of self-destructive behaviour, and the lack of theoretical models. Despite this state of affairs, the NIMH group did isolate two instruments, designed for populations across the life-span, that have some potential in predicting suicide risk (i.e., the intent to kill oneself). They are as follows: *Beck Suicide Intent Scale* (BSIS; Beck et al., 1979a; Steer & Beck, 1988) and the *Lethality of Suicide Attempt Rating Scale* (LSARS; Smith et al., 1984). My own impression agrees to date: Each test, *by itself*, has little utility (Garrison et al., 1991). Maris, and colleagues (1992) drew the same conclusion, namely, that one could not reduce the richness and diversity of suicide and destructive behaviour to *the* test. Furthermore, any procedure to predict suicide cannot be divorced from a clinician's understanding.

There are, of course, other tests that have utility in understanding a person, including if at suicide risk. The Rorschach, Thematic Apperception Test and Minnesota Multiphasic Personality Inventory are just a few tests that may be used in a battery approach, although not as a single test (Eyman & Eyman, 1992; Leenaars, 1992b). More comprehensive procedures such as the Thematic Guide for Suicide Prediction (TGSP, see Chapter 6; Leenaars, 1992b) may prove to be more useful in the future than specific measures. They are designed to measure the pain in lethality and perturbation, the dynamics of suicide. It should be clear, from any clinical view, that tests should not be used as a single test and a clinician may have little utility for them in an individual case.

UNDERSTANDING SUICIDE AS ASSESSMENT AND PREDICTION

If one attempts to understand suicide, as is already evident by Chapter 2 in this book, one becomes aware over time of its enormous complexity. Suicide is not a psychopathological entity in the DSM-III-R (American Psychiatric Association, 1987) or the DSM-IV (American Psychiatric Association, 1994); nor is it likely to be an entity in subsequent editions (or in the ICD). It is not merely a reaction towards external stress, although a recent traumatic downhill course (e.g., drop in income, sudden acute alcoholism, being bullied, disgrace at work or office, separation, and divorce) can often be identified. Rather, suicide is best defined as an event with biological (including biochemical), psychological, interpersonal, situational, sociological, cultural, and philosophical/existential components. Each of these components can be a legitimate avenue to assessment.

Within the biopsychosocial *meta-frame*, let me state that I agree with Shneidman's arboreal metaphor, that the psychological dimensions of suicide are the "trunk" of suicide. This is the focus of this whole book. From the psychological point of view, I would like to offer some critical observations on suicide with the understanding that these are not exhaustive. The ideas, as noted in Chapter 2, are gleaned from the most significant suicidologists in our clinical history, that have some empirical support (Leenaars, 1988a).

A THEORY OF SUICIDE

Suicide, as we learned in Chapters 1 and 2, is an intrapsychic drama on an interpersonal stage. From a psychological view, I believe that it is helpful to clinically understand suicide from at least the following patterns (or templates or concepts), with specific protocol sentences in each pattern. The protocol sentences are testable hypotheses that must be subjected to verification in the person's words, notes, and so on.

Intrapsychic

I *Unbearable Psychological Pain*
  1. Suicide has adjustive value and is functional because it stops painful tension and provides relief from intolerable psychological pain.
  2. In suicide, the psychological and/or environmental traumas among many other factors may include: incurable disease, threat of senility, fear of becoming hopelessly dependent, feelings of inadequacy, humiliation. Although the solution of suicide is not caused by one thing, or motive, suicide is a flight from these spectres.
  3. In the suicidal drama, certain emotional states are present, including pitiful forlornness, emotional deprivation, distress and/or grief.
  4. S appears to have arrived at the end of an interest to endure and sees suicide as a solution for some urgent problem(s), and/or injustices of life.
  5. There is a conflict between life's demands for adaptation and the S's inability or unwillingness to meet the challenge.
  6. S is in a state of heightened disturbance (perturbation) and feels boxed in, harassed, especially hopeless and helpless.

II *Cognitive Constriction*
7. S reports a history of trauma (e.g., poor health, rejection by significant other, a competitive spouse).
8. Figuratively speaking, S appears to be "intoxicated" by overpowering emotions. Concomitantly, there is a constricted logic and perception.
9. There is poverty of thought, exhibited by focusing only on permutations and combinations of grief and grief-provoking topics.

III *Indirect Expressions*
10. S reports ambivalence; e.g., complications, concomitant contradictory feelings, attitudes and/or thrusts.
11. S's aggression has been turned inwards; e.g., humility, submission and devotion, subordination, flagellation, masochism, are evident.
12. Unconscious dynamics can be concluded. There are likely more reasons to the suicide than the person is consciously aware.

IV *Inability to Adjust*
13. S considers him/herself too weak to overcome personal difficulties and, therefore, rejects everything, wanting to escape painful life events.
14. Although S passionately argues that there is no justification for living on, S's state of mind is incompatible with an accurate assessment/perception of what is going on.
15. S exhibits a serious disorder in adjustment.
    (a) S's reports are consistent with a manic-depressive disorder such as the down-phase; e.g., all-embracing negative statements, severe mood disturbances causing marked impairment.
    (b) S's reports are consistent with schizophrenia; e.g., delusional thought, paranoid ideation.
    (c) S's reports are consistent with anxiety disorder (such as obsessive-compulsive, post-traumatic stress); e.g., feeling of losing control; recurrent and persistent thoughts, impulses or images.
    (d) S's reports are consistent with antisocial personality (or conduct) disorder; e.g., deceitfulness, conning others.
    (e) S's reports are consistent with borderline personality; e.g., frantic efforts to avoid real or imagined abandonment, unstable relationships.
    (f) S's reports are consistent with depression; e.g., depressed mood, diminished interest, insomnia.
    (g) S's reports are consistent with a disorder (or dysfunction) not otherwise specified. S is so paralysed by pain that life, future, etc., is colourless and unattractive.

V *Ego*
16. There is a relative weakness in S's capacity for developing constructive tendencies (e.g., attachment, love).
17. There are unresolved problems ("a complex" or weakened ego) in the individual; e.g., symptoms or ideas that are discordant, unassimilated, and/or antagonistic.

18. S reports that the suicide is related to a harsh conscience; i.e., a fulfilment of punishment (or self-punishment).

Interpersonal

VI   *Interpersonal Relations*
19. S's problem(s) appears to be determined by the individual's history and the present interpersonal situation.
20. S reports being weakened and/or defeated by unresolved problems in the interpersonal field (or some other ideal such as health, perfection).
21. S's suicide appears related to unsatisfied or frustrated needs; e.g., attachment, perfection, achievement, autonomy, control.
22. S's frustration in the interpersonal field is exceedingly stressful and persisting to a traumatic degree.
23. A positive development in the disturbed relationship was seen as the only possible way to go on living, but such development was seen as not forthcoming.
24. S's relationships (attachments) were too unhealthy and/or too intimate (regressive, "primitive"), keeping him/her under constant strain of stimulation and frustration.

VII   *Rejection–Aggression*
25. S reports a traumatic event or hurt or injury (e.g., unmet love, a failing marriage, disgust with one's work).
26. S, whose personality (ego) is not adequately developed (weakened), appears to have suffered a narcissistic injury.
27. S is preoccupied with an event or injury, namely a person who has been lost or rejecting (i.e., abandonment).
28. S feels quite ambivalent, i.e., both affectionate and hostile towards the same (lost or rejecting) person.
29. S reports feelings and/or ideas of aggression and vengefulness toward him/herself although S appears to be actually angry at someone else.
30. S turns upon the self, murderous impulses that had previously been directed against someone else.
31. Although maybe not reported directly, S may have calculated the self-destructiveness to have a negative effect on someone else (e.g., a lost or rejecting person).
32. S's self-destructiveness appears to be an act of aggression, attack, and/or revenge towards someone else who has hurt or injured him/her.

VIII   *Identification–Egression*
33. S reports in some direct or indirect fashion an identification (i.e., attachment) with a lost or rejecting person (or with any lost ideal [e.g., health, freedom, employment, all A's]).
34. An unwillingness to accept the pain of losing an ideal (e.g., abandonment, sickness, old age), allows S to choose, even seek to escape from life and accept death.

35. S wants to egress (i.e., to escape, to depart, to flee, to be gone), to relieve the unbearable psychological pain.

In concluding this section, it should be clear that what these elements mean is a seed for an extensive project. Of course suicide is more. These common elements, however, at least highlight that suicide is not only due to one factor such as external "stress". The common consistency in suicide is with lifelong adjustment patterns (Shneidman, 1985). Suicide has a history. Hopefully this synthesis will provide a useful clinical perspective on suicide risk, however.

A FEW NOTES ON TRANSFERENCE AND COUNTERTRANSFERENCE IN ASSESSMENT

Although the issues of transference and countertransference are critical, even in assessing suicide risk, they are so broad that space here only allows a brief note (Eyman, 1991; Freud, 1974d; Heimann, 1950; Maltsberger & Buie, 1974). Yet, every clinician must be fully aware of these concerns.

Transference is a process arising in any therapeutic situation and involving reactivation of the patient's previous experience, recollections, and unconscious wishes regarding (often early) significant people (object relations). Such processes in object relations must be identified in treatment, beginning at the assessment stage of intervention.

Suicidal people, for example, could feel angry, injured or rejected in the following situations: After premature termination of the evaluation; with excessive waiting for the evaluation (even one hour, or one day!); when assessment time was short and they felt "cut off"; if referred to others; dealt with too directively; given inadequate rapport, interest, etc.; disappointed by a clinician who forgets important details during the interview; confronted by a clinician about an issue too early or too late in the evaluation; contacted by a person other than the assessing clinician.

Countertransference comprises all the clinician's unconscious reactions to the patient and the patient's transference. These reactions originate in the evaluator's own conflicts and/or real objective relationships (object relations). These may not necessarily be negative; indeed, they can be most constructive in developing an understanding of our patients (and us). It is, however, the negative ones that can be not only problematic but also suicidogenic. The following reactions in the clinician may arise if confrontation with the suicidal patient provokes feelings of guilt, incompetence, anxiety, fear and anger, and when these feelings are not worked through: underestimation of the seriousness of the suicidal action; absence of discussion of suicide thoughts, attempts, etc.; allowing oneself to be lulled into a false sense of security by the patient's promise not to repeat a suicide attempt (such as in the use of a simplistic written suicide contract, until treatment is begun); disregard of the cry for help aspect of the suicide attempt and exclusive concentration on its manipulative character in the evaluation; exaggeration of the patient's provocative, infantile, and aggressive sides; denial of one's own importance to the patient;

failure to persuade the patient to undergo further treatment; feeling of lacking the resources for the evaluation required by a particular patient; exaggerated sense of hopelessness in response to the patient's troubled social situation and abuse of drugs or alcohol; being pleased when the patient claims to have all problems solved after only a brief time period during the assessment, without reflecting closely on the plausibility of this statement; feeling upset when the patient shows resistance after a brief course of enquiry, despite the clinician's initial profound commitment. Obviously, issues of transference and countertransference are complex and the clinician experiencing them can benefit from contact with a supervisor or consultation with a colleague, as well as consideration of the broader literature on such reactions written for psychotherapists.

CASE ILLUSTRATION: VINCE FOSTER JR

To return to the "trunk" of suicide, which is the current basis of clinical evaluation, let me present a case, Vincent Foster Jr. Case presentations have an important place in suicidology (Allport, 1942), and despite limitations will be my main mode of illustration in this volume. Vince Foster Jr was President Bill Clinton's deputy White House counsel who shot himself, with his father's gun, on 20 July 1993. Vincent Foster was also Clinton's friend. He was, 48, married and had three children. Foster had been in Washington for six months, when he was found dead in a park on the Northern Virginia side of the Potomac River. Here is his suicide note:

> I made mistakes from ignorance, inexperience and overwork
> I did not knowingly violate any law or standard of conduct
> No one in the White House, to my knowledge, violated any law or standard of conduct, including any action in the travel office
> The FBI lied in their report to the AG [*attorney general*]
> The Press is covering up the illegal benefits they received from the travel staff
> The GOP has lied and misrepresented its knowledge and role and covered up a prior investigation
> The Ushers Office plotted to have excessive costs incurred, taking advantage of Kaki [*White House Designer*] and HRC [*Hilary Rodham Clinton*]
> The public will never believe the innocence of the Clintons and their loyal staff
> The WSJ [*Wall Street Journal*] editors lie without consequence
> I was not meant for the job or the spotlight of public life in Washington. Here ruining people is considered sport.

What can we learn from Vincent Foster Jr's note? Utilizing the model outlined, we propose the following hypotheses:

- *Unbearable Psychological Pain*—Vincent Foster's mind, based on the note, was permeated with pain—the pain of pain. The suicide was seen as an escape. Although there were many likely motives, the accusations by the FBI, Press, GOP and so on, of violating the law or standards of misconduct overwhelmed him. Mr Foster was forlorn and distressed. He could neither endure nor cope with the injustices, feeling so hopeless and helpless.

- *Cognitive Constriction*—Vincent Foster's mind was a constricted mind. He was "intoxicated" with the trauma—"ruining people is considered sport". His note is only permutations of that trauma.
- *Indirect Expressions*—Vincent Foster Jr was overwhelmingly angry. Yet, the anger eventually turned inward. Indeed, it is quite clear that the manifest aspects of his note imply much more latently. One must speculate on unconscious dynamics as the driving force to his death.
- *Inability to Adjust*—Vincent Foster could not cope; he saw himself too weak to adjust to "the spotlight of public life in Washington". He is, in fact, so passionate in his reverie of that topic. Indeed, his state of mind was indicative of a mental disorder. Vincent Foster probably suffered from, at least, a depressive disorder.
- *Ego*—Vincent Foster's ego was weakened; he lacked constructive tendencies. There is such pain over his unresolved problem—the accusations. He feels so punished.
- *Interpersonal relations*—Mr Foster was weakened and defeated by the FBI, the *Wall Street Journal*, and even the public. Indeed, Vincent Foster lists a long history, experiencing the world as traumatic. Vince Foster committed suicide because of a frustration of needs—these included attachment, affiliation (the White House), autonomy, defendence (to defend), harmavoidance, and infavoidance (to avoid humiliation) (Murray, 1938).
- *Rejection–Aggression*—Vince Foster felt so rejected. Indeed, the rejection was a narcissistic injury—narcissism, of course, is central to this type of executive suicide. Vince Foster, and individuals like him, struggles against narcissistic catastrophes. Foster is so angry but so weakened by the lies of the Press, GOP, and the public. Indeed, he is so weakened that he turns the aggressive impulses against himself. He kills himself, although his suicide, especially the note, was calculatedly written to have an impact on the Press, the FBI, and so on. Vince Foster wanted revenge.
- *Identification–Egression*—Vincent Foster Jr was so attached to the Clintons, the White House, law, standards of conduct. These were deep ideals and identifications. With the loss of these attachments (ideals), he needed to escape, egress. Death became the *only* solution.

The actual protocol sentences from this chapter (or see Chapter 6) that were verified in Foster's note are as follows: Unbearable Pain: 1, 2, 3, 4, 5, 6; Cognitive Constriction: 7, 8, 9; Indirect Expressions: 11, 12—no ambivalence (10); Inability to Adjust: 13, 14, 15; Ego: 16, 17, 18; Interpersonal Relations: 19, 20, 21, 22; Rejection–Aggression: 25, 26 (narcissism), 27, 30, 31, 32; Identification–Egression: 33, 34, 35.

Can we learn more? Fortunately, because of Mr Foster's relationship to then President Clinton, a psychological autopsy was undertaken and a brief synopsis appeared in Maris et al. (2000). This autopsy, as we will learn in detail in Chapter 10, allows us to place the note and its analysis within the larger context of Foster's life (I borrow here from records, keeping in mind that the note and above analysis were undertaken well before I read his autopsy). One can see how the analysed note is mirrored in the psychological autopsy.

Vincent Foster Jr's life was described as one of "success and distinction". This included president of his high school class, first in his law class, top score on Arkansas bar exam, partner of a top law firm, and so on. He was listed in "Best Lawyers in America". He was a success and had a reputation of high standards, something quite obvious in his note.

Vincent Foster Jr was narcissistically attached to his ideals, law and standards of conduct. One's reputation was everything—he needed to be first in his class. Public self was self. He spoke a few months before his death about one's public image at the University of Arkansas Law School:

> The reputation you develop for intellectual and ethical integrity will be your greatest asset or your worst enemy. You will be judged by your judgement. Treat every plead-ing, every brief, every contract, every letter, every daily task as if your career will be judged on it.

Those statements made the note and his death more understandable. Days after his speech at the law school, the accusations by the FBI, Press, GOP, and so on, began. "Travelgate" occurred; he began to be judged about financial misuse of travel, the use of the FBI, and so on. *The Wall Street Journal* even questioned his public behaviour, and on 17 June wrote an editorial "Who is Vincent Foster?". A narcissistic injury occurred. Vincent Foster Jr had been described as "The Rock of Gibraltar" and then, in Washington, he was defeated. He is said to have been disgraced. He became "intoxicated" with the loss of his ideals. In his presentation at the law school, he had said, "Dents to reputations are irreparable". There was a dent, an unbearable pain. He became forlorn and distressed. Foster looked "blue", "down", "out of it", and "frustrated" (e.g., his needs, i.e., infavoidance, were frustrated). Foster, in his constricted mind, even believed that he was a liability—a dent—to President Clinton. Vincent could not cope. He, as the note reveals, was depressed. He could not cope—a man who always got A's, got an F. Death became the only solution—as noted in the psychological autopsy, he could not return to Arkansas. Suicide became the only solution.

Yet, his life, like the note, reveals unconscious dynamics. For example, what does it mean to use his father's gun—a 1913 Colt Army service revolver? Did Foster feel a dent or, as he said, "a blemish on (his) reputation"? And his family, what more could we learn? And President Clinton: what did Clinton mean to Foster? Did Foster see a dent in President Clinton, who we later learned suffered in his public reputation as in the Monica Lewinsky affair? The notes, like his psychological autopsy, reveal much—but does it say it all? And could we, aspiring to rescue, have saved Foster? Would psychotherapy have helped?

ASSESSMENT OF SUICIDE RISK: A PROLOGUE

The ideas presented here for understanding of suicide, and by implication, assess-ment and prediction of suicide risk, are only a prologue, a beginning. Predicting suicide is complicated. Suicide assessment and prediction should be ongoing in our treatment of suicidal people. Vincent was obviously at risk. He was depressed, having a weakened ego. There was a lack of sound personal (ego) functioning. He had been at risk, but he did not reach out for help, for psychotherapy.

It is likely that no one behaviour, including a test score or an interview, will provide all of the information needed to assess and predict suicide. Vincent's or anyone's suicide risk cannot be assessed at one time by one test, one interview, etc. Each bit of information (like a test score, an observation) will have to be placed in the context of that person's life. It is likely that a number of tests, interviews, and scales will be needed to *ongoingly* predict such a complex human behaviour as suicide. No one test or behaviour or observation may be the answer. There is no one "bump on the head" that will tell us whether a patient is suicidal or not, much less how suicidal that person is. Furthermore, all predictions ultimately depend on the skill of the clinician. In that sense, suicide prediction is a task like many others that a clinician faces: a problem of understanding a number of evaluations of the same person.

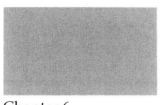

Chapter 6

THEMATIC GUIDE FOR SUICIDE PREDICTION (TGSP)

(Copyright © 1998 by Antoon A. Leenaars)

THEMATIC GUIDE FOR SUICIDE PREDICTION
Antoon A. Leenaars, PhD, CPsych.

I PATIENT DATA

Date: _____

Name: _____ Age: _____ Sex: _____

Date of Birth: _____ Marital Status: _____

Education Status: _____ _____
                    (years)   (degrees)

Current Employment: _____

II SUICIDAL EXPERIENCE

1. Has the patient ever seriously contemplated suicide? (If yes, note particulars)

   _____

2. Has the patient ever attempted suicide? (If yes, note particulars)

   _____

3. Does the patient know anyone who attempted suicide? (If yes, indicate family, acquaintance, etc.)

   _____

4. Does the patient know anyone who committed suicide? (If yes, indicate family, acquaintance, etc.)

   _____

III   REFERRAL DATA

1. Purpose _____

2. What is the referral question? _____
   _____

3. What is the presenting problem(s)? _____
   _____
   _____

IV   INTERVIEW SITUATION

1. Observations _____
   _____
   _____

2. Other procedures (e.g., tests, interviews) _____
   _____

V   INTERPRETATIONS

1. Perturbation rating: Low   Medium   High
   scale equivalent   1 2 3   4 5 6   7 8 9

2. Lethality rating: Low   Medium   High
   scale equivalent   1 2 3   4 5 6   7 8 9

3. Guide summary:
   scores: I: 1, 2, 3, 4, 5, 6;   II: 7, 8, 9;   III: 10, 11, 12;
               IV: 13, 14, 15;   V: 16, 17, 18;   VI: 19, 20, 21, 22, 23, 24
               VII: 25, 26, 27, 28, 29, 30, 31, 32;   VIII: 33, 34, 35

Conclusions: _____
_____
_____
_____
_____

VI   REMARKS

_____
_____
_____
_____
_____

Include on back any other relevant data.

INSTRUCTIONS

Your task will be to verify whether the statements provided below correspond or compare to the contents of the patient's protocols (e.g., interview, written reports). The statements provided below are a classification of the possible content. You are to determine whether the contents in the patient's protocols are a particular or specific instance of the classification or not. Your comparison should be observable; however, the classification may be more abstract than the specific instances. Thus, you will have to make judgements about whether particular contents of a protocol are included in a given classification or not. Your task is to conclude, yes or no.

Intrapsychic

I   *Unbearable Psychological Pain*   Circle/Check
  1. Suicide has adjustive value and is functional because it stops painful tension and provides relief from intolerable psychological pain. (P)[1]   Yes   No
  2. In suicide, the psychological and/or environmental traumas among many other factors may include: incurable disease, threat of senility, fear of becoming hopelessly dependent, feelings of inadequacy, humiliation. Although the solution of suicide is not caused by one thing, or motive, suicide is a flight from these spectres. (P & D)   Yes   No
  3. In the suicidal drama, certain emotional states are present, including pitiful forlornness, emotional deprivation, distress and/or grief. (P & D)   Yes   No
  4. S appears to have arrived at the end of an interest to endure and sees suicide as a solution for some urgent problem(s), and/or injustices of life. (P)   Yes   No
  5. There is a conflict between life's demands for adaptation and the S's inability or unwillingness to meet the challenge. (P)   Yes   No
  6. S is in a state of heightened disturbance (perturbation) and feels boxed in, harassed, especially hopeless and helpless. (P)   Yes   No

II   *Cognitive Constriction*
  7. S reports a history of trauma (e.g., poor health, rejection by significant other, a competitive spouse). (P & D)   Yes   No
  8. Figuratively speaking, S appears to be "intoxicated" by overpowering emotions. Concomitantly, there is a constricted logic and perception. (D)   Yes   No
  9. There is poverty of thought, exhibited by focusing only on permutations and combinations of grief and grief-provoking topics. (D)   Yes   No

---

[1] The letter P refers to a specific highly predictive variable, whereas the letter D refers to a specific differentiating variable of the suicidal mind.

III *Indirect Expressions*
10. S reports ambivalence; e.g., complications, concomitant
    contradictory feelings, attitudes and/or thrusts. (P & D)   Yes No
11. S's aggression has been turned inwards; e.g., humility,
    submission and devotion, subordination, flagellation,
    masochism, are evident. (P)   Yes No
12. Unconscious dynamics can be concluded. There are likely
    more reasons to the suicide than the person is consciously
    aware. (D)   Yes No

IV *Inability to Adjust*
13. S considers him/herself too weak to overcome personal
    difficulties and, therefore, rejects everything, wanting to
    escape painful life events. (P)   Yes No
14. Although S passionately argues that there is no justification
    for living on, S's state of mind is incompatible with an
    accurate assessment/perception of what is going on. (P)   Yes No
15. S exhibits a serious disorder in adjustment. (P)   Yes No
    (a) S's reports are consistent with a manic-depressive
        disorder such as the down-phase; e.g., all-embracing
        negative statements, severe mood disturbances causing
        marked impairment.   Yes No
    (b) S's reports are consistent with schizophrenia; e.g.,
        delusional thought, paranoid ideation.   Yes No
    (c) S's reports are consistent with anxiety disorder (such as
        obsessive-compulsive, post-traumatic stress); e.g.,
        feeling of losing control; recurrent and persistent
        thoughts, impulses or images.   Yes No
    (d) S's reports are consistent with antisocial personality
        (or conduct) disorder; e.g., deceitfulness, conning
        others.   Yes No
    (e) S's reports are consistent with borderline personality;
        e.g., frantic efforts to avoid real or imagined
        abandonment, unstable relationships.   Yes No
    (f) S's reports are consistent with depression; e.g.,
        depressed mood, diminished interest, insomnia.   Yes No
    (g) S's reports are consistent with a disorder (or
        dysfunction) not otherwise specified. S is so paralysed
        by pain that life, future, etc. is colourless and
        unattractive.   Yes No

V *Ego*
16. There is a relative weakness in S's capacity for developing
    constructive tendencies (e.g., attachment, love). (D)   Yes No
17. There are unresolved problems ("a complex" or weakened
    ego) in the individual; e.g., symptoms or ideas that are
    discordant, unassimilated, and/or antagonistic. (P)   Yes No

18. S reports that the suicide is related to a harsh conscience; i.e.,
     a fulfilment of punishment (or self-punishment). (D)   Yes   No

Interpersonal

VI   *Interpersonal Relations*
19. S's problem(s) appears to be determined by the individual's
     history and the present interpersonal situation. (P)   Yes   No
20. S reports being weakened and/or defeated by unresolved
     problems in the interpersonal field (or some other ideal such
     as health, perfection). (P)   Yes   No
21. S's suicide appears related to unsatisfied or frustrated needs;
     e.g., attachment, perfection, achievement, autonomy, control.
     (P)   Yes   No
22. S's frustration in the interpersonal field is exceedingly
     stressful and persisting to a traumatic degree. (P)   Yes   No
23. A positive development in the disturbed relationship was
     seen as the only possible way to go on living, but such
     development was seen as not forthcoming. (P)   Yes   No
24. S's relationships (attachments) were too unhealthy and/or
     too intimate (regressive, "primitive"), keeping him/her
     under constant strain of stimulation and frustration.
     (D)   Yes   No

VII   *Rejection–Aggression*
25. S reports a traumatic event or hurt or injury (e.g., unmet love,
     a failing marriage, disgust with one's work). (P)   Yes   No
26. S, whose personality (ego) is not adequately developed
     (weakened), appears to have suffered a narcissistic injury.
     (P & D)   Yes   No
27. S is preoccupied with an event or injury, namely a person
     who has been lost or rejecting (i.e., abandonment). (D)   Yes   No
28. S feels quite ambivalent, i.e., both affectionate and hostile
     towards the same (lost or rejecting) person. (D)   Yes   No
29. S reports feelings and/or ideas of aggression and
     vengefulness towards him/herself although S appears to be
     actually angry at someone else. (D)   Yes   No
30. S turns upon the self, murderous impulses that had
     previously been directed against someone else. (D)   Yes   No
31. Although maybe not reported directly, S may have calculated
     the self-destructiveness to have a negative effect on someone
     else (e.g., a lost or rejecting person). (P)   Yes   No
32. S's self-destructiveness appears to be an act of aggression,
     attack, and/or revenge towards someone else who has hurt
     or injured him/her. (P)   Yes   No

VIII *Identification–Egression*

33. S reports in some direct or indirect fashion an identification (i.e., attachment) with a lost or rejecting person (or with any lost ideal [e.g., health, freedom, employment, all A's]). (D)   Yes   No
34. An unwillingness to accept the pain of losing an ideal (e.g., abandonment, sickness, old age), allows S to choose, even seek to escape from life and accept death. (D)   Yes   No
35. S wants to egress (i.e., to escape, to depart, to flee, to be gone), to relieve the unbearable psychological pain. (P)   Yes   No

Chapter 7

TGSP: PRACTICE ON SUICIDE NOTES, PSYCHOTHERAPY PROTOCOLS, AND POEMS

There is no better source to understand a suicide than the words of that suicide—whether Mary or Bill. Suicide notes are an example, but so are poems and the patient's own narratives. They give us a window into the suicidal mind. Below, I have chosen a few key poems of Sylvia Plath, a suicide (see Chapter 8 for a detailed presentation), a series of suicide notes and some actual patient protocols from psychotherapy sessions—the latter made available by Dr Konrad Michel. Not only do these documents provide a window into the mind, but the analysis with the TGSP will provide an understanding of the suicidal mind (and brain). Your task will be to verify whether the protocol statements in the TGSP (see Chapter 6) correspond or compare to the contents of the poems, notes, and actual protocols. The standard instructions are as follows:

Your task will be to verify whether the statements provided below correspond or compare to the contents of the patient's protocols (e.g., interview, written reports). The statements are a classification of the possible content. You are to determine whether or not the contents in the patient's protocols are a particular or specific instance of the classification. Your comparison should be observable; however, the classification may be more abstract than the specific instances. Thus, you will have to make judgements about whether or not particular contents of a protocol are included in a given classification. Your task is to conclude, Yes or No.

You will have to apply the TGSP to each poem, note, etc., and you will have to make judgements (see Chapter 5 for details of the TGSP). This is the homework to this volume. (I can only induce the reader to think of their school years; homework was essential to getting A's, or B's.) The data, followed by the suggested scores, will be presented for some of Sylvia Plath's poems, some suicide notes of the famous and not so famous, and an array of therapy notes. David Lester, when he reviewed the volume, wondered why this material was not in an appendix. The simple reason for placing it here is to have the reader understand the suicidal mind better, before proceeding to the intervention section of this book. The principle is: You need to understand what you are treating.

SUICIDE NOTES

Suicide Notes: 1

Marc Etkind (1997) collected a unique array of suicide notes. In his book one finds a wide array of notes from the past, literature, Hollywood, the rich and the famous. The notes range from Adolf Hitler to Kurt Cobain to Vincent Foster Jr. Here is a very small array of the notes in Etkind's book.

1. Sylvia Plath, the poet, killed herself on 11 February 1963. Here is her short note to her nurse for Dr Horder, her psychiatrist:

    Please call Dr Horder.

2. Adolf Hitler killed himself on 30 April 1945. Here is an excerpt from his suicide note:

    My wife and I choose to die in order to escape the shame of overthrow or capitulation. It is our wish for our bodies to be cremated immediately on the place where I have performed the greater part of my daily work during the twelve years of service to my people.

3. Kurt Cobain and his band invented the grunge sound. On 5 April 1994, he shot himself. An excerpt from the note reads:

    This note should be pretty easy to understand. All the wording's from the Punk Rock 101 . . . I haven't felt the excitement of listening to as well as creating music, along with reading and writing too many years now . . . I've tried everything.

4. Vincent Foster, as noted in Chapter 5, was President Clinton's deputy White House counsel who shot himself on 20 July 1993. Here, again, is his note for you to score:

    I made mistakes from ignorance, inexperience and overwork
        I did not knowingly violate any law or standard of conduct
        No one in the White House, to my knowledge, violated any law or standard of conduct, including any action in the travel office,
        The FBI lied in their report to the AG [attorney general]
        The Press is covering up the illegal benefits they received from the travel staff
        The GOP has lied and misrepresented its knowledge and role and covered up a prior investigation
        The Ushers Office plotted to have excessive costs incurred, taking advantage of Kaki [White House Designer] and HRC [Hilary Rodham Clinton]
        The public will never believe the innocence of the Clintons and their loyal staff
        The WSJ [Wall Street Journal] editors lie without consequence
        I was not meant for the job or the spotlight of public life in Washington. Here ruining people is considered sport.

Scores
1. No score
2. 1, 2, 4, 7, 9, 12, 13, 15, 20, 21, 25, 26, 31, 32, 33, 34, 35
3. 1, 2, 4, 5, 7, 8, 9, 13, 15, 16, 20, 21, 25, 26, 33, 34, 35

4. 1, 2, 3, 4, 5, 6, 7, 8, 9, 11, 12, 13, 14, 15, 16, 17, 18, 19, 20, 21, 22, 25, 26, 27, 30, 31, 32, 33, 34, 35

Suicide Notes: 2

Of course, it is not only the rich and famous that leave a last letter. Here is a sample of suicide notes, selected from my personal archive of over 2000 notes.

#2   Hello Sweetie

I just wanted to tell you i still love you very much Sweetie I'll always love you very much.

My God i don't know how all this happen but it did. I wish it never did happen. All i know it hurts real bad just thinking of it makes me cry and say why. I never thought you would do this to me.

Byi my Lady I love you forever,

P.S.   talk

Byi

You're always be
part of me and thought
Betty I just want you to know I love you very much You know I still love you sweetie, I don't understand how all this happened, but you know what, I wish this would never have happened. Betty It hurts me very much. Just thinking of what happened makes me wonder why. I never thought you would do this to me! Sweetie I miss you.

respectfully
Mary

PS. I love you Sweetie

#5   Mary,

You can have your student card back. Give it to the next guy in line. I'm curious to see who's next. I hope he doesn't get hurt easy. I don't know about you but I find it hard to hurt someone.

Why don't you figure out exactly what you expect from a guy. Then shop around to find one. Good luck at finding one. There aren't too many total jurk-off guys who will tell you that they love you and then let you do whatever you want (and not even tease you once). You had this with John and you made him sound like a fuckin idiot. That's how I felt. How does a guy keep you happy?

Do you enjoy people sucking up to you and do you enjoy fuckin everyone's life up?

I think you're the one who needs to grow up.

See you in Hell.

Bill
Thanks for the chocolates but you can have them back.
Why do I still love you?

What does it take to Fuckin grow up?
How many times do you have to be Fuckin hurt?
What do you have to do to Fuckin please someone?
Doesn't anyone give a shit?
Don't the words I LOVE YOU mean anything?

I have nothing left to experience in life.
My conclusion is, Life Sucks and I'm getting the fuck out.
One last thing. I hate every fuckin one of you. So creamate me and dump my ashes over the town dump where I belong with everything else that nobody has a use for. (*I'm so childish.*)

Just give me what I want and I'll be happy, shit.
I don't want fuck all. Okay!
Bill

I knew I'd Die before I got old.
            Ha!   Ha!
I was a drugging teen
                      okay
I admit.
I enjoyed it for a while at least.
Bill

#6   Dearest Bill,
      No matter what you think I've loved you so completely me life is over now that you're going. Just the thought of you coming home from work, you gave me a thrill walking in the house. And not to have you with me anymore is more than I can bear. Forgive me, if you can. It has all been my fault for not being a wife first, a mother second. Because I would end up, embarrasing you, as you say, because I want you with me forever and I know that's no more for me. I love you so much.
                                  Mary

Honey,
Sue is a very good and lovable child. Give her a chance to love you as she has me. Take good care of her, please.
                                  Mary

Joe,
Call Frank over to get me up.
                                  Mom

Dear Sue & Joe & Tom,
      I'm sorry for all the trouble I've caused. I would love to be here for the baby, but I would be no good for any one any more. I love all my children so much. Sue, Joe, Tom his birth certificate and all the other certificates are on the shelf in the closet in my room in the insurance envelope. I wish I had something to leave you besides grief. Forgive me. I love you.
                                  Mother

#12 I'm sorry for this and so much else—I have no backbone—have always been weak & lazy—life for me has been a living death—it is my fault—for the few I have been close with & hurt deeply & still hurt just by being a fearful, stupid, self-centered one year old crybaby—I'm tired of crying—I'm tired of myself— I'm tired of seeing my closest & oldest friends & having nothing to say but— yes—I must be queer—I am but not in the way it would seem—I am happy when asleep—when alone—I think I've never been happy since my brother was born & whom I tormented constantly throughout our growing up—I always wanted to be spoiled so I went to people who would spoil me—There is no one to blame—no one to feel guilty—no one to blame themselves in any way for what has happened—I fell in love like a little boy—never wanting or able to take responsibility for the words that fell so easily from my lips

---

People (all those who love themselves & love their parents & relatives as well) I am a beast . . . for 10 years I felt sorry for myself & made things as easy for me & difficult for others as possible. I never knew who I was or what I was, I never tried & hence took little pride in myself, I never broke loose & had fun . . .

I am a homosexual who has never wanted to

#14   My baby,

I know why you left me this time and I wish there were some way it could have been avoided but I guess thats one of life's more unfortunate facts—men will never completely understand woman and vise-versa. I also know this is all there is now because I just can't go on any further like this. The last time you left me and we got back together again, you wondered where the writing paper had gone to. Well; I told you I had written a couple of letters and not to ask me any questions about them in hopes that you would gather yourself what they were. I don't know if you did or not but they were both letters of my last words. One to my family and the other to you. Well, on the night I wrote them you called, so I through them away. I knew I might be writing the same type of letter again but I didn't care as long as you and I were together again. You see honey, you really are the only person I have every really loved and I know I just can't except another love again the way I did yours. You were very foolish to think I only wanted you here for such petti reasons as having someone with a licence to get me around or because I needed someone for sex. You did please me as far as sex or a good housewife goes but what really hurt me the most is that you didn't really need me. Not being wanted is a bad feeling but not being needed by the person you love most is something entirely different and very hurting. I'v hurt you by phisical means but you just can't understand that I loved you too much to hurt you any other way, yes—I'v hurt your feelings too, but I've never stoped loving you or needing you, I couldn't. I needed and need you now so much as always but for some damned reason you just don't need me. I guess you never really did need me because it's always been so easy for you to do without me. I can't go without you so now I won't. Without you I have no reason to go on because everythink I lived for and had to look forward to was because I had you. Every day I looked forward to coming home to you and was always happy to have you with me for whatever I did. Just as I told you befor a couple of times, I just don't want to do anything or go anywhere without you. I'm not happy going out with the boys like most every other man is, I only wanted to spend every minute with you. You're such a darling but you just dont know how much I love you and most of all need you. Please honey, don't misunderstand me, I'm not saying these things just to make you feel bad, maybe it seemed like I think you were all wrong but I don't because I know I have been wrong too. a man writing his last words doesn't lie. I wish right now that you would walk in here and stop me from doing this. I dont want to go now but always the same, I just dont have anything to go on for now. Some people might say-ah-come on now, you're just a young man yet and you have everything ahead of you. Well I dont believe that. Not that I don't think I have a lot I could gain by living my life through, but I just don't have the same reason I had befor. I truly hope you never intended for us to get back together again because now we _____ _____ this letter and I wish I had never met such a beautiful person because if I hand't I would never be faced with the problem of having to give you up. I almost wish I could take you with me but I know that isn't right either.

Mary, please my daring—don't ever give yourself to another. I never will & love you.

I'm still only yours,
Bill

To the police—please see that my family gets both, my letters to them and my wifes. My sisters address:

88 Peach St. Orchard
Ph. 000-0000   xxxxxxxxxx
                  xxx, xx

I don't know where my wife is so my family will hold her letter for me. Please try to contact her and have her contact my family. She may have gone to Canada, Toronto or Niag. Galls or she may even be in the states yet but please see that she knows there is a letter for her and not to be afraid to call my sister because my family is not going to hold anything against here. Her mother and father live at xx xxxxx, xxx. Please do not give my letter for her to her mother and father as they dislike me very much and would through it away instead of giving it to here.

Please respect my last wishes. Please don't blame my darling for this. I love her and don't want her hurt in anyway. She has no one to turn to now, she gave up her family for me. Please see that she gets my letter. Also I want my body burned and if she wants my ashes, let her have them, if not then do as you would like. These are the last things I ask of you, please respect them and I don't want your religion involved in any way. I love you all,

Bill

P.S. I hope the day never comes when you need someone as much as I need you because its too painful to find out that the person you love and need so much doesn't need you. I hope you are never caught in that situation.

Honey, the poem you wrote is truly the most beautiful thing ever said to me by anyone in my life. I've been reading it over and over. If I were poeteck enough that I could write something as beautiful maybe you then would understand my love for you. But I guess I'm not very good at that sort of thing so I can only say that every word in it is just what I feel also. Please keep it and don't every let anything happen to it. I love you so *very very very* much.

Bill

#22   My dear dear family,

I do not really know how to word this. Please, I beg of you, do not blame yourselves, please. You have done everything possible for me. Your love—all of you—has been everything & now I wish I could hold you all in my arms and kiss you tenderly—for I love you all so.

I have tried & tried to overcome my unhappiness: but in the end have always failed. It seemed I always was to heavy or too flashy, or underflashy or too thin or something. I never have really achieved anything except for Bohemian items like my earrings etc. & we all know that I am 24 & have not even been loved truly by a boyfriend or husband. Everything I have desired has been so close—yet so far.

It has not been anyone's fault—only a quirk of fate or work of God. I hope that God understands & receives me into his Kingdom for is it possible for one to deserve two hells in succession. Perhaps reincarnation is true, then I shall certainly succeed in my second life.

Mother, I love you so please do not weep tears of sorrow for me. I would have suffered all my life & you would have suffered, too. I love you beyond words, be happy that I am at last at peace. You have never failed me, it is only I that has failed. Keep your love alive for you have a complete and wonderful family now. I love you so.

Dad, you have been wonderful and now I know that you have loved me also. Please stay as you are & never return to you "old way of life". You have now found the "secret" of life, and God bless you. We have never really been close, but the love has always been there.

Bill, you are so beautiful & elegant & sweet & unspoiled by modern trends & influences—stay that way. I have always loved & admired you & know you will find an excellent place in life.

Bill, I have no words for you because I love you so. I have even carried your picture everywhere with me. Please, Bill, try your best in school, & make everyone happy. I have always felt so close to you. We both have similar emotions—a little nervous, very sensitive & you are very handsome too. I love you very much be good.

Sam, you are a little devil. You're darling & fun to be around. Take care of yourself & be good.

Mom, I love you always remember our love. Joe, don't cry, instead you re-member our love too.

I am much better off as I am because I have only thru the years, become pro-gressively worse & sick. You have all tried your best, so do not blame yourselves. I love you all.

I hope you do not cry. You can't understand the pain of fighting & failing time after time. Here, at the hospital I see people fail & degenerate before my very eyes. to think that someday I would be one of them. I do not fear for myself, but I can't put you thr that pain for years to come. Mother, I love you too much for that. This, you will overcome someday, my continuing illness you could not.

I do not regret being my life, only the joy (incomparable) of your company mother, the strength of yours dad, the pride I have for you Joe, the laughter of you Bill & Sam—the everything of you. I love you all so.

When you think of my name, think only of love.

Love forever & beyond,
Mary

#28   Dear Bill:

Sorry I have to leave you, but I am suffering so much, just can't go on.

Don't get sick and grieve over me. I don't want you to. Will be much better, I will never be well, all this time.

Bye
with love
Mary

The Lord will help you along.

Dear Betty, Marie, Alice, Dora and friends.

Just can't go on my health is very bad. My illness doesn't improve, just can't take it. Sick all the time.

Please forgive me - Will be much better off.

Love
Mary

Dear [five names]

Please forgive my for what I have done. And also God forgive me. I just can't go on, my health doesn't improve. The doctors can't seem to help me and I am in misery. Very depressed and unhappy. It is much better this way. I hope you understand. I will be much better off. So please forgive me. I will join our loved ones. Please don't grieve over me. I don't want you to. Will be so much happier, no pain, problems to worry about.

Bye
Aunt Mary

#30   Honey, I love you very much as you know. Thank you for the beautiful years you have given me. Tell Dad how much I have appreciated all he has done for me much more than I deserved. Tell Mary how much I love, here. Mary-Anne, Dave and Anne and gloria Jockie, and the kids. Tell any everybody all of the family how much love them. Joan, tell your mother and father and everyone how I love them and miss them. Thank-you Joan for the trials and tribulations. I have put you thru, by my stupid drinking. I have known blew this job to honey. I was warned but never told you. Sorry for how much hardship I have caused you.

---

to ever finds me.

my telephone—No. (000)—AB-0-0000 is disconnected. she is there trying to sell the house. She has done so much I so little. I would prefer if some mean to contact her. rather my fathers No. a direct shock is so much he is an old man.

I worked for xxxx, form section 000-0000

Mike & Hal: thank you for all you have done for me sicerely. It was all my fault. Please will you help Joan, with things up here. Tell Mary & Cal that don't feel in anyway, that it was their fault. The fault lies with me. The car is parked around the corner keys on table. Please help *Joan*—take every effort to try to have the school lessen.

But this is the end. I can't go on struggling, shifting, make excuses I will change. I can't face life any more.

> Joan—I really love
> Dad—I really love
> Mary—I really love

and every member of the family.

#31   Dear Mary

I am so sorry to say good-bye but I can't stand bye and see you with some other man. I love you and I always will love you. I am sorry to hurt those who have tried to help me but I feel that no one or thing (cancer) will ever hurt me again. I have loved my wife while living and shall continue to do so during death. I believe God can forgive me and will some day let me live again in happiness. I refuse to live and hurt my wife and those who care. I can't face reality and I'm sorry to mess up 3 years of our life.

Love,
Bill

#33   Actually I already died on Sunday morning. What will die tonight is only (finally) my body and my damned heart will finally stop beating like mad! Since Sunday morning my heart seems to be saying to me nonstop: "Mary you're still alive!" But I have been thinking the whole while, damned heart why don't you stop beating so wildly? I don't want to go on, because I no longer know what for and why. I loved Bill for 3 months, 3 short months and yet everlasting months. I don't want to go on any longer without him. I just say "Adieu, you (beautiful) life!" All over with pain and anxiety and vegetating and all that shit. It just occurs to me, my sign is Scorpio and I have something in common with real scorpions: When they see no way out, they poison themselves with their own stinger!! Incidentally, a behavior unique to them in the animal kingdom!

I am getting away from the subject again, I know. But there is really nothing more to say.

I would like David to get in touch with Bill to tell him that he needn't have a bad conscience, because it's not his fault that I love him so and can't come to terms with the fact. And that it was the most beautiful and meaningful time of my life, 3 months with Bill!

That was it!

#36   Life isn't worth the bother. I know I am a coward for taking the easy way out, but it isn't easy too kill yourself. About a month ago I told Bill that I was going too kill myself. I was drunk at the time. I am slightly drunk now. He talked me out of it. I gave him my Army ring mainly so I would remember that he had a worse life than I have so far. It is too late.

#37   Perhaps I am being cowardly by just departing from life like this, but I see no other solution. I am afraid of disappointing even more people that I have already. I don't want to go on, I have simply had enough. It was bad enough for me not to have been at Mother's funeral. Since Mother's death I haven't known what I am doing. But one more thing—it is not true that I hit Mother, that was a lie. I have just been a very bad person, but now you are all rid of me.
Mary

#43   Mary
Hi There

I just wan't to say. That I still love you and the baby so heres $50.00 and I'm sorry what I did it's to late to say I'm sorry I always said this to you when I was with you. I know I'm a asshole to you. I'm gonna miss you Shelley. I thought I was gonna make it with you. but I Guess not because I'm a asshole you know that I drink alot. I wish I could see the baby. why did I do this to myself. I guess I'm fucked up. will Mary I got to cut her off for now.

Please take care of the baby plus you. I still love you Mary
Love Bill

#49   No P-M please

| Police | This is suicide. drugs from |
| Coroner | Canada when I came just in case _____ here. |

I have lost everything
Nothing in life remains.
Only depression all my life
Call my brother 00 00 00 Peach Rd.
Toronto 000–0000
or my aunt Mrs. M. Aunt
000 ? xxx Dr.
Bill Toronto
Morphia 150 ×g 1/4
phenobarb 150 ×g $1^{1/2}$

#51   Dear Grandma
I am sorry for what I'm going to do, but your daughter is driving me crazy with her running around with Dee across the street. I am now on the brink of a nervous breakdown because she think's I dont know about her. I am going to shoot her & Dee because Dee started it. I have some money in the BSB so make

sure the kids get it. I have a lot of insurrance too. Please take care of our kids Give them to Diane not Joyce because Joyce is no good either.

Bill

#56   Your wedding band is in my radio, give it to Beverly.
This is the cheepest devoroce you can get
I'm going to wear my wedding band.

Here is all I got take it and be happy

#57   I had a stroke Feb; 19 ___. Aug. 19 ___ I heard of good news from the milkman. I have had arthritis, hardening of arteries ever since. Arthritis is getting worse. I just about can stand the pain. To whom it may concern. I want to thank you for the propaganda. I have a nice reputation. I want to thank you again for the kind words you said about me.

The next time you hear anything, keep your god damn mouth shut. I've been on this earth 5 years on borrowed time. I don't want to go to a Hospital or Home. I want keep the bills down, we haven't that kind of money 35.00 a day. I sooner be dead than alive.

Give me a cheap funeral. No flowers.

Bill

Dr. Smith—you have been good to me. I have been a poor patient

---

Eddie:
Put screws in cabinets before they come down and somebody gets hurt. There only hanging up there in the kitchen.

PA

#58   Della—

Im heartsick First grnma the Otto—then my home—my car—my eyesight— now my apartment. The last few days my sight is getting worse. I can only write by (*one word*)

Love
Mary

Thanks for everything to everyone
Alice & George: so long to two good friends.

Mary

#59   Barbara—

If I can't have you for the rest of my life than my life is not worth living anymore. You really know how to hurt a guy.

Scores

#2	F, 29	7, 9, 11, 12, 21, 25, 26, 31, 22, 2, 3
#5	M, 16	1, 2, 3, 4, 5, 6, 8, 11, 13, 14, 15, 17, 20, 21, 22, 23, 25, 26, 28, 29, 31, 21
#6	F, 40	1, 2, 3, 7, 11, 16, 21, 24, 25, 27, 28, 33, 25
#12	M, 23	1, 2, 3, 5, 6, 8, 11, 12, 13, 14, 15, 17, 18, 20, 21, 22, 23, 25, 26
#14	M, 24	1, 2, 3, 4, 5, 6, 7, 8, 10, 13, 14, 15, 16, 17, 19, 20, 21, 22, 23, 24, 25, 26, 27, 28, 29, 32.
#22	F, 24	1, 2, 3, 5, 6, 7, 10, 12, 13, 15, 16, 17, 21, 25, 35

#27	F, 17	2, 3, 4, 5, 9, 10, 12, 19, 22, 31, 32
#28	F, 67	1, 2, 3, 5, 6, 7, 13, 14, 15, 20, 25, 34
#30	M, 55	1, 2, 3, 4, 5, 6, 10, 13, 14, 15, 17, 20, 21, 22, 26
#31	M, 25	1, 2, 3, 5, 7, 11, 12, 13, 15, 16, 17, 18, 19, 21, 22, 23, 25, 27, 31, 32, 34, 35
#33	F, 17	1, 2, 3, 4, 5, 10, 11, 12, 14, 15, 16, 19, 20, 21, 25, 26, 27, 29, 31, 32, 33, 35
#36	M, 18	1, 2, 3, 4, 5, 6, 10, 13, 14, 15, 17, 20,
#37	F, 16	1, 2, 3, 5, 6, 7, 11, 12, 15, 8, 20, 21, 22, 25, 29, 32
#43	M, 17	1, 2, 3, 4, 5, 6, 7, 10, 11, 12, 13, 15, 16, 17, 18, 19, 20, 21, 25, 26, 27, 28, 29, 31, 32, 35
#49	M, 59	1, 2, 3, 5, 6, 15, 17, 20, 21
#51	M, 34	1, 2, 3, 5, 6, 7, 8, 15, 17, 19, 22, 23, 25, 26, 27, 29, 30, 31, 33, 35
#56	M, 42	1, 3, 4, 7, 10, 12, 19, 21, 25, 27, 28, 29, 32, 35
#57	M, 72	1, 2, 3, 4, 5, 6, 12, 13, 15, 19, 20, 21, 22, 29, 31
#58	F, 65	1, 2, 3, 4, 5, 6, 9, 14, 15, 20, 21
#59	M, 41	1, 2, 3, 5, 6, 7, 10, 12, 16, 19, 24, 25, 27, 28, 29, 31, 33, 35

PSYCHOTHERAPY PROTOCOLS

Konrad Michel, one of Switzerland's most noted suicidologists, has worked over the years on developing effective psychotherapy. He is head of the international training group on intervention in suicidology, The Aeschi Gang (of which I am honoured to be a member). As it would be obvious that I cannot present my protocols (i.e., "I see what I see"), Dr Michel was kind enough to assist this book with providing an array of psychotherapy protocols. We begin with a few vignettes, with the scores found below.

Patient 3, Mrs M

Pat: In the evening I was very agitated. My sister had a terrace to which the door was open, and I thought that the door should be closed, because I had the feeling that I was like being pushed out through this door. And always this thought—you can't live with the children if you end up in a psychiatric hospital. And then I knew that I had to keep myself occupied, because of this restlessness. So, I started to do some mathematics and I thought, you know this already, and it was soon finished, and the agitation was still there, and it was as if I was driven without knowing where to and what for. It seems that I also spoke to my mother on the phone and she said something about suicide and that I shouldn't harm myself, but somehow it didn't reach me. And my daughter said something but I couldn't concentrate and I thought it would be best if nobody said something because I couldn't follow any more.
I tried to eat a yogurt to keep occupied.

Psy: What happened then?

Pat: and then—it was like a rupture, I can't remember anything after that. They say that I got up and walked straight out to the terrace and jumped over it as if this had always been my plan. My sister saw me in the last moment and asked what I was doing and in that moment I jumped.

Patient 18, Mrs W

Pat: I had the feeling that I had done something forbidden. I had a bad conscience. But at the same time I felt very free. It is a strange feeling. It is like a race for freedom.
. . .
I also don't know exactly if at that moment I still felt pain. I can't remember. It is as if the memory is deleted.
. . .
Simply—sometimes I do things that in fact I don't want to do. For instance when I take drugs, part of myself says no, because really I don't want to do this. But I still do it. Then I have no trust in myself any more.
. . .
Mostly I feel fear only after I have done it. Before, I am like dead. There is nothing left inside. I don't feel anything any more. This is scary. But then the fear comes.
. . .
It all feels alien to me. I have the feeling that it wasn't me, that this was another person. This is strange.

Psy: Is it as if you were distant from it, as if it wasn't really you?

Pat: Yes. In fact as if it wasn't really myself. In those moments I always have the feeling as if I was another person.

Psy: When you do something like this, or when?

Pat: Yes.

Psy: A person who is also part of yourself or really some other person?

Pat: No, it is part of myself. But maybe like the child which is in a person. Something of this kind, like that. Then, I always have the feeling that I do something which I don't want to do. It is as if I am driven. It is not really planned.

Patient 11, Mr B

Pat: Drugs are not my thing any more. First I watched TV, then I went to the toilet. Then my parents came and started to make a scene. They were very angry. And I have weak nerves, anyway. I just couldn't bear it any longer. I fell into a kind of trance-like state. I don't know how else to call this state. Suddenly you don't realize what is happening around yourself.

Psy: Is it similar to shutting down consciousness?

Pat: Yes, exactly. But totally and completely. And this is not the first time that I experienced such a state. I have had this several times in the past.

Patient 33, Mrs N

Pat: It was not the first time that this kind of thing happened. But in the recent years, I had thought that I wouldn't take my pills again. But still, I did it again.
. . .
Well, I happened to have another argument with my friend. Really, it was nothing unusual. But, with me, it is like this, that I don't usually know any more what is

going on, when I freak out. I quite often have these black outs. Often I can't recall what it was all about in such moments.

...

With me, this is like an episode in which I don't care about anything. In such a moment I could stand in the middle of the road. I wouldn't care if a car came. I would take things the way they come ... Everything is like this in these moments. I couldn't care less.

Psy: OK. Can I remind you once again of the moment when you took the tablets? Were you really at this moment not afraid of death? Were you really oblivious to everything?

Pat: At that moment I was totally oblivious to anything. I guess in such a moment the brain shuts down. I couldn't think properly any more.

...

I can't even remember what I said.

Psy: In what kind of situations does this occur?

Pat: This happens when I have too much alcohol. But it does not always have to be alcohol. In fact, I don't know what triggers it. I become verbally aggressive. The worst thing is that afterwards I can't remember. And it must be like that, because many people have told me the same thing. I guess they don't all invent this.

...

Then there is something else. My friend told me that there was something strange with me. Sometimes I get these cat-eyes, and then he can't communicate with me any more. In these moments people don't understand what I say. However, if people leave me alone for 10 mins. I am OK again.

...

I can remember that during my high school years, I often wished that I was dead. But at that time I didn't know how to kill myself.

Psy: Yes.

Pat: In the past I didn't succeed because I didn't know how to do it. Sometimes I simply lied on the floor and I imagined that I was dead. I simply switched off until I was ice cold.

Patient 1, Mrs H

Pat: I did not see any way out. I could not go any further.

Psy: And what did you do afterwards?

Pat: Afterwards I went to the bathroom. (*Patient describes how she took the razor blades*) It looks terrible, but it works well and then I tried at first here (*upper lower arm*) and it did not hurt. Then I watched how it was bleeding and it was nothing special. And then I cut myself at the lethal places (*wrist*) ... and put the arm into water and watched the rings, which looked pretty. I was more or less simply watching myself. In the previous months, I had drawn boundaries around myself, and I had often observed myself as if from outside and I did the same then (during the suicide attempt).

Psy: The way you tell it, it sounds as if you were separated from your feelings.

Pat: Yes, completely. I was watching myself even then, I know it sounds schizophrenic but it was like that—"it's simply bleeding now". And then I cut again. First, I cut three times and then once more ... and suddenly I was not outside myself any more.

Psy: Then you were what?

Pat: Not outside myself any more. And it was this last deep cut and it really did not look nice any more and I knew, if I did not do anything, I would die. As stupid as it sounds.

Scores

Patient 3:   1, 3, 4, 5, 6, 8, 12, 13, 15(c), 17, 20, 21, 26, 34, 35
Patient 18: 1, 3, 5, 6, 8, 11, 12, 15(g), 16, 17, 18, 21, 35
Patient 11: 2, 3, 4, 5, 7, 8, 12, 13, 15(g), 16, 17, 19, 20, 21, 22, 25, 26, 29, 30, 31, 32, 35
Patient 33: 1, 2, 3, 4, 5, 6, 7, 8, 11, 12, 13, 15(g), 16, 17, 19, 20, 21, 22, 23, 25, 26, 27, 28,
             29, 32, 34, 35
Patient 1:   1, 3, 4, 6, 8, 12, 15(g) 16, 17, 26, 35

POEMS

Sylvia Plath, the well-known American poet, killed herself. Her poems, especially those from the last six months of her life, are windows to her suicidal mind. The reader needs to find a text of her poems (Plath, 1981) and read and analyse, at least, the following ones: *Daddy* (12 October 1962); *The Jailer* (17 October 1962); *Lady Lazarus* (23–29 October 1962); *Totem* (28 January 1963); *Balloons* (5 January 1963); *Edge*, (5 February 1963).

Scores

Daddy   1, 2, 3, 6, 7, 8, 11, 12, 18, 20, 21, 22, 23, 24, 25, 27, 32, 33, 35
Jailer   1, 2, 3, 6, 7, 8, 11, 12, 15(g), 18, 20, 22, 24, 25, 26, 27, 28, 33, 35
Lady Lazarus 1, 2, 3, 5, 6, 7, 8, 12, 15, 16, 17, 19, 21, 22, 32, 35
Totem   1, 3, 6, 7, 8, 12, 15(a), 35
Balloons   15a, 15b
Edge   1, 3, 6, 9, 11, 15(a), 18, 21, 30, 34, 35

CONCLUDING REMARKS

I hope that the homework on the analysis of the actual words, poems, notes, and so on, helps you to understand the suicidal person better. I hope that the narratives have provided you (the reader) with some special revelations to the suicidal mind. If so, I once more attest to the special virtues of understanding personal documents. There is much one can learn from them.

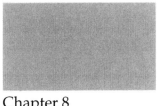

Chapter 8

SYLVIA PLATH: A PROTOCOL ANALYSIS OF HER LAST POEMS

(Dying is an Art; Like Everything Else I Do It Exceptionally Well)

As we have learned, the main problem in suicidology is how can we understand the suicide? What data can we legitimately use to understand the suicidal mind? Unlike most other areas of practice (and research) regarding pathological human acts, we cannot ask questions of the deceased person. This fact alone forces us to look elsewhere. Shneidman and Farberow (1957a) suggested that this fact forces clinicians to rethink the basic problem about a clinical data source. I believe that personal narratives or documents form some of the most valuable data sources; for example, therapy notes from attempters/ideators, case studies (or what the field calls psychological autopsies), suicidal diaries or poems, and—perhaps the most valuable, life-saving and revealing—suicide notes.

Over a century ago, John Stuart Mill (1892) had proposed that we make distinctions about the general and the particular in science. He showed that both the general and the unique are critical for science's development, although some object strongly to the study of individual cases to develop guides for treatment. Allport (1962) noted that the real concern in science, whether idiographic or nomothetic in approach, is developing methods that are rich, flexible, and precise, that "do justice to the fascinating individuality" of each individual. I, in fact, believe that people live a life of stories, not statistics. Suicide notes and other personal documents allow us to meet the challenges of Mill, Allport, Shneidman, and Farberow. People's narratives do, indeed, contain special revelations.

SUICIDE NOTES AND OTHER PERSONAL DOCUMENTS

Allport (1942) makes a clear case for the use of personal documents. One is here reminded of Maslow's view (1966) that much of scientific psychology is "mechanistic and ahuman". Most researchers only know the controlled quantitative experiment, but, according to Maslow (1966) and Shneidman (1980), if we want to know the person, we have to be more open-minded. The experiment (such as used in statistical studies, third-party interviews, and studies of attempters) has an important place, but so do other methods (and questions). Maslow (1966) noted, for example, that we can use subjective reports in psychology as well as "covert communications, paintings, dreams, stories, gestures, etc.—which we can interpret". Personal documents provide such an invaluable source of data. As an interesting footnote to his trail-blazing work, Allport wrote about diaries, memoirs, logs, letters, and autobiographies, but it did not occur to his capacious mind to think of perhaps the most personal documents of all: suicide notes.

As has been historically well established (Benjafield, 2002), we do not need to be defensive about the use of personal documents or pleading for their occasional admissibility in suicidology and psychology in general. On the contrary, Allport, Shneidman, and many others have emphasized their special virtues and their special power in doing the main business of psychology: The intensive study of the person and, by implication, how to intervene effectively.

A common criticism in the field is that personal documents, such as therapy notes or logs, are open to different formulations. Runyan (1982a), for example, has noted that "it is claimed that Freud's case studies suffer from the critical flaw of being open to many interpretations". The studies of most people's lives are, in fact, open to any number of theoretical templates. Gergen (1977) has gone so far as to argue that the events of people's lives allow the investigator freedom to simply support his or her formulations. I would agree that such misuse is possible; yet, Runyan (1982a) suggested that misuse could be avoided. One must "critically evaluate alternative explanations and interpretations". This multiple perspective approach has been one of the richest contributions in the field (Leenaars, 1988a) and, as outlined in detail in Chapter 2, is the essence of the approach in this volume. Indeed, from a phenomenological view, as humans, we cannot but make formulations about events (Husserl, 1973), including those of our suicidal patients.

A related issue is that theory should not play any role in treatment. This view holds that psychotherapy should be atheoretical. Theory, explicit and implicit, however, plays some role in psychotherapy, whether solving a specific problem, modifying irrational cognitions, or investigating the person's past psychological abuse. The problem is that frequently the theory is not stated. Yet, we need empirically supported theory to sort out the stories of many people and that person—such as Sylvia Plath.

OTHER PERSONAL DOCUMENTS

Suicide notes are not the only valuable personal documents. Indeed, there is a host of personal documents worthy of psychological digs: diaries, poems, novels, and so on. A most fascinating kind of personal document left by suicides is the suicide diary. A suicidal diary is a suicide note with a history. It meets the following criteria: It is a lengthy, literate document kept over a fairly long period of time, often years; the diarist writes explicitly about suicide, including his or her suicidal thoughts, impulses, reflections, and resistances; and, the diarist commits suicide. The suicidal diarists are but one subgroup of people who keep books about their lives. Rosenblatt (1983) notes that diaries "allow one to see . . . clearly day-to-day changes, long-term trends, and the effects of specific events". A diary is a document about how life is lived. Most of us are as curious about diaries as we are about suicide notes. To cite a diarist, Evelyn Waugh, "the routine of their day properly recorded is always interesting". The personality of its keeper is richly found within a diary—a document not only of events but of the very writer him/herself.

Why do people keep such a document? Mallon (1984) cites Virginia Woolf, who later drowned herself, reflecting on her diary, "I wonder why I do it . . . Partly I, think, from my old sense of the race of time 'Time's winged chariot hurrying near'. Does it stay it?" Anais Nin notes that the diary is a personal document, an exploration, a growth, a meaningful personal relationship and much more. Both Mallon (1984) and Rosenblatt (1983) point out that a large variety of diaries are written for various reasons—all diarists wanting to write "it" down on pages, like the writer of the suicide note. Both the diary and the suicide note are rich personal documents left by their writers—something they wanted to communicate to themselves and, almost always, to specific and/or unknown others.

Diaries, like suicide notes, sometimes show us the wretchedness and unbearable pain as it unfolds day to day for the keeper. Kafka, as he worked on *The Castle* and *The Trial*, contemplated and wrote about suicide in his diary. Others write about their own suicide attempts. Mallon, for example, cites Lee Harvey Oswald, who attempted suicide and later wrote, "I decide to end it. Soak wrist in cold water to numb the pain, then slash my left wrist . . . I watch my life whirl away." Some diaries are about extremely inimical life-styles, such as *Go Ask Alice*; a diary by a 15-year-old runaway girl, who finally died of a drug overdose. Few diarists write about their death, one fascinating example being the Arthur Inman diaries (Aaron, 1985; Leenaars & Maltsberger, 1994; Shneidman, 1994b). Mallon (1984) provides a detailed account of suicide diaries—of Sylvia Plath, Dora Carrington, and others, all worthy of intense study.

A most insightful account of the suicidal mind, much because of its literary style, is the exegesis by William Styron, in his book *Darkness Visible* (1990). He writes, "For some time now I have sensed in my work a growing psychosis that is doubtless a reflection of the psychotic strain tainting my life." These are a few lines of a note Styron wrote minutes before standing at the suicidal abyss. William Styron's book, which he painfully subtitles, " A memoir of madness", is an essential read for any practising and/or aspiring suicidologist.

William Styron is no stranger to writing and is a most respected author. He is author of *Lie Down in Darkness, The Long March, Set This House on Fire, The Confessions of Nat Turner, Sophie's Choice,* and *This Quiet Dust*—books which themselves give expression to the desolation of melancholia and suicide. He has been presented with numerous awards, including the Prix Mandial Cinco del Duca, which itself played a special significance in William Styron's malaise. It is his literary skill that makes this document rich. One can learn much from this document. It also is—not just can be—rewarding to our patients.

After his survival in balancing the life and death scale, William Styron advises those who suffer depression: "Chin up." He quickly adds that although this is "tantamount to insult", "one can nearly always be saved". In encouraging prose, he notes that when depression is at its "ghastliest", and one is in a state of unbearable pain and unrealistic hopelessness, then others—family, friends, lovers, etc.—must "persuade the sufferer of life's worth". He reveals, as suicide notes have, that it is the attachment to people (and/or other ideals) that are so critical in siding with life when one is facing one's final egression.

Styron's own memories are most revealing. On a cold bitter night, "when I know that I could not possibly get myself through the following day", after his wife had gone to bed, William Styron planned to kill himself. Fortunately, however, he forced himself to watch one of his own plays. At one point in the play a piercing passage occurred from Brahms' *Alto Rhapsody*.

This sound resulted in a flood of recollections of his home: "The children who rushed through its rooms, the festivals, the love and work, the honestly earned slumber, the voices and the nimble commotion, the perennial tribe of cats and dogs and birds, 'laughter and ability and Sighing/And Frocks and Curls'." It was *this* that he could not leave. And, as many survivors painfully feel, Styron knew that he could *not* inflict pain on "those, so close to me".

William Styron also reveals a deeper identification with attachments, which were not only relevant to one's choice of death, but of life—and that his choice of life "may have been belated homage to my mother". She had sung to him, when he was young, the passage from the *Alto Rhapsody*.

Documents have often had therapeutic value in and of themselves. To illustrate, let me cite two of my patients who have brought in Styron's book. The first, a woman diagnosed with a menopausal depression, noted, "Few people understand my pain. This book reveals what it is like for me." She has since had her family read this book. The second, a woman diagnosed with Bipolar Disorder, equally found the book helpful and, even more importantly, became more open to the idea of hospitalization if needed—something that William Styron found for himself, a necessity (see Chapter 19). There is no doubt that many of our patients will resonate to this book. Styron has done suicidology a significant service by writing about his own unbearable pain.

William Styron's book also raises questions about how professionals intervene. He makes us reflect on the utility of even psychotherapy for those who endure "the despair beyond despair". His therapist, he reports, helped him little. (Do we?) Ultimately, it was his attachments that saved his life, as they so often do for our patients. *Eros* won over *Thanatos*. There is obviously much one can learn from Styron's book and other personal documents, such as diaries and notes about suicide.

THE SUICIDAL POEM

A related document—and in many ways a personal one—is the poem. Poems have always been seen as a looking glass, being open like the diary and suicide note to understanding the human mind. This is especially true about the poems left by suicides, although, of course, they have probably been written to be more public than the note, but not as public as many diaries. There is a host of poets who have killed themselves, including: John Berryman, Hart Crane, Cesare Pavese, Anne Sexton, Sara Teasdale and, of course, Sylvia Plath (Lester, 1993). These poets' lives, as evident in their poems, diaries and other documents, were full of pain, depression and suicidal behaviour.

Cesare Pavese is an illustrative example of the poet's inimical life—a life that was characterologically suicidal (Shneidman, 1982b). Pavese's childhood was, by his own words, a desolate existence (Pavese, 1961; Shneidman, 1982b). His father died when Pavese was 6 and his mother was described as "spun steel, harsh and austere". He was haunted by pain all his life. Even in adolescence, he wrote about suicide ("You should know that I am thinking about suicide"). He did so deeply in his life, and at the age of 42 on 27 August 1950 he committed suicide. His writings are reflective of his pain, as one can read in the last words in his diary:

> August 18th, 1950. The things most feared in secret always happens.
> All it take is a little courage.
> It seemed easy when I thought of it. Weak women have done it. It takes humility, not pride.
> All this is sickening.
> Not words. An act. I'll write no more.

Anne Sexton's life was equally marked by suicide. Lester (1993) lists the following attempts: 1949, November 1956, May 1957, November 1961, July 1966, August 1970, September 1973 (twice), Winter 1973–1974 (twice), February 1974, Spring 1974—and eventually killed herself with car exhaust in 1975. Dorothy Parker, a well-known American poet, was suicidal for years, although she never killed herself (Keats, 1970). Once, she wrote these most revealing lines:

> If wild my breasts and sore my pride,
> I bask in dreams of suicide;
> If cool my heart and high my head,
> I think, "How lucky are the dead."

Of course, the poetry and writing of these poets are often projective of their unbearable pain. Cesare Pavese, for example, once wrote that he fought the pain "every day, every hour, against inertia, dejection, and fear". He and the others in the end chose death, leaving their poetry as documents to their suicidal mind. And like diaries and suicide notes, they are open to analysis by placing them in the context of broad theoretical formulations about suicide and personality functioning in general.

SYLVIA PLATH

Sylvia Plath may well be the best-known American poet who killed herself. She killed herself at the age of 30 in 1963 in England by putting her head in a gas oven.

Sylvia was born on 27 October 1932. There are a host of factors in her history that have been associated with her suicide (Butscher, 1976; Lester, 1996). The rejection and final loss of her father, her ambivalence towards her father and identification (attachment) to him were central. There was also the abandonment by her husband for others. Her life has been described as painfully unbearable. Of note, she distrusted her own ability to write, seeing herself as a failure even here. Yet, she wrote voluminously, despite continued rejection of her manuscripts. She suffered deep depression. There was a psychiatric breakdown in 1953. Butscher (1976) makes special note of her being weakened, presenting to the world a mask, something that often occurs in suicidal people (Leenaars, 1997; see Chapter 9). There were other symptoms (see Lester, 1996), all pointing to her inability to adjust to life's demands. In the end, she chose death.

Sylvia Plath's death is not simply due to a situational event, even the death of her ambivalent father is not sufficient to understand her suicide. To understand Sylvia Plath's suicide, we must take a multidimensional perspective, as outlined in this volume, i.e., unbearable psychological pain, cognitive constriction, and so on. These elements, common to suicide, highlight that suicide is not only due to external "stress" or pain or even rational choice—not to one event. The common consistency in suicide is, as noted earlier, with lifelong adjustment patterns (Shneidman, 1985); something that is evident in Sylvia Plath's life—as in the lives of Cesare Pavese and Natalie. These suicidal people have experienced a steady toll of life events; i.e., threat, stress, failure, loss and challenge—pain—that undermined their ability to adjust and they chose death.

The intent of this chapter is to analyse Sylvia Plath's (Plath, 1981) last six months of poems by way of the theory of suicide, outlined in Chapters 2 and 5, to hopefully help us to better understand her choice. In this way, her poems will be approached as personal documents that are open to empirical study, much like suicide notes or diaries. The actual data to be presented here are Plath's poems written in the last six months of her life, utilizing Carnap's logical and empirical procedures for analysis (1959). The TGSP will be used to score the themes in Plath's last poems. From an archival perspective, it is of note that in the first month, September, there is only one poem and then there is a flood of poems, emanating from her suicidal mind. As caveats, the analysis here is more clinical than experimental. There is inter-rater reliability only by the author and Susanne Wenckstern, an issue that is critical in science (Leenaars, 1988a). Equally, the task of rating the poems is even more difficult than suicide notes. Sylvia Plath's poems, in fact, are pulsing and very raw, and some are even terrifying. Personal documents, like all data, have shortcomings as well as benefits. I present the analysis of her last poems to aid in a better understanding of her life—and suicidal lives. (Some of Plath's most revealing poems are noted in Chapter 7.)

PLATH'S PROCESSES TO DEATH

The role of writing, whether a note, a diary, a novel, fiction and so on, may be "a death facilitating process in certain author's lives" (Shneidman, 1982b). This was certainly true of Sylvia Plath in her last six months, with the final poem reading like her own obituary. Often in such writings, patterns or "unity thema" (Murray, 1938) emerge; i.e., recurrent psychological themes in the death-facilitating process. Sylvia

Plath's themes, based on the protocol analysis, are the following: unbearable pain; an emotional state of forlornness, deprivation and distress; heightened disturbance; overpowered by emotion and mental constriction; a serious disorder in adjustment; frustrated and unsatisfied needs; and wanting, if not needing, to egress. These themes are not that different, for example, from Pavese's where themes of pain, frustration and the desire to be dead equally emerge (Shneidman, 1982b).

The themes or patterns of Plath seem omnipresent in the last half year of her life. They are there constantly in her poems; and, by implication, in her suicidal mind. Of note, the protocol analysis revealed that all the protocols presented in the TGSP in Chapter 6 were present at least once in her poems; yet, the following protocols were most evident: 1, 3, 6, 8, 15, 21, 35 (see Chapter 6). Thus, we can tentatively conclude that the following mental processes highly contributed to her death.

Unbearable Psychological Pain

Forlornness, deprivation, distress and grief were constant themes in her mind. Sylvia Plath was perturbed and boxed in. She was hopeless and helpless. In the poem, *Jailer*, she writes: "I have been drugged and raped. Such pain." Further she writes: "His high cold masks of amnesia. How did I get here?"

Plath writes about "Hung, starved, burned, hooked". Such imagery is evoked, and then to ask: "How did I get here?" Pavese (1961), in a similar vein, once wrote: "The richness of life lies in memories we have forgotten" (13 February 1944). Imagine wanting to forget, to have amnesia, to not feel the pain. The need to stop the pain, to stop the suffering, is so pervasive in suicidal people. In the *Jailer*, there is such hopelessness and helplessness. She writes what would freedom do "... do, do, do without me?".

The actual protocols of the *Jailer* are as follows: 1, 2, 3, 6, 7, 8, 11, 12, 15(g), 18, 20, 22, 24, 25, 27, 28, 33, 35.

Cognitive Constriction

Sylvia Plath was probably overpowered by her emotions. Her logic, as Shneidman (1982) also noted about Pavese, was constricted.

Plath's poems are full of mental constriction. The *Jailer* is. One also finds it in the poem, *Lady Lazarus*. Not only does she use words that intoxicate (such as "only") but imagine the state of mind to write:

> Dying
> Is an art, like everything else
> I do it exceptionally well.

The protocols of this poem are 1, 3, 5, 6, 7, 8, 15, 16, 17, 19, 21, 22, 32, 35.

Inability to Adjust

Sylvia Plath, as we know, and as her poems reveal, was probably suffering from a mental disorder. Her poems would suggest that the most likely disorders were as follows, and particularly the first: manic depressive disorder, anxiety disorder, and depressive disorder. Sylvia Plath's poems are clearly reflective of being paralysed by pain. All was colourless.

In the autumn of 1962, there appears in her poems a notable increase in painful themes, e.g., death/morbidity/mutilation, blood, depressed thoughts, violence to self and others, hurt, pain, sexual abuse. One gets the impression of an emergingly disturbed mental state, most likely manic depression (i.e., Bipolar Disorder). The earlier poems in her last six months were more frequently reflective of depression and/or a colourless life (15(f) and (g)). It is later that the poems reflect more the depth of psychosis (15(a) and (c)). In the poem *Totem*, she writes:

> In the bowl the hare is aborted,
> Its baby head out of the way, embalmed in spice.

She later writes about blood and death, themes that continue to be omnipresent, concluding "Death with its many sticks".

The actual protocols were 1, 3, 6, 7, 8, 14, 15(a), 35.

Her second last poem, *Balloons*, was only scored for the "inability to cope" content and, of course the last poem, *Edge*, is clearly reflective of her malaise (see below).

Interpersonal Relations

Sylvia Plath's poems are reflective of unsatisfied and frustrated needs. The deeper we go into her poems, we suspect that much is related to attachment. After all, she had just been abandoned by her husband. This is much like many suicides, including Pavese (Shneidman, 1984) and Natalie (Leenaars, 1993b; see Chapter 7). There is such a bitter quality in their lives.

Pavese (1961) once wrote, "If you were born a second time, you should be very careful, even in your attachment to your mother. You can only lose by it" (22 January 1938).

People bear such heavy costs. The loss is ceaseless. Probably, nowhere is this expressed as well as in Sylvia Plath's poem, *Daddy*. She writes:

> Daddy, I have had to kill you
> You died before I had time—

She writes about her terror — "scared". The loss, the rejection, the abandonment is so deep; she writes: "There's a stake in your fat black heart."

Pavese had loved a woman, Constance Dowling, an American actress. In one year, 1950, he loved her, lost her, and killed himself. Sylvia Plath had a similar history. Both parents, in fact, rejected Inman before he was born (Leenaars & Maltsberger,

1994). One wonders why Pavese wrote about mother and Plath about father. What does it mean to say "Daddy, daddy, you bastard, I'm through". Plath was through a few months later.

The actual protocols of *Daddy* are: 1, 2, 3, 6, 7, 8, 11, 12, 18, 20, 21, 22, 23, 24, 25, 27, 32, 33, 35.

Identification–Egression

Sylvia Plath wanted to egress. She wanted to flee. Her first lines of her last poem, *Edge*, read:

> The woman is perfected
> Her dead.

Imagine to be perfected is death. *Edge* reads not only like an obituary, but also like a Greek tragedy. The word "dead" is used twice; she says "it is over". She needed to be gone . . . to be dead.

The actual protocols of *Edge* are: 1, 3, 6, 9, 11, 15(a), 18, 21, 30, 34, 35.

CONCLUDING REMARKS

Sylvia Plath's suicidal death became inevitable. Her poems allow us to look into her mind; yet, I believe not all her mind. They provide a few snapshots; yet, when placed into the context of her life, we can see a full-length movie. This chapter, as part of this larger volume, does show a movie. It allows us a better understanding of her suicidal mind.

It is likely that Sylvia Plath killed herself in order to cope with her malaise. Pavese (1961) wrote "One does not kill oneself for love of *a* woman, but because love—any love—reveals us in our nakedness, our misery, our vulnerability, our nothings" (25 March 1950). That was equally true for Plath. The poem *Daddy* is so clear about these themes; the associations to Auschwitz and a Fascist, as examples, in all probability are representations of her German father. One gets the impression that she felt greatly abandoned—a theme that also occurs in Natalie, who also lost her father early in life and her husband before her death (see Chapter 7). Did Natalie or Plath count? Did Plath validate herself in death? Did the poetry become "the counting for something" as Pavese and Inman noted?

One's attachments are so deep. As Litman (1967) stated, our "ego is made up in large part of identifications". These identifications are especially associated with our earliest attachments (e.g., father in Plath, mother in Pavese) and significant people (e.g., Plath's husband, Pavese's Constance). With loss, rejection, and so forth, the energy (libido) in this attachment is withdrawn and experienced as abandonment. As Fenichel (1954, p. 400) noted, "The loss is so complete that there is no hope of regaining it. One is hopeless . . . and helpless". Plath reveals the conclusion (see Leenaars, 1993b) of many suicidal people: No love, no life.

Plath's malaise can be equally gleaned from her other personal documents. In her last letter (Plath, 1975) to her mother, dated 4 February 1963—a few days before her death—she writes:

> I just haven't written anybody because I have been feeling a bit grim—the upheaval over, I am seeing the finality of it all, and being catapulted from the cowlike happiness of maternity into loneliness and grim problems is no fun.

The loss was, as her poems reveal, so tragic. In the letter of 4 February, she also identifies with her daughter, Frieda, and associates the following:

> I appreciate your desire to see Frieda, but if you can imagine the emotional upset she has been through in losing her father and moving, you will see what an incredible idea it is to take her away by jet to America. I am her one security and to uproot her would be thoughtless and cruel, however sweetly you treated her at the other end. I could never afford to live in America—I get the best of doctors' care here perfectly free, and with children this is a great blessing. Also, Ted sees the children once a week and this makes him more responsible about our allowance . . . I shall simply have to fight it out on my own over here. Maybe someday I can manage holidays in Europe with the children . . . The children need me most right now, and so I shall try to go on for the next few years writing mornings, being with them afternoons and seeing friends or studying and reading evenings.

How ironically prophetic these last thoughts came to be. For her children, there would now be even greater loss.

In the end, Sylvia Plath appeared to be so preoccupied with her pain. Her last lines of poetry read:

> She is used to this sort of thing.
> Her blacks crackle and drag.

What does she mean? What does this final looking glass reveal? Sylvia Plath does, indeed, have a post-self (Shneidman, 1982b). Pavese did, and so did Arthur Inman, Anne Sexton, and so on. Yet, imagine to count in death. Sylvia Plath's death was such a loss to all of us.

Chapter 9

RICK: A SUICIDE IN A YOUNG ADULT
(*And No One Knew Who Rick Was*)

"Suicide happens without warning." This is a myth that Shneidman challenged around 1952 and incorporated into a number of publications (e.g., Shneidman & Mandelkorn, 1967). He stated that, in fact, "Studies reveal that the suicidal person gives many clues and warnings regarding suicidal intentions." Another fact, according to Shneidman, was "Of 10 persons who kill themselves, 8 have given definite warnings of their suicidal intentions." However, is "Suicide happens without warning" really a fable?

Studies by McIntosh et al. (1983) and Leenaars et al. (1988) supported the general belief that "Suicide happens without warning" is a myth. Yet, clinically, if 8 out of 10 people give warnings, what about the other two? Goldblatt (1992) and Litman (1994) have separately stated that a small but noted percentage of completed suicides left no clues. A minority of these people are most perplexing to even the most veteran suicidologist. How do we understand and predict their suicide?

The classical case, albeit a literary one, is Robinson's *Richard Cory*. The poem describes Richard Cory as a "gentleman from sole to crown". He was "human", "rich", "favored", "schooled", and, in fact, people "thought that he was everything". Then, as the poem ends, Richard Cory, unexpectedly puts a "bullet through his head". Here is Edwin Arlington Robinson's classical poem, one that many of us read in high school:

RICHARD CORY

Whenever Richard Cory went down town,
We people on the pavement looked at him:
He was a gentleman from sole to crown,
Clean favored, and imperially slim.
    And he was always quietly arrayed,
And he was always human when he talked;
But still he fluttered pulses when he said,
"Good-morning", and he glittered when he walked.
    And he was rich—yes, richer than a king—
And admirably schooled in every grace:
In fine, we thought that he was everything

> To make us wish that we were in his place.
>   So on we worked, and waited for the light,
> And went without the meat, and cursed the bread;
> And Richard Cory, one calm summer night,
> Went home and put a bullet through his head.

That suicide happened without warning. The Richard Cory type of patient is, in fact, a person whom many of us experience in our clinical career. Bongar and Greaney (1994) in their studies, have found that the odds are greater than 50% for psychiatrists, and greater than 20% for psychologists, to lose a patient to suicide over the course of their careers. A patient committing suicide is, thus, not a rare event, although the Richard Cory patient does not comprise all of them. The fact is that over 80% of the patients who killed themselves did leave clues. The other 20% raise our anxiety, with the Richard Cory type being even more infrequent. A much publicized Canadian case is Dr Suzanne Killinger Johnson who, in August 2000, jumped to her death with her infant at a subway station in Toronto. She was a therapist who managed to hide her spiralling depression from her medically trained family. She was discussed on the front page of Canada's national newspaper, *The Globe and Mail*, over and over, and in every other media. She was what I call a Richard Cory type of suicide. I will here discuss such a patient who did not give a warning before his death in the hope of understanding the Richard Cory type patient better.

RECONSIDERATION OF CLUES

Shneidman (1994a) had in the 1990s reconsidered his perspective on clues to suicide. He asked, "How it is that some people who are on the verge of suicide ... can hide or mask their secretly held intentions?" Shneidman suggests that many clues are veiled, clouded and guarded, and some are even misleading. He argues that there are individuals who live secret lives and do not communicate. On the Rorschach, as an example for clinicians, they would score a high Lambda (Exner, 1986). These people do not process and/or mediate the stimuli in the usual way, having a defensive intent, conscious and/or unconscious, to avoid the situation, and this often reflects a basic coping style, with conscious and unconscious elements in the process (Leenaars & Lester, 1996). Shneidman calls it *dissembling*. To dissemble means to conceal one's motives—to disguise or conceal one's feelings, intention, or even suicide risk. These people wear "masks". They present a false-self. It is a masking. The story they tell is that they DO NOT tell their story; indeed, they themselves may be unaware of the dissembling or masking. Often, unconscious processes are involved (see Chapter 3). In their dealings with potentially suicidal patients, most clinicians encounter such people. Their stories are invalid; sometimes, they even intentionally produce or feign a behaviour (or symptom). Shneidman (1994a) stated:

> We suicidologists who deal with potentially suicidal people must ... understand that in the ambivalent flow and flux of life, some desperately suicidal people ... can dissemble and hide their true lethal feelings from the world. (p. 395)

I believe that this is especially true with our adolescents, and perhaps even more with young adult patients. These young people often dissemble with their parents, girl/boyfriend, therapist, everyone.

YOUNG ADULTHOOD

Young adulthood is a discrete time-line in development (Frager & Fadiman, 1984; Kimmel, 1974). It has its unique biological, psychological, cultural, and sociological issues. I tentatively support the position in limiting this time-line from 18 to 25 (Kimmel, 1974; Neugarten et al., 1965). Of course, no developmental period can be rigidly defined chronologically, and at best the 18 to 25 range approximates what can only be defined developmentally, i.e., some people mature earlier, others later than the mean.

Adolescence, as explicated in Chapter 2, is a stage marked by the development of a sense of identity. The young adult continues to develop this sense of identity, evolving a finer and more discrete sense of who he/she is in relation to others. Not distinct from this process, the demand to master the challenge of intimacy emerges as the central issue of young adulthood. Erikson (1963, 1980) was one of the first to pioneer work on intimacy (Intimacy vs Isolation) in young adulthood, noting that one must have a sense of who one is before one can appreciate the uniqueness of another. Although the capacity to relate to others emerges earlier, "the individual does not become capable of a fully intimate relationship until the identity crisis is fairly well resolved" (Kimmel, 1974, p. 23). Often, before such development, the individual can only avoid genuine closeness or engage in narcissistic relationships. As Frager and Fadiman (1984, p. 152) note:

> Without a sense of intimacy and commitment, one may become isolated and be unable to sustain intimate relationships. If one's sense of identity is weak and threatened by intimacy, the individual may turn away from or attack whatever encroaches.

I would add, even oneself!

RESEARCH ON SUICIDE IN YOUNG ADULTS

Research regarding any psychological area of young adulthood is scarce (Kimmel, 1974), and studies on suicide in this group are even scarcer. Even the volumes on suicide that are apparently directed to include this age group (e.g., Klerman, 1986), disappoint us, for they only take note of our lack of knowledge about this group of individuals. Insights are often generated from general developmental issues, but we do not find specific information about suicide (see Levinson, 1986). Often young adults are classed together with adolescents, a taxonomic manoeuvre both theoretically and empirically unsound. There have been exceptions to the overlapping taxonomy in the field (e.g., Leenaars, 1989a, 1989b, 1991b; Rickgarn, 1994); however, clearer definitions are required in the research of young adults, which needs to be integrated into life-span perspectives (Leenaars, 1991a). Thus, the clinicians working with young adults are cautioned about using current research, and need to be clear and distinct about age, cultural issues and more in their clinical applications.

IDIOGRAPHIC APPROACH

Case studies have an important place in suicidological history (Allport, 1962; Shneidman, 1985). I will present here a clinical case of a Richard Cory type patient that, through a psychological autopsy, I was able to reconstruct. I will not address treatment, only the psychological assessment of understanding an individual. I will primarily provide the material from the therapist's notes, with other data as needed from the autopsy.

THE CASE: INTAKE

Rick was a 23-year-old male who first arrived at the office of the therapist quite distraught. He was agitated and perturbed. The therapist asked, "What is wrong?" Rick reported that he had been charged with allegations of sexually harassing an unknown female. He was primarily focused on the arrest, fearing conviction and jail.

He reported that the charge was upsetting him, presenting initially only permutations of that crisis. He denied other problems. Further enquiry, however, revealed that he had experienced a rejection by a girlfriend, Sally, about two years earlier. They had dated for two years and planned to marry. One evening, however, when he went out with some friends despite Sally's objections, he learned that Sally had a sexual relation with one of his few friends. She broke off her relationship with Rick, and he had not dated since the break-up. Having found an unknown female attractive, he had made suggestive remarks to her. When asked about the harassment, he admitted that he had been making such remarks for a few years, and earlier before dating Sally. He reported that he had never been charged, questioning the therapist about possible consequences.

Rick's mood was depressed, exhibiting a markedly diminished interest. There was no weight loss although he complained about insomnia. He was agitated and exhibited mild problems in concentrating. When asked about suicide ideation or any attempts, he denied any suicidal intent. However, he did reveal that his mother's brother had killed himself many years earlier. Rick identified his parents as problematic for him, suggesting a stressful history at home. He admitted to use of steroids (which, according to records, were not used subsequent to the arrest).

Rick had no previous mental health history and denied any disturbances or treatments. However, he did report that he believed that his mother was disturbed (although he was initially vague about what he meant). Rick's medical history was unremarkable. He had the usual childhood illnesses. Rick's parents, both of British ancestry, met at high school, and had been married for 28 years. Rick described their relationship as empty, stating "they never talk". Rick's father was in sales, and was often away from home. His mother had never been employed outside the home. Rick had one sister, Susan. Susan was one year older, having married at 17. He did report, however, that his mother was too involved in her life, much like his own.

Rick's personal history, according to him, was generally unremarkable. He was an average student. He reported no problems at school, completing grade 12. He did, however, suggest that problems increased after school. He became more isolated, primarily associating with one good friend, David. He reported only one female relationship in the past, i.e., Sally.

THE CASE: THE PROCESS

Utilizing a time sequence format, let me outline the complexity of the case as it is recorded in the treatment notes:

When asked about his reason for seeing the psychologist, he stated "the charge". He reported that he had been told to see a psychologist by the arresting officer. Fearing jail, he followed the suggestion. The therapist noted that there was likely no personal motivation for treatment, only being propelled by the crisis.

The records indicate that he attended five sessions, missing a number of appointments. The missed appointments were explained as forgotten. Rick had discussed, upon enquiry, his ambivalence about seeing the therapist. He expressed that it made him anxious although jail was expected to be worse. Of note is the fact that Rick was anxious about everything. Avoidance was a general pattern. He talked about deep shyness. For example, going to grade 9 had been a devastating event. He simply withdrew, becoming very isolated in his first year of high school.

The anxiety and ambivalence further hindered the treatment. Rick often lacked focus, asking the therapist to focus. The notes often raise questions about dissembling. The therapist also noted that the first "no show" occurred after Rick received a letter from the therapist for his lawyer. Rick had requested the letter to assist in the pending trial. The content of the letter reflects Rick's ambiguity to treatment, but clearly states the need.

A number of aspects of Rick's life were learned.

Sally had been his best friend. The relationship was "everything". It was his first and only sexual relationship and he described the sex as binding. They were always together. One night, his friend David asked him to go drinking. Despite Sally's request that he should not go, he went. He then discovered that Sally met with one of his other friends that night, engaging in sex. That was the end of the relationship.

He described the event as painful, building an even higher "wall" around him. He had mentally collapsed, although he denied any suicidal reaction. He stated that he had met other women but "always found something wrong with them". He remained alone, insulating himself from other relationships. The therapist noted that Rick associated the current symptoms to that trauma (and more). Of critical note was Rick's relationship to his mother. She was described as an adult child of an alcoholic, having been herself prone to alcohol abuse.

His mother was overly obsessive, often negative. A diagnosis of depression is likely. She was described as critical and overly controlling, exhibiting extreme panic reactions if things were not her way. He stated, "Everything had to be right." For example, if he arrived home 10 minutes late, she panicked. As another example, if one moved any of her over 100 Royal Dalton figurines, she would rage mercilessly. The family life, in fact, revolved around her wants, following what he called "strict British rules". The family, according to Rick's report, was dysfunctional. His mother controlled his sister and father and him, instilling guilt in everyone. It is, in fact, the guilt induction that is relevant to his verbal harassment; after the statements, he would be very harsh and self-critical.

The harassment was probably related to a cycle of depression, describing boredom before making such statements. He would fear the female and then be excited by the sexual nature, only to subsequently self-punish himself. It was suspected that at a deeper level the harassment was related to his anger towards his mother. Of note is the fact that Rick admitted that he knew that he would get caught, suggesting that he often did things knowing that he would be punished.

The last session of the first series of visits involved discussing his dysfunctional family. Rick and the therapist focused not only on his mother but his father. His father, the son of British immigrants, was described as very passive, following his wife's wishes. The father often spent the little time that he had at home cleaning the house because Rick's mother wanted it "spotless".

Rick returned to the therapist after six months without a scheduled appointment. He was extremely upset, having just returned from court where he had been found guilty. Rick was not jailed but the judge had ordered Rick to seek treatment as a condition of probation.

When Rick returned for a scheduled appointment, he indicated that he had to be here, still lacking self-motivation. Rick's probation officer contacted the therapist from time to time. The issue of participation was figural; "no shows" were frequent. There were a number of hiatuses in the contact. He attended 17 sessions every other week, which met the legal condition. Yet, the notes are full of questions about his lack of communication and openness. The therapist asked from time to time about termination; yet, Rick stated that he had to attend. Obviously, such situations are not optimal and one would question whether there even was a therapeutic alliance.

When Rick first returned, he reported that he was dating Gloria, who was a friend from his high school years. Gloria and Rick quickly bonded. Rick described the sex as more mutual than with Sally. He now described the former relationship as negative, always having to make the advances. He stated that he was now "always happy". However, at home, his problems remained.

The discussion in subsequent sessions focused on his relationships, such as with Sally, describing her as controlling and castrating. He now also saw his harassing statement as his way to control women. He associated those insights to his mother. Yet, his relationship with Gloria was different, stating "I don't want to be _____ whipped". Rick often associated these discussions to insecurity—not only his, but the insecurity of men in general. That was especially true about his father, someone with whom he identified. That identification was likely deeply problematic for Rick. Discussion occurred about his mother's narcissism, much like Sally's. However, insight into his own narcissism was lacking. He reported to the therapist that he needed a mask, "a false self" to cope, suggesting that his mother would not accept him otherwise. Obviously, as the therapist noted "the not being able to move the figurines in the house" issue was only the conscious tip of the iceberg.

According to Rick, he needed to avoid and dissemble. He stated that it allowed him to cope with his mother. He described, for example, his mother's confrontation about Sally, "Did you have a good _____?" Although Rick held that that question was inappropriate, he felt guilt. Again, the therapist associated these guilt inductions to his own criminal charge.

Equally, Rick associated his mother's sexual inquisitiveness to his parents' marital problems. He reported that they did not sleep together. He questioned the relation, suggesting divorce would have been best, including for him and his sister.

After a few months, a long hiatus occurred in therapy. Upon Rick's return, the therapist noted that the defenses were stronger. The walls were often there with only a few specific breaks occurring. On one occasion, the therapist noted that "Rick talks. That is unusual." Rick, in fact, reported that no one talked in his family, stating that it is "the British" way. "No one speaks," he said. The anger towards his passive father was especially noted and the therapist and Rick identified a circular system. They discussed that Rick's father's passivity actually reinforced the rage of his mother. Rick concluded that it caused a lot of pain as did Sally and the harassment, describing it all as "hopeless".

The father's role, subsequently, became figural. Rick reported that he never talked to his father; even worse, he "never went to a ballgame, nothing". That, too, was described as painful. Much later, Rick revealed that his father had been an abused child, having been removed at the age of 8 from his home by the Child Protection Agency, shortly after the family's immigration to Canada. His father's relationship to his family of origin ceased to exist, never seeing his siblings. Despite those insights, Rick deeply lacked a closeness to his father and that lack was critical.

The notes in the next few months suggested that the relationship to Gloria was developing. One issue that emerged, however, was Rick's lack of openness. Rick reported that Gloria "wants more discussion". However, there was even greater dissembling. Rick never invited Gloria to his home; indeed, the parents subsequently revealed that they never knew that she even existed. Yet, Rick felt positive, talking about a future. Rick saw Gloria increasingly as his only attachment. More and more he saw his mother—and Sally—as negative. He explored issues of marriage and children. Their sexual relationship was discussed equally positively, describing it as "more healthy" than with Sally.

Gloria was accepting of Rick, whereas other women were not. His mother especially was not so. He once stated "Nothing is okay". He suggested, however, that his mother acts like the victim, that she blames him, his sister, and her husband for everything. Only with Gloria did he describe a closeness. He noted that being in therapy allowed him to be more open, being so different from at home. One time he stated, if mother communicates "she'll say it through the door".

In the last few months, Rick's attendance was more sporadic, attending only once per month. The therapist noted that Rick went on vacation, travelling with his friend, David. Of particular note about that relationship was David's relationship to his own girlfriend. Rick described them as opposite, not talking. He described David's girlfriend like his mother, wanting very little sex. There were a lot of issues; yet, David married her. Rick's reaction was one of fear, asking "Is that what happens?" Of course, the association to his parents is obvious.

The records indicate that the crime was only figural when the probation officer contacted the therapist. There were no subsequent charges and Rick denied any involvement in harassment. However, the issue was always associated to acute anxiety and some relapse prevention work is documented in the treatment. (Rick continued throughout "therapy" to refuse any suggestion for medication, even for the anxiety.)

During Rick's penultimate visit, the therapist noted that Rick's defensiveness increased. They spoke about his motivation for treatment. Rick stated, "it is a parole condition as needed". His probation officer continued to ask about his attendance. However, probation would cease in six months. The therapist noted, "So, he'll be here till the end of probation."

Rick did, however, reveal new consequences to his charge. He had always wanted to be a police officer and had learned that that option was now closed—a painful recognition. Indeed, Rick expressed anger at the charge, the lawyer, and the system.

During his last visit, Rick reported that he was doing well (Dissembling?). He focused only on his relationship to Gloria. They had gone out for lunch and she had told him that she loved him but he questioned his love. Indeed, he stated that his parents did not love each other, asking if anyone did. Rick was especially intellectual in the discussion about relationships, citing that David's was a failure too. He asked questions like "What is love?" and "Is there love?" Most important, he asked if he was capable of love. Rick was especially and unusually inquisitive about the therapist's thoughts. What did he think love was? Did the therapist love? Did he think people did? At the end of the session, Rick reflected on a movie about a mother's love for her son. It was, of course, something that he wanted; yet, it was something that he never felt.

The next session was not kept. The therapist was called by Rick's sister announcing that Rick had "passed away" of a heart attack (Familial dissembling?). Later, the therapist learned that Rick had killed himself.

PREDICTION AND ASSESSMENT

Could Rick's suicide have been predicted? As we have learned, suicide is generally difficult to predict and assess. Two instruments that have some potential in predicting suicide risk (i.e., the intent to kill oneself) are: Beck Suicide Intent Scale (BSIS) and Lethality of Suicide Attempt Rating Scale (LSARS). Would these tests have assisted in predicting Rick's risk? Both of these instruments would, I believe, have resulted in a low score for Rick. Indeed, it is unlikely that a test will allow us to predict a Richard Cory type suicide. Most assessment is based on some direct or indirect clue and when people dissemble, there is no such clue.

Probably the best approach to assessing risk with patients is the simple question: "During the last 24 hours, what were the chances of you actually killing yourself: Absent, low, moderate, high, very high?" Rick's records indicate that the therapist approached the issue twice with Rick. At intake, the therapist asked the question but suicide intent was denied. There was no reported ideation and no plan, only that the mother's brother had killed himself (although that itself is, of course, a risk factor). The question arose on one other occasion. The therapist explored suicidal risk during the session when the mask came off. ("Rick talked. That is unusual.") Rick had discussed feeling depressed and "hopeless". The hopelessness was about the loss of Sally, yet he denied any suicide risk.

UNDERSTANDING SUICIDE

From a psychological view, Rick, I believe, can be clinically understood from, at least, the following concepts:

Intrapsychic

I *Unbearable Psychological Pain*
The common stimulus in suicide is unendurable psychological pain. Rick's life was full of pain. Despite his dissembling, he clearly felt pain. He was distressed, depressed and boxed-in. Yet, there is no suggestion that it was unbearable. He did describe the situation at home as hopeless, not bottomless. The trauma with Sally was equally catastrophic; yet, he escaped from that by his harassment. One wonders, what became unbearable. In all probability, it was likely that the relationship with Gloria had failed. Was he again rejected? Or did he terminate the relationship? Did he believe that he could not love? Or did he harass other females again?

II *Cognitive Constriction*
The common cognitive state in suicide is mental constriction. Rick was constantly constricted. His vocabulary was full of words like "always", "never". He was intoxicated with the loss of Sally, even two years later. Again, however, there is no suggestion in the records that suicide had been *the* solution, until he killed himself. Be that as it may, he had a propensity towards mental and psychological blindness.

III   *Indirect Expressions*

Complications, ambivalence, redirected aggression, unconscious processes are often evident in suicide. Rick was deeply ambivalent towards his mother, Sally, maybe even Gloria. His harassments were redirected aggression; he was deeply angry with Sally and his mother. Submission, subordination and flagellation were evident. Yet, there was more. At a deeper level, there were painful attachments to Sally, his mother, and a yearning for a father who was psychologically absent. Indeed, I suspect that the unconscious processes in our dissembling patients are more important than the conscious ones.

IV   *Inability to Adjust*

People with all types of disorders, problems, pain, and so on, are at risk for suicide. Rick was depressed. His mood/behaviour and verbal expression reflected that state of mind. He felt dejected, being hesitant in social contacts. He often isolated himself; in fact, his sexual harassments can be seen as primitive forms of seeking out contact. There were obsessive–compulsive features, and thus, an identification with his mother. Rick also had some narcissistic features, something Goldblatt (1992) has associated to the Richard Cory type suicide.

I once consulted a friend, Harvard psychiatrist Terry Maltsberger, on the question of psychopathology, dissembling, and suicide. Dr Maltsberger associated with a clinical finding of Fawcett (1997). Fawcett had noted that in 78% of inpatient suicide cases, severe anxiety was evident, what Shneidman calls perturbation. Maltsberger speculated that clinicians need to be aware of the heightened risk factor of anxiety, especially in cases such as the Richard Cory type of suicide. Of research note, the very denial of suicidal ideation in an at-risk inpatient population was the last communication of 64% of those who killed themselves (Busch et al., 1993). Maltsberger (2000) has further noted: "Your letter set me to thinking how normal it has become in American psychiatric units to make decisions about readiness for discharge on the answer the sometime suicidal patient, admitted a short time before, gives to the question, 'Are you feeling like harming yourself now?' Clinicians are remarkably naïve about this question—how many of us are prepared to take these patients at their word! There are lots of reasons for telling your doctor, 'No, I am not suicidal now.' One of them is to fool him and get out of the ward, which of course many patients dislike in the first place. Yet there are others. Patients know we want to hear that suicide is no longer an option, and tell us so because they don't like it if they don't get better quickly. Yet another is that the patient really may think he/she is no longer suicidal, overestimating his/her capacity to endure suffering and not reckoning on how bleak life can be on the outside without a supportive therapeutic team to help" (p. 154).

Maltsberger's lesson: "The lesson is that we should pay more attention to severe anxiety and agitation in our depressed patients than we do to denial of suicide intent if we want to save lives" (p. 154).

As one examines the notes of Rick's therapist, anguish (or anxiety) was clearly evident. Rick, on his last visit, was uncontrollably worried about whether he could love. His mother, for example, had not; so, he concluded with the belief, "I can't love." Whether it is anxiety or some other element of perturbation, clinicians need to consider Maltsberger's lesson carefully in evaluating risk.

V   *Ego*

The suicidal person's ego, the part of the mind that reacts to reality and has a sense of individuality, is a critical aspect in the suicidal act. Rick lacked ego strength. Ego strength is a protective factor against suicide. He had experienced a steady toll of rejections, even the charge resulted in a loss of a dream of becoming a police officer.

Interpersonal

VI   *Interpersonal Relations*

The suicidal person has problems in establishing or maintaining relationships (object relations). Rick's object relations were problematic. The relationship with Sally was a calamity, resulting in self-destructive behaviour (i.e., the harassment). Equally, his family was dysfunctional. There was insufficient individuality, being controlled by his mother. Such symbiotic relations, in fact, occur frequently in suicidal people. The system was inflexible, lacking open communication. Rick's needs, especially attachment, were frustrated. Yet, the relationship with Gloria was seen as a possible way to go on. Yet, on his last visit, he confessed that he could not love.

VII   *Rejection–Aggression*

Loss is central to suicide. Rick felt rejected. Loss was related to his pain; it is likely that the rejection by Sally was a narcissistic injury. That fact makes it more probable that the loss of Gloria occurred. Be that as it may, much of Rick's pain was self-directed. He was deeply angry, and even the harassment was aggressive.

VIII   *Identification–Egression*

Intense identification with a lost or rejecting person or, as Zilboorg (1936) showed, with any lost ideal (e.g., health, youth, career, freedom) is crucial in understanding the suicidal person. Rick was deeply bonded to Sally and even more so to his mother. Those emotional ties were critical in Rick's behaviour. His father, of course, was overly absent from his identification. Yet, the *essential* key to suicide, "I will kill myself", the egression, was not stated. Without this, lethality is difficult to evaluate. We do know subsequently that the death was calculated to be discovered by his mother.

THE CASE: INTERPRETATION

Thus, it can be concluded that the TGSP is a useful avenue to understanding suicide. Yet, even the best of suicidologists may have casualties. This is especially the case with patients that dissemble—such as Rick. Rick was highly perturbed at times; however, his lethality was low. Rick exhibited many of the outlined psychological commonalities of suicide; however, he equally lacked some of the key characteristics. None of our patients fit completely into our templates/frames (Goffman, 1974).

It is of importance that Rick's profile fits, according to research, some essential characteristics of young adults who killed themselves. The suicide of young adults is most different from other adults across the adult life-span (Leenaars, 1989b). Although there may be other differences, Leenaars (1989b) isolated critical differences in inability to adjust, ego, and interpersonal relations.

Even more than other adults, suicide in young adults is related to psychopathology, their lack of ability to cope (Leenaars, 1989b). They more often exhibit a psychological disorder. Rick was weakened, depressed, and exhibited a history of maladjustment. Not completely distinct from the inability to adjust, young adults are also more likely to exhibit a relative weakness in their capacity to develop constructive tendencies (Leenaars, 1989b). They lack ego strength. Like all too many young adults, Rick did not overcome his personal difficulties. His ego, already at his young age, had been weakened by a steady toll of pain.

Consistent, however, with theory (Erikson, 1963), the most important observation documented by Leenaars (1989b) is that the suicide of young adults more than other adults is related to a disturbed, unbearable, interpersonal situation. This is an observation of more or less, not of presence or absence. Relationships are central in almost all suicides. It is, however, especially with young adults, that intimacy vs isolation is figural. It was for Rick. He had problems developing intimacy, even questioning if he could love. With rejection, especially from Sally, he isolated. He attempted to be intimate with Gloria but probably failed at the end. At home, he was isolated. He felt deeply alone. Maybe even his harassments were attempts at making connections. From his last session, however, one hears about a young adult painfully alone, much like his own father.

Thus, we can conclude that lack of attachment was an unbearable anguish for Rick. Intimacy is the core conflict of young adults. If a narcissistic injury occurred before his death, it would have added to the lethal mix of a lonely, anxious young man and allowed him to jump into the abyss. Theoretically, it is known that such injury would have heightened the lethality.

To frame these observations more deeply, I would like to offer the following more general observations about suicide across the life-span, not only of young adults.

Suicide is an intrapsychic and interpersonal event. However, the most significant unconscious processes in suicide may well be interpersonal (Leenaars, 1993b; Maltsberger, 1986). This, I believe, is very true for suicide in young adults. Freud (1974i), as outlined in detail in Chapter 3, had already speculated on the latent interpretation that leads someone to kill him/herself:

> Probably no one finds the mental energy required to kill himself unless, in the first place, in doing so he is at the same time killing an object with whom he had identified himself and, in the second place, is turning against himself a death wish which had been directed against someone else. (p. 162)

People need to develop a strong identification with other people. Attachment, based upon an important emotional tie with another person, in a person's earliest development, was Freud's (1974j) meaning for the term of identification. The person (or other ideal) does not merely exist outside; rather, the object becomes introjected into one's own personality. Although the word identification has different meanings in the literature (see Hartmann, 1939; Meissner, 1981), I have here retained Freud's use of the term as attachment. Freud speculated:

> Identification is known to psychoanalysis as the earliest expression of an emotional tie with another person . . . There are three sources of identification. First, identification is the original form of emotional ties with an object. Secondly, in a regressive way it becomes a substitute for a libidinal object tie, as it were by means of introjection of the object into the ego, and thirdly, it may arise with any new perception of a common quality shared with some other person who is not an object of the sexual instinct. (Freud, 1974j, p. 105)

Freud's (1974n) own use of the concept was divergent. In his later writings, he frequently used the concept of identification as a mechanism of structuralization, namely the superego. Although I am not suggesting that these views are not relevant, I wish to preserve identification to mean a deep primary attachment to significant people (e.g., parents) or some other ideal. Identification is a means of identifying with an object consciously and/or unconsciously, making it part of one's own internal world. It has a psychic existence in the mind.

Identification becomes a hallmark of one's early development; the attachment is deep within one's mind and is all too frequently symbiotic. As Litman (1967), noted, our "ego is made up in large part of identification" (p. 333). These identifications are associated primarily with one's parents, especially the primary caregiver. With loss, abandonment, excessive dependency and other traumatic experiences in the relationships, especially if symbiotic, the attachment becomes dysfunctional. These identifications often get repeated in other significant relationships and the person experiences ongoing pain, becoming hopeless and helpless (Fenichel, 1954). This was true for Rick and was critical to his suicide.

RICHARD CORY: RECONSIDERED

Rick, of course, is not Richard Cory. Individuals are different. However, by the very fact that we are all human beings, there are commonalities. I have attempted to isolate some of these characteristics in the suicidal individual.

Shneidman (1994a) wrote, "If it is true that all the world's a stage, then some players, on occasion, may wear masks. And then, to paraphrase Melville—if man will help, reach through the mask!" (p. 397).

That is difficult with some players such as Rick—or Richard Cory. They constantly dissemble, namely from themselves. However, like Rick's therapist, we have to "reach through the mask".

Within the tradition of my idiographic study of Rick, Hendin and his colleagues (2001) undertook a large-scale nomothetic and idiographic study of a number of surviving psychotherapists. Data from therapists who were treating 26 patients when the patients committed suicide, indicated that two of these patients clearly dissembled. They intended to kill themselves and not only said nothing, but they lied to their therapists just before killing themselves. When Hendin (2001) presented his study at a psychoanalytic congress in Hamburg in August 2001, I asked about further data on dissembling. He informed me that they had not gathered these data, but he agreed that they would assist. We need to be more aware of the mask.

Once I was asked to do the psychiatry rounds at a large hospital (I was going to present Rick at the grand medical rounds later). A staff member presented me with a case of a bright 40-year-old female who had been depressed and treated as an outpatient by a psychiatrist. The patient was known to have a suicidal history. On one visit, the psychiatrist asked how she was. She said fine, left the office and jumped immediately in front of a train. She survived, was hospitalized and treated, and after some months reported that she was well. She appeared well and was to be released if she agreed to outpatient care. The same psychiatrist was to see her. She arrived for her appointment, said she was well, walked to the train station and once again jumped, to the horror of the people waiting on the platform. This time the train stopped. The woman was again hospitalized and the question posed to me was, "What do we do?" I was silent for a few minutes; the organizer looked at me, puzzled. I was thinking. I then said, "Thanks, could you not give me a typical patient to discuss? This woman dissembles. She is a mask." I then began to talk about Rick and the suicidal mask. We need to know the mask if we are to treat such people. As a psychotherapist, I have learned not to underestimate the many masks of suicidal people.

Individuals like Rick are people of mystery. Litman's psychological autopsies (1995) of the Richard Cory type of suicides revealed that people often knew little about them. No one knew who Richard Cory was. People only saw the "glitter", "the grace"—or, to use Shneidman's term, "the mask". Litman (1995) noted how even wives and partners knew little about such people. That was true about Rick's parents. When they were subsequently interviewed they did not even know about Gloria. Litman described the Richard Cory type as autonomous, independent, self-sufficient, and help rejecting. That was true for Rick although the self-sufficient, independence, and autonomy are false; they are, in fact, people with the opposite characteristic. The self-sufficient, etc., are self-believing masks. The help rejecting, of course, is a hallmark, as Freud (1974m) had documented, of a person with a weak ego, not being able to cope. Denial, inhibition, forgetting, avoidance, and phobia are negative ways to cope with life's demands (Freud, 1974m). Despite being at the therapist's office, Rick was not in treatment. There was a lack of attachment (Leenaars, 1994). He rejected help, being only there because of a court order. He rejected everything.

Litman (1995) noted that people have a hard time accepting the Richard Cory suicide as a suicide. That was true with Rick. His therapist, the probation officer and his friends did not accept it, despite the physical evidence. Rick was a mask; he dissembled. Yet, did he kill himself without warning?

CONCLUDING REMARKS

Is it possible to help Rick or Richard Cory? Can we reach through the mask (see Leenaars et al., 1994b)? Shneidman's (1994a) guidance here may assist:

> How can the helper reach inside, except through the mask? What this means in practice is that if we have the least reasonable suspicion that a friend or a patient is dormantly suicidal, we have a responsibility to reach behind social and public masks and to touch the real face of suffering. In such a case, the key questions—those that reflect our interest (and paradigmatically, our lifesaving concern)—are "What is going on?" and "Where do you hurt?". The challenge is to resonate to the other's hidden psychache (Shneidman, 1993) to reassemble what the others have dissembled. (p. 397)

Rick's therapist asked "What is going on?" and "Where do you hurt?" Yet, despite aspiring rescue, Rick felt doomed. Sadly speaking, there will be casualties. There are hazards to doing psychotherapy with suicidal people (Jobes & Maltsberger, 1995).

Only 8 out of 10 people leave clues about suicide risk. In the other 2 out of 10, suicide happens without warning. It is generally difficult to predict suicide because it is rare. Most suicidal patients do not dissemble, probably less than 20% do—but this is still a significant number. Thus, we need constantly to address the dissembling in this small but lethal group of patients.

Chapter 10

SCOTT: SUICIDE OR HOMICIDE?

(He Loved Her a Lot, But Not Wisely)

John Scott Dell was born on 3 March 1951 to parents Myra and John. He died on 29 December 1995. His death certificate is shown in Figure 10.1.

What was the mode of death? Was it a suicide or, as some believed, a homicide? This is the question in this chapter. Suicide and homicide are interwoven; to assess one is to eliminate the other—although sometimes we meet a person who is both homicidal and suicidal. The homicide–suicide presents a special task for risk assessment. To answer the question in the case of Scott Dell, I will follow the principle of *res ipsa loquitur*. The facts—personal documents, letters, psychological autopsy notes, court testimony, and the verdict—will be presented verbatim. It is a "Whodunit?".

The data convey their message. I assembled them here, some two-banker boxes, as the case unfolded to me, beginning with a history of Scott Dell. Next, I present a note and the analysis of the note. There are, however, limitations, as you will read, to a note. To determine the mode of death, one has to address the central question of intent. Did the person intend to kill him/herself? One cannot conclude from a note alone that this is a suicide. The specific procedure within suicidology that would assist is called the psychological autopsy. In the psychological autopsy, data are obtained—personal documents, reports, letters, and third-party interviews. The note is valuable—sometimes essential—within this larger procedure of the psychological autopsy. The note, when placed in the context of that person's life, allows us to answer the question: "Is this a suicide or not?" This is the question about Scott Dell (and is not uncommon in our day-to-day clinical practice).

An outline of the psychological autopsy is provided, following Shneidman's perspective on the technique. There are standard questions. The data, beyond the note examined, include newspaper accounts, police reports, letters, and court testimony. The most important technique in the psychological autopsy is the third-party interviews. I plan to present abbreviations of the interviews of Myra Dell, mother; Loretta McCarthy, aunt; Elsa Steenberg, friend; Sue Kwast, friend; and Paul O'Dell, physician. Scott's own story, his autobiography, is presented next, followed by some pre-trial accounts. Finally, my court testimony and the verdict are presented in detail. The data are immense, perhaps my truncated presentation is too brief,

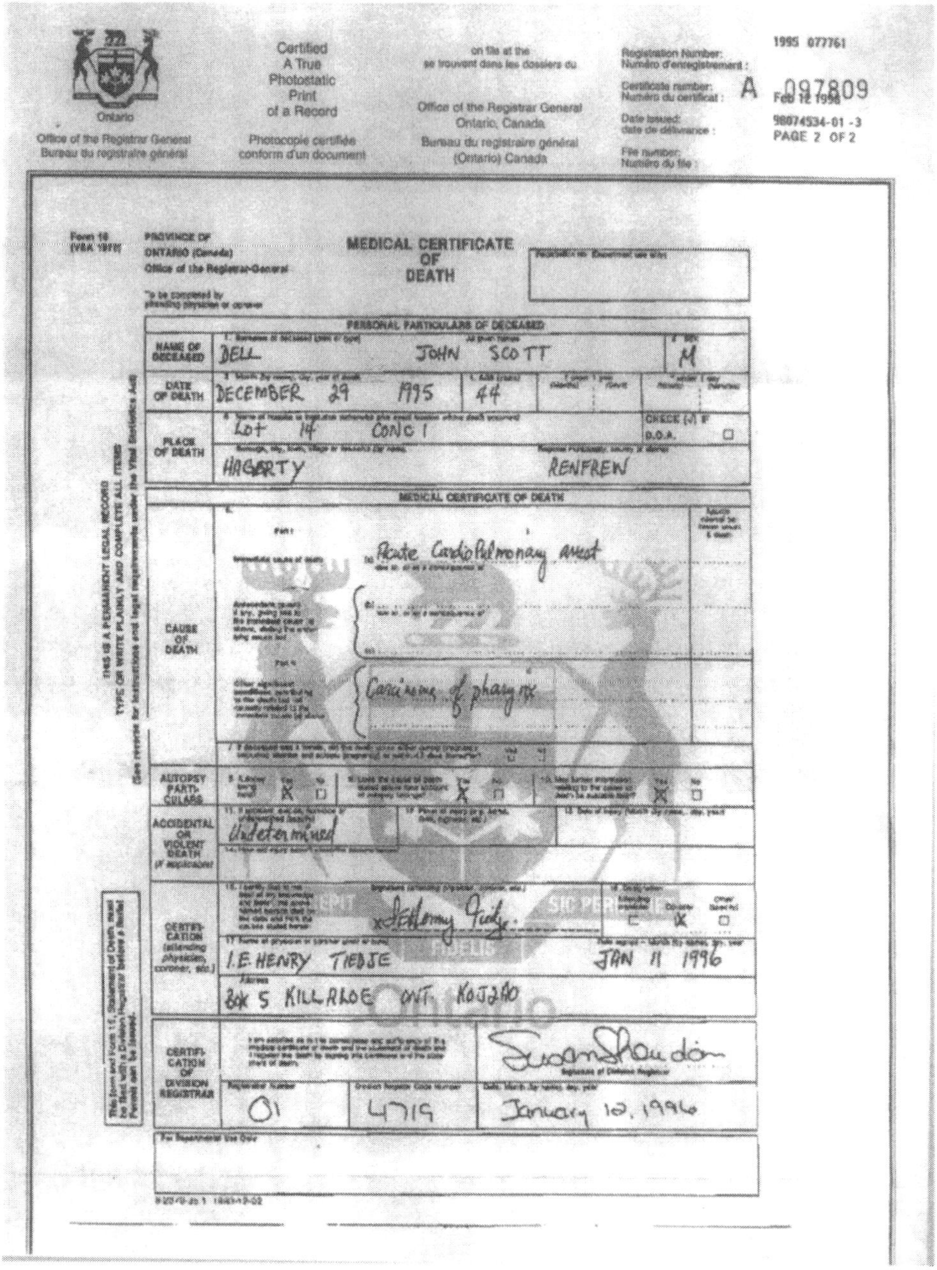

Ontario
Office of the Registrar General
Bureau du registraire général

Certified A True Photostatic Print of a Record
Photocopie certifiée conforme d'un document

on file at the
se trouvent dans les dossiers du
Office of the Registrar General Ontario, Canada
Bureau du registraire général (Ontario) Canada

Registration Number: Numéro d'enregistrement: 1995 077761
Certificate number: Numéro du certificat: A 097809
Date issued: date de délivrance: Feb 12 1996
File number: Numéro du file: 98074534-01-3
PAGE 2 OF 2

MEDICAL CERTIFICATE OF DEATH

PROVINCE OF ONTARIO (Canada)
Office of the Registrar-General

PERSONAL PARTICULARS OF DECEASED

NAME OF DECEASED: DELL JOHN SCOTT M
DATE OF DEATH: DECEMBER 29 1995 44
PLACE OF DEATH: Lot 14 CONC I — HAGARTY — RENFREW

MEDICAL CERTIFICATE OF DEATH

CAUSE OF DEATH: Acute Cardio Pulmonary arrest
Carcinoma of pharynx

AUTOPSY PARTICULARS

ACCIDENTAL OR VIOLENT DEATH: Undetermined

CERTIFICATION: I.E. HENRY TIEDJE JAN 11 1996
Box 5 KILLALOE ONT K0J2A0

CERTIFICATION OF DIVISION REGISTRAR: Susan Shaudon
01 4719 January 10, 1996

Figure 10.1

although others may see it as too long. David Lester, when he read the chapter, noted, "The biggest point and most interesting is your court testimony verbatim. A verbatim account is most rare." The testimony was an interesting and historical experience, especially the cross-examination by a Mr Bumble (Mr Selkirk). On a final note, Dr Lester suggested that I should mention the judge's decision beforehand—but to do so would be to deviate from the classical, "Whodunit?".

It would also detract from the reader's clinical task, i.e., to put the pieces of data together to make his/her own assessment: Is it homicide or suicide? That is the purpose of this chapter. I hope that the case illustrates the clinical process of suicide risk assessment.

Let me begin with more history.

HISTORY

Scott Dell was married to Cherrylle Dell. Cherrylle was born on 15 November 1954; at age 17 she met Scott in Wilberforce, Ontario, Canada, in 1970. They married on 31 December 1971.

To place Scott's death in the context of his life, here is a brief biography of Scott's life: In October 1974, Scott and Cherrylle moved to Toronto; Cherrylle separated from Scott in April 1975, while she was employed as an exotic dancer. During the separation, Cherrylle became pregnant by another man and Eden was born in 1976. Scott and Cherrylle reconciled; Scott raised Eden as his own daughter and became employed at General Motors in Oshawa.

In May 1978, Scott and Cherrylle applied and were approved to be foster parents. They moved to Millbrook in November 1985 and began a home for special needs children. In 1987, Megan was adopted. In November 1988 Scott and Cherrylle purchased a farm called Stony Hill Farm near the village of Killaloe. In 1989, their biological son, Frank, was born and Scott left employment with General Motors.

In July 1992, Cherrylle left Scott, moved in with her female lover, Gay Doherty, and commenced a petition for divorce from Scott. Between July and December 1992, Cherrylle repeated allegation of physical assault by Scott upon her, allegations of physical assault upon a special needs foster child, and allegations of sexual abuse by Scott upon their children. In January 1993, the assault charges against Scott were withdrawn; all abuse allegations made by Cherrylle were determined to be fabrications. In May 1993, Scott was awarded sole custody of the children. Cherrylle continued to make allegations of sexual abuse which were again determined to be false. Scott owned the farm at this time.

Early in 1994, Scott developed throat cancer. Cherrylle then became pleasant towards Scott in public. Scott underwent traditional treatment under the care of Dr Paul O'Dell as well as exploring spirituality and medication. He underwent surgery on his throat cancer in September 1994. This surgery, combined with radiation treatment and Scott's own efforts, resulted in complete remission; however, he completely lost his sense of taste. Scott and his family and friends were happy.

In November 1994, Gay Doherty left Cherrylle, remaining first in the area, although she moved to Texas in April 1995. Scott hoped for reconciliation and transferred the farm into joint ownership. In July 1995, Cherrylle met Nancy Fillmore and they moved into Cherrylle's home. Scott met Susan Kwast in August 1995 and started dating.

On 14 December 1995, Scott attended the clinic of Dr O'Dell. There were no signs of cancer and Scott was described as having a positive attitude.

Despite dating Susan, Scott was still quite attached to Cherrylle. Scott had planned to have Susan come to the farm for Christmas, but, despite Scott having custody, Cherrylle was upset and stated that he could not have the children if Susan was there. Around 18 December, Susan terminated the relationship with Scott. Scott continued to plan a Christmas dinner with the family, planning the event for 30 December.

On 28 December 1995, Gay Doherty returned for a visit to Killaloe. She called Scott and went to visit Cherrylle and Nancy. While there, Cherrylle was talking to Scott on the telephone and did so, almost continually, from early evening to 4:00 a.m. on 29 December. Scott was reported to be drinking wine. On 29 December, Gay returned to Cherrylle's house, picked up the children and returned around 4:30 p.m. Scott had planned to pick up the children, but did not show. While waiting, Cherrylle told Gay that Scott's cancer had returned and that he had finally admitted to the sexual abuse. At around 5:00 p.m., Cherrylle called the farm, but received no answer. Gay decided go to the farm; upon her arrival, she found the door ajar. Gay left the property and returned to Cherrylle's home, asking for help. Cherrylle and Nancy refused, but Cherrylle called a friend, who, together with another man, returned to the farm with Gay. A short time later, Scott's body, half-naked, was found. They discovered a partially full bottle of wine, Le Piat D'Or, with a partially full glass of wine. A note was found. The Ontario Provincial Police (OPP) were called.

OPP officer, Wayne Carmaly, arrived at the farm at approximately 11:55 p.m. on the 29 December. The note, wineglass and bottle were seized. The coroner was called. Dr Tiedje viewed the body the next day and issued a death certificate listing the immediate cause of death as Metastatic Carcinoma of the Mouth.

Upon being notified of Scott's death, his parents and family became suspicious. Cherrylle had told everyone that the cancer had returned; however, they contacted Dr Paul O'Dell who stated that that was not possible. Cherrylle continued to tell people that the cancer had returned and requested a cremation. Yet, because of the family an autopsy was performed by Dr. Archarya and it was learned that the cause of death was acute ethylene glycol poison (or more commonly known as antifreeze). The antifreeze had been found in the bottle of wine. The autopsy report reads as follows:

Synopsis:

This 45-year-old male with a previous carcinoma of the pharynx with recent recurrence and surgery on the right side of the neck related to the carcinoma was doing heavy work on the day of death, which was January 2, 1996. He was shoveling the snow off the roof and also drinking wine.

The exact cause of death is not clear but is thought to be cardiopulmonary. The body of the deceased which was frozen was referred to the Ottawa General Hospital for a post mortem. The date of death was January 2, 1996.

Cause of Death:
 1. No residual primary or metastatic carcinoma.
 2. No definite anatomical cause of death.

Scott's mother, Myra, was informed of the coroner's office decision on 16 April 1996. The letter read as follows: "I am unable to state with any confidence that his death was a suicide. I have elected to mark the death certificate as undetermined."

A NOTE

The cause of death was listed as "Undetermined"; yet questions remained—was it suicide or homicide? The note, found at the scene, was called a "suicide note". The coroner and police officer, for example, had called the note a "suicide note". The note read as follows:

SCOTT DELL NOTE—29 DEC 95
Dear Mr Fantasy
Carmelita—Linda Ronstadt—Debbie Quinn
Fun—life would go on forever. Death—suicide
The truth is simple but seldom ever seen.

If Truth is Purity can it ever exist in such an impure world. If it can't what does that mean. Are we all living in the shadows of

I feel like holding you close to me like never before I feel like making love to you I feel like all the bad stuff would go away.

You and I are stuck because of all the bad stuff that has happened to us last 3 years. We need to make it go away.

I'm trying not to think about things I want to think about. I don't know if that is what I should do or not. I can't help it. I don't want to want you. I don't want to be rejected

If we don't get back together we maybe shouldn't see each other very much.

I thought maybe this wasn't a good night because I was too tired but I think the truth is revealed no matter what.

Sun—before

Lying on a beach with you

We forget all time that our life is a gift that has been given us to enjoy not to waste.

I doesn't last long. It is not a sin to be happy but it may be to be unhappy.

What did you think was going to happen if I drank a bottle wine listening to music we used to listen too

I'm going to think about you and me together

Maybe that's the only way you can except to thru a spiritual vision.

I seems true that is not a sin to be happy so maybe that means that it is to be unhappy

You will have to listen to your heart not your head.

I had a vision of you very briefly you were like some neophyte Angel floating in the air but you were disconnected you head from your body.

1. Mary Akroyd.
2. I was probably supposed to die
   But my life was spared
   I don't know why. That bothers me.
3. Let go theres nothing that you are holding onto now is going to help you

4. Let go. You are holding on tight.
5. Our lives are going by really fast

THE ARREST

Stories continued. Then, beginning in August 1996, Cherrylle contacted the OPP with a series of suspicious fires; later it was learned that these were fabrications. In March 1997, the relationship between Cherrylle and Nancy Fillmore ended and Nancy, by arrangement on 18 March attended the Killaloe OPP detachment to meet with Sgt Ken Leppert. She later returned on the 18th and 27th of the same month. In April 1997, Cherrylle learned that the OPP were investigating Scott's death. Cherrylle continued to contact the police, making allegations of fraudulent behaviour of Nancy Fillmore, fires, and so on. A number of harassments occurred towards Nancy, including a fire in the backyard of her apartment. By the summer of 1997, Nancy became more agitated and feared that Cherrylle intended to kill her. She told, for example, Sgt Leppert that she feared for her life. On 18 August 1997 she told a number of people about her fear, and then, on 19 August 1997 it is alleged that a 16-year-old street youth entered Nancy's home, where she had passed out because she had consumed a lot of alcohol. He set a fire and Nancy died. The cause of death was determined to be carbon monoxide poisoning.

On 20 December 1997, Sgt Ken Leppert, charging her with a number of offences, most importantly first degree murder, arrested Cherrylle. Yet, questions remained in the case against Cherrylle, most notably the note that was alleged to be a suicide note. Subsequently Sgt Leppert contacted me and asked for my opinion: Is the note a suicide note or not? The specific referral question was: Is the note found at the scene of Mr Dell's death on 19 December 1995 a suicide note?

THE ANALYSIS OF THE NOTE

The documents and data reviewed was the note found at the scene. The case, thus, presents a unique opportunity. To postdict a communication as representing suicide risk or not, the TGSP will be used. In performing my analysis, I first looked at the note before any background information was known. The note had the following characteristics of suicide notes:

Intrapsychic

  I *Unbearable Psychological Pain* (1 out of 6 protocol sentences, PS)
     • In the note, certain emotional states are present, including pitiful forlornness, emotional deprivation, distress and/or grief.

  II *Cognitive Constriction* (1 out of 3 PS)
     • S reports a history of trauma (e.g., rejection by significant other).

  III *Indirect Expressions* (1 out of 3 PS)
     • S reports ambivalence; e.g., complications, concomitant contradictory feelings, attitudes and/or thrusts

IV *Inability to Adjust* (1 out of 3 PS)
- S exhibits a serious dysfunction in adjustment. Unable to specify.

V *Ego* (1 out of 3 PS)
- There is a relative weakness in S's capacity for developing constructive tendencies (e.g., attachment, love).

Interpersonal

VI *Interpersonal Relations* (3 out of 6 PS)
- S's problem(s) appears to be determined by the individual's history and the present interpersonal situation
- S reports being weakened and /or defeated by unresolved problems in the interpersonal field.
- S's suicide appears related to unsatisfied or frustrated needs; e.g., attachment.

VII *Rejection–Aggression* (3 out of 8 PS)
- S reports a traumatic event or hurt or injury (e.g., unmet love, a failing marriage).
- S is preoccupied with an event of injury, namely a person who has been lost or rejecting (i.e. abandonment).
- S feels quite ambivalent, i.e., both affectionate and hostile towards the same (lost or rejecting) person.

VIII *Identification–Egression* (1 out of 3 PS)
- S wants to egress (i.e., to depart, to flee, to escape, to be gone), to relieve the psychological pain, associated to the traumatic event.

Based on the foregoing analysis, I reached the following primary opinions:

- Based on my training, experience and research in the field and my review of approximately 2000 suicide notes, there is no doubt in my mind that this is *not* a suicide note, i.e., a note written by someone with suicide intent in mind.
- The specific protocols scored in the TGSP are as follows: 3, 7, 10, 15(g), 16, 19, 20, 21, 23, 25, 27, 28, and 35.

LIMITATIONS OF A NOTE

More generally on the question raised, based on an analysis of an alleged suicide note alone, one cannot conclude, "This is a suicide" (Leenaars, 1999b). One needs to know one's limitations. Be that as it may, the suicide note is of particular interest and import to forensic scientists/clinicians. To illustrate, I present another much-publicized coroner's inquest case in Canada, Daniel Beckon.

Daniel Beckon, Canada's premiere jockey, died on 2 July 1987. His death resulted in one of Canada's most publicized inquests. Two notes written by Daniel Beckon were found at the scene of his death. The notes were: (1) to Sue Beckon and (2) to the couple's son Tom.

(1) I hearby leave everything to my loving wife Sue Beckon Farm Ltd. Stocks in REFF house
    Sue I wish that I could be the husband you deserved for what it's worth I only loved you.
    Forgive me for all the hurt.
    Love
        Daniel

(2) Tom I love you so much you are the only thing I can be proud of.
    Never do drugs son they only hurt the one's you love. For give me for what Im going to do.
        Loving only You's
        Daniel Beckon

The question raised in this case is whether Daniel Beckon's death was a suicide. This case was complicated by the fact that a social scientist, with no known expertise in suicide notes and suicidology in general, reported the following to the inquest: "Based upon an analysis of the content and ideation of the two communications, it is my judgement that they are precisely what they manifestly appear to be; namely messages in certain contemplation of suicide." The expert goes on to say, "The content is archetypically consistent with a state of mind . . . " of shame, self-blame, and enduring hopelessness. He concludes, therefore, that "Mr. Beckon's death was in all likelihood, self-inflicted".

How was this judgement made? The expert testified that, "Both experience and research" led to his conclusion: a note, therefore, suicide. However, there was no reference to research in his testimony, despite frequent reference to "research indicates". A descriptive procedure, utilizing a patchwork of information, appears to have been used; one that is not documented in the literature. Of even more concern is the fact that the final conclusion was based on an analysis of a note alone. The point being that if one wants to present an analysis of a suicide note in the court, there are a variety of methods in the literature to understand them and, even then, one needs to know their limitations.

An important aspect of the issue at hand is that suicide is an intentional act. As Litman (1984, p. 88) notes:

> The concept, which defines a death as suicide rather than an accident, is intention. For example, we assume that when a man shoots himself in the head with a gun, he intended to die. Therefore the death was a suicide. However, if in fact, he intended to survive, for example, if he thought the gun was not loaded, the death was accidental.

In cases where it is difficult to evaluate a dead person's intention, the death is called *equivocal*. For example, the facts surrounding the case are not known, or because the person's intentions were unclear, or—if the author might add—the only datum is a note alleged to be a suicide note.

In the Beckon case, there were other data questioning whether it was suicide. It may have been a murder. Daniel Beckon may have been forced to write the note. If that is true, it means that a suicide note does *not always* indicate a suicide (Litman, 1984). The case of the actor Freddie Prinze is an example in point. Freddie Prinze shot himself in the head one night while his manager was present. Mr Prinze had called several people, stating, "I'm going to do it". He wrote a note in which he stated "no one is responsible". Even if he left a note: Was the death intentional? A few other facts were critical, according to Litman (1984). Freddie Prinze was a drug user and had used drugs that night; he also played with guns, often pretending to shoot himself. The decision in that case, at least for insurance purposes, was that he did not intend to kill himself. To conclude, the question to determine the mode of death as a suicide is: Did the person intentionally kill him/herself?

To address the question of intent, the suicide note must be placed within the context of other forensic data. The specific procedure within forensic suicidology that would assist in such situations is called the *psychological autopsy*. The psychological autopsy may include the following: Why did the individual kill him/herself?; How did the individual die and when—that is, why at a particular time?; and, What is the most probable mode of death?

In the psychological autopsy, data are obtained through interviews with persons close to the deceased, including, for example, family, friends, doctors, and associates at work. Facts and circumstances from anatomical autopsy, suicide notes, and police records are obtained and other procedures are utilized. It is on this basis that one can begin to answer the above questions and, specifically here: Did Scott Dell (or Daniel Beckon) kill himself? All this should not be construed to mean that the suicide note has no place in forensic cases. On the contrary, a suicide note is a "window" to the mind of the decedent. For example, if a note of a decedent is determined, by a scientific method of analysis, to be a suicide note, one can conclude that in all probability at the time of writing the note the person had suicide on his/her mind. The note is, indeed, an extremely valuable (invaluable) bit of datum within the larger procedural framework of the psychological autopsy to assess intentionality and to conclude that, in all probability, the death was a natural death, accident, suicide or homicide (NASH; and, of course, undetermined).

Returning to Scott Dell's case, his writing had a few characteristics of a suicide note, having 12 out of 35. The 12 protocol sentences relate primarily to an interpersonal trauma; i.e. unmet love, rejection. It lacks in the intrapsychic characteristics; for example, unbearable psychological pain is almost absent and it is *the* stimulus to suicide. There is a lack of mental constriction and so on. I will outline in more detail my testimony at the trial. Let it suffice to conclude here: This is not a suicide note.

THE PSYCHOLOGICAL AUTOPSY

After the initial analysis and decision, I subsequently looked at the OPP's condensed synopsis of John Scott Dell Murder, 25 April 2000, which was the basis for most of the background information presented earlier.

In addition to the earlier opinion, I reached the following opinion:

> Mr Dell's note is consistent with the experience of and preoccupation with a traumatic event, the break-up with, who in the Condensed Synopsis is identified as his ex-wife, Cherrylle Dell. The "bad stuff" in "last 3 years" was painful for Mr Dell. Mr Dell

has been frustrated and ambivalent. He wished for a positive development in the relation, but feared rejection. Thus, there is a history and a current circumstance that are the focus of the writing. He wished to have relief from the "bad stuff". The note is primarily a note about trauma, i.e., the relationship, but it is not consistent with other aspects of a suicide note.

Subsequently the following question was asked: Did Scott Dell intentionally kill himself? This question is on the mode of death; i.e., the question of intention: Did this person intentionally kill himself? To address this question, as noted earlier, this case must be placed within the context of further information about Scott's life and death. The specific procedure is the psychological autopsy.

SHNEIDMAN'S PERSPECTIVE ON THE PSYCHOLOGICAL AUTOPSY

How is the psychological autopsy conducted? As this is the work of Edwin Shneidman, I will here quote him from my edited volume of his selected works, *Lives and Deaths*:

> How is a psychological autopsy performed? Talking to some key persons—spouse, lover, parent, grown child, friend, colleague, physician, supervisor, and co-worker—who knew the decedent, does it. The talking to is done gently, a mixture of conversation, interview, emotional support, general questions, and a good deal of listening. I always telephone and then go out to the home. After rapport is established, a good general opening question might be: "Please tell me, what was he (she) like?" Sometimes clothes and material possessions are looked at, photographs shown, and even diaries and correspondence shared. (On one occasion, the widow showed me her late husband's suicide note—which she had hidden from the police!—rather changing the equivocal nature of the death.)
>
> In general, I do not have a fixed outline in mind while conducting a psychological autopsy, but inasmuch as outlines have been requested from time to time, one is presented below with the dual cautions that it should not be followed slavishly and that the investigator should be ever mindful that he may be asking questions that are very painful to people in an obvious grief-laden situation. The person who conducts a psychological autopsy should participate, as far as he is genuinely able, in the anguish of the bereaved person and should always do his work with the mental health of the survivors in mind.
>
> Here, then, are some categories that might be included in a psychological autopsy (Shneidman, 1977):
>
> (1) Information identifying victim (name, age, address, marital status, religious practices, occupation, and other details)
> (2) Details of the death (including the cause or method and other pertinent details)
> (3) Brief outline of victim's history (siblings, marriage, medical illness, medical treatment, psychotherapy, suicide attempts)
> (4) Death history of victim's family (suicides, cancer, other fatal illnesses, ages of death, and other details)
> (5) Description of the personality and life-style of the victim
> (6) Victim's typical patterns of reaction to stress, emotional upsets, and periods of disequilibrium
> (7) Any recent—from last few days to last twelve months—upsets, pressures, tensions, or anticipations of trouble

   (8) Role of alcohol or drugs in (a) overall life-style of victim, and (b) his death

   (9) Nature of victim's interpersonal relationships (including those with physicians)

 (10) Fantasies, dreams, thoughts, premonitions, or fear of victim relating to death, accident, or suicide

 (11) *Changes* in the victim before death (of habits, hobbies, eating, sexual patterns, and other life routines)

 (12) Information relating to the "life side" of victim (up-swings, successes, plans)

 (13) Assessment of intention, that is, role of the victim in his own demise

 (14) Rating of lethality

 (15) Reaction of informants to victim's death

 (16) Comments, special features, and so on.

In conducting the interviews during a psychological autopsy, it is often best to ask open-ended questions that permit the respondent to associate to relevant details without being made painfully aware of the specific interests of the questioner. As an example: I might be very interested in knowing whether or not there was a change (specifically, a recent sharp decline) in the decedent's eating habits. Rather than ask directly, "Did his appetite drop recently?", a question almost calculated to elicit a defensive response, I have asked a more general question such as, "Did he have any favourite foods?" Obviously, my interest is not to learn what foods he preferred. Not atypically, the respondent will tell me what the decedent's favourite foods were and then go on to talk about recent changes in his eating habits—"Nothing I fixed for him seemed to please him"—and even proceed to relate other recent changes, such as changing patterns in social or sexual or recreational habits, changes which diagnostically would seem to be related to a dysphoric person, not inconsistent with a suicidal or subintentioned death. (Leenaars, 1999a, pp. 399–400)

RES IPSA LOQUITUR

Following Shneidman's lead (see Shneidman, 1999a), the chapter will follow the principle of *res ipsa loquitur*: The facts speak for themselves. The documents, newspaper accounts, letters, autobiography, investigation reports, third-party interviews, court testimony and so on—speak for themselves. Let me begin with a few letters that Scott had written, to Cherrylle in cards, with a letter, well before his death

> Whenever we are apart,
>   I think back
>   to how you came into my life . . .
>   like a sunrise
>   bright and magical.
>   Setting me aglow
>   with your love
>   I know when we're
>   finally together
>   it will feel just like
>   that first time . . .
>   You'll never know
>   how much I miss you, babe.
>   No matter what happens, you'll
>   always be my most Precious Angel
>   Love forever Scott

Cherrylle
      I guess you know how I feel about you. Milestone events tend to bring out the reflective side of me. Also tends to emphasise that loss I feel I guess when we don't celebrate together I don't usually look at the past with regrets but last couple of days found me thinking about our past wishing I hadn't taken so much for granted, wished I had realised how precious and fragile real love is and held on to you with all my might
    I really wish you happiness,
    Just wish I could share it with you
Love Scott

These two cards, with letters addressed to Cherrylle, suggest that there is a history to the traumatic relationship to Cherylle Dell. The content and themes in the note and earlier letter are consistent. The note was not a new communication. From the note, letters and other data, it can, indeed be concluded that Mr Dell loved Cherrylle a lot, but not wisely.

Subsequently, the following question was raised: Did Scott Dell intentionally kill himself?

This question is on the mode of death, i.e., the question of intention: Did this person intentionally kill himself? To address this question, as we noted, this case must be placed within the context of further forensic data, beyond the note (Litman, 1988; Shneidman, 1999a).

- For the psychological autopsy, the following people were interviewed:

Myra Dell, mother
Lauretta McCarthy, aunt
Elsa Steenberg, friend
Sue Kwast (by telephone), friend
Paul O'Dell (by telephone), physician.

- The following records were requested and reviewed:

Dr Harris—Statement and Transcript from Prelim
Dr O'Dell—Statement and Transcript from Prelim
Myra Dell—Statement
Elsa Steenberg—Statement and transcript from Prelim
Sue Kwast—Statement and Transcript from Prelim
Loretta McCarthy—Statement and Transcript from Prelim
Blair Voyvodic—Interim Report from OPP
Francis Murphy—Interim Report from OPP
Nancy Peplinskie—Interim Report from OPP
Statement of Death
Medical Certificate of Death
Letter re: Scott Dell by Henry Tiedje, Coroner
Anatomical Pathology Report
Report of the Centre of Forensic Sciences
Scott Dell Transcript from Divorce Petition

Scott Dell Transcript CAS and Children
Scott Dell Autobiography from Durham CAS file
CAS Foster Home Study
Scott Dell Chronology from Peter Sammon file
Scott Dell GM Employment Records
Scott Dell Records from Dr O'Dell
Note written from Scott Dell to Eden Dell 27 October 1992
Christmas Card to Eden from Scott Dell 1995
Two cards with letters, addressed to Cherrylle Dell from Scott Dell
(Exhibits seized from 18 Mill Street, Killaloe)
Poetry, addressed to Sue Kwast
Photographs, Scott Dell and others
Photographs, Farm
Photographs, Scene of Death

THE INTERVIEWS

Let us begin with the interviews, utilizing Shneidman's basic outline, although I have tended to add after #9, a question about the nature of the person (i.e. his/her ego), eliciting an array of descriptions to the person. Be that as it may, I routinely conduct the autopsy in a standardized fashion as Dr Shneidman taught me, although in an open-ended fashion. It is not like a police investigation. Here are the verbatim answers as recorded:

Question 2: Tell me about the death

MYRA DELL: Well Cherrylle, his wife, her phone call Saturday morning, said that Scott's body had been found the night before, he died . . .

And Cherrylle added to my daughter, Scott had a bad report at the last visit to the hospital, December 14th or 16th. And he and Eden, oldest daughter and a friend in "Killaloe", Elsa had met at Cherrylle's house, and Scott told them that things looked bad, a bad report. But keep it quiet, and we believed that. So we went up to the funeral and this is what happened. He had a heart attack.

LORETTA McCARTHY: Well, there were specifics that he had been cleaning snow off the roof, and overdid it, himself, because he had cancer. There was a rumour about that he had a bad report about cancer.

SUE KWAST: I found out through Elsa, she and, she called me and they found him a few days after Christmas. He'd been drinking wine, a friend found him. And then they thought it was cancer. That didn't make sense to me.

Question. I just didn't think that, he was fine, you will not go so sudden. He had been planning for Christmas; he was seeing the kids. He was planning to go to school in Ottawa and go to Scotland. It didn't make sense, and because his cancer was in remission. It didn't make sense. The suicide thing, it will be so far from what Scott would do.

PAUL O'DELL: I learned about it from a physician in the hospital, who knew the aunt. The aunt had called about the status of the cancer. The doctor called . . . Yes, cancer was under control. The death was, thus, under unusual circumstances.

Question 3: Outline the victim's history

MYRA DELL: Mother is Myra, 77. Father is John, 79. Retired, he was a grounds keeper. Children six. Richard '52, Catherine '54, Stephen '56, Patricia '58, Marion '60, and Sterling '64. Scott was the oldest, born in '51 . . .

Was he ever suicidal?
No.

Did he ever make a suicide attempt?
Never, no.

Was he depressed?
I don't think so. He did say, after the cancer, I've got different priorities now. It makes you see what is important and not.

LAURETTA MCCARTHY: Scott, mild-mannered man, a thinker, loved music. Was up on a lot of issues. Loved politics also loved land. He was a vegetarian . . . growing on the land. We talked music things, he loved to talk and discuss things. I remember one at the Cuban embassy, we talked with people. He had left US because of Vietnam, the war. Loved discussions . . .

ELSA STEENBERG: Lots, he's a friend, a close friend, very supportive friend, especially, very supportive family, especially his mom, except in his teens years, when rebelling. But he had a real strong commitment to his family, regarding his mom . . . He felt Cherrylle couldn't be with him. He couldn't deny her. She was so manipulative . . .

What was he like when he found out about the cancer?
He was very distraught. He was worried about the kids. Who would look after them? Where will the kids go? That was initially, he just found out. He went to see a social worker for that, he did that . . .
   . . . he talked to me about Cherrylle, and her affair, her silicone breasts and, exotic dancing, getting pregnant by someone else, and pretending it was Scott's child. He was always saying, she couldn't help it that it's the way she is. Always making excuses. She would dress very provocative. He would say, fine, but she would push, he would say it's fine, including the affair. Scott wanted her to get it out of her system, and renew the marriage and fix it. His biggest regret was his marriage, didn't work out.

Was he ever suicidal?
Never.

Did he ever make a suicide attempt?
Never. He was more determined to stay alive because of the kids.

Was he ever depressed?
Like depressed? No. I don't think more than a person would be about the cancer. He was upset, depressed about the cancer, but he worked at it.

SUE KWAST: . . . He told me about Cherrylle, difficult, not easy. She appeared to have him wrapped around her finger, manipulative. He was helpful. He still loved her. He knew she was troubled . . .

The relationship?
We got along fine . . . Broke up at the time? just before Christmas. I thought it was the best, not a good idea. It was a long distance relationship. I dislike getting in between Cherrylle and Scott.

Reaction to?
He was really sad, later he was upset, left a message, angry. He said, "okay, I'll get on with life". I felt good, better to be angry and I hoped that he had a good Christmas . . .

PAUL O'DELL: He had cancer . . . being on the tongue and in lymph nodes, had treatment, including radiation . . . operation. The response to treatment was excellent, completion . . . cancer not detectable . . . some residual effect? Well. None. He did have a support system. He did have symptoms, dryness of the mouth, due to post radiation, operation of mouth. No evidence of cancer. No evidence of cancer progressing. In Mr Dell's mind, he was "well".

Question 4: Details of victim's family

MYRA DELL: *Was anyone ever suicidal?*
No . . .

Were there any deaths of cancer?
Lots of people. It's very prevalent in the family.

Were there any unusual or catastrophic deaths?
No.

Motor vehicle accidents?
No.

Question 5: Description of personality and life-style of the victim

MYRA DELL: Can you tell me something about Scott?
He came up to Canada to avoid the Vietnam War. It was a lottery, he was never chosen. He went through American school, but we came to Canada in the summer. He stayed in Canada. He was very political . . . He had lots of friends. Loved sports. Did well in school. Found it very easy, and did well . . .

Tell me about the kids.
Eden, not his. Cherrylle left and came back pregnant. He said, "I think a lot of her." Adopted a girl Megan, 13. Had a child, Frank, 11.

ELSA STEENBERG: *Describe his personality.*
He's quiet. Once you get to know him, he never stops talking. He was very intellectual. He was open-minded. He'd think about a situation and see it in different ways. He wouldn't be judgemental . . .

PAUL O'DELL: He was pretty upbeat, very robust, big physical man. Had children he felt committed to.

Question 6: Victim's typical pattern of reaction to stress

MYRA DELL: *What were the typical patterns of reacting to stress or emotional upsets?*
He probably kept it inside. Never told anything.

What about Cherrylle?
Most stressful. Yes.

What kind of reaction?
He was very frustrated. He didn't understand why. She just went out one day, took the car, cleaned out the house and went to Toronto with a woman.

LORETTA MCCARTHY: *What were his typical patterns of reactions to stress or upsets?*
I think he would internalize them

How did he react to the cancer?
Strongly, well he'd take it in stride. He was facing it. About suffering, he wasn't a complainer. He had to get through it, and this is how he dealt with it. He had researched it, thinking that he was going to do, he had read and dealt with it.

ELSA STEENBERG: *What were his typical patterns?*
He would call me; he'd talk to me for hours. I know, little sleep and he'd still be talking.

Anything else?
He'd talk, go on and on about Cherrylle . . .

What was he upset about?
Cherrylle, Nancy Fillmore, they were together. He didn't like that. He felt Nancy was trying to manoeuvre the kids away. She had said bad things and, everything he felt...and problems with Cherrylle, he once picked up the kids and Cherrylle was under dressed. Put some clothes on, she said and she just laughed...

What about the cancer?
He talked about it, beating it...

PAUL O'DELL: I think he had taken his treatment, his radiation and did well...He accepted that he was good.

Depressed? I can't think of any signs of clinical depression. When first presented himself, he had advanced cancer, it was a great concern. He went into treatment. He was not depressed...and responded well.

Depressed? No. As a doctor I see many patients with clinical depression. I am not an expert, but I see discouragement... in people and then refer to psychiatrist to evaluate.

Question 7: Any recent upsets, pressures?

MYRA DELL: Well the cancer, he was fighting cancer, recovering from it.

LORETTA MCCARTHY: The cancer, and just the ongoing relationship with Cherrylle. They had been separated for awhile.

ELSA STEENBERG: *Any recent or upsets in the last 12 months?*
The cancer.

Anything else?
The Nancy and Cherrylle thing in the relationship. Cherrylle and Scott were becoming friends again, during the summer before Nancy moved in. It was for the kids. He wanted to make sure there was a positive relationship for the kids...The cancer, it was gone in early December, positive. It was clear that it was under control.

Was he upset?
No, he was happy.

In December?
Yeah, early December.

SUE KWAST: Cherrylle, he had a lot of problems with her. I we talked a long time, it was about Cherrylle...That's the reason why we broke up. I didn't want to get involved. There were so many problems with Cherrylle. I didn't want to get involved it.

Anything else about the break up?
He was upset, like anyone would be.

Question 8: Role of alcohol or drugs

ELSA STEENBERG: *Any drugs or alcohol in his lifestyle?*
Occasionally he'd smoke pot, but stopped, once sick. He had an occasional beer, Sleeman, but after the cancer he stopped, only occasionally...

Question 9a: Nature of interpersonal relationships

MYRA DELL: *Tell me about his interpersonal relationships with anyone.*
He got along. A lot of people admired him. He was the big brother. My kids thought he was great.

ELSA STEENBERG: He wasn't that outgoing. People listened; he had lots of friends. He was a part of a group, a co-counselling group...

Question 9b: Nature of ego

MYRA DELL: Outgoing.

LORETTA McCARTHY: *How would you describe his personality?*
Sensitive, protective, tenacious, courageous, hard working

ELSA STEENBERG: One of the most intelligent people that I ever met

SUE KWAST: Gentle, kind, humble.

Secretive?
I'd think about his health

Cherrylle?
He spoke about her past history, a bit.

Family?
Yes.

His health?
Yes.

Question 10: Fantasies, dreams, thoughts...

LORETTA McCARTHY: Well we would talk about dreams, about how they relate to our lives. That they were special, how the dreams affect us, if we pay attention to them.

ELSA STEENBERG: He wanted to go to Ottawa to take a chef's course. Talked about success.

Ever talk about death?
No.

SUE KWAST: To go to Scotland, to go to learn to find out his history, Scotland and Ireland. That's what he wanted to do.

Death?
No.

Suicide?
No.

Question 11: Changes in the victim before death

ELSA STEENBERG: No.

Question 12: Information relating to the life-style of the victim

MYRA DELL: He bought the farm, he grew up on a farm.

Was he happy?
Yes. He spoke to us at Christmas about the kids. He wanted to buy a plough to clean the snow so that the kids could get to the school bus... He loved the farm.

ELSA STEENBERG: The cancer check, he was excited about it.

Question 13: Assessment of intentions

MYRA DELL: *You think there's any reason why he may have intentionally played a role in his death?*

No. For two reasons. Why would he? He was so happy that he had a good report. He looked at life differently... If he had, he would have talked and talked. He never left without talking and talking.

LORETTA McCARTHY: No. There wouldn't have been any sense after what we had gone through.

Elsa Steenberg: No. We had planned to go out for New Years. He had too many things to do, to talk.

Paul O'Dell: No. If record of any suicidal indications, it would be documented and referred to someone...

Question 14: Lethality

Myra Dell: *Did he behave in any kind of destructive fashion?*
No.

Paul O'Dell: No. Not a violent type of person, a passive person, upbeat, not violent. I mean pacifist, not passive.

Question 15: Reaction to information of death

Loretta McCarthy: *Any reactions to his death?*
I was shocked. I couldn't believe it, because he went through so much. He went through all this and then to be dead. It made no sense at all. Why did this happen, all the pain and then die?...

Elsa Steenberg: I didn't believe it. Scott's death, it couldn't be right. We had planned to go out on New Years. I had talked the night before. Later, I called his number but no answer...

Paul O'Dell: I just saw him within two weeks. I examined him, x-rays, etc. and there was nothing. There was no evidence of cancer. This was complete inconsistency about the cancer story. You can't do assumptions. There was no clinical evidence. He was 2 to 2½ years past treatment...

AN AUTOBIOGRAPHY

I believe that the interviews speak for themselves; yet, there was much more information. I had requested a long list of documents, cited earlier. And here we learn more; let me begin with an autobiography that Scott had written on 24 April 1987:

AUTOBIOGRAPHY: SCOTT DELL

I was born in Toronto in 1951 and moved to Connecticut with my family near the end of 1954. My earliest memories revolve around living in Toronto and the subsequent events leading up to our move. I am the oldest of seven children, and my brother Richard and sister Catherine were also born in Toronto before we moved.

One of my earliest memories is living on Winter Avenue in Scarboro, which at that time was very rural. As a matter of fact the small house we lived in had no indoor toilet. Two memories from this house are my father accidentally running over our dog in our driveway, and a recurring occurrence which was our neighbour who was a truck driver coming over to our house with his guitar and singing Hank Williams' Song's with my Dad. When we decided to move to Connecticut we sold this house and we moved in with my aunt in subdivision in Scarboro. My aunt had just lost my uncle and I remember that things were quite strained. One vivid memory I have of that time is of my older cousin who had been mildly stricken with Polio. When we moved in he was in the process of starting to walk again. Another memory I had was my father, who had left to work on our house that we would live in Connecticut, returning with a brand new 1954 Green Ford Pick Up Truck. As soon as he came home he took me out for a ride around the block. I remember also taking the train to Connecticut with my mother and my brother and sister. My dad drove the truck with what belongings he could carry. I remember repeatedly asking my mother where he was, all the time looking out the window of the train for him.

I have very warm feelings about my childhood. I remember always feeling very secure and loved by my parents. I have a very close relationship with both my parents and brothers and sisters today still, even though separated physically by the distance between Millbrook and Connecticut.

As far as the three main lessons my parents taught me, I would have to say they would be honesty, the ability to share (necessary with six brothers and sisters) and the concept of equality. My parents were very liberal politically and they really stressed the equality of all races and creeds.

My early school years were quite enjoyable as I found schoolwork to come very easily. I got quite bored with school by the time my high school years came to an end. I had a fairly active social life, Scout's when I was younger and Sports and Dances when I was in highschool.

I left school after Grade 12 though I had thought of going to University. By the time my Grade 12-year came around I just couldn't bear the thought of sitting in a classroom for 4 more years.

I met Cherrylle up in Wilberforce, where my parents had a summer cabin. I had gone up with my family that summer and had decided to stay, because it was my draft year in 1970, and the Vietnam War was at its height.

What has been good about marriage has been having someone to share life's dreams, hopes and concerns. What not so good I suppose is always having to temper your personal wants and desires to be compatible with your mate. Unless you want to lead a totally narcissist existence, I don't suppose that's so bad though.

The biggest problems I have had to face were probably first deciding at nineteen to leave home and evade the US military draft. It is a decision that I sometimes still question myself. Another problem after being married for only a couple of years agreeing to an abortion for Cherrylle, even though I did want the child. I felt my marriage was more important though ... Another big problem we had to face, as a family was the death of a foster daughter, Stacy who died in our home last year.

I am already a parent, but I feel that I would enjoy more children, and have more love to give other children besides our daughter. I see some differences in adoption as opposed to natural parenting. As you will be having children with perhaps hostilities, fear and insecurities from very possibly bad experiences.

As far as faith, I was raised a Roman Catholic, though not in a terribly dogmatic fashion. I suppose any faith I have now is very loosely defined fairly flexible. I find myself constantly looking at and questioning spiritual beliefs and very interested in other's beliefs. On that sense it is not the same as when I was a child because it is always changing to some extent. Growing I hope. What I would teach a child is I think as much as possible about many beliefs and what I believe, and to try to install the ability to search for themselves to find their own truth.

Pleasant changes would of course be the addition to our family, which would be more the physical presence, but of collective sharing. Unpleasant could of course be the working out of problems, which a child may bring to us from the past. The positive thing about this of course is that by working through these problems it should bring us all closer together.

A FEW PRE-TRIAL DOCUMENTS

The information on Scott is now two banker boxes full (and the police have even more boxes). I can thus only highlight a few observations here, in the hope of providing a few snapshots of the events.

Dr Bruce Harris was Scott's family physician since February 1989; Dr Harris frequently saw Mr Dell and his family. In his statement to the OPP and Preliminary, we read:

Mr Dell was seen as an attentive parent with a sincere interest in his children. His personal visits to my office were relatively infrequent, as he appeared to be healthy. He was seen in July of 1993 requesting support regarding family issues. At that time he was estranged from his wife. His wife had accused him of sexually abusing their three children. The patient suffered intensely over these accusations. The degree of stress was very severe and resulted in considerable sleep disturbance and weight loss. The patient stuck by his children and was able to endure the emotional crisis of this accusation, which was eventually decided to be unfounded. Throughout this the patient remained committed to his children. Despite the stress involving this accusation and the disruption of his family the patient never displayed any signs to me of depression.

(1) In February of 1994, he was noted to have a sore throat. This eventually led to the referral of an ears, nose and throat specialist who found a carcinoma at the base of his tongue. The patient applied himself intensely to getting better. He was referred to literature; in particular, a book by Dr Bernie Siegel entitled *Love, Medicine and Miracles*, which encourages people to dedicate themselves positively to overcome the illness of cancer. Scott did this in earnest and underwent radiation therapy at the Cancer Clinic in Ottawa.

He did very well, going into complete remission. Throughout this time Scott remained very committed to getting well and seems quite inspired in his commitment. He stated that he had to get better in order to meet the needs of his children. Again, at no time was there any suggestion of depression, although, he certainly was under considerable stress and strain, not only from the illness but from the alienation within his family.

Scott worked with his former wife to develop a mutual custody agreement in order that his children were able to see their mother. Again, his commitment was very consistent to his children.

Scott was last seen in my office on 14 September 1995. At that time I could see no indication of depression or suggestion that he was suicidal.

And in the Prelim in respect to questions by the Crown (Prosecuting) Attorney, Peter Barnes, we learn:

Q. Was there any indication at that time or any concern that you had that the discomfort that he was suffering was in fact possibly result of cancer returning?
A. There was no indication of that.
Q. And, again, as of the date of that visit was there any indication of him being depressed?
A. No, there was no indication of that.

We learn, from Scott's family doctor that there are no records of mental illness, depression or suicide risks. We also learn that despite Scott having been described as "secretive", he sought help and counselling for traumatic issues in his life; e.g., sexual abuse charges, cancer.

From Paul O'Dell's Prelim, we learn the following:

Q. During the time that you saw him then were there any significant milestones chronologically, or dates which would be of particular significance to you in that you might use those occasions then to discuss any change in his prognosis or expectancy?
A. There are no significant milestones to make in following a cancer, but as I said in earlier questioning, the statistical . . . surviving the first year is a definite plus and each year after that brings in it, and if you're looking at survival from cancers it's not a linear thing. It's more logarithmic and so that getting through that first year is a very definite positive step. We will usually mention that to patients and we'll,

but usually be realistic. They always want to ask the question "Am I cured yet?" We never said that to him.

Q. At what point would you have been in a position to tell Scott Dell that he appeared to be disease-free?

A. Well, he is always clinically disease-free because that is a term that we use.

Q. Would you, given the nature of the disease that you treat, have any concerns with respect to the patients that you see as to depression or clinical depression, or any suicidal thinking, or ideation?

A. Well, clearly that's a problem. People do get depressed with . . . there are many things that cause you to be depressed. When a diagnosis of cancer is made, just the diagnosis would be a source of depression for, to some extent, for many of us. The treatments that you have to go through and some of them quite arduous are a further source of depression. I'm not in the business of, on a day to day basis, recognizing clinical depression, not being a psychiatrist, but in medicine we do see people who are depressed and most of us will recognize significant clinical depressions. Now, what happens in an office encounter is different that what happens when the person goes home and they are in the confines of their own home, and you know, clearly we could miss depression, but in my experience and exposure to this individual, he did not exhibit clinical depression.

Dr O'Dell's testimony is entirely consistent with my interview material. Briefly, Scott was cancer free, not depressed and focused on getting well. At the last office visit, on 14 December, a few weeks before his death, Scott was most positive. Scott knew he was well. Dr O'Dell had made a follow-up visit in three months. Of note, Dr O'Dell's reaction of concern to the unexplained death of one of his success stories makes clear sense, once you learn about Scott and speak to Dr O'Dell directly. He is clearly a bright and learned physician.

The statements and Prelim Deposition of Elsa Steenberg and Sue Kwast present basically only more detail to what had been learned in the interview. Ms Steenberg revealed that Scott was positively involved in meditation and visualization (something he shared with Cherrylle), and this fact may make the reference to a vision in his last letter more explainable. Both Elsa Steenberg and Sue Kwast emphasize Scott's obsession with Cherrylle, and Ms Kwast was quite specific that this was the stimulus for Scott's break-up with her. We also learn that Cherrylle was quite upset at Sue's existence. There were a number of writings from Scott to Sue; here is a sample:

> Can't wait to see you again!
> Out of the blue a warm wind blew
> You to me around me surrounding me
> A warm blue wind that carried me to this place
> I needed to be This place that is you
> Your warm blue eyes like clear coral waters
> Calling me Home This place that is you
> A home I have been missing all my life
> Home
> To this place called you
> Love Scott
>
> Sue
> I knew you were gone
> Tonight

When I went to bed alone
And smelled you on my sheets
And almost felt you pressed up close
Against me
Your hair all in my face
I knew you were gone
Tonight
When I could almost see you
On top of me
Riding slow up and down up and down
I knew you were gone
Tonight
When I could almost hear you
Moan
And laugh
And tell me once again
You love me
I knew you were gone
Tonight
When I went to bed alone

The content and themes in the letters to Sue are not consistent with those to Cherrylle (as presented earlier). As stated, Scott's last note and previous letter were similar and different from those to Sue (to provide a George Kelly type of personal construct to the event). This is critical because the defence had argued that Scott was overwhelmed by the loss of Sue, resulting in the stimulus of his alleged suicide.

CHERRYLLE AND SCOTT

Scott's history is full of positives. For example, even his GM application, when he first began to work there, states "Strong appearing applicant". These descriptions appear consistent (sameness) throughout his history.

The court material in this case is, from my experience, not common (although it does occur). Here we learn a large array of facts, all made under oath. One fact appears obvious; Cherrylle lied about everything, even in court. She, for example, had lied that she had a degree from the University of Toronto; indeed, records showed that she completed grade 8 and only started grade 9. And of course, all the allegations about Scott, such as the sexual abuse, were ruled to be fabrications. Although it is not my purpose to detail Cherrylle's life, a few facts are critical.

Cherrylle's family was described as "severely dysfunctional". Cherrylle's grandfather molested her and, of note, her father was charged and found guilty of sexual molestation of children. Cherrylle's father's guilt is stated to have sparked a major regression in Cherrylle and was the beginning of all the sexual abuse allegations towards Scott.

Cherrylle suffered from mental illness; she was troubled and had already been hospitalized as a teenager. At least three suicide attempts have been recorded. Cherrylle is described as suffering from low self-esteem, being very, very sensitive to criticism, having a really bad temper and having physically assaulted Scott on occasion. She accused Scott of physical assault, such as attacking her with a knife;

all allegations were judged to be fabricated. Scott did admit to one incident, when he grabbed Cherrylle, after she left him for the first time in 1975, and pushed her against the wall of her father's house. On that occasion Cherrylle was with her lover and Scott was upset. In the court recording, it is noted that Scott immediately let go. There are no other records of physical abuse, despite Cherrylle's statements to the contrary. Cherrylle, it is believed, lied about everything, even under oath (dissembling). Cherrylle had many problems, including some with her children. They preferred Scott and the oldest two testified against their mother at the murder trial of their father. Based on the data, I believe that Cherrylle probably had recurrent Depressive Episodes, and had a history of suicide attempts, and a Narcissistic Personality Disorder.

Scott, on the other hand, is described as coming from a healthy family, although Cherrylle labelled them as dysfunctional. He is seen as quiet, having a slow temper and being very bright. He was a family man, having strong interest in his children. He often took care of the children; one was described as difficult and Scott often cared for the child, as Cherrylle would get quickly frustrated. For example, he would spend hours with the child in a Fisher Price swing to soothe the child. As another example, during a sexual assault to one of the children by an older boy, he was seen as most supportive (an event that is seen as having added to Cherrylle's regression). He was known to be determined to beat his cancer for the children.

Just before his death, he was planning to buy a snowplough for his truck to clear the snow to the road to make walking easier for the children. He was described as "excellent" with children. He had interests and hobbies (e.g., gardening, enjoying music, playing the guitar, and reading). He had future plans; for example, he had bought a New Year's ticket to celebrate with Elsa Steenberg and other friends at a local establishment, the Wilno. His main problem was constantly stated to be "Cherrylle". He was aware of this fact, but felt that he was so in love with Cherrylle. Scott believed Cherrylle needed only support, not criticism.

Based on the psychological autopsy, I developed the following opinion on the question: "Did Scott intentionally kill himself?" "No." Utilizing standard profile from the TGSP as well as Shneidman's commonalities (see Table 10.1), Scott showed few of the characteristics of suicide; indeed, the note's scores were the same for his life. If one uses Shneidman's prodromal clues in his Terman's studies of gifted

Table 10.1 Shneidman's Ten Commonalities/Standard Profile of Suicide

    I. The common purpose of suicide is to seek a solution.
   II. The common goal of suicide is cessation of consciousness.
  III. The common stimulus in suicide is intolerable psychological pain.
  IV. The common stressor in suicide is frustrated psychological needs.
   V. The common emotion in suicide is hopelessness-helplessness.
  VI. The common cognitive state in suicide is ambivalence.
 VII. The common perceptual state in suicide is constriction.
VIII. The common action in suicide is egression.
  IX. The common interpersonal act in suicide is communication of intention.
   X. The common consistency in suicide is with lifelong coping patterns.

suicides, one comes to the same conclusion (Shneidman, 1971). These include some 10 items: early evidence of instability, including dishonesty; rejection by the father; multiple marriages; alcoholism/drug abuse; an unstable occupational history; ups and downs in income; a crippling physical disability; disappointment in the use of one's potential; any suggestions of self-destruction; a competitive self-absorbed spouse. Again, Scott had some markers, but not the large majority. Shneidman in his review of the Terman cases, looked at trauma, instability, recent downhill course, controls (inner and outer) and so on. He was able to identify successfully four of the five most potentially suicidal cases that had, in fact, committed suicide (the fifth case was Shneidman's number 6 selection). The probability of this result would be 1 in 1131. That is prediction! Thus, I espouse the use of more than one common or standard profile in determining whether a death is natural, accident, suicide, or homicide.

Based on the psychological autopsy, here are a random number of other opinions that I reached:

- There is no history of mental disorder.
- There is no history of depression.
- There is no history of suicide risk.
- There is no history of depression or suicide in Mr Dell's family-of-origin.
- Mr Dell does not have a history of depression or suicide risk.
- Mr Dell does not appear to have had a mental disorder, although he did have a problematic relationship (adjustment problem) to Cherrylle Dell.
- Mr Dell did experience a number of traumas in his life (e.g., marriage/loss of Cherrylle, carcinoma, false accusation about sexual abuse by Cherrylle).
- Mr Dell adjusted to traumatic events without signs of depression or suicide risk, although reactions were evident, e.g., very severe degree of stress to the (false) accusation of sexual abuse.
- Mr Dell was diagnosed and treated for carcinoma of the base of the tongue. Mr Dell adjusted well and positively to the diagnosis and treatment. There was no indication of depression or suicide risk.
- Mr Dell did not have "persistent cancer" at the time of his death. There was no indication of depression or suicide risk prior to his death, regarding cancer or any other physical condition.
- Mr Dell did not suffer from depression or suicide risk during the last 12 months before his death.
- There is no indication of recent depression or suicide risk before his death.

Thus, there is no doubt in my mind that, in all probability, at the time of his death Mr Dell did not intend suicide. Therefore, my answer to the question, "Did Scott Dell intentionally kill himself?" is "No".

A NEWSPAPER'S STORY

By the time Cherrylle Dell's murder trial came to court, the case had become a national event. The following account appeared on the front page of Canada's national newspaper, *The Globe and Mail*, on Saturday 18 November 2000:

THE VILLAGE VAMP AND HER TWO LOVERS
By Erin Anderssen
Crime Reporter, Killaloe, Ont.

There once lived in Killaloe, a place of aging hippies, herbal marijuana bust, a comely woman whom most everyone considered charming, if a little odd for the fur coat and high heels she favored on trips to the post office.

Years from now, when they talk of Cherrylle Dell, as they most assuredly will, the story may start this way, with what everyone first noticed: the Barbie Doll looks and flashy clothes that made her a small-town original even before two of her lovers turned up dead.

She'd married an American, Scott Dell, when they were still teenagers. They lived outside town in a log farmhouse, raising a family and taking in disabled children.

About 10 years ago, Cherrylle left her husband for a woman, which, though this was the conservative Ottawa Valley, did not engender the reaction you might expect and was generally accepted among friends.

It's what happened later that truly earned Ms Dell her place in valley folklore.

Just after Christmas in 1995, Scott Dell was found half-naked in an upstairs bedroom in the farmhouse, poisoned, the authorities would allege by antifreeze-laced wine—quite possibly by his own hand, although in the village there were whispers of something else.

Cherrylle had, by then, moved in with Nancy Fillmore, a social worker who a friend says answered an ad to be caretaker to Cherrylle's kids. In 1997, after the two had separated, the apartment building where Ms Fillmore paid rent, and from where she would have been able to see the red brick of Cherrylle's house across Brennan's Creek, burned to the ground. Trapped inside, Ms Fillmore died....

Police eventually arrested and charged a teenage boy with murder in connection with the fire, but their investigation continued . . .

Five months later, the authorities decided that Scott Dell had not committed suicide after all, but had been poisoned intentionally; Ms Dell, now 46, was arrested and charged with first-degree murder . . .

She'd been in jail awaiting trial for more than two years when the police came calling again. She was accused of instructing the teenager to set the fire that killed her one-time lover and was charged for the second time with first-degree murder . . .

For pure titillation, the case of Cherrylle Dell has it all: a beautiful defendant, sex and betrayal and a strange, small town rumbling with chatter.

Gay Doherty, the former lover who discovered Mr Dell's body, has said she's considering a book, and a Toronto film company has already expressed interest.

Residents here can be expected to tune into the trials, the first of which, for her husband's death, is scheduled to start on Monday.

COURT TESTIMONY

Before court, I read the testimony of key witnesses. These did not change my opinion; yet, I did learn from Gay Doherty that Cherrylle was writing while she was on the telephone and Elsa Steenberg testified the following:

Q. So she phoned you between the time of Scott's death and the funeral?
A. Yes, she did.
Q. How long did the conversation last?
A. Not very long.
Q. Tell us what you remember of the conversation?
A. She told me that she had told Scott that he could let go now and her angel would take him to heaven.

Q. What do you mean she said that he could let go now? What context was that?
A. Well, I was under the impression that she was giving him the right to let go.
Q. When did she say that had happened, that she had said that to him?
A. The last time they had spoken together on the telephone.
Q. Well, perhaps I've missed it, but I don't think you've told us about a conversation on the telephone.
A. Cherrylle told me that she had been talking with Scott on the telephone.
Q. When did she say she had been speaking with him?
A. I don't remember the day. However, I do remember her telling me that "You can let go. My guardian angel will take you to heaven."
Q. During that conversation, do you remember her saying anything else to you?
A. I remember her saying to me, "Now that Scott is dead, I want to be your friend, I want to take Scott's place."
Q. Prior to Scott's death, had you ever been to her home before?
A. I've never been to her home.
Q. Okay. I want to ask you about some pieces of information. Did Scott ever tell you, at the beginning of 1995, that his cancer was no longer in remission?
A. That it was no longer in remission?
Q. Yes.
A. That his cancer had come back?
Q. Yes.
A. Never, his cancer had not come back.
Q. Did Scott ever tell you or did you ever become aware in 1995, in the last year of his life, that he was throwing up?
A. Never.

Keeping in mind that I had been asked about Scott, not Cherrylle, I enquired about these facts, the police provided me with the following notes. These were alleged to be written by Cherrylle on the night of 29 December. What is obvious is that the content and themes are identical to Scott's note. Not only is Scott's note not a suicide note, but there are also questions about the author of the note (as there were with the Daniel Beckon case). Did Scott or Cherrylle author the note or parts of the note? I will return to this point in my testimony. Here is Cherrylle's note:

> The sun as a life
> Source
> Staying in the sun
> Laying on the
> Beach
> Staying in the light
> Were not meant to be
> Happy
> It's not sin to be
> Happy
> Maybe it's a sin to be
> Unhappy
> Should live in
> Environment your
> Happy in.
> Looking for guidance
> Not doing this right
> Something's wrong.
> If it's the spiritually right thing to
> Do theirs nothing to
> Be afraid of

Something has to change
Mini-brief vision
Cherrylle floating almost
Like an angel—but not
Really an angel—head
Was not connected to
My body. Flash vision—
Wasn't connected.
Close to each other but
Not connected.
I need to let go of something
I need to let go of something
How fast our lives are going.

MY TESTIMONY

To turn to my testimony, I will again use the principle of *res ipsa loquitur*:

1766.
R. vs *Cherrylle Dell*
Tuesday, 16 January 2001
—Upon commencing at 9:30 a.m.

Mr Barnes: Good morning, Your Honour.

The Court: Mr Barnes.

Mr Barnes: Your Honour, the purpose of course this morning was for the Crown to call Dr Antoon Leenaars. Mr Selkirk has indicated that a Mohan type of *voir dire* will be required ...

Mr Barnes: Your Honour, perhaps I can just articulate for the Court then the purpose that I'm calling Dr Leenaars. Of course, it's for him to be permitted to give expert opinion evidence in two areas in particular. First, as to the application of a technique to the facts of this case that is widely or generally accepted and used in the fields of psychology, psychiatry and suicidology—Dr Leenaars will tell us what suicidology is—and used to distinguish between genuine and non-genuine suicide notes or what are purported to be suicide notes ...

Mr Barnes: Secondly, Your Honour, I anticipate his giving evidence as to the application of a technique known as a "psychological autopsy" to the case ...

Q. Can you just briefly describe the subject matter in a little more detail with respect to your thesis? ...

A. Yes. Part of the problem in suicide is trying to understand the suicidal person because of course he's deceased, and so one looks at alternative information, trying to understand the person. And suicide notes have always been considered one window to the mind of the deceased.

Studies in this area began much more empirically in the 1950s with Shneidman and Farberow. Through contacting them ... So what we developed was a way of looking at suicide notes through protocol, by that I mean protocol sentences, which is a—empirical, it's a positivist procedure where falsifiability, which is so important in science, is possible ...

Q. Are you currently involved or recently involved with respect to the training of any medical health professionals?

A. Yes .... You see, suicide prediction is very difficult. There aren't very simple scales available. If you will, there's an old notion of phrenology, looking for a bump on the head. You're not going to find a bump of suicide on the head. So it's complex . . . .

So what we do is we try to train psychiatrists and psychologists into this kind of understanding, trying to understand the suicidal person from commonalities rather than simply whether they have depression or not . . .

Q. Now, is there—in the literature of suicidology, have there been any empirical tests—testing that has been done and published with respect to the analysis of suicide notes or the technique that you employ?

A. Yes. The very beginning of suicide studies actually sort of coincides with the modern suicidology beginning. Dr Shneidman had been sent to the V.A. from the V.A. Hospital to a coroner's office, and to his surprise he discovered some 700 suicide notes . . .

A. And he's a good scientist, and what he decided to do was not read these notes but rather he decided to use the technique of science to look for falsifiability by comparing them to non-genuine notes. This was the very first beginning studies scientifically of notes . . .

Q. When was that that Shneidman had started this work?

A. This started in the 1950s. They published a book in 1957 called "Clues to Suicide". He called on his friend Norman Farberow, who is also one of the grandfathers of the field. And they started publishing the first study showing that indeed genuine notes and non-genuine notes were very different, that if you ask people to simulate a note, that they're not the same, that there are actually distinguishing features . . .

Q. Have there been any tests of the ability of lay people to distinguish between genuine and non-genuine or simulated notes?

A. Yes. This has been one of the questions from the very beginning. In one of the first studies that is published in a journal by Arbeit and Blatt, he had taken 93 judges with four different levels of clinical training, and . . . what he found is out of that group only 13 were able to distinguish genuine from non-genuine notes . . . basically what it showed is that, according to Arbeit, only those with clinical training could distinguish genuine from non-genuine. Subsequently, David Lester . . . and I have looked at a series of studies, trying to see, you know, what allows people because we've also found that most people, even undergraduate students in psychology, cannot distinguish genuine from non-genuine notes.

What we did is, for example, we gave the sample of genuine and non-genuine and tried to see whether there was some way of distinguishing what is it that allows a person to decide a note is genuine . . . And basically we couldn't find any . . .

. . . And basically what we found is that people have very idiosyncratic theories about suicide, their own very personal belief.

Now, there was one common thing that people quite consistently looked for in a suicide note, and that was a trauma, that there was some event that was quite traumatic for the person, an unmet love, a physical disease, et cetera. But, of course, when you ask people to write non-genuine or simulated note, you also find people being able to simulate or to say "put that into the note". So it doesn't really distinguish a genuine from a non-genuine note very well . . .

. . . Generally, what can be concluded is that there are a lot of myths about suicide and suicide notes that people have.

Q. On the other hand, in terms of the employment of the 35 protocol sentences and the methodology which you say you've developed and which has been peer reviewed, what do you say as to the ability of somebody trained in that method to distinguish between genuine and non-genuine notes?

A. Quite good actually . . .

Q. What are the limitations, in your opinion, in individual cases, in trying to apply these protocol sentences and this methodology to the analysis of individual notes which may or may not be genuine suicide notes?

A. Well, if I may, part of the problem, of course, in the whole field is that in science, whether it's sociology or psychology or psychiatry, we're looking at the general. This is the nomothetic approach. Here you get general patterns, common patterns, and of course when you look at the individual case, the idiographic approach, if you will, it can be quite different. This is sort of like—more like what I do clinically with each individual patient than some of the research ...

   You have to look at the individual note and be cautious about, you know, what you're concluding because there have been cases where people in court—for example, in the Daniel Beckon inquest that I was involved in, which—

Q. That's the Ontario inquest?

A. Yes, that was the Ontario inquest where the late Sopinka hired me to take a look at this conclusion where someone said, you know, "If there's a suicide note, therefore the person killed himself." From my point of view, of course, you can't conclude that. What you can conclude from a note is that, you know, the person's mind may have had suicidal intent, there may have been characteristics of suicide, but then to jump that the person killed himself seems to me to be a little erroneous. You have to know the limitation of the data. That's, for example, why a psychological autopsy comes into play, to give you a wide array to answer the question, "Did the person commit suicide or not?" ...

Q. Doctor, in this particular case, in July of 2000 you were approached by the Ontario Provincial Police.

A. Yes.

Q. And you were provided with a note?

A. Yes.

Q. And were you at that time provided with any material other than a note?

A. Yes. I was provided with a synopsis of the case. However, it should be important for the Court to note that I did not read the synopsis. In fact, I never read anything that anyone sends me until after I do the note. I let it be, I score it again, and then I might, after I make my conclusion, start reading the other material ...

Mr Barnes: Q. And do I take it that—I think we've covered this, but I take it that you were asked by the police, first of all, as to whether or not you had an opinion as to whether or not the note in front of you, Exhibit 8 in the trial, was a genuine or non-genuine suicide note essentially.

A. Yes. I concluded that it was not a genuine note, that the person who wrote this did not have suicide intent, did not have characteristics of a suicidal mind in this note.

Q. All right. And did you reach that opinion, then, by applying the protocol sentences that has become Exhibit A?

A. Yes. I had scored this note, then left it, and then scored it again not knowing my previous scores, to develop some consistency. And again concluded that, although it had a few characteristics that you might find in a note, specifically about a trauma ...

Q. All right. And perhaps we will go into the protocol sentences, then, and the basis of the formulation of your opinion. When you say that you looked for the presence of protocol sentences—

A. Uh-huh.

Q. —that is you looked for each of the 35 protocol sentences being present or being evidenced in the note.

A. Yes, that's basically the technique ...

Q. Go ahead when you're ready.

A. Yes. In terms of the various aspects that I find in the note, that you might find in a suicidal state, the first one relates to—in the suicidal drama, certain emotional states are present.

Q. Could you just refer to the protocol sentence as well to make it easier for counsel to follow what you're saying?

A. Yes, number 3.

Q. Yes.

A. In the suicidal drama, certain emotional states are present, including pitiful forlornness, emotional deprivation, distress, ... or grief.

Clearly in this note—keep in mind it says "and/or", so it's not necessary, and these are including, so they're examples, if you will. But clearly there's distress in this note and there's deprivation, the loss of the relationship, which subsequently, with the synopsis, I concluded was in terms of Cherrylle....

Q. Go on.... Are there any elements that you found to be consistent in this note with a mental disorder?

A. Well, there's an item under this category, number 15(g), which is sort of like when people communicate that there's something wrong, that there may be a disorder or a dysfunction, but you can't really specify it. You know something is wrong, but it might be a situational distress. It's sort of like the category that you use if none of the other ones apply.

Q. Is a situational distress different than a mental disorder?

A. Yes, it would be ... what we find is more discussion about the situation, the context for Scott. For example, 19, the subject's problems appear to be determined by the individual's history and the present interpersonal situation. He talks, for example, about a history, three years of bad stuff, so there's a history to this, plus the current situation. If we can't get together again, maybe we should leave, you know, maybe we shouldn't see each other so much.

Q. And the reference to the three years of bad stuff, and if we can't get together again, perhaps we shouldn't see each other. Are those phrases that appear in the note?

A. Yes. Then 20, he discussed being weakened and/or defeated by the problems in the interpersonal field. This is that, you know, if we can't really get back together, then maybe we shouldn't see each other that much because, you know, all the bad stuff, et cetera, that he just seems that he can't solve this, and if we can't get back together, maybe we shouldn't see each other.

21, the suicide appears to be related to unsatisfied or frustrated needs. Clearly, that's evident in his need for attachment to Cherrylle, and it's frustrated. It's been thwarted, if you will, unsatisfied.

23, a positive development in the disturbed relationship was seen as the only possible way to go on living, but it was not seen as forthcoming. Again, he talks about the relationship, if they get back together, but if they can't, and it's likely not going to happen, maybe we shouldn't see each other.

Then under "Rejection–Aggression", we find 25. Again, this is that there is a traumatic event, again, the unmet love kind of thing.

And then 27, that he's preoccupied with the event or injury, namely, the letter is about his preoccupation or obsession, if you will, with Cherrylle.

And then 28, he's quite ambivalent, both affectionate and hostile, angry if you will if we can't get together. So there's an ambivalence towards this. But there's none of the anger or aggression, the hatred in some of the other protocols. If I may, it's not only what is in this note, it's what's not in the note that makes it so important to distinguish as a genuine or non-genuine.

And the last one, in terms of identification, egression, he says he wants to egress, to escape. Basically, what he says is, again, maybe we shouldn't see each other so much, but he never says the ultimate that we find in a suicide note, "This is the only way out; I need to kill myself. Please forgive me", et cetera. There's none of those kinds of wishing to escape. It's just simply not to see Cherrylle if they can't get back together.

Q. Now, if I can, just in perhaps—further, the protocol sentences have subheadings.

A. Yes, they do.

Q. The first deals with the general heading "Unbearable Psychological Pain", and as I've been counting, there are six protocol sentences, and you found evidence of one of the six protocol sentences under the general heading "Unbearable Psychological Pain".

A. That's correct. It doesn't have the kind of pain that we look for in a note where the person says, "It's intolerable and the only thing I can do is escape to kill myself." It doesn't have the hopelessness and helplessness, for example, that we find...

Q. With respect to the second half of the protocol sentences, then, "Interpersonal Relations".

A. Four of—I think there's four, yes, four of six. The ones that are missing is that, you know, the frustration is to a point that he can't tolerate it anymore, and there isn't an indication from this note that he's under constant kind of strain or that he's too unhealthy or that he can't do anything about it. He says basically, you know, "If we can't work this out, let's not see each other."

Q. And to what degree are the ones present, in your opinion, under this heading?

A. Well, the four that I find are clearly evident, that there is an interpersonal problem, and that there's a history, and that he's been frustrated by his needs in this. However, you know, if I would write a forlorn love letter, I would also find these elements in any forlorn love letter . . .

The final cluster "Identification–Egression" . . .

—that he wanted to escape from the difficult relationship, but there is none of that in the sense of "I'm going to kill myself, this is the only way out", which we classically find in suicide notes. And we also might find, you know, "Please forgive me, this is the only thing I can do." There's none of those kinds of things. There's also no suggestion that, you know, he's unwilling to accept this. He's just basically saying, "If we can't work this out, then let's not see each other so much." . . .

Q. In any event, as a result of your examining this note on those occasions, are you, by employing these protocol sentences and the methodology that you have described, able to express an opinion with respect to whether or not it is a genuine suicide note?

A. I believe it's a non-genuine note. By that I mean this note does not seem to be consistent with having suicide intent in mind.

Q. Now, if I may, I'll just move along. And subsequent—now, you provided that opinion in a letter, doctor. You provided that opinion in a letter?

A. Yes . . .

Q. All right. And, subsequently, then, you were contacted by the Ontario Provincial Police and asked to do a further analysis of additional materials.

A. Yes. They asked me whether I could determine whether the person killed himself or herself, and I said from the note alone, as I've written in some of my articles like Suicide Notes in the Courtroom, that you cannot determine that from a note alone, and that the procedure that's generally accepted in the field is a psychological autopsy that would allow us to give you an answer to that question . . .

Q. All right. What is a "psychological autopsy"?

A. A psychological autopsy is a generally accepted procedure in the field . . . This is a retrospective investigation, a psychological investigation, where you take a look at what occurred. You would examine the coroner's reports. You would examine the autopsies. You would interview typically three or more people who may have known the deceased. You would read, anything, material that the person might have left, court documents, police records, school records, employment records, maybe they've been hospitalized, looking at clinician notes, whatever. You gather a wide array of information trying to determine whether this person intentionally tried to kill themselves.

Q. Now—

A. Let me go back again. This first started back in the 50s when the coroner in L.A., Curphey, who by the way was a Canadian, asked Shneidman, Dr. Farberow and Dr Litman—he had a number of cases that were undetermined, and he asked them, "Could you assist me here in whether these cases, because it could not be determined based on the more forensic investigation or police reports, whether they were actually suicides or not." And they assisted Curphey in this kind of technique since the 50s to try to analyse and give a perspective about intention, whether this person intended.

Now, keep in mind people often ask, like bereaved families, "How could you kind of determine that the person intended to do something after they're dead?"

Well, we all make assumptions about people's intentions. We don't see them. We constantly, in our relationships, make inferences based on what people say, and maybe what they wrote, et cetera. We do that all the time. The psychological autopsy, the trained person simple in terms of this knows how to do that better. They're trained as a psychologist or a psychiatrist or some related field to analyse and understand the intention.

So it's been used, the psychological autopsy, since the 50s, but not only in terms of individuals cases like what was—occurred since the 50s, and some cases are famous like the Marilyn Monroe case that Litman did, but also in terms of research . . .

Q. Now, are the protocol sentences that you've described to us applicable to the psychological autopsy?

A. Yes, absolutely, because these are sort of like the common characteristics that you might find in suicide. Ed Shneidman, for example, talks about 10 commonalities. They're embedded in these protocols . . . So it allows you, if you will, with these protocols or Shneidman with his commonalities, or et cetera, to frame, to try to understand the intent to determine these equivocal cases: Was it a suicide or not? . . .

Q. May I stop you there for a moment, please, and just ask you this. When you were asked to do this by the police, that is perform a psychological autopsy with respect to Scott Dell, did you employ the 35 protocol sentences?

A. Yes, I constantly have them in my mind. They're constantly—they're sort of my protocols. They're my hypotheses. They're the things that I look for. But certainly would not be the only things that I would look for. I mean, there's much more to suicide, and each case, each individual case is unique . . .

Q. Other than in the fact that in the psychological autopsy that the individual is deceased, what then are the similarities or differences between the psychological autopsy and the diagnosis or treatment of the individual patient?

A. Actually, in the psychological autopsy it's easier because what you are doing is postdiction. When you're treating a person and trying to predict, you may not have all the information in front of you. They may not be giving all the information. You may not be able to speak to their Minister or Rabbi who may be a support system.

So when you're trying to work with a clinical patient, it's actually even more difficult. When doing a psychological autopsy, you can gather all sorts of information . . .

Q. In this particular case, that is relating to the death of Scott Dell, when the police asked you if you would be prepared to do this, did you have an opportunity to tell them what data or what interviews you would like to conduct?

A. Yes. I chose the interviews myself, who I wanted to see. I was very explicit about wanting to speak to Dr O'Dell and . . .

Q. Doctor, the questions that you asked during the interviews, did they cover a specified or pre-specified list of topics?

A. Yes, they do.

Q. And did you record the answers from the interviews in any way?

A. Yes. There's a fairly standardized kind of questioning that Dr Shneidman taught me . . .

Q. You preserved the list of questions?

A. Yes.

Q. And your answers.

A. Yes . . .

Q. The purpose of asking these questions during the interviews and looking at these materials was to answer certain questions, if possible.

A. Yes. It would be basically: Did the person intend to kill themselves? Was this a suicide? That's the basic question.

Q. And having conducted that psychological autopsy, was the information that you were able to gather sufficient, in your opinion, for the purposes of answering those questions?

A. Yes ...
Q. And, again, when you were looking at these documents, do I take it that you're relating them in some way to the protocol statements with respect to state of mind, that is intrapsychic as well as interpersonal relations?
A. Yes, you constantly look for these common features, whether it's, you know, Ed Shneidman's or these protocols, something that gives you some sort of consistency. Again, Maris's notion of suicidal career, if you will ...
Q. As a result of conducting this psychological autopsy with these materials, were you able to form an opinion as to whether or not Scott Dell was suicidal?
A. Yes.
Q. And what was that opinion?
A. That he was not suicidal, that he had never been suicidal, that he was not suicidal at the time of his death.
Q. You've indicated that subsequently you had an opportunity to review further materials, that is between the time that you formed that opinion and reported upon that opinion and today's date in January of 2001.
A. Yes. ... presented me with some notes that were alleged to have been written by Cherrylle Dell. I was most interested in this because Gay Doherty, for example, in her testimony said that that night Cherrylle was on the phone until four o'clock in the morning with Cherrylle, which made me curious. Also Elsa Steenberg reported that she had—Cherrylle had been speaking to Scott about "letting go, letting go", which is part of what appears in the suicide or what was alleged to be the suicide note, the non-genuine one, if I may.
Q. The suicide note that's attributed to Scott Dell.
A. Yes.
Q. All right. And just if you could, what passages in that note are you referring to about letting go.
A. "Let go, let go." These were things that Elsa Steenberg in this court had said that she had told Scott on the phone. It's concerning to me——
Q. That is that Cherrylle Dell had said?
A. That Cherrylle Dell had said "letting go". It concerns me because "letting go" can mean all sorts of things. For example, some of us may have known people who have a terminal cancer or disease, where we kind of provide guidance, where we kind of assist, you know, "let it go", "it's okay", "relax, be peaceful". You allow the person, if you will, to go peacefully into their death. It's—I mean, I don't see many, but I do work with cancer patients, in helping them assist in their dying.
Q. And those lines that you're talking about are in fact the last lines on the last page of the note.
A. Yes. There's also something else in the note, though, that had always puzzled me, but then Gay Doherty sort of supports it. When he writes:

> What did you think was going to happen if
> I drank a bottle of wine listening to the
> music we used to listen to. I'm going to
> think about you and me together.

I mean, it makes then sense that, of course, these notes are notes he's taking probably from the telephone conversations because obviously he's communicating to Cherrylle, and we know from Gay Doherty that she was on the phone that night all night.
Q. So were the Court to find that the notes in fact were the product or made during that conversation, making that assumption, are there any other matters that—would that change or vary your opinions that you've previously expressed in any way?
A. No, it would not change my opinion that this note is not a suicide note, but it would raise the issue of who's the author of this note, which goes back, for example, to the questions that I've been asked for, like Sopinka asked me in the Daniel Beckon case, is "Who's the author of the note?"

CROSS-EXAMINATION BY MR SELKIRK:

Q. Now, I gather at some point in time, quite recently, that there is a doubt in your mind as to whom authored what we've been referring to as Scott Dell's note.

A. Yes.

Q. There is a concern that Mr Dell, if we accept the fact that Mr Dell was on the phone with Cherrylle Dell at the time of the writing of this note, there is a concern that Scott Dell was simply writing down what Cherrylle Dell told him, was saying on the phone.

A. If I may, I think there are certain lines in there, because they're consistent with other writings that I've had from Scott such as about the relationship with Cherrylle, I think is clearly his writings, his statements.

Q. Which writings are those, please?

A. When he's writing about:

> I feel like holding you close to me like
> never before I feel like making love to
> you ...

The areas of being preoccupied with an object, in this case a person, and being rejected or abandoned by that person or object. That's a classic scenario for a suicide, I'll suggest to you. Dr Shneidman will suggest that to you.

He will suggest to you that it's more than simply a trauma. All sorts of people have traumas, rejections but don't kill themselves. That's the situation around the event. What you have to look at is the suicidal mind, the events, not simply whether somebody has a disease, lost employment or rejection. You always have to go to the commonalities, the kind of pain, the frustration of needs, the hopelessness and helplessness. The rejections are part of the limbs of the tree, to use that analogy; the core is the trunk. So you're always looking at the mind part, but you also look at the situation around it.

All sorts of people have traumas, difficulties and don't kill themselves. It's not sufficient. It's certainly part of it, although sometimes even for you and I it would make no sense. Like the person in California who wrote a note, killing himself because there's a scratch on the car. For you and I it makes no sense; for him it did ...

Q. And, of course, whether or not a person left a note or not is determinative of whether the person committed suicide.

A. It should be, at least from my point of view, one part of determining—one part of the facts to determine that.

Q. But if a person did not leave a note, that does not mean—you would not conclude, "Oh, the person did not commit suicide."

A. That's correct.

Q. And if he did leave a note, you would not conclude, "Oh, that person committed suicide."

A. I would want—

Q. Based on the note.

A. Just simply based on the note, I would want more evidence. It might be, to use a metaphor, a "smoking gun", but you still want the body and how that body was killed or how he died, if I may say so. Sorry about the word "killed". It's how the person died ...

Q. Well, let's go back to Scott's family situation. If the situation is that his family home is broken, to use the common terminology, it's a broken home, the family split up; if it's found that the eldest daughter moved out without even telling Scott, snuck out; if it's found that there are significant custody access problems and in fact Scott might be losing, gradually losing custody of the children; if Scott's ex-wife is living with a lesbian partner who strongly dislikes Scott and made it obvious; in terms of just that one aspect of family, Scott is not coping very well.

A. What we know is that he had a series of traumas, difficulties, but you certainly would also, before you look at that family, look at the family of origin. For example, in his life, the ground that we all have, the building blocks of who we are, that's where you begin in terms of the suicidal career. You look at——

Q. Let's just stay with your opinion as to whether or not Scott appeared to be coping, contending successfully with his family life.

A. I think he was doing quite well given the circumstances. He was seeking help. He went to speak to Dr Harris about the problems. He spoke to Dr O'Dell. He sought other people for assistance. He spoke to some friends about his problems. He got help. He persevered. The court cases that he was involved in show that he was receiving support from the Children's Aid. The Children's Aid tested him. The psychologists didn't have any concerns. There was a whole host of support systems, markers. He also had interests, hobbies, the vegetables—the gardening I should say and the guitar and other things that would be on the positive side, the protective aspects. So, again, it's not simply the events but how we cope with them, how we adjust to them.

Q. Objectively looking at Scott Dell's family life, he was not coping very well.

A. I disagree.

Q. Because you want to read subjective things into Scott Dell's mind, which you have no idea about, right? You want to say he got this help, therefore he was helped.

A. I, you know, listened to people, I read the case material of the court and other things which——

Q. And if one gets help for a problem in 1992, that doesn't necessarily have any relevance to the person's situation in 1995.

A. It shows a career in terms of him getting help ...

Q. People who are coping well are not experiencing trauma at the same time, are they?

A. They're not the same.

Q. Of course not, but he can't say, "If I'm being—if I'm walking down the street, coping very well walking down the street and people are hitting me on the head", it is the same, "I'm not coping with going down the street very well because people keep hitting me in the head."

A. It depends on your state of mind, on how you cope with things. Most——

Q. Right, but that's the subjective element which you know nothing about.

A. But that's the core of what you look at in terms of the various data on how we adjust. We also know that he saw various doctors. He saw——

Q. And if Scott comes to Dr O'Dell and says, "My social situation has improved", it's not very helpful as to what Scott did or did not do eight months later because his situation could have unimproved.

A. Yes, of course.

Q. Sure. In fact, that's the problem with relying on all of this stuff from '92 and '93, that his situation could have changed.

A. But you also look at the beginning of his life, the consistency over time. That is, again, the life-long coping patterns, the consistencies, or the suicidal career, if you will, or coping career. You never take one thing, Mr Selkirk, in isolation. You look at ...

Q. Okay. When you are doing a psychological autopsy, the validity of your findings is determined by the reliability of the information that you receive, is that fair to say?

A. Yes, in that sense it's sort of like what we do everyday. Whether a psychiatrist or a psychologist, you're kind of trying to make formulations and ideas, and of course in the everyday clinical world, there's always issues of reliability and the amount of information. This would not be any different except in this case we have even more data than usually we get, you know, working as a psychologist or a psychiatrist ...

Q. And his relationship with Cherrylle and/or other females, it would appear that he could not be with the one he loves, and he doesn't love the one he's with, and no suggestion that that situation is going to change or improve.

A. I think he always maintained hope about Cherrylle. There's no question that he was very obsessed or, if you will, in love. I think he loved Cherrylle a lot but not wisely.

Q. And if the evidence is that he was aware that Cherrylle was simply manipulating him and that the opportunity or chances for reconciliation are slim and nil, then again helpless, hopeless.

A. Not necessarily. He had coped with this problem with Cherrylle from time to time. It wasn't the first time. I mean, already early on in their marriage, et cetera, they had been separated. So again looking at that, I mean, he sought people out, he talked to people about it, he tried to cope. Again, you'd have to look at each individual and the actual data, whether they're hopeless or helpless or what their state of mind is . . .

Q. . . . Thoughts of suicide or death, that's another symptom?

A. Yes.

Q. And clearly in Scott's note, if he wrote it, authored it, he writes "suicide/death".

A. Death/suicide.

Q. Death/suicide. Thank you.

A. Yes. But that doesn't mean necessarily he's thinking about suicide. I mean, Shake-speare wrote about——

Q. Not necessarily.

A. Shakespeare wrote about suicide. He wasn't necessarily suicidal. So people write about it——

    All I'm saying is people write about it. It doesn't necessarily mean that they're suicidal . . .

Q. Would you agree that on this area of cancer and suicide, that literature on the subject seems to indicate that the incidents of suicide in males with cancer are increased in the immediate period following diagnosis and extending perhaps for as long as five years?

A. I've read that in that book. They also said that the data is ambivalent in that section . . .

    They say themselves that—in this, that there is some ambivalence in terms of—however—"Overall however the literature is ambiguous" they say. So it's not clear. Although generally it would be the case that many medical conditions, including cancer, place a person at higher risk. Again, those are the things around, the branches, et cetera, of each individual person. We've long known since Sainsbury that certain medical conditions place people at risk. I mean, we even debate here in this country about terminal illnesses, you know, and suicide . . .

Q. Well, the text goes on to say: Cancers of the head and neck have an 11-fold increase in suicide rates, as opposed to cancer generally which has a relatively modest twofold increase.

A. Yes, but they also go—say elsewhere that gastrointestinal cancers have the highest rates. So the fact is, yes, cancer is a risk factor, but so are diabetes, so is Lou Gehrig's disease, so is spinal cord injuries . . . It's axiomatic that medical conditions put us at risk. That doesn't mean, though, that everyone with cancer or diabetes kills themselves. Again, it's how their mind is, how they cope with things . . .

Q. Now, when you're doing the psychological autopsy and interviewing people that could be described as survivors, is it fair to say that the survivors can only give their point of view?

A. That's correct . . .

Q. They have a tendency to see the deceased in a positive light.

A. Yes, or a very negative light. You always, in the autopsy but even in your everyday interviewing, have to judge people in terms of that it's their point of view. We do this in the clinical setting everyday, constantly . . .

Q. Nonetheless, is it your recollection from what they told you that Scott was secretive about his feelings *vis-à-vis* Cherrylle and about his health? Is that your understanding from which you based your conclusion on, or is it something different?

A. Most of them did not use the word "secretive". I think that the mother might have used the word, but most of them basically said that he did not talk about, did not want to share about these kinds of things. He wanted especially, for example, with Cherrylle, to try to keep a positive appearance of who Cherrylle was. He didn't want to focus—continually, even in his court appearances, he discussed about—that she had this bad background, and he just wanted her to get help and be well. ... but he talked about other things. He talked about his health to doctor——

Q. Unimportant things.

A. No, he talked about his health to Dr Harris, Dr O'Dell, to some of the other people. He certainly talked about the relationship to various people, including Dr Harris.

Q. He talked about his relationship with Cherrylle?

A. Yes. The issue of the sexual abuse charges, according to the deposition.

Q. People have killed themselves for less.

A. People kill themselves for a scratch on a car. The death of a canary is another example. It depends on the person. I'm serious about the canary.

Q. No, I fully appreciate that ... Now, let's add to the suggestion that he would not speak about his feelings or his health. A psychiatric or psychological testing, I guess—did you see Dr McLean's report on Scott?

A. No, I did not.

Q. This is done in—the report is dated January 13th, 1994. This is a full family clinic assessment of Scott, Cherrylle and the children. This is something you would have appreciated seeing had you known of its existence?...

MR SELKIRK: Q. Well, Dr McLean is a psychiatrist practising in the City of Ottawa here and has done Family Court Clinic for many years. His conclusions were that:

Personality testing suggested that Scott was quite concerned about presenting an unrealistically positive image of himself. In day-to-day living, he would invest a lot of energy to maintain an appearance of adequacy, control, and effectiveness. He may tend to utilise denial to overlook faults or insecurities in himself or his life situation.

Resultantly, he would likely have a serious lack of personal insight into or understanding of his own behavior. His need to look good may have lowered the clinical scales to make him appear better adjusted psychologically. Nevertheless, the testing did suggest that Scott be somewhat immature and self-centred. He would demand attention and approval from others and would be sensitive to rejection. He would likely blame other people for his difficulties and if angry would tend to express his anger indirectly. Most of the time he would appear to be overcontrolled but brief episodes of more aggressive behavior could occur. Although Scott appears outwardly socially conforming, inwardly he may tend to be rebellious.

This would have been information that should have been provided to you, in your expert opinion?

A. I would have appreciated seeing it...

Q. And only Scott can tell us if that pain was unbearable.

A. Well, I think in a psychological autopsy we can get a fairly good concept of that ...

There is evidence that he had trauma, crisis, that he had had these since, I think, the early parts of the problems in the relationships, but it also shows that he coped with these, that he handled them that he sought out help support, et cetera. You can't simply determine, because this person has a crisis, that they're suicidal or in unbearable pain ...

Keep in mind, when you're looking at anybody, whether it's in my office or in this kind of situation, you look at the positives and the negatives. You're always going to find some negatives in anybody's lives, but overall you look at the positive. He clearly, I don't believe, had a mental disorder or an underlying mental disorder. I don't think it was discerned or assessed by anyone that he did so. So I think generally he seemed to have good coping abilities. There are other people, site documents, like even the job application where he's called a "strong applicant". I think all of that is relevant. Again, you look at the person's history over time, how they coped, adjusted.

Q. Would you—in terms of being called by some unknown person in GM in the 70s a "strong applicant", would you not agree that that has little relevance to Scott Dell in 1995?

A. Oh no, it's relevant. It would be relevant when you do a psychological autopsy because you don't simply look at the current event. You look at the person's personality and coping style throughout their life.

Q. People change.

A. People change but they stay enormously consistent as well. I mean, the Shneidman study that I mentioned where by the age of 30 he already, from reading the material, could determine which ones would kill themselves by the age of 50 with quite an accuracy...

... It's a trained element, it's the professional training that make the difference. Even in Arbeit and Blatt's discussion, what is it that allows people to distinguish genuine from non-genuine was the clinical training that these people had...

Q. There is no standardized form established by the scientific community to do a psychological autopsy?

A. There's a fairly standard procedure, for example, that Ed Shneidman would teach me, and the kind that they've been using since the 1950s that many of the people use. I don't know what other people are using, but this is the one that I use that is most published and discussed...

Q. But it is not standardized to the point or in a way to give reproducible results.

A. I think that, from my point of view, this is fairly standardized. The person may ask the questions differently, but generally the psychological autopsy would be looking at the person's intention, looking at precursors, looking at the history, looking to see whether there's been attempts, looking at the people's family of origin, how they cope with stress, whether there's been a mental disorder, et cetera. I think how they might go about it would be different, but generally there would be similar questioning, I think, standardized...

Q. And the testing or analysis that you did, you did not subject it to any form of peer review or independent review to see if others would come up with similar opinions as you?

A. One would never do this in a specific individual case. You do that for research, in terms of whether people can use this or whether it's peer reviewed. Typically——

Q. As far as you're aware, you have not asked anybody else to review your work on this case to see if they would come up with a similar opinion.

A. I did not give this case or ask Dr Shneidman to interview the people...

Q. Right. There is no standard profile for a suicide?

A. I think there is general—it depends on what you mean by "standard profile". If you mean sociological, like male, divorced, if you mean the sociological phenomena, I would say, no, there isn't a standard kind of profile. If you mean in terms of pain, hopelessness, helplessness, ambivalence, yes, I think there's a fairly common agreement about many of the factors...

RE-EXAMINATION BY MR BARNES

Q. Thank you. During the recess, then, you had an opportunity to look at the report of Dr McLean in its entirety, the 29 pages.

A. Yes, I did.

Q. And having had an opportunity to look at the entire report but more particularly the eight pages that pertain to Scott Dell, has anything that you've read in the balance of the material resulted in your wishing to qualify any of the answers that you gave to my friend and the passage that you were referred to?

A. Well, from my point of view, Mr Selkirk only read part of the report and only part of the psychological testing, not the concluding impression. And so he's just giving me part of that report that I had not seen. His conclusion is:

It was the writer's impression that Scott Dell suffers from no major psychiatric illness. I did feel he tends to be a rather controlled and guarded individual who is perhaps not as open about his emotions and feelings as Cherrylle, somewhat inwardly rebellious [he says]. Appears to be less impulsive or likely to act out on these tendencies as compared to Cherrylle. Although Scott has some personality difficulties, they appear to be less significant than Cherrylle's.

He then says:

Scott does seem to have an emotional attachment with the children, and also it seems they have done well since being in his primary care over the last eight months. It would also seem that Scott would be more supportive of the children's relationship with their mother's and vice versa...

Q. And does that opinion, and giving that opinion credit, cause you to modify any of the views that you've expressed today?

A. No, it actually continues to support my belief that, you know, during his career, his life, he did not suffer from a major psychiatric illness as opposed to Cherrylle Dell who he says did...

VOIR DIRE

My testimony was a *voir dire*. The main question was: Is this testimony admissible? This is important because no expert in suicide has ever testified on such issues in a Canadian criminal court. The *Ottawa Sun* on 17 January 2000, printed the following article:

WITNESS MAKES HISTORY

While Dr Antoon Leenaars has twice testified in California, yesterday marked the first time a suicide expert has ever taken the stand in Canadian court.

It's the opinion of the clinical psychologist that the 1995 death of Scott Dell, 44, was no suicide and that his final hand-written letter was no suicide note.

The Crown is trying to introduce the expert evidence in the murder trial of Cherrylle Dell, 46, accused of poisoning her estranged husband.

Not reliable

But defence lawyers argue the doctor's findings are not scientifically reliable. Moreover, the Supreme Court of Canada has recently cautioned lower courts against allowing expert witnesses to do the judge's job, which, in this case, is to determine the cause of Scott Dell's death.

Leenaars, who has a practice in Windsor, is the past president of the American Association of Suicidology and a member of the International Association for Suicide Research and Prevention. He's also an author and long-time researcher who has examined more than 2000 suicide notes.

The doctor said he believes Scott Dell had been coping with life's problems around the time of his death by trying to maintain a positive attitude, despite his inability to romantically move on after his wife dumped him.

Caroline Murray

Psychological autopsies have a long history in the United States, not Canada. Shneidman, Litman and Farberow are generally credited with introducing the technique in the 1950s to civil matters and coroner's inquests. They are now widely accepted in civil cases (Litman, 1988). This standardized technique was first introduced into criminal cases in Arizona in 1976 (Lichter, 1981).

In the Arizona case, Wendy Jones's murder of her husband Michael appeared to be a simple act of first degree murder (Lichter, 1981). At trial, defence counsel employed the autopsy technique to show that Mr Jones had been a sadistic paranoid who beat his wife. The jury relied on the autopsy to make a decision. Since then the autopsy has been employed in civil cases in the United States, and also by the author. In a most interesting clinical case (Jacobs & Klein, 1993), *Jacobs* vs *State of Florida*, the appellate ruled:

> The expert psychiatrist specialized in suicidology and, for purpose of this trial, performed a psychological autopsy on the appellant's seventeen-year-old daughter who had committed suicide in March of 1986. His testimony explained that a psychological autopsy is a retrospective look at an individual's suicide to try to determine what led that person to choose death over life. In order to make that determination, in this case, the expert reviewed the child's school records, the police records surrounding the case, including all of the state's evidence and all of the defendant's statements and medical records, an incident report from an earlier suicide by the child and various testimony from the witnesses appearing at this trial. However, he admitted that he did not personally interview any of the witnesses who appeared at trial nor did he ever meet or interview the suicide victim. His opinion, bounded by reasonable psychiatric certainty, was that the nature of the relationship between the defendant and her daughter was a substantial contributing factor in the daughter's decision to commit suicide.
>
> Having reviewed the record, we are satisfied that the state presented sufficient evidence to establish that the psychological autopsy is accepted in the field of psychiatry as a method of evaluation for use in cases involving suicide and that the trial judge acted within his discretion in admitting this evidence at trial. Sections 90.402; 90.403; 90.704; Fla.Stat. (1987).
>
> With regard to the concerns of the defense that the psychological autopsy was not established as reliable before it was admitted as evidence, we note that such opinions are subjective and therefore the issue of reliability is best left to the jury. Further, we perceive no distinction between the admission of the expert's opinion in this case and, for example, admitting psychiatric opinion evidence to establish a defendant's sanity at the time of committing an offence or to prove the competency of an individual at the time of executing a will. See *Morgan* vs *State*, 527, So.2d 272 (Fla. 1202), *United Stated* vs *Edwards*, 819 F.2d 262 (11th Cir. 1987); see also *Krusa* vs *State*, 483 So.2d 1383 (Fla. 4th DCA 1986); *Terry* vs *State*, 467 So.2d 761 (Fla. 4th DCA 1985); In re *Estate of Hammerman*, 387 So.2d 409 (Fla. 4th DCA 1980).
>
> There being no merit to the other arguments raised, we affirm the judgment of conviction.

The technique has also been accepted beyond the court; for example, the congressional hearing of the explosion on the USS *Iowa* on 19 April 1989. Whereas in the US, the technique is widely accepted, not so in Canada. Bob Selkirk, the defence lawyer deemed it "junk science" and the judge, James Chadwick, agreed.

My testimony was not allowed, which is of interest, because the trial was by judge. This then raises a problem: How could Chadwick not have a memory, for example, for what I said suicide is? I fully understand that there are issues in expert evidence (Paciocco, 1999); yet, both my suicide note analysis and the psychological autopsy meet not only the Frye test of general acceptance (or the McIntosh test in Canada) but also the Daubert criteria, set in *Daubert* vs *Merrill Dow Pharmaceutical, Inc.* (No. 92–102 (US 06/28/1993). Once more Canada lags behind.

In the US courts, suicidology (including analyses of notes, psychological autopsies) have been accepted under rules of evidence. The autopsy approach, as I noted, in criminal court dates back to 1976 (Lichter, 1981). The science is not seen as novel, passing the classical Frye test of "general acceptance" (although it is the Federal Rules of Evidence, not Frye, that provide the standard for admitting expert scientific testimony in a federal trial). *Daubert* vs *Merrill Dow Pharmaceutical, Inc.* set out a reliable foundation for opinion. The foundation calls for a theory or technique to be scientific, i.e., "can be falsified" (citing Hempel, 1966), "The statements constituting a scientific explanation must be capable of empirical test". For a science to have a reliable foundation, it must meet the following criteria: (1) theory or technique can be and has been tested; (2) theory or technique has been subject to peer review and publication; (3) a standardized technique or method (there has to be a potential for error); and (4) Frye test of general acceptance. In the US, suicidology has passed all these tests; but not in Canada (nor in many other countries).

The place for science of any kind in Canada is most problematic (the situation probably differs in each nation). Behavioural sciences, such as suicidology, fare the worst. A danger is seen in relying on expert opinion (Paciocco, 1999). The classical Canadian equivalent to the Frye test is the McIntosh Test, in which the subject of testing must be generally accepted scientific knowledge. However, *R.* vs *Mohan* ([1994] 2 SCR 9) was the leading case on the criteria for admission of expert evidence. The Mohan formula is as follows: (a) relevance; (b) necessity in assisting the trier of fact; (c) the absence of an exclusionary rule; and (d) a properly qualified expert. Mohan raised, for example, the issue of novel science; to be not novel, a science had to be generally accepted in a respected field (e.g., the psychological autopsy in suicidology). Behavioural science, after Mohan, became less accepted. Although the issues are detailed, a consequence of a recent ruling of the Supreme Court of Canada, a warning has been issued about expert testimony (*R.* vs *D.D.* [2000] SCC 43). That case was about child sexual abuse; yet, since the ruling, few social scientists have been granted permission to testify in federal court. In Mohan, the late Chief Judge Sopinka stated:

> There is a danger that expert evidence will be misused and will distort the fact-finding process. Dressed up in scientific language which the jury does not easily understand and submitted through a witness of impressive antecedents, this evidence is apt to be accepted by the jury as being virtually infallible and as having more weight than it deserves. As La Forest Jr stated in *R.* vs *Beland* [1987] 2 SCR 398 at p. 434, with respect to the evidence of the results of a polygraph tendered by the accused, such evidence should not be admitted by reason of human fallibility in assessing the proper weight to be given to evidence cloaked under the mystique of science. (p. 21)

The decision has created considerable controversies (Oglaff & Cronshaw, 2001). Mohan was, however, to be applied on a case by case basis—since D.D., it has changed. In *R.* vs *Dell*, Judge Chadwick ruled the following:

R. vs DELL

The crown seeks to introduce the evidence of an expert, Dr Antoon Leenaars. Dr Leenaars is a PhD in psychology, with a defined speciality in suicidology. Suicidology was defined by him as "the study of suicide and suicide prevention".

Approximately 75 to 80% of his practice is clinical. The balance of his practice relates to analysing suicides and providing professional opinions as to whether the deceased met his or her death by suicide. He uses a method involving protocol sentences to analyse suicide notes and to prepare a psychological autopsy of the deceased.

In this case he has studied the notes found on deceased, Scott Dell's desk shortly after his death. In addition he has prepared a psychological profile or protocol of Scott Dell.

The psychological protocol was based upon reviewing statements and transcripts of a number of people, most of whom gave evidence at trial. Dr Leenaars also reviewed a number of documents, some of which were made exhibits at trial.

Counsel for the Crown and the defence reviewed with me a number of the leading authorities dealing with the admissibility of expert evidence. In their submissions they also reviewed Dr Leenaars' evidence.

The Supreme Court of Canada in their most recent decision on the admissibility of expert evidence, have set forth the criteria a trial judge should apply to determine admissibility. In *R.* vs *J*. 148 c.c.c. (3d) 487, Binnie J., in a unanimous decision of the court, reviews a number of previous cases, in particular, *R.* vs *Mohan*. Binnie J. emphasizes that the trial judge should take seriously the role of a "gatekeeper". He goes on to establish the criteria the gatekeeper should apply to determine the admissibility of evidence.

1. Subject Matter of the Inquiry.
2. Novel Scientific Theory or Technique.
3. Approaching the Ultimate Issue.
4. The Absence of Any Exclusionary Rule.
5. A Properly Qualified Expert.
6. Relevance of the Proposed Testimony.
7. Necessity in Assisting the Trier of Fact.
8. The Discretion of the Trial Judge.

My concerns rest with criteria numbers 1, 2, 3, 6, and 7.

Whether the case is being tried by a judge and jury, or by a judge alone, in my view does not make any difference. The same considerations apply. In this case there is ample evidence, to date, to assess the state of mind of Scott Dell and to determine if he committed suicide. Although Dr Leenaars' evidence was interesting and informative, a trier of fact would apply many of the same signs in reaching their conclusion.

The field of expertise practised by Dr Leenaars has not been recognised to date in the Canadian courts. It has been accepted in a limited number of United States courts. Mr Selkirk refers to it as "junk science". I would not go that far. New scientific theories have to be carefully scrutinized.

The ultimate issue to be decided is whether the accused Cherrylle Dell killed her husband. If it is found that Scott Dell committed suicide, that would dispose of the ultimate issue. As stated in *R.* vs *Mohan*, this requires the application of "special scrutiny". As Sopinka J. stated in Mohan: "The closer the evidence approaches an opinion on an ultimate issue, the stricter the application of this principle."

The last concern is whether this evidence is necessary to assist the trier of fact. In this case I am satisfied there is sufficient evidence for the trier to decide the question, without the assistance of an expert.

January 19, 2001

THE VERDICT

Chadwick deemed the science of suicide not to be acceptable science in Canadian court. There is, in fact, considerable time consumed these days about whether expert testimony (especially those of psychiatrists, psychologists, and other social scientists) is admissible, especially those said to approach the "ultimate issues" (as in the case of Dell). Yet, other judges would differ from Chadwick. Judge J. Saunders (2001) noted that social science experts have an important place in court, quoting Chief Justice Scott (*R.* vs *D.D.* ([1998] MJ No. 322).

> ... The opinion evidence is deemed necessary not so much because the area is outside the common knowledge of the trier of fact, but because common sense may be wrong! In other words, the evidence is necessary to counteract myth, stereotypes, prejudices and biases lay people and judges may have regarding certain classes of persons or subject.
>
> (*R* vs *D.D* [1998] para. 60)

Thus, Saunders (2001) claims—and I agree—that expert evidence is necessary because the trier of fact could draw wrong conclusions. This would certainly be true about suicide. No trier of fact, whether jury or judge (as in the Dell case) could draw the right conclusion beyond doubt. These issues are well beyond this volume, but will need to be resolved in Canada (Ogloff & Cronshaw, 2001) and other countries, whereas they appear to be resolved in the US for some time. As for my testimony in the Dell case, it is lost to history. It is here presented as a most insightful learning case for the aspiring and veteran psychotherapist. It has, at least, a value.

On 2 February 2001, Cherrylle Dell was found guilty. I will not comment further; however, it is of note that about the suicide note, Judge Chadwick stated: "This is not a suicide note." How was that judgement made? How was it made beyond a reasonable doubt? Science tells us that the judge cannot make such a decision; Bob Selkirk would state, "That is a junk decision." (It is of note that Judge Chadwick was featured in the *Ottawa Citizen* on 3 February 2001 as a knight of justice.) Yet, I believe that, as a clinical case, Scott Dell's is most useful. On the decision, the *Ottawa Citizen* on 3 February 2001 presented the following:

"ANGEL" OF DEATH GETS LIFE IN PRISON
"Cherrylle Dell wanted Scott Dell out of her life forever"
By Peter Hum

Cherrylle Dell was found guilty yesterday of murdering her husband, Scott, by poisoning him with antifreeze, to the surprise of onlookers who packed a tense Ottawa courtroom.

"I don't believe it," said Mr Dell's mother, Myra, immediately after Ontario Superior Court Justice James Chadwick gave his reasons for convicting her daughter-in-law.

"We went in with misgivings. We thought it would go either way . . . even though we knew she was guilty," she said.

The first-degree conviction, which meant that Mrs Dell was immediately sentenced to life behind bars with no chance of parole for 25 years, concludes a two-month trial that has held rapt the Ottawa Valley, where the Dells lived, because of its bizarre details. It had also been the buzz of the Ottawa courthouse because, to many onlookers, including Mr Dell's relatives, it seemed that Mrs Dell might be acquitted.

The defence had argued that Mr Dell, 44, who was found dead on Dec. 29, 1995, in his Killaloe farmhouse, and who had ingested wine laced with antifreeze, had committed suicide in a fit of depression. The Crown's circumstantial case was so bizarre and full of holes as to be unfeasible, the defence argued.

But Judge Chadwick, who presided over the non-jury case, was satisfied beyond a reasonable doubt that Mrs Dell duped her husband into drinking what he called a "lethal cocktail".

Reading a summary from his 89-page decision, Judge Chadwick said: "I find that from 1992 onward Cherrylle Dell expressed hatred towards her husband Scott Dell and wished him dead.

"She wanted the exclusive custody of the children, the sole occupation and possession of the farm, and wanted Scott Dell out of her life forever.

"There is seldom a case where we hear such strong and consistent evidence about the character of a deceased person. Scott Dell . . . was very positive about his life and his love for his children. He wanted to live for his children.

"I am satisfied beyond a reasonable doubt that Scott Dell did not commit suicide but was murdered by poisoning."

Part III

APPLICATIONS AND PSYCHOTHERAPY

Karl Menninger taught that "The patient is always right". Much of our treatment of suicidal people is figuring out how they are right, even if they wear a mask (dissembling). The way to understand how the patient is right is in the natural progression from understanding to application and to practice. Once one knows the person, then therapy comes naturally.

The proof of the suicidal pudding is in the "ventions"—as in prevention, intervention, postvention—and here most focused on intervention, specifically, psychotherapy. In other words, the main payoff of all our research and training activities, which I hope includes this volume, lies primarily in making our clinical efforts more effective. That is what counts in the psychotherapy room. The chapters in this section repeat some of the earlier ideas, but approach the topic from a different direction—idiographic or case study—showing some of the special aspects of psychotherapy with suicidal patients. They cast some new light, based on our theoretical understanding—both the general and the unique—of the suicidal person.

Let me here repeat a favourite story. When I asked Edwin Shneidman, what I should tell my readers about psychotherapy with suicidal patients, he offered the following:

> Our treatment, psychotherapy, whatever, should address the person's story, not the demographic, nosological categories or this or that fact. It is not what the clinician knows. It is the clinician's understanding of the person's story, each individual's own story. It says, please tell me who you are . . . and what hurts.

The first two chapters outline the application of our theory for crisis intervention and for psychotherapy, both person-centred. The latter chapter is the core of the pudding. It is what I have learned to be useful and life-saving in the psychotherapy room.

I am a developmentalist; I make no apology for this fact. In my day-to-day practice, I see children, adolescents and adults (I even have a playroom, with my toys, to see the younger kids). The youngest suicidal patient (Justin) that I saw, was 4; the oldest was 92. The works of E. Erickson, A. Freud, S. Freud, and J. Piaget, among others, have given me some of my best education. The cases in this book reflect the life-span, from Justin to Joe, who at age 65, when he finally retires and loses his wife, falls into the suicidal abyss. I will never forget his pain, stated in a few words in his narrative, "When my wife was alive, I could dance, now I can't even walk." The studies are as follows: Justin; Jeff, a youth who kills himself; Jennifer, a teen who attempted suicide; Susan, a young adult, who, while attempting to survive her pain, must cope with her father's suicide; Peter, a man who must cope with narcissistic loss; and Joe.

These cases, I hope, will allow one to progress from conceptualization to understanding and then to psychotherapy. I hope one will learn that psychotherapy, echoing Shneidman, "is concerned with what kind of person that individual is". It is person-centred. Yet, the chapters promise to do more. They are a unique window to my clinical mind. I am the therapist. I apologize here for my obvious countertransferences (and maybe, the not so obvious ones). One learns, thus, not only about the suicidal patient, but also about some suicidological insights. The hope is that the clinical remarks will allow for better intervention.

No psychotherapy with suicidal people can be isolated; intervention may require medication, hospitalization, and direct environmental controls. The final chapter in this section provides a few ideas on each of these topics. Psychotherapy with suicidal people must use a multicomponent (or multimodal) approach.

Chapter 11

APPLICATIONS FOR CRISIS INTERVENTION WITH HIGHLY LETHAL SUICIDAL PEOPLE

Crisis intervention is a systematic process of problem resolution and it occurs in a relationship. Within the context of the relation, the interventionist attempts quickly to focus on and address a presenting problem, whether the patient is presenting suicidal or other traumatic experiences.

Crisis intervention is not "magic". Instead, what is needed is systematic, model-guided intervention. Crisis work of any kind requires a structure to allow one to intervene not only constructively but also professionally.

True suicidal crises involve highly suicidal people, those who would be assessed as high on lethality as distinguished from someone of moderate or low lethality. In understanding suicidal people, the concept of *lethality* as well as the concept of *perturbation* are not only helpful but also essential (Shneidman, 1973, 1985). When intervening with highly lethal people, one must stay alert to both concepts. Lethality kills. In practice the distinction may be difficult to draw because lethal states are often associated with high perturbation (but not necessarily vice versa).

Crisis intervention affords immediate avenues of response to individuals poised between living and dying and is not to be confused with the usual psychotherapies appropriate for less lethal individuals. Of course, a suicidal act (deed, occurrence, event, threat, attempt) of whatever lethality is always genuine in its own light and merits serious considerations. Thus, in crisis intervention, there is almost no place for hostility, anger, sardonic attitudes, pejorative comments, daring the person, pseudo-democratic indifference, or other aversive behaviour.

Crisis intervention with highly suicidal people differs from other human relation-ships (see Hoff, 1984; Leenaars, 1991c; Mackinnon & Michels, 1971; Parad, 1965). The goal is simple: to keep some person alive. The procedures are often not sim-ple, however. Working with such people demands a different kind of involvement from the usual psychotherapy, which we will examine in Chapter 12. The activity that crisis intervention requires can be compared to that of a cardiologist in an emergency unit. It is more assertive than what transpires in a routine office visit. The focus is to sustain life. In crisis intervention we actively work to increase the patient's psychological sense of possible choices and sense of emotional attachment (Leenaars, 1993b).

A CASE

Peter and Rita, a married couple, having been referred by their family physician, arrived at my office both dishevelled, and looking depressed. Rita, unlike Peter, was also agitated. She could not be still; her speech was racing. Rita was overly distraught. Peter, on the other hand, was quieter, withdrawn, but deeply distressed. I learned that Rita had just returned from a trip to San Francisco with her lover, David. Peter wanted me to make Rita stop seeing David.

Since the focus in crisis intervention is not personality change, but problem resolution, I will say little in this chapter about Peter and Rita except the following: (1) Peter came from a dysfunctional family; his only brother had killed himself two years earlier. (2) Rita came from an even more dysfunctional family; her father was an alcoholic and her mother had a major affective disorder. (3) Rita had been on antidepressants since she was 16; she was now 36 (he was 40). (4) Peter and Rita had two children in late adolescence, both of whom were experiencing social and academic problems. I later learned that both had often been physically abused by Rita.

The focus of the intake was on the marriage. As is so commonly the case, the couple's perception of the problem was different. Rita described Peter as controlling, dominating, and rigid. Peter was beside himself over Rita's infidelity, and was overwhelmed that Rita had run off. Both denied any suicidal thoughts or plans. An appointment was made to return in a few days.

Two days later, Peter arrived for their appointment by himself. Rita had gone to David and had not returned the previous night. He was extremely perturbed, agitated, and very angry. He saw the situation as hopeless. Upon enquiry (see Leenaars, 1992b; Maris et al., 1992; and Kral & Sakinofsky, 1994) it became quite clear that Peter was moderately suicidal. He refused a referral to either a psychiatrist for medication or to his general practitioner who had first referred him. He refused hospitalization. He had refused earlier similar suggestions from the referring physician, reluctantly accepting a referral only to a psychologist for marital counselling. As in other such cases I did not insist on hospitalization; where a therapeutic relationship is developing, the alliance can be destroyed by involuntary commitment (see Chapter 19). The therapeutic relationship may be essential in keeping the person alive, although each case needs to be evaluated on an individual basis. Yet, Peter was willing to return the next day—a plan probably not optimal but the only one to which he would agree. I felt that the patient would be safe until our next meeting. Thus a crisis intervention plan was initiated.

The next day Peter returned with Rita. She reported that Peter had been emotionally abusive during the previous night, demanding sex. She announced that she was going to leave him, whereupon Peter became quite upset. Both were seen individually; Peter continued to refuse additional assistance and left the room.

Alone with me, Rita declared that she was in love with David and that they intended to live together. Although she had only met David (a man 10 years younger) a month earlier, she saw no problem in this plan and said when I questioned it, "It is none of your business." She said the same when I questioned her about anything. Nevertheless, she was worried about Peter. Though he had earlier denied the availability of a weapon, I now learned he had a collection of guns. With the assistance of the police, Rita had removed the guns from the home the night before.

Suggestions that Rita needed help were dismissed; she insisted, "I'm okay." I never saw her again. She promptly moved out of the house and left Peter and the children in tears.

That night, the police were called back to Peter's house. He had gone to the car and attempted to kill himself; however, before he went to the car, he telephoned a friend and informed him of his suicidal plan. (He was strikingly ambivalent.) The friend called the police. Peter was taken to an emergency unit of a local hospital and treated, but again refused admission and signed himself out. He assured the hospital that he would see me the next day and left with his friend.

Peter arrived the next day at my office, less agitated, with his friend. He was much more verbal and open than before. In light of the ongoing developments, we continued with a modification of our crisis plan, the basis of which will be outlined below. It is important, however, to emphasize that crisis intervention with highly suicidal people is best not attempted in isolation; we therefore included his friend, family, general practitioner, and others in the evolving plan.

Peter's trauma is not unusual in cases that we meet as crisis interventionists. He was suicidal, but responded to intervention positively. No further suicide attempts occurred, although ideation, with plans, continued. He was seen for over two years in psychotherapy. Indeed, good crisis intervention with suicidal people should lead to long-term psychotherapy. Interventionists who do not offer good follow-up care with their highly suicidal patients leave themselves open to questions about their mode of care in the event of a later suicide (Bongar, 1991).

THE MODEL

Here are some organizing questions: What is Peter's problem? What is he feeling? What does Peter want? What is Peter going to do? Why is he in my office? What does Peter want from me? A therapist, a crisis-line volunteer, and any interventionist in high-risk suicidal situations, must ask not only these questions but permutations and combinations of them. Therefore, a model is essential, i.e., a planned conceptual construction of interaction. Such a model is a framework. For example, questions such as the above allow us to approach the situation rationally and, simultaneously, reduce our own anxiety. Without a model, one is "slippery" in approach.

Although there are other models, here are five steps in mine:

1. Establish Rapport
2. Explore

3. Focus
4. Develop options and a plan of action
5. Terminate.

The model here is not unique; it is a common framework found in intervention.

No one response can be isolated to be life-saving in all suicide crises; but, a clear understanding of suicide allows us to state certain general guidelines for crisis intervention and therapy. The response must vary depending upon the unique individual; we should never mimic the suicide's all too often narrow perception. Our thinking, planning, and action do not need to be constricted.

Establish Rapport

Crisis intervention begins in the first encounter. The patient talks, and the interventionist listens. It requires the development of an active, non-judgemental rapport or therapeutic alliance. Rapport is a process, not a thing. Rapport is the ability to relate mutually in a human encounter. A capacity for good object relations is of crucial importance in establishing rapport. Tarachow (1963) has defined good object relationship as a "strong interest in, affection for another person, a willingness to give up something for another person, a willingness to assume responsibility for another person. It is quite an achievement to have a real interest in someone else..." (p. 103). This is empathy. In a sense, to establish rapport, love predominates over hate. If an interventionist has difficulties expressing attachment, he or she would do best by not doing crisis intervention (or therapy). From my view (Leenaars, 1988a, 1993b), the key to working with suicidal people is the relationship, the therapeutic alliance. This is not an everyday relationship, however. It is a special therapeutic relationship and it is vital. This was certainly true with Peter; fortunately rapport was quickly established. He looked forward to the visits. No rapport ever developed with Rita, a circumstance extremely problematic for an interventionist.

Response to an intensely suicidal person is a special task. It requires a special relationship marked by a genuine caring and a non-judgemental response. It is not just traditional therapy and demands a different kind of involvement. The goal is different; namely, to keep a person alive. The goal of treatment is quite simple. It consists almost by definition of lowering the lethality; in practice, this amounts to decreasing or mollifying the level of perturbation. We defuse the source of the person's constricted focus on suicide. We create community interest around the person. We make that person's temporarily unbearable problems and/or injustices just sufficiently better so that he/she can stop to think and reconsider and discern alternatives to suicide. The way to decrease lethality with the individual is by dramatically decreasing the felt perturbation—a process in which the relationship is the key.

The intervening psychotherapist can focus on any number of emotions (distressing feelings of pitiful forlornness, deprivation, distress, grief and especially hopelessness and helplessness). He/she works to improve the external and internal situations related to these emotions and other aspects of the suicidal state, to achieve a JND (Just Noticeable Difference). This can be accomplished initially through ventilation, interpretation, instruction, and realistic manipulation in the outside world, and requires a heightened level of interaction and rapport during the period of heightened lethality. The therapist needs to work diligently, always giving the suicidal person realistic transfusions of hope until the intensity of the pain subsides enough to reduce the lethality to a tolerable, life-permitting level.

Explore

A perception; i.e., the way an individual construes his/her circumstance defines a crisis. A B grade in an examination is acceptable to many but to others it may occasion unbearable pain. After reading thousands of suicide notes, I am struck by how divergent crises often are, but the patient's perception is critical in the total suicidal scenario (Leenaars, 1988a). Peter and Rita, obviously, had very different views of the marital crisis. Rita saw Peter as *the entire* problem; Peter saw the affair with David and the subsequent separation as painfully problematic. The two children, whom I saw later, also gave the contretemps a different reading.

The belief that a crisis is defined by a subject's perception does not mean that one accepts the person's view of the problem without question. Given the person's view, suicide has adjustive value. It abolishes pain. For example, Rita's announcement that she was leaving made the situation *unbearable* for Peter. Since Rita's return was highly improbable, Peter would be dead if we had accepted the proposition that preserving the marriage was the only solution. One must translate the patient's perception into a wider adaptive view. One has to widen the blinders. One does not talk only about the low grade or the lost spouse. Despair over a low grade, for example, can be translated into a need for perfection. With Peter, we reached beyond the anguish of his immediate abandonment. We must explore a wider array.

As we explore, we redefine to the individual the trauma as painful but tolerable. We develop the adaptive potential of the person. If the intervener accepts the perspective, "I can't live with this" then we tacitly collude with the person's decision to die and the patient cannot survive. We have to handle the drama better than the patient does. Yet, we cannot simply provide naive reassurance by simply saying, "You can too"! A better response would be something like, "When you say I can't live with *this*, what is *this*?" The interventionist can then redefine (reframe) the problem in terms of, say, a need for perfectionism, or another limiting, intolerable value (view).

We may be tempted in crisis intervention to take away the person's responsibility. A rule of thumb, including the early stages of crisis intervention, is never to take away the person's responsibility. Statements like "Don't worry—I won't let you hurt yourself" or "I will help you and you won't have to kill yourself" are inappropriate and, indeed, may be deadly. Yet, one needs initially to assume some responsibility by fostering life-sustaining action (not thought alone). We need to assist in the development of some constructive behaviour; the person's state of mind makes it imperative.

Two further points are relevant to the exploration phase of the model:

1. The pain of the suicidal person relates to the frustration or blocking of important psychological needs, that is, needs deemed to be important by the person (often attachment, as in the case of Peter). It should be the therapist's function to help the individual in relation to those thwarted needs.
2. The suicidal individual is ambivalent. He/she wants (needs) to die and yearns for intervention, rescue and life. For example, minutes before his attempt, Peter called a friend. Rescue often implies improvement or change in one of the major details in the person's world such as the wish to have Rita back, and so on.

Focus

It is imperative for the crisis intervener to understand how the suicidal person defines the trauma; i.e., what it is that cannot be endured. A crisis is a perception, not a thing-in-itself. These patients often cannot concentrate; they are too perturbed. It is therefore useful to bear the question in mind: "What is it that we are going to focus on?" Although the intervener assists, the suicidal person should do the focusing. Typical questions when focusing are: "What is the problem?"; "What were you hoping to accomplish?"; "What would be most helpful?"; "We've talked about a lot, what do you want to discuss?" The focusing allows not only the patient to focus but also the interventionist so that clarity can emerge. It allows for a good consensus and collaboration.

We do not exacerbate the crisis by talking about it. The patient is already angry and hostile (and also hopeless and helpless). This was certainly the case with Peter. At first he could only talk about Rita; he was hurt, angry, agitated and hopeless. He said, "Without Rita I'm nothing", adding that he now understood the words in his brother's suicide note. The brother had written: "No one loves me. Mom hates me. I'm all alone. I have no reason to live."

With help, Peter quickly focused on these feelings, addressing his need for attachment. (The dynamics with his mother were explored much later.) Ventilation, lightening of angry feelings, adequacy of expression and need for contacts have a critical place in crisis intervention—all with the intention of focusing on the trauma. The rule is: Reduce the elevated perturbation and the lethality will come down with it.

Develop Options and Constructive Action

The purpose of crisis intervention is to assist the patient with problem resolution, not personality change.

Suicide is an effort by an individual to stop unbearable pain. Suicide is the solution. Suicidal people need prompt relief and want action. To save some person's life, we have to do something! This may include putting information that the person is in trouble about something into the stream of communication, letting others know about it, breaking what could be a fatal secret, proffering help, and, always showing interest and deep concern.

Three things should be borne in mind when exploring options and constructive action. (1) A key to intermediate and long-range effectiveness with the suicidal person is to increase the options of actions available. (2) When the patient is no longer highly suicidal, the usual methods of psychotherapy can be usefully employed. Do not leave the patient with a weakened, inadequately developed, ego; he/she needs therapeutic assistance. (3) Given all that, we need to be reminded that work in suicide prevention is risky and dangerous and there are casualties. In the case of Peter, actions (1) and (2) were implemented. His family and the friend were involved, and his father uncharacteristically helped, although he was overwhelmed with guilt about his other son. Peter and his children entered therapy, and were seen for over two years.

A primary goal, when one explores options, is to reduce the patient's sense of perturbation. The aim is to decrease the pain to a level just below the traumatic degree (a JND). One assists the person in making the pain bearable, but *not* to deny, repress, deflect, etc.

Suicidal patients are all or nothing thinkers. Something is either black or white (or "A or non-A"). To presume that the suicidal individual either wants to kill him/herself or doesn't want to kill him/herself is an extremely limited point of view, even if the person generates *only* such permutations and combinations in his own options. Peter wanted to be dead or have Rita back (with "back" meaning before the affair with David). However, it is not necessary to work within a view of the world as "black or white" considering only permutations and combinations of one option. To adapt this all-or-nothing logic is to foster a limited and harsh view of life, one which neither the suicidal person nor the interventionist has to accept. Thus, the task is to increase the options, and to widen the range of possible cognitions.

The main point with a suicidal person is to increase that individual's psychological sense of possible choices *and* his/her sense of being emotionally supported. Relatives, friends, and colleagues should, after they have been determined to be on the life-side of the individual's ambivalence, be talked about in the total treatment process—as options for providing direct assistance (as in the case of Peter). The person needs other objects (people) with whom to identify and on whom to depend. Being so perturbed, Peter could not give up even a negative part of his identity, nor could he search out objects on his own. He was simply in too much pain and too pessimistic to do this. Yet, support was there. As Peter eventually realized: "I'm not alone."

The highly suicidal person wants out. It follows that, when possible, the means of exit should be blocked (see Chapter 19 for details). A practical application of this view is to "get the gun" in a suicidal situation where it is known that the individual intends to shoot himself and has a weapon. The explosive situation needs to be defused until that person no longer has the need for a suicidal weapon (see Berman, 1990). Maltsberger's consultative words (Berman, 1990) on such cases may guide us here:

> I would consult as much to avoid charges of negligence as to deal with my own anxiety. I think that any time I get into a difficult case, where I am concerned that somebody is imminently suicidal...I would want to be careful. It is enormously helpful to ask a

colleague to help to monitor one's own judgement when in a tense, anxiety-provoking situation. (Berman, 1990, p. 118)

Clearly, consultation is needed in some crisis cases. When a suicidal person has access to a lethal weapon, one may in some cases even want to speak to a lawyer. In the case of Peter, the guns had already been removed, although the fact that he had such means needed to be monitored. What would happen, for example, if the police returned the weapons? He had a permit and could easily have them returned.

As we have learned, the focus in crisis intervention with highly lethal people should not be on "why" suicide has been chosen as the method of solving the problems. This is probably better addressed in more usual psychotherapy, once the lethality is lower. Instead, the focus should be on solving the problem(s), so that pain becomes mollified. The problems are discussed and addressed in terms of what can be done about them. One talks about practical items—job, rent, sickness, food, whatever. The individual needs immediate partial reduction of the urgently felt suicidal impulses or wishes. To allay these impulses, the patient's unmet needs must be addressed, and this is done not only in the consultation room but also in the real world.

The interventionist should always guard against "buying into" the overpowering emotions and constricted logic presented by the suicidal individual. It is vital to counter the suicidal person's constriction-of-thought by attempting to widen the mental blinders and increase the number of options, certainly beyond the two options of either having some magical resolution or being dead, such as Peter having Rita or being dead. In this sense, with Peter as with all suicidal patients, we invite them into our inner world, to help them to solve problems, to cope, etc.

The question for the patient is: "What is it that you are going to do?" The answer needs to be active, not passive (if passive, one must go back to steps (1), (2) and (3) above). Active contact, letting others know about it, encouraging the person to talk to others, getting loved ones involved, interested and responsive, and creating action around the person are all examples of active intervention. (See Shneidman, 1981c and 1985, for example, for details.)

As a note, one must limit one's caseload to crisis intervention with only a very few highly lethal individuals. It is impossible to deal effectively with many highly lethal individuals without risking therapist "burnout" or emotional withdrawal from the demands of such patients.

Termination

Before terminating the treatment, one should summarize, rehearse, develop planning skills, identify resources, make referrals, identify emergency procedures, and establish follow-up, to identify but a few essential steps before ending contact with the patient in crisis.

Crisis intervention does not completely fix situations. Once the lethality is lowered, once the difficulties are more bearable, one moves towards more usual therapy—psychoanalytic, cognitive, behavioural, whatever. In a professional psychotherapeutic exchange the focus is on feelings, emotional content, negative cognitions and unconscious meanings, rather than the immediate crisis difficulties. The emphasis is on the latent significance of what is being said, more than on the manifest and obvious difficulties. The brief descriptions of Peter, including his brother's suicide note, raise many latent questions. However, these endeavours usually come after the lethality is lowered, although it is sometimes possible to embark on these efforts in one's earliest interventions. (See, for example, Chapter 12; Leenaars et al., 1994.)

Finally, in any intervention it can be difficult to terminate. One should always affirm the person (i.e., provide ego strengthening) in such a process. When one concludes, one asks, "Have you got what you wanted?" If not, one goes back to step (2), and one must leave the door open even if referring the individual for treatment elsewhere. The person may again be in need of crisis intervention.

A FEW NOTES ON TRANSFERENCE AND COUNTERTRANSFERENCE IN INTERVENTION

Although the issues of transference and countertransference have been discussed earlier in Chapter 5 on assessment, they are equally critical in intervention—and will be rewritten, added to, etc., for intervention (for details see Eyman, 1991; Freud, 1974d; Heimann, 1950; Maltsberger & Buie, 1974; I am deeply indebted to them for the following insights). Yet, every crisis worker and psychotherapist must be fully aware of these concerns.

As stated earlier, transference is a process arising in a therapeutic situation and involving reactivation of the patient's previous experience, recollections, and unconscious wishes regarding (often early) significant people (objects). Such processes in object relations must be identified in treatment, and even in crisis intervention.

Suicidal people, for example, could feel angry, injured, or rejected in the following situations: after premature termination or discharge; with excessive waiting for help (even one hour, or one day!); when treatment time was short and they felt "cut off"; if referred to others; dealt with too directively; given inadequate rapport, interest, etc.; disappointed by a therapist who forgets important details; confronted by a therapist about an issue too early; presented with simplistic use of a written suicide contract; contacted by a person other than a crisis interventionist.

Countertransference comprises the therapist's entire unconscious reactions to the patient and the patient's transference. These reactions originate in the therapist's own conflicts and/or real objective interactions (object relations). The therapist must admit to and understand his/her fears, anxiety and so on (especially since these are often denied because they are seen as weaknesses; and is the old problem that the doctor must be perfect and strong). The following reactions in the therapist may arise if confrontation with the suicidal patient provokes feelings of guilt, incompetence, anxiety, fear and anger, and when these feelings are not worked through:

- underestimation of the seriousness of the suicidal action;
- absence of discussion of suicide thoughts, attempts, etc.;
- allowing oneself to be lulled into a false sense of security by the patient's promise not to repeat a suicide attempt (such as in the use of a simplistic written suicide contract);
- disregard of the cry for help aspect of the suicide attempt and exclusive concentration on its manipulative character;
- exaggeration of the patient's provocative, infantile, and aggressive sides;
- denial of one's own importance to the patient;
- failure to persuade the patient to undergo further treatment;
- feeling of lacking the resources required by a particular patient;
- exaggerated sense of hopelessness in response to the patient's troubled social situation and abuse of drugs or alcohol;
- being pleased when the patient claims to have all problems solved after only a brief contact, without reflecting closely on the plausibility of this statement;
- feeling upset when the patient shows insufficient progress after brief course of assistance, despite the therapist's initial profound commitment.

If these feelings are not addressed, acknowledged, and so on, it will activate destructiveness, even rage. The therapist's own hate may destroy the suicidal person (Maltsberger & Buie, 1974). All good therapists—Shneidman, Maltsberger and, if I may, Leenaars—must admit to such feelings and reactions if they occur. It is not, as Maltsberger and Buie (1974) point out, that one feels hate, but how it is expressed in the therapy room. Obviously, issues of transference and countertransference are complex and the interventionist experiencing them can benefit from contact with a supervisor or consultation with a colleague, as well as consideration of the broader literature on such reactions written for psychotherapists. Once more, I can only emphasize how the patient can sense our fear, helplessness, and so on. (He/she says something like, "Oh, even the therapist cannot help. No one can help.") Even the therapist can dissemble and, at such times, there is nothing better than a good consultation.

CONCLUDING REMARKS

Ultimately, we must understand that there are no universal formulations regarding how to respond to a highly lethal person. We can speak of understanding, but never with precision. When our subject matter is crisis intervention, we can be no more accurate or scientific than the available ways of responding that our subject matter permits. Yet, the yearning for universal suicidological laws, understandably, persists. A sweeping psychological statement with a ring of truth becomes a dictum. I believe that the search for a singular universal response to suicide is a chimera, an imaginary and non-existent conceptual fabrication—our own negative countertransference. The search for a singular universal response is a foolish and unrealistic fancy. There is no one method for intervention. There is no cookbook!

I wish to add several concluding ideas: One should use all measures with highly lethal individuals. These include support, behavioural techniques, psychodynamic interpretation, hospitalization, medication, etc., . . . and especially the involvement of others, not only others to whom the patient was (or is) attached but also "social" agencies—teachers, priests, elders, the Chief, doctors, social workers, anyone—all of whom serve, directly or indirectly, to mollify the pain. Peter is alive today not only because of his therapist but also because of the many people who helped to make his life hopeful and more bearable (although not perfect).

In summary, intervention in the trenches, as for the cardiologist, is not as clean as described. Crisis workers constantly must adjust, widening their formulations and actions to meet the needs of those they try to assist.

Chapter 12

APPLICATIONS FOR PSYCHOTHERAPY WITH SUICIDAL PEOPLE

Suicide, we have learned, is a human, multidimensional malaise. Too few have utilized a theoretical-conceptual analysis to understand the malaise, despite, as we have learned since the first empirical psychological study of suicide, that such contributions offer a rich potential (Shneidman & Farberow, 1957a). A recent task force of the International Academy for Suicide Research (IASR) has made the same conclusion (Leenaars et al., 1997). They state: "There is no substitute for theory in research. There is no data without interpretation" (p. 139). And I would add there is no substitute for theory in psychotherapy.

Briefly, as we read in Chapter 2 and beyond, the theoretical model presented in this volume was the following:

Intrapsychic

I   Unbearable Psychological Pain
The common stimulus in suicide is unendurable psychological pain—*the pain of pain*. The suicidal person feels especially hopeless and helpless. Although other motives (elements, wishes) are evident, the person primarily perceives that he/she wants to flee from *a trauma, a catastrophe*. The suicide is functional because it abolishes unbearable pain.

II   Cognitive Constriction
The common cognitive state in suicide is constriction; i.e., rigidity in thinking, narrowing of focus, tunnel vision, concreteness, etc. The suicidal person only construes his or her trauma.

III   Indirect Expressions
The suicidal person may see his letter as a clear and obvious communication but it is a confusing, contradictory message. Complications, ambivalence, re-directed aggression, unconscious implications are often evident.

IV *Inability to Adjust*
Depressed people are not the only ones who kill themselves; other disorders have been related to some suicides. The suicidal person perceives him/herself as unable to adjust.

V *Ego*
The person him/herself is a critical aspect in the suicidal act. Often a relative weakness in the person's capacity to develop constructive tendencies and to overcome his/her personal difficulties is evident.

Interpersonal

VI *Interpersonal Relations*
The suicidal person very frequently has problems in establishing or maintaining relationships. The suicide is often related to unsatisfied or frustrated affiliation (attachment) needs although other needs may also be evident.

VII *Rejection–Aggression*
Suicide may be the turning back upon oneself of murderous impulses (wishes, needs) that had been directed against a traumatic event, most frequently someone who had rejected the person. Suicide may be murder in the 180th degree.

VIII *Identification–Egression*
An intense identification (attachment) to a lost or rejecting person or to any ideal is critical in understanding the suicidal person. If this emotional need is not met, the suicidal person experiences a deep discomfort (pain) and wants to egress. Suicide is the *only* solution.

Focus

My initial studies in suicide have focused primarily on understanding suicide and suicidal phenomena, an aim of science in general. Yet, I also hold to the tenet that understanding is a—if not *the*—key to prediction and control. The very aims of science are understanding, prediction, and control. The purpose of this chapter is to outline the applications for intervention, specifically psychotherapy from the theoretical model presented. I believe that this is important because, as one reviewer of my early book, *Suicide Notes*, noted:

> The reported research is an interesting attempt to approach suicide notes from a quantitative and qualitative vantagepoint, but the reader asks what the conclusions are for preventive work. The author himself says that he hopes "that researchers will continue to develop models to interpret suicide that can be logically and empirically tested and, most importantly, can be made useful and life-saving". (Battegay, 1990, p. 75)

Thus, I hereby provide some useful and hopefully life-saving responses for psychotherapy. Yet, before I begin, let me be explicit about my debt to Dr Edwin Shneidman in this chapter (and this book).

No clinician invents psychotherapy. This is true for my work and this volume. Many grandparents in the field influence it; yet, as you read, the influence of Dr Shneidman will be obvious—especially in this chapter. His influence and work can be found on every page—and what I do on a day-to-day basis in my office. His own work on the topic has been diverse, but not detailed; Shneidman's best voice on psychotherapy can be found in two short papers, "Psychotherapy with Suicidal Patients" (Shneidman, 1999b) and "Aphorisms of Suicide and Some Implications for Psychotherapy" (Shneidman, 1999c)—both represented in my volume of Shneidman's selected works, *Lives and Deaths* (Leenaars, 1999a). These papers contain prescriptive advice for psychotherapists; the second paper repeats several ideas of the first but approaches the topic from a different direction and shows some of the special aspects of psychotherapy with suicidal patients from a new light. If one reads these papers, one will see the immediate influence on what I do with suicidal people and I thank Dr Shneidman for his kind permission—and encouragement—to use his ideas, but, of course, the words and conclusions herein are my own.

By way of an addendum to this introduction, Shneidman (Leenaars, 1999a) has, since he took courses in logic as a college freshman at UCLA in 1934, been keenly interested in making explicit the latent logical (cognitive) components of everyday thought. Later, he realized how useful it is to examine the cognitive styles exhibited in *each* suicidal person. For example, in a terse but insightful paper, "On 'Therefore I must kill myself' " (Shneidman, 1982), he shows how vitally important it is for a psychotherapist to understand the patient's idiosyncratic logical style—and then not agree with that patient's major premise when the premise is the keystone to the patient's lethal (suicidal) syllogistic conclusion. ("People who have committed a certain sin ought to be dead; I am a person who has committed that sin; *therefore*, I ought to be dead.") Or stated simply, the therapist needs to know the suicidal person's world, not necessarily agree with it. Shneidman's view is that psychotherapy contains these cognitive components and it is often prudent, if not necessary, for the therapist to make them explicit and to deal with them (Leenaars, 1999a). Shneidman's psychotherapy is in many ways a dynamic cognitive therapy.

Recently, Shneidman (2001) named his approach to therapy as Anodyne Therapy (I do not follow his lead here). The intention of Shneidman's therapy—and this is most important—is to reduce the patient's psychological pain. He writes:

> If the villain is psychological pain then we need something that fights that pain. There is a word for that: *anodyne*. An anodyne is a substance that (or an agent or person who) assuages pain. Psychotherapy in general ought to be anodynic. But with a highly suicidal patient—with *perturbation* and, even more seriously, high *lethality*—the anodynic function of the therapist is vital.
>
>   The most famous essay on anodynes is Thomas De Quincey's nineteenth century *Confessions of an English Opium Eater* (1821/1986), a brilliant piece on the role of anodynes in alleviating suffering. (p. 182)

For Shneidman, the main task of therapy with suicidal patients is as follows:

> ...assess and address the patient's psychache that stems from unfulfilled psychological needs. The therapist should serve as an anodynic agent—to relieve the pain so

that the patient's *raison d'être* for suicide is mollified and the need to end the inner suffering is no longer pressing. (p. 182)

Psychotherapy should be person-centred.

BACK TO THE PREFACE

There is nothing like a good consultant. There is almost no instance in a therapist's professional life when consultation is as important as when he/she is dealing with a suicidal patient. I have been most blessed as I often discussed my patients with Dr Shneidman.

Let me begin with some discussions on 4–6 November 2001 in Shneidman's home. We were talking about this very book; and we spoke about my last case to write (someone Shneidman knew from our conversations). I asked on that occasion whether he had any further thoughts about psychotherapy with suicidal people. He offered a preamble, something he had recently written:

> Suicide prevention is about a person, a person wanting to be helped to stop their pain, what I call psychache.
>
> In a sense, suicide prevention tries to mollify the whole person. Psychotherapy is concerned with what kind of person that individual is. What works is a view held by Sigmund Freud, William James, Erwin Stengel, not Pavlov or Skinner or any reductionist view. [I would, of course, add Shneidman to the list—Author.]
>
> Our kind of treatment, psychotherapy and so on, should address the person's story, his/her narrative, not the demographic, nosological category or this or that fact. It says, "Please tell me who you are . . . what hurts?" Not, "Please fill out this form . . . and give me samples of your body fluids."
>
> Of course, the practical disadvantage of this approach is that it requires more than a few minutes per patient. Suicide prevention is not an efficiency operation. It is a human exchange.

Suicide prevention is based on a humanitarian approach to life. The psychotherapy, I believe, that works with suicidal people is a person-centred therapy—or, if you prefer, a patient-centred therapy; what Martin Buber (1970) called an "I–Thou" relationship, not "I–it". It is of note that research shows that what works with suicidal people is, in fact, clearly associated to the relationship itself. I will go further. I believe that it is the relationship. What we have known for a long time is that patients who persevere and benefit from psychotherapy are the ones that have developed a good working relationship (Dyck et al., 1984; Luborsky et al., 1985). These patients feel heard and understood. This is person-centred.

The relationship (attachment) that the therapist develops is central in effective psychotherapy. Spirito (2001), for example, presented a study with a group of suicidal people receiving a cognitive-behavioural approach (a specific task-oriented treatment) and the other suicidal group receiving a non-directive approach. What these researchers learned is that it did not matter what treatment the patients received. Patients in both groups showed positive response. It was, thus, hypothesized that the relationship was critical. Suicidal people were telling their narratives and someone was listening (after all, these patients were important; they were part of a research study). Keep in mind that in this study the same seven therapists did both treatments; perhaps they were just good therapists. Psychotherapy is the attachment, not this or that technique. This is person-centred. What works is mollifying that person's pain. What works is quality care.

One further study on the importance of the relationship is worth noting. Wasserman (2001), in a long-range follow-up study, found that suicidal patients with multiple contacts with different people over years had a much higher rate of suicide than expected. They were the suicidal patients that had most frequently been seen by different people over time, after various attempts. These people, in fact, received the not-too-unusual practice, when people find their way to clinics or hospitals. They are never assigned to *the* doctor, nurse, therapist, and so on. According to Wasserman (2001), these suicidal people never received the attachment that they needed to traverse their pain. They remained detached. Once more, our relationships are highly important.

"Suicidal people", says Shneidman, "need a human exchange." They need to tell their stories. It is not the clinician who knows best. Suicidal people are the experts of their own story. This is not armchair speculation, but evidence-based practice. A task force of the American Psychological Association (APA), Division of Psychotherapy (Task Force on Empirically Supported Therapy Relationships, 2001) identified the following elements of effective therapy relationships: therapeutic alliance (or rapport), therapist empathy, and patient–therapist goal consensus, and collaboration. The patients are a "Thou".

Finally, as a researcher, we need much more research on what works: what works with a 4-year-old, a 65-year-old, a male, a female, a Dutch person, and so on. What works with people and their diversity? What works with that unique individual? This, too, was a recommendation of the Task Force on Empirically Supported Therapy Relationships (2001). Efficacy in treatment depends on individually tailoring therapy to the unique characteristic of each patient. Furthermore, the task force—and this book—recommended the concurrent use of empirically supported relationship factors within the context of research-based understanding of the person to generate the best clinical outcome. This is multicomponent psychotherapy at its best.

Prolegomenon: Jonathan Swift, the great Irish ironist, concluded, " No man values the best medicine if administered by a physician whose person he hates or despises."

IMPLICATIONS FOR RESPONSE

There is no one response that could be isolated that would be life-saving for all would-be suicides. However, as one begins to understand suicide, it becomes apparent that one can reasonably infer some implications for assessment, rescue, intervention, and therapy. The response would vary depending upon the unique individual. We should not mimic the suicide's all too often narrow perception. Our own actions do not need to be constricted. The purpose of this chapter is to provide some associations for intervention, based on our empirical data. These implications are not limited to the suicidologists researched to date for we can cast a wider net and include other suicidologists who have specialized in psychotherapy with suicidal individuals and crisis intervention in general (I especially need to note Aaron T. Beck). It is, however, largely reflective of a metaview.

The *a priori* assumption in this book: The reader already knows. He/she already knows something about psychotherapy, counselling, crisis intervention, and so on. No one book can teach a person to be a therapist; it requires an education and experience. Thus, this book provides a person-centred metaview and assumes that the reader is, or is aspiring to be, a therapist, whether cognitive-behavioural, psychodynamic, relational, problem-centred, psychoanalytic, whatever. It does not teach a therapy; rather, it charts the howling seas of anguish to address the archetypal rage in the suicidal person. It offers an empirically supported definition, with applications across age, gender, historical time, and so on, as well as countries (few explanations of suicide exist globally). This understanding of suicide provides, by inference, the implications and applications for response in this book. Psychotherapy follows understanding the unique person—Natalie, Sylvia, Scott, and any suicidal person that you will meet in the fight to stay alive (Eros over Thanatos).

My intent is to provide specific implications for intervention from the theory outlined earlier. Each implication will begin with a significant protocol sentence, divided into the eight clusters, keeping in mind Shneidman's two concepts of perturbation and lethality (1973, 1985).

It is important to understand that the focus of this chapter is on responding to perturbed and to moderately and highly lethal people. It describes some avenues to respond with individuals who are at their life/death decisions and is not intended to replace more traditional psychotherapies that are more appropriate for less lethal individuals. Of course, as I noted in Chapter 11, a suicidal act (deed, occurrence, event, threat, attempt) of whatever lethality is always genuine in its own light and should be treated, at the very least, as an important problem. Thus, in responding to a suicidal person, there is almost never any place for the therapist's hostility, anger, sardonic attitudes, pejorative comments, daring the person, or pseudo-democratic indifference.

Intrapsychic

I   *Unbearable Psychological Pain*
1. *Suicide has adjustive value and is functional because it stops painful tension and provides relief from intolerable psychological pain.*

Pain is the enemy of life; the person wants relief from intolerable psychological pain (e.g., a lost spouse, a low grade). Questions such as "What is going on?"; "Where do you hurt?"; and "What would you like to have happen?" can usually be asked by the therapist trying to help the suicidal person. The person needs to tell you what hurts. We listen to his/her story of pain. Suicide is *the* solution to that pain.

We do not, however, have to accept the person's solution to the problem, his/her pain, namely suicide. Given the suicidal person's view (or beliefs, or cognitions) suicide does have adjustive value. It abolishes pain. It allows the person to escape. Rather, one has to translate the person's value into a (wider) adaptive value (and view) something more than stopping painful tension. Somewhat restated, depending on one's clinical orientation, one translates cognitively (reframes) the person's constricted beliefs into a wider belief or the person's manifest language into a less constricted language (etc.). Do not talk only about a low grade, a lost spouse, whatever. The concern over the low school grade, for example, can be translated into talk about a need for perfection.

One redefines to the individual the trauma as painful, but tolerable. One develops adaptive value in the person. If you accept the statement, "I can't live with this" then the person does not have to survive. Don't respond "You can too"! A better response would be something like, "When you say I can't live with this, what is *this*?" ... redefine (or reframe) the problem in terms, of say, a need for perfectionism, or other limiting, intolerable values (or views).

2. *In suicide, the psychological and/or environmental traumas among many other factors may include: incurable disease, threat of senility, fear of becoming hopelessly dependent, feelings of inadequacy, humiliation. Although the solution of suicide is not caused by one thing, or motive, suicide is a flight from these spectres.*

Suicide is an effort by an individual to stop unbearable anguish or intolerable pain. It is anguish or pain usually related manifestly to only one thing but latently to much more. It is a response to do something. Knowing this usually guides us. To save a person's life, "do something"! This may include putting information—that the person is in trouble about "a thing"—into the stream of communication, letting others know about it, breaking what could be a fatal secret, proferring help, and, if possible, showing interest and deep concern (all protective factors—see Grad, 2001). I do not agree with those individuals who argue for a no rescue stance in this field. One should have, at least, a provisional rescue approach with moderately lethal individuals, and always an action plan with highly lethal individuals. (See, for example, L. A. Hoff's (1984), *People in Crisis*; and H. Parad's (1965), *Crisis Intervention* and my own volume, with J. Maltsberger & R. Neimeyer, *Treatment of Suicidal People* (1994b).)

3. *In the suicidal drama, certain emotional states are present, including pitiful forlornness, emotional deprivation, distress and/or grief.*

The psychotherapist can focus on any number of emotions, notably the distressing (painful) feelings such as pitiful forlornness, deprivation, worthlessness, guilt, distress, or grief. It is essential to improve the external and internal situations related to these emotions and other aspects of the suicidal mind—a JND (Just Noticeable Difference). This can be accomplished through a variety of methods: ventilation, interpretation, instruction, and realistic manipulation in the outside world. All this implies, when working with a highly lethal person, a heightened level of interaction during the period of heightened lethality. The therapist needs to work diligently, always giving the suicidal person realistic transfusions of hope until the intensity

of forlornness, deprivation, distress, grief (in short, pain) subsides enough to reduce the lethality to a tolerable, life-permitting level. Shneidman's question from
the "Shneidman Psychological Distress Questionnaire" (PDQ, see Appendix 12.1),
that will assist, is as follows.

My psychological pain relates mostly to my *feelings* of (check three):

( ) abandonment	( ) dread	( ) jealousy
( ) anger	( ) emptiness	( ) loneliness
( ) anguish	( ) fear	( ) powerlessness
( ) anxiety	( ) guilt	( ) rage
( ) bad conscience	( ) hopelessness	( ) shame
( ) confusion	( ) humiliation	( ) worry
( ) disgust	( ) inadequacy	( ) Other:

4. *The person appears to have arrived at the end of an interest to endure and sees suicide
   as a solution for some urgent problem(s), and/or injustices of life.*

Response to an intensely suicidal person is a special task. It requires a special relationship; in fact, a genuine, emphatic, non-judgemental relation to the individual is
critical in responding to him/her. It is not just traditional therapy. It demands a different kind of involvement. The goal is different; namely, keeping the person alive.
It is, in fact, straightforward to meet an evidence-based practice, patient–therapist
goal consensus (Task Force on Empirically Supported Therapy Relationships, 2001).
Collaboration follows.

The goal of treatment is quite simple. It consists almost by definition of lowering
the lethality; in practice, decreasing or mollifying the level of perturbation usually
does this. In short, we diffuse the source of the person's constricted focus on suicide;
we create familial and/or social (community) interest around the person. We make
that person's temporarily unbearable problems and/or injustices just sufficiently
better so that he/she can stop, think, reconsider and begin to see alternatives. The
way to decrease lethality with the individual is by dramatically decreasing the felt
perturbation.

The question, from Shneidman's PDQ, to evaluate the intensity (to see if it is the
end) is as follows:

The *intensity* of my psychological pain is (circle one number below):

1	2	3	4	5	6	7	8	9
Little psycho- logical pain; almost non- existent	Mild	Moder- ate	Some- what bother- some	Present but manage- able between moder- ate and severe	Definitely hurtful	Harsh; rather severe	Definitely rather severe	Unbear- able; the worst discom- fort a person can ever experi- ence

Appendix 12.1 presents the complete version of Shneidman's Psychological Distress Questionnaire (PDQ; Shneidman, 1993). (The PDQ may be copied with the permission of Dr Shneidman.) The PDQ is Edwin Shneidman's attempt at quantifying the pain that drives up the lethality. Of course, Shneidman believes that the assessment of pain is *the* most important aspect of suicidality to assess, although the assessment of suicidality requires obviously more than one test.

5. *There is a conflict between life's demands for adaptation and the person's inability or unwillingness to meet the challenge.*

Take the side of adaptation and, in a kindly but focused way, remind the person of the fact that life often involves the choices among lousy alternatives, (or pains). A wise adaptation to life itself is often to choose the least lousy alternative that is practically attainable. Give him/her a challenge that he/she can meet—something not perfect. Pain does not have to be ended. It does have to be bearable.

6. *The person is in a state of heightened disturbance (perturbation) and feels boxed in, harassed, especially hopeless and helpless.*

One decreases the elevated hopelessness and helplessness by doing anything and almost everything possible to mollify the infantile idiosyncrasies, the sense of being harassed and unsuccessful, the feelings of hopelessness and helplessness that the individual is experiencing. It is, in fact, so important how we manage the inner/intrapsychic phenomenology of our patients. We need to address the impotence. However, we should not make the person non-hopeless. One should not attempt to establish an impossibly perfect situation. Indeed, one needs the hopelessness to psychologically move the person. Yet one should initially provide some transfusion of sound hope, self-help and not feeling boxed in.

II *Cognitive Constriction*
7. *The person reports a history of trauma (e.g., poor health, rejection by significant other, a competitive spouse).*

Borrowing from crisis intervention, it is imperative that the reader be reminded that the suicidal person defines the trauma. A trauma is a perception, not a thing in itself. One of Shneidman's educational examples depicts the man who always wanted the perfect car. He saved his money and bought a Ferrari. Then the car got a scratch; his response was to write a suicide note, stating "There is nothing to live for", and shoot himself. For almost all, the scratch appears—to use a popular expression—to be small stuff, but not for him. Another Shneidman example is the elderly woman, who killed herself after her canary died. Thus, therapists must remember that trauma for both these individuals—and all suicidal people—was/is a perception, not "objective" reality.

8. *Figuratively speaking, the person appears to be "intoxicated" by overpowering emotions. Concomitantly, there is a constricted logic and perception.*

Although the person defines the trauma (situation), one cannot buy into the overpowering emotions and constricted logic presented by the individual. They all too often are in a dissociative state. It is, thus, vital to counter the suicidal person's constriction of thought by attempting to widen the mental blinders and increase the number of options, certainly beyond the two options of either having some magical resolution or being dead. We do not increase the perturbation. We do not agree with the person's constriction. The person did not come to us for us to agree with his/her intoxication.

Let us here cite a case example; it is prototypical of what one does:

A middle-aged businessman, forlorn, rather traumatized, was referred to me. He was recently separated, although the "event" that brought him to my office was the loss of his job. He was a bank manager who had worked for the same bank for 18 years. He was suicidal with a formed suicidal plan. His demand of me was that I somehow, magically, had to obtain his job back. Losing his job resulted in overpowering emotions and constricted logic and perception. He simply could not "bear to live". Suicide was his only alternative.

I did several things. I attempted to begin to "widen his blinders" and said something like, "Now let's see. You could look for another job." ("I couldn't do that.") (It is precisely the "can'ts" and the "won'ts" and "have tos" and "nevers" and "always" and "onlys" that are addressed with highly lethal individuals.) "You could hire a consulting firm to help us look for a job." ("I couldn't do that.") "You could involve the help of your business friends." (He was well respected and perceived to be quite competent.) ("I couldn't do that.") "We can look for alternatives." ("I couldn't do that.") "We could call your wife." ("I couldn't do that.") "We could contact your family." ("I couldn't do that.") ... and "You can always commit suicide but there is obviously no need to do that today." (No response.) "Now let's look at our ideas and rank them in order of your preference, keeping in mind that not one of them is perfect."

The very making of the list within the context of our non-threatening and non-judgemental relation had a calming influence on him, a JND. Within a few minutes he was less figuratively intoxicated. His emotions were less overpowering and we began to deconstrict his logic and perception. What was important was that suicide was no longer ranked first. We were then simply searching for a broader action plan.

The point is not how the issue was eventually resolved; let it suffice to say that the contact with his estranged wife was ranked first and this subsequently led to family therapy. What is important is that it is possible to lower his lethality by reducing his perturbation. We could widen his range of visible and realistic options, other than suicide.

9. *There is poverty of thought, exhibited by focusing only on permutations and combinations of grief and grief-provoking topics.*

A common premise is that something is either black or white. Something is either "A or not-A". To presume that the suicidal individual either wants to kill him/herself or not is an extremely limited point of view, even if the person generates *only* such permutations and combinations in his/her thoughts. It is not necessary to require a view of the world as "A or not A" (e.g., "job or not job"); that is, a view (or belief) of the world exhibiting only permutations and combinations of one content. The individual may only think of grief-provoking content but he/she can also have other fantasies, or cognitions. To suggest such an "A and not-A" world is a limited and harsh view of life, one which neither the suicidal person nor we have to accept. Thus, the task is to increase the permutations and combinations of the individual's thoughts (or to reframe), and widen the range of possible cognitions, beliefs and fantasies, beyond "A or not-A". All this is critical in keeping the highly lethal individual alive. (See Watzlawick, Beavin & Jackson's (1967) *Pragmatics of Human Communication* for further clarifications about the pragmatics of change.)

III   Indirect Expressions

10. *The person reports ambivalence; e.g., complications, concomitant contradictory feelings, attitudes and/or thrusts.*

The suicidal individual is often ambivalent. A suicidal person usually has the deepest ambivalence between wanting (needing) to be dead and yearning for possible intervention or rescue. The rescue often takes the form of improvement or change in one of the major details—one thing—in the person's world such as the wish to have an A+, to be loved, to have that job, and so on, regardless of how the person had defined the situation. In general, the therapist should work with the life-directed aspects of the ambivalence without, of course, being timorous about touching upon the death-oriented element in that person.

11. *The person's aggression has been turned inwards; e.g., humility, submission and devotion, subordination, flagellation, masochism, are evident.*

A highly suicidal state is characterized by its transient quality. Intense aggression turned outwards or inwards is usually of brief duration. Therapists are, thus, well advised to minimize those probably well-intended writings in this field which speak of an individual's "right to commit suicide"—an individual's "right to turn his/her anger towards him/herself" or masochism or any other Ahab-like rage against oneself—a right which in actuality cannot be denied.

12. *Unconscious dynamics can be concluded. There are likely more reasons to the suicide than the person is consciously aware.*

Suicide should not be regarded as a crime or a sin. The focus of action is on the individual in both his/her conscious and unconscious mind. The focus is on the person in his/her totality, not simply his/her stated conscious perception. This implies that one must see the individual with a decentred, theoretical frame. There is much more than just the manifest content (e.g., the scratch on the car). The mind is deep, deeper than the conscious mind realizes—especially if constricted.

Finally, since the suicide has unconscious implications, one may be tempted to take away the person's responsibility. A rule of thumb is never take away the person's responsibility. Statements like "Don't worry, I won't let you" or "I will help you and you won't have to kill yourself", are inappropriate and, indeed, may be deadly. Yet, one initially needs to assume some responsibility by creating action (not thought alone). We need to assist in some constructive behaviour; the person's state of mind makes it necessary.

IV   Inability to Adjust

13. *The person considers him/herself too weak to overcome personal difficulties and, therefore, rejects everything, wanting to escape painful life events.*

Once the lethality is lowered, and once the difficulties are more bearable, one must move towards more traditional therapy—psychoanalytic, cognitive, existential, behavioural, etc., but in a person-centred way. Brief crisis work with such people is insufficient to address their needs. They need long-term psychotherapeutic intervention (a protective factor), and such efforts are sometimes life-long. In a professional psychotherapeutic exchange the focus is on feelings, emotional content, irrational cognitions, spontaneous unhealthy beliefs, and unconscious meanings, rather than the immediate difficulties. One focuses on the "weak" and "inferior" cognitions or feelings. The emphasis is on the latent significance of what is being said, more than on the manifest and obvious difficulties. However, these endeavours usually come after the lethality is lowered, although it is sometimes possible to embark on these efforts in one's earliest interventions. (See Cantor, 1991; Leenaars et al., 1994; Maltsberger, 1990.)

14. *Although the person passionately argues that there is no justification for living on, the person's state of mind is incompatible with an accurate assessment/perception of what is going on.*

One takes the person seriously but one does not accept his/her view. The only way to come back from a suicidal abyss and to develop relatively firm logic is to grow and become hopeful. In this regard, following Dr Shneidman, I have a rather decentred view. I use a multicomponent (or multimodal) approach. I endorse psychotherapy, medications, behavioural modification, counselling, outreach groups, healing circles, agencies, living in a home that provides love, living in a loving foster home—in short, anything that develops the person's perspective and will allow him/her to perceive life as not just hard, bitter, futile, painful, unjustified, and hopeless. All these efforts can be protective factors.

15. *The person (S) exhibits a serious disorder in adjustment.*
   (a) *S's reports are consistent with a manic-depressive disorder such as the down-phase; e.g., all-embracing negative statements, severe mood disturbances causing marked impairment.*
   (b) *S's reports are consistent with schizophrenia; e.g., delusional thought, paranoid ideation.*
   (c) *S's reports are consistent with anxiety disorder (such as obsessive-compulsive, post-traumatic stress); e.g., feeling of losing control; recurrent and persistent thoughts, impulses or images.*
   (d) *S's reports are consistent with antisocial personality (or conduct) disorder; e.g., deceitfulness, conning others.*
   (e) *S's reports are consistent with borderline personality; e.g., frantic efforts to avoid real or imagined abandonment, unstable relationships.*

(f) *S's reports are consistent with depression; e.g., depressed mood, diminished interest, insomnia.*

(g) *S's reports are consistent with a disorder or dysfunction not otherwise specified. S is so paralysed by pain that life, future, etc., is colourless and unattractive.*

Suicide is best understood by going beyond nosological categorization, although such classification may assist in identification and even in treatment. In treatment, however, we need to keep in mind that it is the individual who commits suicide, not some category. Psychotherapy should be person-centred, not this or that disorder-centred. We do not treat, for example, the schizophrenic disorder, but rather the individual. Thus, emphasize what is unique; and at the same time, look for what is common or ubiquitous (sameness) regarding suicide, psychopathology, and personality functioning in general. The therapist, in fact, must have a sound understanding of psychiatric/psychological disorders (pathology) and personality in general and, at the same time, must keep in mind that he/she is treating a person. Simply stated, we have to balance the unique and the general in any psychotherapy. If not, the therapist will not be able to intervene adequately and professionally with such people.

In terms of response, I also believe it is essential to comment upon category (d)—the antisocial (a psychopathic) disorder. If one is fed up with the patient "He's manipulating me", "She's just trying to get my attention", "He's a sociopath"—it is time to transfer the patient. This is an issue of countertransference. If one doesn't transfer the patient, one should redefine the problem or the issue and see where the patient hurts.

Finally, I would like to provide as an association a list of some special features that were derived from discussions with Dr Shneidman (see, for example, Shneidman, 1981c, 1985, for details):

- *Monitoring*. A continuous, preferably daily, monitoring of the patient's lethality.
- *Consultation*. There is almost no instance in a therapist's professional life when consultation with a peer is as important as when he/she is dealing with a highly suicidal patient. The items to be discussed might include the therapist's treatment of the case; his/her own feelings of frustration, helplessness or even anger; his/her countertransference reactions in general; the advisability of hospitalization for the patient, etc.
- *Hospitalization*. Hospitalization is always a complicating event in the treatment of a suicidal patient, but it should not on these grounds be eschewed. Obviously, the quality of care—from doctors, nurses, and attendants—is crucial.
- *Transference*. As in almost no other situation and at almost no other time, the successful treatment of a highly suicidal person depends heavily on the transference. The therapist can, for instance, be active, show his/her personal concern, increase the frequency of the sessions, involve the "magic" of the unique therapist–patient relationship, be less of a *tabula rasa*, and give "transfusions" of (realistic) hope and succorance.
- *Careful modification of the usual canons of confidentiality*. Admittedly, this is a touchy and complicated point, but the therapist should not ally him/herself with death. Statements given during the therapy session relating to the patient's overt

suicidal (or homicidal) plans obviously cannot be treated as a "secret" between two collusive partners.

V   Ego
16. *There is a relative weakness in the person's capacity for developing constructive tendencies (e.g., attachment, love).*

The key to intermediate, and long-range, effectiveness in suicide prevention is to increase the options for action—something more constructive than the wish to die. One has to widen the constriction beyond the only solution. Keep in mind that the suicidal act is an effort by the person to stop unbearable pain by the individual's "doing something", one made out of weakness, not strength. This knowledge usually guides us to what treatment should be: increase the constructive tendencies (or protective ones) and decrease the destructive one(s).

17. *There are unresolved problems ("a complex" or weakened ego) in the individual; e.g., symptoms or ideas that are discordant, unassimilated, and/or antagonistic.*

Working with highly suicidal persons borrows from the goals of crisis intervention in general, that is, not to take on and attempt to cure all the complexes in the person's personality immediately but simply to keep the person alive. This is the *sine qua non* of responding to the would-be suicide. However, it is critical that if one has to respond to this, or any, crisis effectively, one has to assess if something discordant, unassimilated, or antagonistic exists in the person. One must be skilled in assessment and prediction. We have to evaluate that person's complexes, anxiety, and other important aspects of his/her dynamics, psychopathology, and reaction patterns. Simply stated, you have to know the person to treat him/her effectively. Thus, it follows that a crisis responder must know something about suicide and personality functioning in general; otherwise, he/she will not know how to keep that person alive.

18. *The person reports that the suicide is related to a harsh conscience; i.e., a fulfilment of punishment (or self-punishment).*

This implies: Don't punish. Don't moralize. Don't preach. Don't pass judgement. Above all, don't agree with the person's major premises (e.g., "All evil people deserve to die. I am evil; therefore, I deserve to die").

Practically (when working with suicidal persons), we do what we can. We see people in consultation; we make interpretations; we write prescriptions, and so on. We also—which is critical—throw in our energies against punishment, and that proves often to be life-saving. Our positive attachment in intervention is, in fact, so critical and often life-saving. We need to reinforce the patient's ego.

Interpersonal

VI   Interpersonal Relations
19. *The person's problem(s) appears to be determined by the individual's history and the present interpersonal situation.*

Suicide is not just determined by the present; it has a history. Regrettably, the clues to suicide are usually not seen, heard, or even responded to before the act. People—spouse, parents, teacher, siblings, elders, and so on—have not seen the history. It follows, as a more general implication for response, that the ultimate prevention of suicide is public education about the clues: what to do and so on. Most people would agree that the best prevention is primary prevention. Primary prevention lies in education. The route is through teaching one another and the community that: (1) suicide can happen to anyone; (2) it has a history; (3) there are clues that can be looked for (if one but has the ability to see and hear them when they occur); (4) the interpersonal dynamics are critical, both for generating and preventing the event; and (5) help is available. Perhaps our main task lies in the dissemination of information, especially about the clues to suicide, in our offices, schools, work places, homes for the elderly, etc., and through the public media. The community, especially school systems, can make a major contribution to saving life; they can be protective factors. Prevention should be part of a comprehensive intervention to address suicide. (See A. Leenaars & S. Wenckstern (1990) *Suicide Prevention in Schools*.)

There is no question that education can be effective. Rutz et al. (1992) have, for example, shown that an educational programme for general practitioners on the Swedish Island of Gotland, resulted in a significant decrease in suicide risk. We need to educate all people, not only psychotherapists, in the care of suicidal patients.

20. *The person reports being weakened and/or defeated by unresolved problems in the interpersonal field (or some other ideal such as health, perfection).*

Suicidal people appear so preoccupied with an unresolved problem that they are often unaware of their developmental history and how they have previously adjusted to trauma, whether interpersonal loss or illness. They are fixated in the present pain. Yet, as outlined in Chapter 2, there is a history, their serial way of coping with problems. There is a suicidal career (Maris, 1981). They have often suffered repeated defeat. The problems have often been resolved by, for example, denial, avoidance, repression, and projection. This implies that one widens the adjustment processes including, but not limited to, helping the person to understand the past, the past maladjustment and how to cope better. All of this also implies that one should first resonate to the patient and his/her immediate unresolved problem, and then to his/her long-term needs. One must eventually address the history of unresolved problems in the patient's interpersonal (or some other ideal) field.

21. *The person's suicide appears related to unsatisfied or frustrated needs; e.g., attachment, perfection, achievement, autonomy, control.*

The pain of the suicidal person relates to the frustration or blocking of important psychological needs—that is, needs deemed to be important by the person (see Chapter 2 for a detailed list). It should be the therapist's function to help the individual in relation to those thwarted needs. Even a little improvement can save a life. The person needs some indication of the value of life, an affirmation of self. It is often just the possibility of a small amount of gain in their satisfaction of needs that gives the perturbed individual enough hope and comfort to divert the suicidal course. It provides an increase in self-esteem. In general, the goal is to increase the person's psychological comfort by addressing the frustrated needs. Shneidman's helpful question from his distress questionnaire (PDQ) is as follows.

My psychological pain is tied to my frustrated *needs* for (check three):
( ) *Achievement:* to accomplish the difficult; to master; to overcome.
( ) *Affiliation:* to affiliate with others; to remain a member of a group.
( ) *Aggression:* to overcome opposition; to oppose forcefully.
( ) *Autonomy:* to be free and independent of social confinement.
( ) *Counteraction:* to make up for failure by restriving; to overcome.
( ) *Defendence:* to defend or vindicate myself against others.
( ) *Dominance:* to control or influence others by persuasion or command.
( ) *Exhibition:* to make an impression; to entertain or shock or amuse.
( ) *Harmavoidance:* to avoid pain or injury or illness; out of harm's way.
( ) *Shame Avoidance:* to avoid humiliation or embarrassment or scorn.
( ) *Inviolacy:* to protect myself from others' interference; my own space.
( ) *Nurturance:* to gratify the needs of others; to help or console.
( ) *Order:* to put or keep things or ideas in good order; to be orderly.
( ) *Play:* to act for fun; to laugh or joke for its own sake.
( ) *Sentience:* to enjoy sensuous experiences and comforts of the senses.
( ) *Succorance:* to want to be helped or taken care of by others.
( ) *Understanding:* to want to know the answers; to ask questions; to speculate.

22. *The person's frustration in the interpersonal field is exceedingly stressful and persisting to a traumatic degree.*

A goal is to reduce the trauma—the real-life pressures, the frustrated needs—that is driving up the patient's sense of perturbation. Thus, decrease the distress at least to just below the traumatic degree. One assists the person in making the pain bearable but not to deny, repress, or deflect the pain, for this will serve as the energy for change. The person needs to face his or her trauma, whether interpersonal or otherwise. Suicide is an escape, a way of avoiding the trauma.

23. *A positive development in the disturbed relationship was seen as the only possible way to go on living, but such development was seen as not forthcoming.*

One has to decrease the interpersonal perturbation (or disturbance). One responds, "That sounds bad, what can you do (interpersonally, health-wise, whatever) and stay alive?"

24. *The person's relationships (attachments) were too unhealthy and/or too intimate (regressive, "primitive"), keeping him/her under constant strain of stimulation and frustration.*

One may, at times, have to assist the person in detaching him/herself from a too highly cathected (or sometimes even suicidogenic) person (or other ideal). The person may need to have his/her wishes stimulated and inhibited to a healthier degree. Thus, one may have to both increase and decrease relations. To increase the relationships, one may need to involve others actively in the suicidal individual's system (e.g., relations, family); not too infrequently the suicidal behaviour signals a system distress. (See A. Richman (1986) *Family Therapy for Suicidal People.*) Psychotherapy with suicidal patients often calls for a community approach.

VII   *Rejection–Aggression*

25. *The person reports a traumatic event or hurt or injury (e.g., unmet love, a failing marriage, and disgust with one's work).*

Experience has taught us the important fact that it is neither possible nor practical to respond to an individual who is experiencing an acute trauma by our use of punishment, moral persuasion, confrontation, or the like. The most effective way is by mollifying the felt trauma, reducing the elevated perturbation. It is the elevated perturbation that drives and fuels the elevated lethality; therefore, one tries to reduce the person's trauma—his/her anguish, tension, and pain. Shneidman's rule is: Reduce the elevated perturbation and the lethality will come down with it.

26. *The person, whose personality (ego) is not adequately developed (weakened), appears to have suffered a narcissistic injury.*

This classification implies at least three things: (1) The key to intermediate and long-range effectiveness with the suicidal person includes the following: to increase the options for action available to the person, to increase awareness of adjustment processes, to widen the angle of the blindness, to address the irrational (spontaneous) beliefs; and to increase objects available (beyond the narcissistic ones). (2) When the person is no longer highly suicidal, the usual methods of psychotherapy can be usefully employed. One does not leave the patient with his/her "weak", "primitive", and inadequately developed ego—he/she needs therapeutic assistance. (3) Finally, given all that, we need to be reminded that the work in suicide prevention is risky and dangerous, and that there are casualties. We can all cite more than one person whom we attempted to rescue (even hospitalized), but who killed him/herself (even in the hospital), as he/she found the narcissistic injury to be so pervasive.

27. *The person is preoccupied with an event or injury, namely a person who has been lost or rejecting (i.e., abandonment).*

The person is often preoccupied with a disturbed relationship (or other trauma). The therapist can say, "Tell me what's happening. Where does it hurt?" The individual, for example, will tell you about his/her loss, rejection, and abandonment, and will tell you his/her story. This implies that to help the suicidal person one must at times go into the real world as an ombudsperson to address the person's loss or rejection. He/she needs to find acceptance from someone. One should do all this without producing an unhealthy dependency, while at the same time recognizing that we ourselves are a decisive element in this therapeutic process, not only in developing family/social (community) interest and relationships, but also in developing that individual's positive identifications (protective factors).

28. *The person feels quite ambivalent, i.e., both affectionate and hostile towards the same (lost or rejecting) person.*

Often the person is ambivalent—he/she is not only affectionate and hostile towards a person, but is also ambivalent about life and death. One works first with the life and death issue on the side of life. Then one works with the affectionate feelings. Practically, however, both are probably responded to simultaneously—siding with life, attachment (affection) is implied.

29. *The person reports feelings and/or ideas of aggression and vengefulness toward him/herself although the person appears to be actually angry at someone else.*

One does not exacerbate the crisis in the sense of making it more real for the person by talking about it. One should not avoid the anger or rage. One should not buy into the taboo of "Don't talk about suicide and death". These people are already angry and hostile (and also hopeless and helpless). One does not create anger by giving voice to the person's pain. Ventilation, lightening of angry feelings, adequacy of expression, and need for contacts have a critical place in psychotherapy. Others, too, need to know that the trauma is "real" for the suicidal person, even if they wish to defend against or deny the crisis. The suicidal person's anger (or other feeling) needs to be heard (rather than introjected and especially not acted out). One has to address the social taboo of talking about suicide.

30. *The person turns upon the self murderous impulses that had previously been directed against someone else.*

The focus with such highly lethal people should not be immediately on "why" the aggression has been turned inward or "why" suicide has been chosen as the method of solving the problems. These are probably better addressed once the lethality is lower. Instead, the initial focus should be on solving the problems, so that the aggression, chosen for whatever reason, is mollified. The problems are discussed and addressed by what we can do about them. The person needs to see some hope (although simultaneously I would agree with some who point out how critical the hopelessness is for therapeutic intervention; see, for example, Smith, 1990). One talks about the aggression with the patient, but one also becomes concerned about practical items—job, rent, sickness, food, whatever. He/she needs at least a partial reduction of the urgently felt impulses or wishes, which were central to the suicidal end of his or her reverie. To address the impulses, including the aggressiveness, one must address the unmet needs. One does this not only in the consultation room but also in the real world.

31. *Although maybe not reported directly, the person may have calculated the self-destructiveness to have a negative effect on someone else (e.g., a lost or rejecting person).*

The therapist should remember that Eros can work wonders against Thanatos. Or, similarly stated, constructive goals can work wonders against destructive ones.

32. *The person's self-destructiveness appears to be an act of aggression, attack, and/or revenge towards someone else who has hurt or injured him/her.*

Suicide is often a dyadic event. The person feels hurt, slighted, or under attack. Revenge is frequently involved. As therapists, we should create activity—something, of course, different from consciously or unconsciously attacking another person. One should also remember a basic of intervention with such highly lethal individuals: Thinking is not a sufficient response.

VIII   *Identification–Egression*

33. *The person reports in some direct or indirect fashion an identification (i.e., attach-*
    ment) with a lost or rejecting person [or with any lost ideal (e.g., health, freedom,
    employment, all A's)].

The person has probably lost someone, a highly cathected person (or some other ideal). The main point with such a person is to increase that individual's psychological sense of possible choices and sense of being emotionally supported. After they have been determined to be on the life side of the individual's ambivalence, relatives, friends, and colleagues should be considered in the total treatment process. Treatment often needs to be a community effort. The person needs other objects (people) with whom to identify. Others can assist in establishing and/or re-establishing positive relations, and all this will help to build constructive tendencies, whether self-esteem, self-support, or some other life-enhancing processes. When so perturbed, the individual cannot simply give up even a negative part of his/her identity, nor can the individual often search out objects on his/her own. The person is simply in too much pain and too pessimistic to do this.

As a further point in relation to the involvement of others, suicide prevention is not best done alone. A combination of consultation, ancillary therapists, social networking, and use of all the interpersonal and community resources that one can involve is, in general, the best way to proceed.

34. *An unwillingness to accept the pain of losing an ideal (e.g., abandonment, sickness,*
    old age), allows the person to choose, even seek to escape from life and accept death.

Centrally, the therapist needs to focus on the "problem" that the individual is trying to solve—the loss, the sickness, old age, etc. Karl Menninger has provided us with an important dictum that is worth remembering: The patient is always right. It is our task to find out even in our earliest efforts of intervention, "how is he/she right?" Then we need to assist in developing an alternative solution(s) to the suicidal act. The person needs to know that something is being done to help him/her through the pain—to block the final egression.

35. *The person wants to egress (i.e., to escape, to depart, to flee, to be gone), to relieve the*
    unbearable psychological pain.

The person wants to escape. It follows that, where possible, the means of exit should be blocked. This is a protective factor. A practical application of this view is to "get the gun" in a suicidal situation where it is known that the individual intends to shoot him/herself and has a weapon (see Chapter 19). The explosive situation needs to be defused until that person no longer has the need for a suicidal weapon.

CONCLUDING REMARKS

Of greatest importance, we must understand that there are no universal formulations regarding suicide. We can speak of understanding, but never with precision. Our subject matter is suicide and we can be no more accurate or scientific than the available ways of investigating our subject matter permit. Our own investigations have not yielded universal laws. Yet, the yearning for universal suicidological laws, understandably, persists. A sweeping psychological statement with a ring of truth becomes a dictum. I believe that the search for a single universal formulation for suicide is an imaginary and non-existent conceptual fabrication—our own projection. It follows that the search for a singular universal response is also a foolish and unrealistic fancy. There is no one implication for psychotherapy.

One should use all measures with highly lethal individuals. These include support, behavioural techniques, psychodynamic interpretation, medication, hospitalization, and especially the involvement of others in the community, not only others to whom the patient was (or is) close but also "social" agencies—teachers, priests, elders, doctors, social workers, etc.—all of whom serve, directly or indirectly, to alleviate the pain. Treatment should be multimodal.

In principle, I do not believe in the solely individual private practice of suicide intervention with highly lethal individuals. Suicide intervention should be optimally practised in cooperation with a number of colleagues, representing various disciplines, and individuals other than the professionals (such as family, friends, crisis line workers, etc.). The community can help. The treatment of a suicidal person should reflect the learnings and response from different points of view; it should reflect a community approach.

Finally, intervention in the trenches is not as clean as has been described in this chapter. Therapists must constantly adjust, widening their formulations and actions.

SHNEIDMAN PSYCHOLOGICAL DISTRESS QUESTIONNAIRE

Name: ————————————— Age: ———————— Sex: ——————— Date: ——————————

Definition: Psychological pain is *not* bodily pain; it is how you feel as a person; how you feel in your mind (your joys or sadness, guilt or shame); how much you "hurt" as a human being, independent of your body. It is mental suffering; it is the opposite of "peace of mind".

1. **My psychological pain relates mostly to my *feelings* of (check three):**

( ) abandonment	( ) dread	( ) jealousy
( ) anger	( ) emptiness	( ) loneliness
( ) anguish	( ) fear	( ) powerlessness
( ) anxiety	( ) guilt	( ) rage
( ) bad conscience	( ) hopelessness	( ) shame
( ) confusion	( ) humiliation	( ) worry
( ) disgust	( ) inadequacy	( ) Other:

2. **The *intensity* of my psychological pain is (circle one number below):**

1	2	3	4	5	6	7	8	9
Little psycho-logical pain; almost non-existent	Mild	Moder-ate	Some-what bother-some	Present but manage-able between moder-ate and severe	Definitely hurtful	Harsh; rather severe	Definitely rather severe	Unbear-able; the worst discom-fort a person can ever experi-ence

3. **My psychological pain is tied to my frustrated *needs* for (check three):**

   ( ) *Achievement:* to accomplish the difficult; to master; to overcome.
   ( ) *Affiliation:* to affiliate with others; to remain a member of a group.
   ( ) *Aggression:* to overcome opposition; to oppose forcefully.
   ( ) *Autonomy:* to be free and independent of social confinement.
   ( ) *Counteraction:* to make up for failure by restriving; to overcome.
   ( ) *Defendence:* to defend or vindicate myself against others.
   ( ) *Dominance:* to control or influence others by persuasion or command.
   ( ) *Exhibition:* to make an impression; to entertain or shock or amuse.
   ( ) *Harmavoidance:* to avoid pain or injury or illness; out of harm's way.
   ( ) *Shame Avoidance:* to avoid humiliation or embarrassment or scorn.
   ( ) *Inviolacy:* to protect myself from others' interference; my own space.
   ( ) *Nurturance:* to gratify the needs of others; to help or console.
   ( ) *Order:* to put or keep things or ideas in good order; to be orderly.
   ( ) *Play:* to act for fun; to laugh or joke for its own sake.

(   ) *Sentience:* to enjoy sensuous experiences and comforts of the senses.
(   ) *Succorance:* to want to be helped or taken care of by others.
(   ) *Understanding:* to want to know the answers; to ask questions; to speculate.

[From Henry A. Murray (1938). *Explorations in Personality.* New York: Oxford University Press. Reproduced with permission].

Chapter 13

JUSTIN: A SUICIDE ATTEMPT IN A FOUR-YEAR-OLD BOY
(*His Mother Often Talked About Hanging Herself*)

> Hello. Dr Leenaars...This is Dr Smith in Windsor. I'm calling to see if you would accept a referral from our hospital. We have a patient who attempted to kill himself by hanging. He needs to be seen as soon as possible...He is a 4-year-old boy, the son of Dr Susanne Jones, one of our psychologists.

That was my first contact with a most extraordinary boy, Justin, who was in deep pain. Indeed, the pain had become so unbearable for him that he wanted to "go away". The case is perplexing and bewildering. Why would Justin, a bright and energetic 4-year-old boy, want to hang himself?

Many people do not believe that a 4-year-old—or even an 8- or 10-year-old—could kill himself. They simply deny the event; e.g., they would say: "Justin did not make an attempt. It was an accident or suicide-like behaviour". Yet, children do commit suicide. Although suicide is rare in children younger than age 12, it occurs with greater frequency than most people imagine. Unlike the relatively low number of children who commit suicide, there is a much higher percentage of children who attempt suicide and an even greater number who think about suicide. Pfeffer (1986) reported in a study of elementary school children that 11.9% of the children had thought about suicide. To my knowledge, there are no figures for completions and attempts.

How do we understand suicide in children? Defining suicide is a complex endeavour, even in adults. Pfeffer (1986) has suggested that the definition of suicide needs to be clarified somewhat for youth, providing the following comment: "It is not necessary for a child to have an understanding of the finality of death but it is necessary to have a concept of death, regardless of how idiosyncratic it may be" (p. 14).

To understand Justin's behaviour, one should keep Shneidman's definition in the foreground, with Pfeffer's clarification about death in mind. Much has to do with children's understanding of death. Although nobody (unconsciously) understands death, people's view of it shifts across the life-span and children have their own perspectives. Research (Nagy, 1948; Pfeffer, 1986) suggests that children's views differ depending on the age. Young children (approximately by age 7) see death as temporary; everything is alive and vulnerable to death. Children around 10 years of age see death as personified and temporary; an outside agent causes death. By the time a child is 12 years old—a young adolescent—he/she sees death as final; internal biological processes cause death. Yet, even older adolescents may misunderstand the finality of death. [A wonderful book to explain death to children is Mellonie & Ingpen's *Lifetimes* (1983).]

To begin to understand suicide in children, I will outline the case of Justin as an idiographic study. Next, I will attempt to show how the concept of the unconscious is necessary to understand his suicide attempt and suicide in children. It is necessary because the child's conscious mind has a large number of lacunae. The consciousness of the child cannot explain his/her suicide any more than in the adult.

Consciousness, as already shown in this volume, affords an insufficient explanation of behaviours. Only by presupposing other processes can one understand suicide. For a person of any age, consciousness is only a small part of the mind. From a developmental perspective, this is especially true in children. The assumption of the unconscious, in fact, is necessary to understand suicide in children. It allows one to better comprehend the enormous complexity of suicide in youth.

THE CASE: AN EXAMINATION

Justin is a 4-year-old boy, attending a pre-school setting. The main reason for referral was the suicide attempt. Justin had attempted to hang himself, still showing the rope marks upon intake. That attempt, however, was his mother's reason for referral, not Justin's. When asked, Justin was unsure initially why he was seeing a therapist (i.e., "a doctor").

Based upon his mother's report, Justin appeared to have been experiencing distress for two years. Justin's behaviour began to be regressive at times. Changes were noted in level of play, sleep patterns, level of activity, and anxiety. The identified stress was marital discord. She reported that Justin's father, Michael Jones, had been abusive, both emotionally and physically, towards Justin and herself. She described these incidents as severe, escalating in the last two months. Yet, the precipitating event was a quite chaotic fight between them four weeks ago. At that time, a chair was broken and furniture was thrown. Mr Jones then left the house and had not returned since that day. Through telephone calls, Dr Jones had learned that her husband had decided to separate and to leave the house. Subsequently, Justin's behaviour deteriorated, becoming quite depressed. The suicide attempt occurred about four weeks later.

Justin has no previous mental health history. Mrs Jones denied any disturbance, treatment, etc.; however, she reported that she now believes that Mr Jones was psychiatrically disturbed, having a "Narcissistic Personality Disorder".

Justin's medical history was unremarkable; he had the usual childhood illnesses. Only the reaction to the abusive father was identified as problematic. She reported that Justin was probably depressed. She knew of no psychiatric illness in her or her husband's family.

Mr and Dr Jones met at university about two years before they married. Dr Jones described the relation as positive, "not like with other men". They were both Catholic and socially established. When married they were financially supported by Mr Jones's family. She reported that there were no problems, until she decided to get pregnant. Mr Jones had wished to delay a family; however, Justin was conceived. She reported that after his birth, things changed, having less time for Mr Jones. She needed to be with Justin. By the time Justin was 2, the marriage was "dysfunctional".

Dr Jones was a psychologist, practising at a hospital. At the hospital, she had a position of responsibility in an adult inpatient unit. She reported no problems at work.

Mr Jones was not seen at intake because, according to Dr Jones, he was not interested in Justin. Dr Jones reported that her husband owned his own clothing store. The business did well, often with Mr Jones's father's support and involvement.

Justin was the only child in the marriage. Dr Jones reported that she was isolated from her family-of-origin with little involvement with them at this time. She did, however, report that Mr Jones's parents were involved in her family, often too much.

Dr Jones's reaction to the attempt was one of distress, reporting that she was overwhelmed. She did not believe that children could make attempts, finding the event highly perturbing. She reported that she was unsure of Mr Jones's reaction, suggesting that he may not care.

Justin's personal history was generally unremarkable until the age of 2 when the conflicts in the home arose. Pregnancy and birth were normal, although Dr Jones reported that her husband did not want children. Early motor and speech development were normal. Dr Jones suggested that Justin began to speak at an early age. Justin began to read by the age of 3. She reported that there were current problems at school, namely relating to other children, not following directions, and being overactive. She reported that Justin had no problems at nursery school earlier. In the last year, Dr Jones reported that Justin was clingier to her when she took him to the school. In fact, for the last four weeks Justin had been even more so. Aside from the abuse and rejection from Mr Jones, Dr Jones saw no other problems with Justin.

THE CASE: THE PROCESS

Utilizing a time sequence format let me outline the complexity of the case as it arose in treatment.

Dr Jones, visibly agitated, brought in her son; the rope marks were evident upon his neck. While Justin played in the playroom, she described the incident, telling me that she and her husband had been separated for four weeks, following a severe conflict in the home. She said that Justin was unhappy about the separation, especially since his father had not seen him during the four weeks. Justin was described as agitated and overactive. He frequently experienced "anxiety attacks", looking numb. "He often doesn't focus for minutes as if he is out of touch with reality", she said. She described frequent crying spells at home and at nursery school. Sleep disturbances occurred, requiring her to sleep with Justin frequently. He had been experiencing school problems lately, often not following directions and just "asking for me". Her diagnosis was a childhood depression as a result of her husband's neglect and abuse. I agreed with the diagnosis, but not necessarily with the reason.

When I saw Justin alone, he was cooperative; he enjoyed the playroom. However, he was unfocused, going from one toy to another. When I asked about how he was feeling he said, "I don't know". I asked if he was happy, he said "no". Upon enquiry, he said he wanted to see his father. I asked if he sees his father, he said, "I don't know"; yet, he revealed that he saw his father "last Sunday".

When I asked about the rope marks, he said, "I don't know." Since I primarily wanted to build an attachment, I allowed him to keep this inhibiting approach. We merely turned to drawing. See Figures 13.1 to 13.3 for some of Justin's first pictures in treatment.

Although my purpose in this chapter is not to address assessment, a few observations about Justin's drawings may assist. The contrast between Justin's picture of

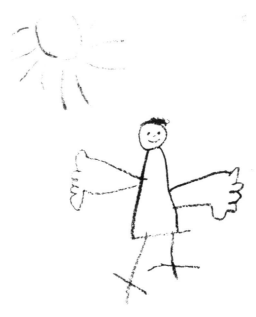

Figure 13.1   Justin's picture of himself

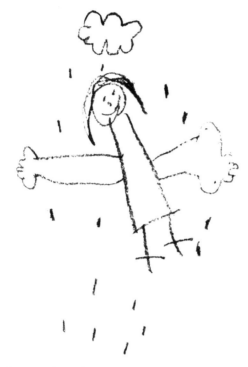

Figure 13.2   Justin's depressed mother

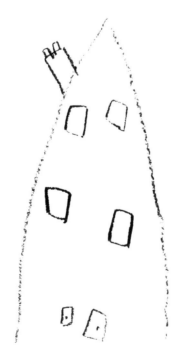

Figure 13.3   A house

himself being happy (e.g., sun) and the picture of his mother being depressed (e.g., rain), is critical. It reflected, largely unconsciously, Justin's perception of who was depressed. One can even note the greater slashes on Dr Jones's neck, something Richman (1986) has associated to suicidal behaviour. Figure 13.3 of the house is not that unusual for a child of Justin's age (although it was more primitive than his ability with words). The house might be remarkable because of the lack of smoke, which, like the inaccessible door, raises questions about what was occurring in the house.

Justin was obviously perturbed; however, how lethal was his act? Understandably, there are no observations or tests that will allow us to know how suicidal Justin was (Maris et al., 1992). Suicide is too complex, and that complexity is even more so with very young children. One needs to use one's clinical skill to evaluate the risk. Many questions arose, such as "What was so traumatic for Justin?"; "What were the dynamics in the family?"; and "What were the unconscious processes that allowed such a young boy to attempt to hang himself?"

Justin returned the next day. He brought me a picture (Figure 13.4), which, like the ones he had drawn for me the previous day, was quite revealing. It was a picture of "a house on fire" that he had drawn at school. The teacher had written Justin's story for me: "There is a fire. It was on Dandurand, in Windsor. The people died. But except the 8-year-old. He got out in enough time." The symbolism about his own family and his pain of isolation is obvious. How was Justin's pain to be addressed? Drawings are windows to the mind.

Dr Jones discussed further with me about Justin. She revealed that he had said, "I am going to see God," before the attempt. These words had been repeated for weeks. Perseveration was a hallmark of Justin's mind. He would often repeat acts and words in treatment. The statement about God had been occurring since the day of the separation, which Dr Jones described as "very violent".

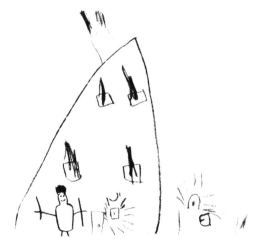

Figure 13.4   The fire

Justin became more familiar with the playroom, and, as he would do every day, he read books. Although he occasionally drew other pictures at my request, the books became our vehicle of communication. Treating children is often that—a relationship within the context of play.

A few days later, I saw Justin and his mother. The mother started to talk about her depression, describing her feelings as reactions to her husband's "abuse". My own impression was, however, that the depression was more endogenous. Justin himself was more perturbed; again, he had not seen his father.

At a next visit, I saw Dr Jones by herself, allowing me to discover more. She appeared to be a very dependent person, who struggled with that need. She described years of abuse by her husband, suggesting that the conflict arose upon Justin's birth. When queried about what she thought the reason might be for the conflict at that time, she said, "Justin needed me." Justin had often experienced verbal and physical conflicts in his family since the day of his birth.

She revealed in response to seeing Justin's picture (Figure 13.2), that she had realized that she was depressed. She said that she had been crying for months, suffering from severe sleep disturbance. She reported increasing isolation, with Justin as her only companion.

The next few weeks, the following events occurred:

(a) Justin arrived for therapy with a fire truck, which he had received from his father. He was most eager to show me the toy, whereas his mother was "having a hard time".
(b) Justin read books. Only after I asked about his father, did he show his agitation. Dr Jones again revealed that his father had not seen Justin.
(c) Dr Jones came in, very frustrated. She expressed extreme anger at her husband. At the same time, she reported that Justin had been acting out at school; for example, he was biting some other children.
(d) Justin arrived happier again, reporting that he saw his father. He talked about people being "mean". However, he was very vague about *who* was mean.

Towards the end of three months in treatment, Justin arrived with some drawings for me, which I believe was an expression of the increasing closeness in the therapeutic relationship. (See Figure 13.5 for a sample.)

For the first time, he spoke about his parents' fighting, stating, "I hate his (father's) butt." Upon this statement, he became more withdrawn, almost frightened. The next session, due to his mother's illness, Justin and I spoke on the telephone. It is sometimes critical to maintain ongoing contact with young children in treatment. The next session Justin said, "I hate it"; the "it" being his parents' fighting. He now began to verbalize more and revealed that he was feeling "sad". Justin, it may be assumed, began to trust me enough to talk about his feelings.

The next five sessions were much the same. Justin began to talk about "divorce", asking, "Who will I live with?" and "What if you/dad get remarried?". Justin also spoke about visits with his father that were more frequent now.

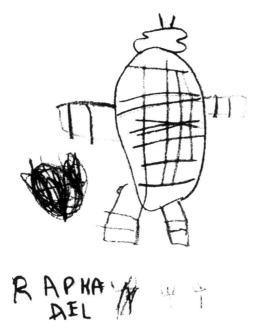

R APKA Y
DIL

Figure 13.5   Justin's hero "ninja turtle"

About $4\frac{1}{2}$ months in treatment, Dr Jones arrived alone, visibly agitated. She reported that "I want to let Michael (her husband) have custody". She wanted to get out of the situation, stating that "everything was too much". She was more willing to talk. She requested to see me alone, an idea that is not so unusual in my practice. Often seeing the parent speeds the child's healing.

The next session Justin decided to read Dr Seuss's "Horton Hears a Who". His favourite line was "a person is a person no matter how small". Justin's self-esteem needed a lot of reinforcement.

The following sessions were unremarkable. However, at the end of five months, Justin informed me that Barika, the class hamster, died. He said, "I felt sad", which led to talk about death. Justin's idea of death was much like younger children. He saw death as temporary; he understandably did not grasp its adult meaning. Throughout his treatment, death was a recurrent theme, something that Pfeffer (1986) has also observed in suicidal children.

About six months into treatment Dr Jones began to reveal more about herself. She reported a very conflictual relationship with her mother. She recalled words such as, "You'll never amount to anything." Her parents were divorced. These issues and others, as well as her own extreme inner anger, became the focus of our therapeutic work, which seemed to result in a just noticeable difference in Justin. The more Dr Jones attempted to work through her own pain, the less Justin's pain became.

One other important shift occurred with Dr Jones's increasing participation in treatment—Mr Jones became more involved with Justin. Justin, in fact, had his first overnight visit with his father, which Justin enjoyed, although he was "lonely" for his mother.

Regrettably, however, these advances were short-lived. Appointments were soon cancelled by Dr Jones. When she finally arrived, she revealed that her husband had a new girlfriend, stating that it was "not moral". Her ups and downs were cyclical.

At about seven months into treatment Justin's work, upon the announcement of a divorce, centred on that event. He talked, for example, about a classmate whose parents were divorced. At school, Justin began to act out more. For example, he urinated on another boy in the washroom. His mother's work in treatment became less productive. Her anger intensified and began to be expressed towards many people. However, she was most angry with Mr Jones, stating that she was often upset at home. She attempted to increase her mental separation from Mr Jones, stating "I've outgrown him", despite her increasing anxiety and insecurity.

Within days Justin's problems at school increased. He described the teachers as "not fair". He stated that he was being punished (with time-outs) "even when I'm good". His agitation increased.

Despite Dr Jones's agitation, she was responsive to my concerns, and those of the school, about Justin's behaviour. She reprocessed the suicide attempt, stating "I don't want him to die." Yet, she said, "There is nothing we can do."

Dr Jones was, in fact, mentally constricted. There was a narrowing of the range of perceptions or opinions or options that occurred to her conscious mind. She used words like "only", "always", "never" and "forever". One had continually to attempt to widen her blinders. She was generally unconscious of Justin's and her own dynamics.

Upon Dr Jones's request, about eight months into treatment, Mr Jones was seen for his first visit. I had previously requested that Mr Jones be involved in Justin's treatment; however, Dr Jones had either refused or indicated that her husband did not want to be involved. When I saw him, he was solely focused on Justin, asking for help. He wanted to know what he could do, suggesting that he wanted to be involved with Justin. Mr Jones was a somewhat anxious individual. He often let things get to him, being too passive and dependent. His father, despite retirement, often ran the business, much like what he described as his parents' overinvolvement in Justin's life. The separation had been very difficult for Mr Jones. Six months after the separation he finally began to socialize and date again.

He genuinely loved Justin, although, when married and after the separation, he was in conflict with Dr Jones over child-rearing practices. The slightest issue resulted in conflict—swimming classes, birthday parties, anything. Mr Jones described Dr Jones as "going on and on" in such situations, demanding her way. Although earlier agreeing to her wishes, in the last few years of the marriage, he began to state his disagreement with her. At such times, he would "lose it", and yell repeatedly. On a few occasions, he reported that he broke objects, including a rocking chair, on the day that he left. He, however, denied any physical violence towards Dr Jones or Justin.

Mr Jones disagreed with Dr Jones about issues of access to Justin (i.e., visitation rights). He reported that he had been refused access. He suggested that he was aware that Justin was upset about the separation and not seeing him on a regular basis. Yet, he said, "I didn't know what to do. She wouldn't let me see him."

After that visit, Justin and I spoke about his father's visit here. However, he would quickly switch topics, wanting only to play. Talking about his father was anxiety producing.

Next week, Mr Jones and Justin were seen together. That visit was productive for them, but Dr Jones, at her next visit, was agitated. We discussed her needs. A colleague had suggested that she was in need of an antidepressant. This suggestion was immediately rejected, with "I have no problems".

Over the next months, Justin and his mother were seen together or individually. Dr Jones was often upset, talking about "the game" Mr Jones was playing. Attempts at providing support became increasingly rejected. Her defensiveness increased and so did Justin's acting out at home and at school. On one such visit Justin arrived upset; he said that his father "broke a promise". He said, "He doesn't keep promises", stating that his father had not called him. He said, "I'm angry at him."

On one of Dr Jones's visits, when she was more introspective than usual, she revealed some tearful memories of her childhood. She described her mother as neglectful, recalling how she got no birthday cake on her seventh birthday. She now revealed that her mother was "a manic-depressive", despite having denied any family history of mental illness at intake. This was to be her last discussion about her mother; thereafter she focused only on her husband's emotional abuse, etc.

Shortly afterwards, Justin revealed that his father had come to the house and moved "his stuff" out. He was visibly agitated. For the first time, in fact, he became angry with me. We were reading a book, and he suddenly grabbed the book and slammed it down. "You did that wrong," he said. His next visit continued to be centred on my reading the book wrong. I asked if he was angry with someone, he said "Yes". He said, "My father is a thief." He suggested that his father stole his mother's money, adding, "You talk to him for six hours. I hate him."

Dr Jones, in her own meetings, expressed similar anger, suggesting that I might speak to Mr Jones. When I saw him, his story was quite different. He was perplexed about the problem, suggesting that the real issue was an attempt at financial settlement in the divorce proceedings. Our focus with Mr Jones became one of how to solve current problems, how to have Justin return for visits, etc.

Next meeting, Dr Jones informed me that Justin had said, "I want to kill dad." Indeed, a visit to his father had been conflictual, "as I predicted", she said. Justin had refused to listen to his father, being very demanding. This resulted in Mr Jones yelling at Justin. Justin, of course, had problems handling his feelings, as did Dr Jones. Dr Jones offered a memory of a girl in grade 4 who had abused her. This experience had been overwhelming, stating that her expressions towards the other girl were like Justin's today. Even today, she harboured homicidal wishes towards the girl.

The next week, Justin and his father were seen. Justin stated, "I don't want to see my father any more." He was quite angry and refused to talk. Later that same day, Dr Jones called, stating that a custody dispute had been started in court.

In our next visit, Dr Jones became focused on the issue of custody, stating that Mr Jones had filed for custody of Justin. However, Mr Jones on a later occasion announced that he was not seeking custody. He suggested that his wife was over-reacting, and that he was only asking for reasonable access to Justin. However, Dr Jones maintained her anger. She stated, "I wish I could kill him."

Despite that focus, for a few weeks during this time she became more relaxed and focused on herself. She described herself as "an insecure, crying little girl". During such periods, Justin was more at ease and visited his father. However, it was a labile situation. Often, the focus was only on her husband's abuse.

During these weeks, Justin's problem at school mirrored the home situation. Questions arose of whether he had an Attention Deficit Disorder—a diagnosis that was not accurate.

Justin's behaviour in my office equally mirrored the home. On one such occasion, he talked about "the fight" that had occurred four weeks before the attempt. He said that his parents were fighting that day. They were pushing each other. "My father grabs a rocking chair," he said. "He breaks it and says, 'Eat this.'" This story, after its first telling, became repetitive. It was quite meaningful to Justin and was symbolic of his broken family. Figure 13.6 shows a picture of Justin in his home. The inner turmoil is expressed by the heavy lines (or chaos) inside his body. Equally the

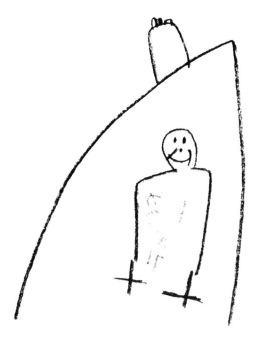

Figure 13.6   A house with Justin boxed in

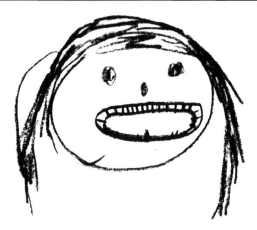

Figure 13.7 Justin's "angry" mother

"Eat this" was reflective of the unresolvable problem—a situation which is beyond a child's ability to solve—something that Orbach (1988) has isolated as a repetitive theme in many suicidal children. Destructive events are a necessary prerequisite to a suicidal solution in a child.

Both parents recalled the event for me in treatment, although quite differently. Neither recalled the statement about the chair, although a chair had been broken by Mr Jones. It was the day that he left. During one of Mr Jones's visits, I confronted him about the event. He agreed that Justin witnessed a lot of "yelling", although he described both his wife and himself as participating in the turmoil that day. He left that day because he felt that the conflicts were destructive for Justin.

Justin announced "I'm angry", talking about the fights between his parents. He vacillated between his father and both parents. It was the first expression of anger, albeit ambivalently, towards his mother. Figure 13.7 shows a picture of Justin's mother. From my view, the picture shows anger. The mother's face with the plentiful teeth and the wide open engulfing mouth lead to being incorporated (chewed up).

Ten months into treatment, in response to Justin's problems at school (e.g., questions about his diagnosis, etc.), a school meeting was planned. Dr Jones and Mr Jones were at that meeting, the only time I ever saw them together. Indeed when Justin saw them, he showed his biggest smile.

Justin was described as very bright; he was estimated to be "gifted". Yet, he was seen as inattentive and unable to concentrate. He was described as "hyper", being aggressive and acting out frequently, especially towards a female teacher.

His diagnosis was explored. The teachers suggested that Justin had an Attention Deficit/Hyperactivity Disorder (ADHD). Reviewing criteria, an alternative was proposed, a post-traumatic reaction within the context of a childhood depression. I discussed the events leading to the separation, the family's conflicts, the evening of the broken chair, etc., and Justin's inability to cope, leading to childhood depressions. Although nosological classifications with children are problematic, they can be useful as a metaphorical communication. The school seemed to accept the post-traumatic label and the ideas about depression.

During the school interview Dr Jones several times became irate, yelling and screaming at Mr Jones. She focused on his lack of support for Justin's swimming classes, a repetitive theme over the last few months. Mr Jones, despite his frustration, remained calm. The meeting ended with satisfaction for the school, not Dr Jones. It was agreed by all that everyone had to work together.

The next appointment for Dr Jones and Justin at my office was not kept. Dr Jones arrived for the following appointment alone, although such visits became rare. She was singly focused on the fact that Mr Jones had abused her, refusing to discuss the school meeting. Subsequent visits alone or with Justin were characterized by the repetitive ups and downs.

Mr Jones, on the other hand, started attending meetings more frequently and asked for a referral for treatment. He suggested that his father was not loving, adding, "I don't want to be like him." Mr Jones said that he wanted to help and work on his relationship with Justin. However, he was at times deflective, avoiding questions about the family's past experiences.

During one of Justin's visits, after his pet bird had died, he asked what would happen if he fell out of the window of my eighth-floor office. He said, "My brain would fallout and I (he) would see this." Death became a preoccupation for Justin. After one visit to his father, Justin's mother was not home to receive him. Justin stated, "Mom is dead." On another occasion he stated to his father, "You hate me. You want me dead." He also asked me on occasion if I would die. Figure 13.8 shows an expression of Justin's wish to be "away". He wanted to be on a spaceship to "go away".

About one year into treatment, Justin's preoccupation with death resulted in Dr Jones returning to see me alone; she had taken a lengthy hiatus from therapy after the visit at school. She was very worried about Justin. She reported that Justin had asked if the rope burns were still on his neck. However, her concern was short lived.

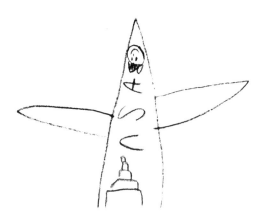

Figure 13.8   An expression of Justin's wish to "go away"

JUSTIN: A SUICIDE ATTEMPT IN A FOUR-YEAR-OLD BOY 243

Dr Jones also announced that she had been dating Dr Clark, a psychiatrist at her hospital, who was being supportive of her. She said that he discouraged the need for her to be at my office. "The problem", she said, "is Mr Jones." Dr Clark had confirmed her belief that she had no problems. When asked about Justin's reaction to Dr Clark, she said, "It's not upsetting." Subsequent meetings were generally cancelled although Justin continued individually.

At the next session, Justin introduced the topic of Dr Clark to me, suggesting generally a vague, non-revealing reaction to him. Justin revealed that he had been told not to mention Dr Clark to me. Dr Jones's lack of participation was increasingly having an impact on treatment. Justin became less active. Mr Jones, on the other hand, became more concerned, focusing on how he could best handle situations.

Dr Jones arrived to see me, announcing that she felt better and had no need for help, except for Justin. On one occasion, Justin said to his mother, "I'm angry at you. You don't let me ... " That proved to be very problematic; Dr Jones became quite upset at Justin. She said, "You don't hate me! You hate your dad."

On a later visit, she stated, "I don't want to be here. I can solve all my problems." However, five days later, she called about an incident with Mr Jones. They again were arguing over Justin. Justin was to go to a birthday party during a visit with Mr Jones. Dr Jones had not told Mr Jones and that resulted in Justin being quite upset. Dr Jones claimed that Mr Jones was being abusive.

A new issue arose about school. Dr Jones wanted Justin to go to a private school, but Mr Jones suggested a public system. This became a very conflictual issue. As in the past, Justin was caught in the middle, similar to the issue depicted by the broken chair. He felt upset. It is likely that, without support, his thoughts would have escalated again towards death.

On one of Mr Jones's visits I confronted him about physical abuse. Despite his defensiveness, he revealed a different story. "She was abusive," he said. He admitted to being verbally abusive but again denied any physical abuse. He said that he was often cornered, feeling helpless. He said, "There was no way out." He said that he felt "castrated", feeling the "push, push" from his wife as unbearable.

Mr Jones also revealed now that Dr Jones had often been suicidal. He stated that she would talk about killing herself in front of Justin. She would say, "I'll hang myself." At other times, she would say, "I'll kill myself." In fact, he described his wife as very depressed at times and aggressive at other times. "She swings up and down," he said.

About 14 months into treatment, Justin and Dr Jones arrived together; it had just been Justin's sixth birthday. We spoke and read his favourite book, *Horton Hears a Who*. He said, "I feel better."

That was the last meeting with Justin. Dr Jones had come to announce that she was moving back to London, Ontario, with her mother. Her relationship with Dr Clark had failed and she felt that she needed a change. "That will solve the problem," she said. She suggested that her family would be supportive, hoping finally to be away from Mr Jones.

Mr Jones continued his contact. He and Dr Jones divorced; he remarried. He continued to see Justin, with access being spelled out in the divorce agreement. These visits were often positive, he suggested.

Six months after Justin's abrupt termination, I was contacted by Dr Berger, a therapist in London. Dr Jones had followed my recommendation for continued treatment for Justin.

Three years after my contact, Mr Jones called. He reported that Justin was doing well, continuing to see his therapist. Dr Jones, however, he reported, had been hospitalized, following a period of highly lethal thoughts of suicide by hanging. The hospitalization resulted in greater intervention. Dr Jones was prescribed lithium and is still being seen for psychotherapy. Mr Jones also carried a message from Justin: "Hello Dr Leenaars. I remember *Horton Hears A Who!*"

CASE DISCUSSION: PRELIMINARY CONSIDERATIONS

It is simply wrong to view suicide from a single perspective. Suicide, regardless of age, is a multidimensional malaise. It is a complex event. I will outline a few comments about Justin's developmental age; present a few notes about lethality and perturbation; provide a general frame to understand suicide; discuss how the unconscious is a necessary concept to explain suicide in children, highlighting attachment; and make a few points about treatment. Finally, I will provide a brief concluding remark.

A DEVELOPMENTAL PERSPECTIVE

People are developing beings. Erikson's outline of human development (Erikson, 1963, 1968) is the best-known developmental perspective although alternative models have been presented (e.g., Carl Jung, Charlotte Buhler, Sigmund Freud). Erikson's model "provides one view of the 'river of life' and its major turning points and forks, so that we might have a sense of what the crucial challenges are for the individual at various points along the stream" (Kimmel, 1974, p. 23). To frame Justin's points on the life-span, a brief outline of Erikson's view will be presented with approximate chronological ages noted, although no development age can be rigidly defined. Some people mature earlier, some later, depending on the ego's structures (as related to familial function, brain damage, etc.).

From birth to approximately the age of 2, one develops a sense of the world. The world is related to the primary caregiver, the mother in America's culture. The experience with the parents is crucial; the child develops either trust or mistrust. It is an early stage of individuation, the early beginnings of an identity. It is also the beginning of a child's experience of pain. The capacity to adjust begins almost immediately and out of that, one's ego—the part of the mind that reacts to reality and has a sense of individuality—begins to form, as does one's earliest structures for attachments. Strength is primarily derived from the ego strength of the parents. With trauma, a growing inability to cope may occur, and one may learn a basic mistrust.

Between approximately 2 and 4, the child matures, exerting greater control over self and the outside world (Frager & Fadiman, 1984). The child develops a sense of autonomy. The child begins to test his/her trust or mistrust. Some children become overly rigid or controlled by developing a demanding conscience with the earliest signs of self-punishment in a few. Rather than adjust, they develop a strong sense of shame or self-doubt. The child feels deficient, having a lack of esteem with weaknesses being constantly exposed. On the other hand, with a supportive environment, even during trauma, other children develop autonomy. The child develops a sound and healthy will. In Justin's case, there is no question about the lack of autonomy. Indeed, one even wonders about the earlier stage; how did Dr Jones and/or Mr Jones address Justin's earliest needs? It is likely that Justin experienced early traumatic events and his needs were frustrated. After all, Dr Jones was focused on her own depression. A climate of detachment must have prevailed.

After Erikson's second stage (i.e., autonomy vs shame and doubt), the child de-velops initiative or guilt. The child experiences greater conscious mobility; one's ability to adjust expands; and one develops mastery and responsibility. Language is a prime example. Equally, the child learns to plan ahead and to have purpose (Ginsberg & Opper, 1969; Piaget, 1970; Piaget & Inhelder, 1969). However, a child's ability to cope can be hampered. The child must do more and his/her learning can be hindered by the parents (for example, as would be experienced in the home of an alcoholic parent). With weakened mobility and inquisitiveness the child develops anxiety, a deep sense of pain. The parents, for example, may support self-guidance and/or self-punishment. If a parent is highly suicidal, the child may equally intro-ject that destructiveness. In some, the anxiety, guilt, etc., is too much to bear, and the pain becomes unbearable. Justin obviously showed such early signs, especially at age 5. He often had, for example, people respond to him as if he was "bad". At the earliest meeting, Justin was self-critical. He knew no direction. Everything had collapsed, symbolized by the "broken chair".

It is important to remember that development does not stop here. Development is continuous, not discontinuous. Development occurs across the life-span (Erikson 1963, 1968; Piaget, 1970). Development is dynamic, ongoing and serial. The suicidal person, even at Justin's age, does not respond anew to each crisis in life but his/her reactions are highly consistent. There is an *elliptical* nature to one's development (Shneidman, 1985).

A FEW PRELIMINARY CONCEPTS

There is no *one* definitive behaviour in children—or people of any age—that is predictive of suicide. As we have discussed, suicide is a multidimensional event across the life-span. Two concepts that are extraordinarily useful and helpful to understand suicide are *lethality* and *perturbation* (Shneidman, 1985) and both concepts are needed in order to understand the depth of pain—or, if one wishes, psychopathology—of suicidal children. All sorts of children are highly perturbed but not suicidal. Lethality is especially difficult to predict in children, in part, because of the time-line. Tests for risk assessment in children have been shown to be of little use to assess lethality (Leenaars & Wenckstern, 1994; Lewinsohn et al.,

1989; Maris et al., 1992). In the case of Justin, his perturbation on quantification scales would be high. His lethality, based on clinical judgement, would be moderate on a few occasions, not high. Overall, his lethality on a day-to-day basis was low.

A PSYCHOLOGICAL THEORY OF SUICIDE

To understand suicide, like any behaviour, one must go beyond general development and even psychopathology in children (Achenbach, 1974; Bemporad, 1980; Cameron, 1963; Eissler et al., 1977; A. Freud, 1965; Horney, 1950). A psychology of suicide is needed (Leenaars, 1988a). Shneidman (1985) suggests that to develop such a model—a psychological theory regarding suicide—one must begin with the question, "What are the interesting common psychological dimensions of suicide?", rather than what kind of people, even as a child, commit suicide. This question, he says, is as true for children as for adolescents, the elderly, etc. (Shneidman, 1991).

Shneidman (1991, p. 40) writes:

> Of course, blacks, females, unemployed, AIDS patients—and, apropos, the human life course—children, youth, adults and oldsters commit suicide, and it is often useful to group suicides under such rubrics. But it is meaningful only if one goes further and looks at underlying patterns. In my analysis of suicide, there are no separate youth suicides, adult suicides, gerontological suicides; there is only human suicide and all of it is to be understood in terms of the same principle.

Most frequently, non-professionals identify external causes as the reason for a child's suicide (e.g., ill health, being abandoned by a parent, divorce) as what is common in suicide. A recent downhill course (e.g., divorce, death of a parent, a suicide) can, indeed, be identified in suicide. However, although there are always situational aspects in every suicidal act, these are only the precipitating events. Suicide is more complex, even in children. Suicide is a multidetermined event. To understand the psychological complexities of suicide in children, let me rewrite what we have learned about suicide, with specific reference to children.

To begin, let me state that I agree with Shneidman (1985) that the psychological dimensions of suicide, even in children, are the "trunk" of suicide. As for all people, for children, suicide is an intrapsychic drama on an interpersonal stage. From this psychological view, I (Leenaars, 1988a, 1989a, 1989b, 1994) believe that suicide in children can be understood from the following components.

Intrapsychic

Unbearable Psychological Pain
The common stimulus in suicide is unendurable psychological pain (Shneidman, 1985). The suicidal child is in a heightened state of perturbation and the child primarily wants to flee from pain. The child feels especially boxed in and that is so painful for many suicidal children. The situation is unbearable and the child

desperately wants a way out of it (even if the child's concept of death is not fully developed). It provides relief from intolerable suffering expressed, for example, as "I can go to sleep" or "I can go to see God".

How is it possible for a 4-year-old child to be in so much pain? Was Justin's pain unbearable? These are obviously difficult questions. Yet, my own opinion and that of others (Orbach, 1988; Pfeffer, 1986) is that children, indeed, can experience unbearable pain. At even younger ages, children experience pain as, for example, in the case of failure-to-thrive infants (Fraiberg, 1980). As young as 8 months, individual differences can be objectively noted in children's behaviour in play (Wenckstern et al., 1984). There are various reasons for such differences including trauma (Fraiberg, 1980), consistent with theory (e.g., Erikson, 1963, 1968). Justin was perturbed, agitated, and troubled. He felt boxed in. Everything was broken. He, as well as his mother, wanted it to go away.

Cognitive Constriction

The common cognitive state in suicide is constriction (Shneidman, 1985). This is heightened in children because of the level of cognitive development (Piaget, 1970). The child is figuratively intoxicated or drugged by the constriction, resulting in dysfunction in emotions, language, perception, and even bodily functions. Significant regression(s) may occur. The suicidal mind is, thus, in a special state of relatively fixed purpose and of relative constriction. This constriction in children is one of the most dangerous aspects of the suicidal state of mind.

Justin was mentally constricted—the constriction was probably associated with his inability to assimilate all of the trauma, e.g., the abuse, the abandonment by the father, the depression of the mother. Justin was often singly preoccupied with one event, such as the fact that I read something wrong. A more concerning example was his preoccupation with death. His emotions, perceptions, language, etc., reflected this state of mind. One often witnessed regression, mainly as a reaction to the state of mind of his mother. Dr Jones was equally constricted: the problem was Mr Jones. Her only solution was to punish her husband, which Justin expressed, for example, in my need to speak to his father for six hours.

Indirect Expressions

Complications, ambivalence, redirected aggression, unconscious implications, and related indirect expressions (or phenomena) are often evident in suicide. The phenomena are oblique. Love and hate clash. Yet, there is much more. What the child is consciously aware of is only a fragment of the suicidal state of mind. Suicide is complex, more complicated than the child's conscious mind had been or can be aware (Leenaars, 1993b). The driving force, as I will discuss below, may well be unconscious processes.

Justin was ambivalent; he often expressed contradictory feelings, attitudes and thrusts towards Mr Jones, his father. Sometimes he was happy, and at other times he was not happy. His love and hate clashed, which, I believe, was equally true with respect to his mother. He expressed his anger towards her on a few occasions. However, Justin was punished for them and although Dr Jones prohibited such feelings she did not succeed in banishing them. Justin needed to repress these emotions, for only love towards her was allowed. Dr Jones was equally ambivalent, even towards Justin. She expressed for a period of time, the wish to abandon Justin—a fact that Justin knew. More frequently, if Justin did not meet her expectations, he was rejected. Her aggression was redirected towards Justin and, obviously, at Mr Jones. However, her deep anger towards her own mother (and an obviously absent father) was buried. The family's dynamics were primarily indirect and, as I will discuss in detail, unconscious.

Inability to Adjust

Although a large percentage of suicidal children exhibit depressive disorders, conduct or behavioural problems, childhood schizophrenia, panic disorders, attention-deficit disorders, learning disabilities—to name a few possibilities—have also been related to suicide in children (Leenaars, 1988b). Most importantly, in fact, suicidal people of all ages do not survive life's difficulties. With children, given their developmental age, they are often insufficiently developed to cope with the pain.

First and foremost, as a relevant aside, it should be understood that not all suicidal children are depressed and that not all depressed children are suicidal. Depression and suicide are *not* equivalent. Yet, Orbach (1988) and Pfeffer (1986, 1993) have noted that depressive disorders distinguish many suicidal children from non-suicidal groups. Depression can be noted in mood and behaviour (ranging from feeling dejected and some hesitancy in social contacts, to being difficult to contact, isolation, serious disturbance of appetite and sleep), verbal expression (ranging from talk about being disappointed, excluded, blamed, etc., to talk of suicide, being killed, abandoned, helpless), and fantasy (ranging from disappointed, excluded, mistreated, etc., to suicide, mutilation, loss of a significant person). Behaviours such as excessive aggressiveness, change in school performance, decreased socialization, somatic complaints, loss of energy, and regressive change in behaviour (e.g., toilet habits, talk) have all been associated with depression (Pfeffer, 1986), although the mode of expression will depend on the child's developmental age (Leenaars, 1991a; Pfeffer, 1993). However, not all depression is overt. Children can exhibit "masked depression" (Leenaars & Wenckstern, 1991). This was certainly the case with Justin, such as in his acting out at school. He was depressed. Data suggested that this had been true for several years, being exacerbated by his parents' separation.

Justin was unable to cope and the break-up of his family was too much to bear. He was, in part because of his age, unable to discern accurately what was going on. Justin was depressed. He had been weakened by a steady toll of trauma. Dr Jones was even more weakened.

If one wishes to use a nosological classification, Justin exhibited a childhood depression. Post-traumatic symptoms were evident, a fact which I have observed in most suicidal children. Justin had experienced an unusual event for him, namely the break-up of the family (American Psychiatric Association, 1987). However, this event was a culmination of ongoing abuse. He persistently experienced intrusive recollections of the broken chair incident. As another example, in the case of

6 year-old David, the recurrent event was an abandonment by the father (Berman et al., 1991). Justin re-experienced his trauma in his play. There was the ever-present fear of losing his mother, as had occurred on the evening that his father returned Justin from a visit and Justin's mother was not at home. Mr Jones took Justin back to his home, and Justin's mother finally called Mr Jones two hours later. During those two hours, Justin was perseverant over his mother's death (which she herself often expressed in the talk of suicide). Justin avoided talking about his pain, often being numb. He had difficulty sleeping, was irritable, and had difficulty concentrating. He often exhibited dissociative behaviours. Needless to say, Justin was traumatized by the age of 4, his depression was so deep. However, Dr Jones's depression (major affective disorder) was even deeper.

Ego

Ego strength is a protective factor against suicide. In children, the ego is often not sufficiently developed. These children have been emotionally deprived of mature growth. Their egos have probably been weakened by a steady toll of traumatic events (e.g., loss, rejection, abuse). This implies that a history of traumatic disruptions, even for a young child, places the person at risk for suicide. It disrupts the child's ability to develop mechanisms (or ego functions) to cope. The weakened ego correlates positively with suicide risk (Jung, 1974). The child's ego, is, thus, a critical factor in the suicidal scenario.

As a child's earliest relationships are critical for the development of an ego (Mahler, 1968), Justin's ego was inadequately developed, offering little strength to cope with events. Even his earliest time-lines were hampered; his mother's own ego strength was lacking. If one examines Justin from Erikson's model of development (1963, 1968) the deficits are obvious. Justin learned mistrust. He lacked autonomy (as did Dr Jones). These earliest years placed Justin at risk; he had not developed the necessary function to adjust. Mr Jones, although more adequately developed, had clear lacunae in his ego, being susceptible to regression during periods of conflict. He would be verbally aggressive at such times. Dr Jones was even more hampered in her development and I suspect, from a generational perspective, that her mother was also troubled.

Interpersonal

Interpersonal Relations

The suicidal child has problems occurring within a disturbed, unbearable familial situation (Sullivan, 1962, 1964; Zilboorg, 1936, 1937). A calamitous relation in the family has likely prevailed. Suicide appears to be often related to unsatisfied or frustrated attachment (affiliation) needs. For example, the child only wants the family to be together. The person's psychological needs are frustrated, exemplified in the often dysfunctional family. Almost always, if not always, the relationships of the parents themselves are disturbed and the children express that dysfunction.

Thus, the family system as supported by ample studies (e.g., Corder & Haizlip, 1984; Corder et al., 1974; Leenaars, 1988b; Leenaars & Wenckstern, 1991; Orbach,

1988; Pfeffer, 1981a, 1981b, 1986, 1993; and Toolan, 1981) is a central factor associated with suicide and suicidal behaviour in children, although by no means do all families of suicidal children display all characteristic patterns of dysfunction. I will attempt to outline these dysfunctions in more detail here because of their central role in childhood suicide. Based on a review of the above references, below are a few common observations regarding suicidal children and their families (although by no means should the list be construed as exhaustive):

1. There is, at times, a lack of generational boundaries in suicidal families. There is an insufficient separation of the parent from his or her family of origin. For example, grandparents take over the parenting role.
2. The family system is often inflexible; any change is seen as a threat to its survival. Denial, secretiveness, and especially a lack of communication are seen in the family. Additionally, such families have strict discipline patterns and limit setting, which restrict the individual in early development. In some cases, even basic behaviours such as eating, toilet use, playing are excessively controlled.
3. At times, there is a symbiotic parent–child relationship. A parent is too attached to the child. Not only is such a relation disturbing, but the parent does not provide the emotional protection and support that a parent usually provides intuitively to a child as he/she grows. Sometimes the parent treats the youth as an "adult". One can see such problems, especially at the ages 4 to 5, when the child needs to separate from the parents. Additionally, it has been noted over and over that if a symbiotically enmeshed parent exhibits an emotional dysfunction, such as suicidal behaviour, the child may exhibit similar behaviour, such as a wish to be magically united with that parent if the parent dies. Indeed, the child may act out the pathology of the parent(s).
4. Long-term disorganization (malfunctioning) has been noted in families of suicidal children, such as maternal or paternal absence, divorce, alcoholism, mental illness. Sexual abuse is more prevalent than in the general population. These problems are often generational.

Justin's family was dysfunctional. People in Justin's family had problems in establishing and maintaining relationships. This was true for Dr Jones and Mr Jones. There was an unbearable, disturbed, familial situation. All was calamitous. There was a lack of individuation in both parents, more so in Dr Jones. The family was inflexible—everything had to be done to suit Dr Jones. Justin's parents lacked communication. Justin's behaviour was extremely controlled. Only certain aspects of his abilities were promoted, e.g., his verbal skills. There was an overly symbiotic relationship between Justin and his mother (which I will discuss in detail below). The Jones family had a history of malfunctioning, e.g., abuse, mental illness. In the familial context, Justin's needs were not met, and, I suspect, neither were the needs of Dr Jones or Mr Jones. Justin's pain was an expression of the family dysfunction.

Rejection–Aggression
The rejection–aggression hypothesis was documented by Stekel in 1910 (Friedman, 1967) and is clearly evident in the suicidal child's family. Loss and rejection are central to suicide; they are often experienced as abandonment. The child is deeply

ambivalent, but because of the anger in such families the child must deny such feelings. Anger is often unacceptable for the child, whether towards a person or in general. Suicide may be veiled aggression—it may be turning back upon oneself some murderous impulses (wishes, needs) that had previously been directed against a traumatic event, most frequently a rejecting or dysfunctional parent (Freud 1974g).

Loss was central in Justin, and not only loss of his father. I believe that Justin experienced an ongoing abandonment in his home. He was often narcissistically injured by his parents (especially Dr Jones) who themselves were narcissistically deprived (Miller, 1981, 1986). There were deep ambivalences. Aggression was often expressed outwardly, especially towards Mr Jones. Dr Jones had murderous impulses towards her husband (and her mother). However, equally, the aggression was turned inwards. Her suicidal behaviour was probably veiled aggression, and Justin's own act, as I will show, was intertwined with her anger.

Identification–Egression
Freud (1974g, 1974i) hypothesized that intense identification—i.e., attachment, with a lost or rejecting person or any ideal, often towards a parent—is crucial in understanding the suicidal person. This is especially true if that parent is suicidal, or had died, killed him/herself, abandoned the family, etc. If this emotional need is not met, the suicidal child experiences a deep discomfort (pain) and wants to escape . . . to be dead, within the context of the child's idiosyncratic concept of death. The child wants, for example, to escape or be magically reunited with the lost or rejecting parent.

Justin was as deeply attached to his mother as she was to him. There was an intense identification (bond). However, this emotional need was doomed since Dr Jones was not able to form a healthy relationship. It is likely that Justin had only partly differentiated himself from his mother so that he was his mother and she was him, to a great degree. Mr Jones, on the other hand, was hindered in developing a close relationship to his wife because of Dr Jones's pathology (as well as the family dynamics generally and his own ego weaknesses). Mr Jones was constantly pushed away as the bad parent (or person), which Anna Freud (1966) has called a splitting of the parents. One parent is bad, whereas the other is good in such families. In such an atmosphere, it would be impossible for Justin to have his emotional needs met. His attachments were deeply troubled and he wanted to go away. Even more so, Dr Jones wanted to egress, to be gone. The suicide attempt of Justin was an expression of both of their wishes.

Of course, in concluding these psychological observations, it needs to be remembered that suicide in children is more than this. These common elements, however, highlight that suicide is not simplistic, even in children. The common consistency in suicide is with the child's development of adjustment patterns (Leenaars, 1991a; Shneidman, 1985). It is not only coping with unbearable pain. It is coping with a history of that pain, consciously and unconsciously, commonly generational.

With the commonalities of suicide in mind, it is possible to structure suicidal phenomena from a developmental point of view. Though suicide is in many ways the same across the life-span as Shneidman (1991) argued, it is productive to consider Justin's behaviour equally from a developmental point of view. Simply put, I believe that it is useful to frame a suicidal child's characteristics within a develop-mental perspective. Yet, the differences that we observe across the life-span may not be the presence or absence of a characteristic, but the mode of expression of that characteristic. The suicide of children is both different from and *the same* as older people.

UNCONSCIOUS PROCESSES

The concept of the unconscious, I believe, is necessary to understand Justin's sui-cide attempt. It is necessary because the conscious has a large number of gaps. The manifest content of the act cannot explain his suicide attempt. It provides an insuf-ficient explanation of Justin's behaviour. Only by including additional factors can one understand Justin. The assumption of the unconscious is, in fact, necessary. It allows us to understand the enormous complexity of Justin's behaviour and his family. It allows us to dig into the deeper aspects of the "trunk".

My perspectives here are largely based on a number of tenets of dynamic psy-chology. It accepts the distinction between conscious and unconscious. It accepts the distinction between manifest and latent, and that there are therapeutic tech-niques for inferring the latent implications from the manifest content. For example, it implies that Justin's representation of the broken chair is an expression of the unconscious. The broken chair has an obvious latent meaning: the broken fam-ily. I do not mean to suggest that the unconscious singly explains suicide (or any behaviour) of a child. My point is that it is possible to understand Justin's suicide attempt from a perspective that includes the unconscious. One needs to go beyond the manifest level, such as his mother's explanation of Mr Jones's abuse. We must put Justin's suicide attempt within the context of his and his family's latent lives.

Research (Leenaars, 1986, 1993b; McLister & Leenaars, 1988) supports this view. This research, as noted in Chapter 3, showed that there are significant unconscious implications in suicide. Specifically, it showed that clinicians judged genuine sui-cide notes to be more frequently reflections of unconscious meaning than control data (i.e., simulated notes). It also showed that latent content (Foulkes, 1978; Freud, 1974f) could be objectively scored more frequently in genuine notes than in simu-lated ones. Although further research is needed, this research established that one can use the concept of the unconscious to understand suicide.

Suicide is an interpersonal event. As noted in Chapter 3, significant unconscious processes are related to the interpersonal aspects (Leenaars, 1986). Indeed, the most significant unconscious processes may well be interpersonal (Leenaars, 1993b; Maltsberger, 1986). Freud (1974i) had already speculated on the latent interpretation that leads someone to kill him/herself:

> Probably no one finds the mental energy required to kill himself unless, in the first place, in doing so he is at the same time killing an object with whom he had identified

himself and, in the second place, is turning against himself a death wish which had been directed against someone else. (p. 162)

The suicidal person, even the child, has had to develop a strong identification with other people. Attachment, based upon an important emotional tie with another person, was Freud's (1974j) early meaning for the term of identification. The person (or other ideal) does not merely exist outside; rather, he/she becomes introjected into one's own personality. Although the word "identification" has different meanings in the literature (see Hartmann, 1939; Meissner, 1981), I have here retained Freud's early use of the term. Freud speculated:

Identification is known to psychoanalysis as the earliest expression of an emotional tie with another person ... There are three sources of identification. First, identification is the original form of emotional ties with an object. Secondly, in a regressive way it becomes a substitute for a libidinal object tie, as it were by means of introjection of the object into the ego, and thirdly, it may arise with any new perception of a common quality shared with some other person who is not an object of the sexual instinct. (p. 105)

Freud's (1974n) own use of the concept changed. In his later writings, he reserved the concept of identification as a mechanism of structuralization, namely the superego. Although I am not suggesting that these views are not relevant, I wish to preserve identification to mean a deep primary attachment to significant people (e.g., parents) or some other ideal. Identification is a means of identifying with an object consciously and/or unconsciously, making it part of one's own internal world. It has a psychical existence.

Identification becomes a hallmark of one's early development. The attachment is deep within one's mind. Regrettably, the attachment is often symbiotic. As Litman (1967) noted, our "ego is made up in large part of identification" (p. 333). These identifications in children are associated primarily with their parents, especially the primary caregiver. With loss, abandonment, excessive dependency and other traumatic experiences in the relationships, the attachment becomes dysfunctional. The development is hampered; the child may develop mistrust, shame and doubt, and guilt. He/she experiences pain and may become hopeless and helpless (Fenichel, 1954). The child, for example, may express the pain as being "boxed in" (Orbach, 1988). The importance of attachment in Justin is obvious. It was his relationship to his mother, Dr Jones, that was especially painful. This relationship was critical in hampering Justin's development and then the loss-abandonment by his father was too much for his fragile ego to bear. Attachment is, I believe, the basic process in suicide in children, although not the only one. A death wish may occur but it is less primary. Although aggressive wishes, directed both inwards and outwards, occurred in Justin, it is primarily identification (i.e., attachment) that is a key to understanding his behaviour. The suicide attempt for Justin was more an outcome of frustrated attachment needs (wishes) than of aggressive ones. The earliest attachments were dysfunctional; the relation to the mother was deeply problematic. Indeed, Justin's family showed many of the familial dynamics that have been related to suicide (e.g., Orbach, 1988; Pfeffer, 1986; Trad, 1990). Then, the loss of his family, experienced as abandonment, at both the broken rocking chair level and the deeper latent level, fuelled both his pain and his mother's pain. His mother could not cope: no family, no life.

Indeed, it was Justin's mother who was especially hopeless and helpless. Her attachments were fragile, obviously related to her earliest relationships. For example, the experience with the cake on her seventh birthday was even now unbearable for her. She continued to exhibit overly painful attachments. She needed the regressive relationship between her and Justin. Justin's and his mother's dynamics were intermeshed. She had been suicidal for years. It is likely that Justin's attempt was more an expression of her death wish than his own. Justin acted out the nature of the relationship.

The dynamics in Justin's suicide attempt, I believe, are thus related to key significant others (i.e., his mother and his father). The need in his relationships was one of attention, approval, validation, affection, love. That was equally true for his mother. According to Horney (1950) such a person evaluates his/her life according to how much he/she "is liked, needed, wanted, or accepted". This type of person is often self-punishing, even by the age of 4. One's development is hampered, and there is a continued need for attachment. In Justin's mind, as in most children of his age, love and family are closely intertwined. His family was everything. Dr Jones equally exhibited such a need, and would sacrifice everything—even her son. Although other needs may be present, it is the need for attachment, within both of their developmental contexts, that was critical in the suicidal behaviour.

It is likely that, as a group, suicidal children are in fact quite pathological in their love, and that is equally true of their caregivers. In his analysis of Freud's speculations on suicide, Litman (1967, p. 370) writes:

> Freud often referred to certain dangerous ways of loving in which the "ego is over-whelmed" by the object. Typically, the psychic representation of the self and others are fused and the other is experienced as essential to survival.

Dr Jones's love of Justin was dangerous. Justin even introjected her suicidal wishes. She was overwhelmed as the case presentation outlined, and her obvious affective disorder was catastrophic in the family. Dr Jones was often intoxicated by her emotions and thoughts. She had problems developing constructive, loving attachments. She needed Justin's existence. She was overly narcissistic, being unable to provide for the development of a sound sense of self or identity for Justin (Miller, 1981). A mental breakdown was an ever-present reality, despite her denial. For her, the problem was often only Mr Jones. She was so constricted. Even more regrettably for Justin, Dr Jones and Justin were emotionally fused by a fusion that was, as is so common, fragile. The broken chair—and Justin's association "Eat this"—was experienced, for example, as an end to their survival. Dr Jones's problems, such as Justin's expression of anger to her in treatment, only added to the pain. Dr Jones and Justin simply could not cope . . . they could not eat the chair.

We term such attachments "symbiotic" (Mahler, 1968) and it is likely that "symbiotic love is a potential precursor of suicide" (Litman, 1967). Justin's family exhibited unhealthy love. For them, love was a trauma, the separation, that Dr Jones and, by identification, Justin could not bear. Dr Jones's pain was probably related to her mother, who sounded equally disturbed. The trauma in the Jones family was so complete that there was little hope. There was an overwhelming level of perturbation and the pain in the family was unbearable.

Suicide occurs in needful children, and in children whose development has been shackled.

> It is difficult to conceptualise an individual committing suicide apart from the individual seeking to satisfy inner felt needs; ... there can never be a needless suicide; ... it focally involves an attempt to fulfil some urgently felt psychological needs. Operationally, these heightened unmet needs make up, in large part, what the suicidal person feels (and reports)... (Shneidman, 1985, pp. 208–209)

This is equally true of suicidal children (Trad, 1990). If we use the perspective of the unconscious, we learn that Justin's suicide attempt is largely related to loving, needing, wanting, liking, accepting. In the suicidal child, love is the driving force. Justin needed love.

TREATMENT: A FEW OBSERVATIONS

Intervention with children will depend on the developmental age of the specific child. Each child has his/her own unique pain, attachments, needs, relationships, etc. Specific interventions are based not only on the child but also on the family. Although I utilize play activities (e.g., Axline, 1947; Caplan & Caplan, 1974) with children in therapy (Reisman, 1973), I almost never just see the child. As the case of Justin shows, even greater complexity is added. One must consider the parents' (and even siblings') pain, needs, etc., which can be complicated by a host of factors such as divorce in Justin's case (or in paternal abandonment in the case that I discussed under the title of David (Berman et al., 1991)). Factors such as long-term instability, alcoholism, imprisonment are just a few other examples of events that can be traumatic and affect a child's pain and development in general.

Often I see the child and parent(s) separately. Often the parents need to discuss the child and the therapist serves as an auxiliary-ego. Even more so, the parents' own pathology, as with Dr Jones, makes such treatment necessary (Leenaars et al., 1994b; Leenaars, 1991c, 1995). Although joint sessions with the parents are desirable for some issues, that may often be complicated as in the separation—experienced as "hate"—in Justin's family (Haley, 1971).

Freud (1974c) was the first to show the utility of seeing parent(s) individually in the case of Hans, a 5-year-old boy. Little Hans's problem was not unlike Justin's. Hans's trauma dated back to the age of 2. At an early stage Hans developed a deep attachment to his mother. At $3\frac{1}{2}$ years of age, several traumatic events occurred for Hans: his mother threatened to castrate him and his sister was born. At age 5, Hans woke up one morning in tears. He had dreamt that his mother had abandoned him. The more problematic the relationship(s) became to his mother and others in the family, the more the attachment became symbiotic at an unconscious level for even the mother. Hans became erratic, very perturbed. The family was dysfunctional, although much less, I believe, than Justin's. Indeed, Hans never exhibited suicidal behaviour; instead, his pain was expressed in a phobia.

In Freud's case, and in my case, the parents needed assistance. In Justin's case the assistance went beyond parenting skills. Dr Jones exhibited a significant affective problem in her life. Indeed, in the case of Justin, I foresaw little gain for him without treatment for Dr Jones. One needed to reduce Dr Jones's pain in order to reduce Justin's.

Extensive family treatment is often required with suicidal families (Richman, 1986). Addressing the family's dysfunctions, as outlined earlier, is necessary. However, despite my attempts, this was difficult with Justin's family as they had separated.

Equally, one may need to address system issues, beyond the family, especially within the school (Leenaars & Wenckstern, 1990). In Justin's case, this became increasingly necessary and the joint meeting at his school was most useful. It allowed the teacher to reframe Justin's problem and introduce better remediation. After all, one uses different techniques with Attention Deficit Disorders than with deep pain. In other cases, such as David's (Berman et al., 1991), a social welfare agency and treatment centre were needed. I strongly believe, in fact, that one should use the help of all people—medical doctors, siblings, the elders, ministers, teachers, etc.,—in the treatment of suicidal children and, indeed, people in general (Leenaars, 1994). Consultation with a peer is often useful, especially when treating suicidal children. One may then discuss one's treatment, the family's dysfunction, one's countertransference, the need for medication and hospitalization, etc. (Shneidman, 1981c).

On the issue of medication and/or hospitalization, each case needs to be evaluated separately, and medication may be necessary if there are medical/physical complications. Hospitalization should not be eschewed, but used only in the very highly lethal cases of the child and/or parent. Of course, hospitalization is always a complicated event in the treatment of suicidal children and the quality of care from doctors, nurses, and others is crucial (Shneidman, 1981c).

The specific implications, outlined in Chapter 12 (based on the TGSP) that applied to Justin were as follows: 1, 2, 3, 4, 5, 6, 13, 15f, 19, 20, 21, 22, 23, 24, 25, 27, 33, and 35. These initial targets for psychotherapy especially involved elements in unbearable pain and interpersonal relations. This is common in the treatment of suicidal children (and young teens). Subsequently, as one reads the transcripts, specific implications *also* included the following: 7, 8, 9, 10, 11, 12, 16, 17, 26, 28, and 32. The cognitive elements become more figural, even with a young child. Justin needed to widen his blinders, and so did the family. Ego development was needed.

The reader should return to Chapter 12 and re-read each implication, thinking how it would apply to Justin. In subsequent chapters, I will outline each implication as it appears in the case and explicate the implications for that individual. This, to some, may seem redundant and too detailed. However, I believe, echoing Shneidman, that is what works: Each individual needs to be treated in the detail of his/her pain. Global responses will be suicidogenic.

CONCLUDING REMARKS

Miller (1981) reports the following account of a patient about her pain as a child in a dysfunctional family:

> I lived in the glass house into which my mother could look at any time. In a glass house, however, you cannot conceal anything without giving yourself away, except by hiding it under the ground. And then you cannot see it yourself either. (p.21)

Even at the age of 4, Justin had buried much. Yet, with the broken chair, he could no longer bear the pain. His attachments were disrupted. He was boxed in and needed to get out. His mother's own suicidal wish was acted out by Justin. Unconscious processes, within the context of unbearable pain, cognitive constriction, egression, etc., were a driving force in the suicidal behaviour of Justin and his mother, who had hid so much from themselves.

To conclude, if one attempts to explain suicide in children at a manifest level, one will understand little. To do so, would, for example, accept Dr Jones's hypothesis of Mr Jones's abuse—a belief that was, in fact, more fantasy than reality. Regrettably a current popular formulation regarding suicide in children, is that it is simply due to an external event or stress such as a divorce, abuse, whatever. Although these events do occur in the lives of suicidal children, there is much more than the manifest level. Suicide is complex and, to understand such complexity, the concept of the unconscious is necessary. Without the unconscious, developmental suicidology will be overly barren.

Chapter 14

JEFF: A YOUTH'S SUICIDE
(*And Then He Killed Himself*)

Suicide is a major cause of death in youth. In Chapter 2, a detailed discussion of this fact from a developmental perspective (i.e., Erickson) was provided. In this chapter we will meet such a teen, Jeff, and, in the next chapter, another young person at risk, Jennifer. The question can be raised whether Jeff should not be labelled a young adult. Jeff was 18 and young adulthood begins at 18; yet, equally, adolescence stops at 18. Indeed, the choice of overlap on the age groupings was intentional, following the literature on the topic (e.g., Kimmel, 1974). Some people mature earlier, some later. Jeff certainly fell into the later group. He was in many ways fixated at a psychological age of 14 or so.

Jeff had a long history of depression and suicidal behaviour. He was isolated, whereas his early life had been filled with happiness, play and friends. By the time he was 14, he had suffered deeply from recurrent depression, had made a suicide attempt, was treated and hospitalized. That was in grade 9. He never got much better, despite a community response—family, friends, doctors, counsellors, ministers, parents of friends, and so on.

BACKGROUND

Let's begin this exegesis at the turn of 2000. On 4 January 2000, Jeff presented himself to a mental health clinic. The intake physician/counsellor, Dr Jill Smith, noted that Jeff exhibited "anxiety, paranoid thoughts, and difficulty concentrating regarding the 'real' world". She noted that Jeff expressed bizarre thoughts of a very negative self-image, for example, perceptions of being worthless. He felt totally isolated, stating, "There are walls between me and my friends."

Jeff described himself as a "messed up kid". He stated, "I'm getting discouraged and just want some help." When asked, "Help with what?", he said "Pain."

Jeff had been prescribed Paxil, an antidepressant, which Jeff reported helped him with his anxiety, but not his painful thoughts. He was started on Zyprexa, 5 mg (an antipsychotic) to be renewed weekly, so as to limit drug availability. Jeff was also referred for a psychiatric evaluation.

Jeff was seen by Dr. Jim Jones. Dr Jones, who was familiar with Jeff historically, did note regression in Jeff's mental status at that time. He noted symptoms of vagueness, very negative self-perception and quasi-paranoid ideation. Yet, the following was most figural: "I was struck by Jeff's marked thought disorder with very tangential thinking and a rambling speech pattern which made it very difficult to conduct an interview." Dr Jones continued Jeff on the Zyprexa and followed up with Jeff on a regular basis.

Dr Smith continued to see Jeff on a very regular basis, sometimes three times per week from January until May 2000. On 14 January, Jeff revealed to Dr Smith that he was not in a good place in his life, stating, "Everything seems all over." He felt anxious, confused, and easily distracted. He experienced depersonalization, feeling that every day he was a different version of himself. He felt so lost and isolated. He expressed that he lost touch with his friends. The paranoid ideation continued, often having to glance over his shoulders. He feared that people could read his mind. His thoughts were scrambled and he thought, "It will all go downhill", adding, "Everything is all over." Jeff continued to be monitored for suicide risk.

Also of note, Jeff had been quite aggressive at times. He exhibited delinquent behaviour. He had broken windows, stolen, and had been involved in multiple drug use, although he often denied (although it was not believed) any drug use.

With regard to his history, we learn that he had no trouble in his early years. He had "good friends", and did well in school. He had no social problems. Then in grade 9, school became "really bad". "Everything got worse," Jeff had reported. He went to alternative school and regressed, being quite depressed and suicidal. His first hospitalization and placement in a treatment centre occurred.

About his family of origin, it was learned that his mother's side had a long history of depression. His mother and sisters suffered from recurrent episodes. Questions about Bipolar Disorders (Manic-Depressive Disorder) were noted. The maternal grandmother suffered from anxiety and the great-grandfather suffered from depression, both having been treated and hospitalized for the same. Jeff's father was described as exhibiting no disorder; however, his paternal grandfather was "troubled" and his great-grandfather had attempted suicide. Two uncles also suffered from depression and other unspecified mental disorders.

By 18 January 2000, Jeff had taken himself off his medication, reporting that he felt no different while on them. He would often regulate his own medication and, I believe, self-medicate with street drugs. On 26 January, he was again taking his medication, reporting "eerie feelings". He stated, "My head is a bad place," wanting relief—to escape from the pain. He was very depressed. On 10 February he was suicidal; yet, Jeff reported that he was puzzled. There was no reason to feel depressed from his view; "Nothing was happening." He was prescribed Lorazepam, 1 mg bid to manage his anxiety. A few days later, he was not thinking about suicide. He reported some joy, was getting along with his parents, and was planning to get a job. He was more revealing about his drug use, reporting use of "marijuana, acid, cough medicine and downers". He continued to use the Lorazepam and reported that he felt better. On 22 February Jeff still felt "up", but was continuing to experience his painful episodes. He reported that his mind "sometimes takes over". He felt a lack of control over his thoughts, feeling that he would get worse. He stated that thoughts trigger a downward slide; for example, "not being in school", "not seeing friends at all", "just in a rut", "just stuck". Jeff now continued, however, to feel good, wanted to do things and went on a "health quest". The following week Jeff took an overdose of Lorazepam, was hospitalized, treated, and released. Dr Smith saw him the next day, 1 March, Jeff reporting to Dr Smith that "I didn't want to live". On 3 March he was still very depressed, describing himself as "very down". Impulsivity was an increasing concern. His medication was changed, with a trial on Effexor, an antidepressant, after terminating the Paxil. On 6 March Jeff reported that he had felt better, but was experiencing problems at home. He had taken his parents' car without telling them and had a single car accident; he rolled the car into a ditch. Jeff reported that this was the second accident, having earlier driven his mother's car into a ditch. Dr Smith marked an "!" about this event and notified Dr Jones, as on other matters routinely. Jeff also started reporting olfactory hallucinations; he smelled something sweet, which put him into a bad frame. He stated, "I feel like I'm stoned," even when not smoking marijuana. There were further meetings with Dr Smith and by 16 March Jeff felt better; he reported "no great worries". (One can notice the cycling.) His medication was continued. On 23 March Jeff continued to do well; his obsessive thought patterns, especially about anger, were discussed with Dr Smith. Again, a review of his medication was undertaken and it was decided to try Risperdal, an antipsychotic agent. On 20 March Jeff again took the car and got it stuck on a gravel road; the police were involved. His cycling continued over the next four months, until 3 May when Jeff tried to hurt himself. Questions about his heightened suicide risk then occurred. He reported that he was quite depressed and arrangements were made for him to see Dr Jones. Jeff was taken to emergency at the hospital.

Dr Jones saw Jeff, noting depression as the reason for referral and also that Jeff had been very depressed for four months. In the mental status examination Dr Jones noted that Jeff was sitting on a stretcher, not responding. His mood and affect were depressed. Thought form was slow; thought content demonstrated no delusion, obsession, phobic or homicidal thoughts. Suicidal ideation was present. On the perceptual examination, there were no auditory hallucinations, but olfactory hallucination for marijuana was noted. Cognitively, Jeff was oriented in three spheres and was described as "normal". Insight and judgement were seen as "poor".

Jeff was admitted to hospital with a diagnosis of Major Depression. He was subsequently in and out of hospital. When first hospitalized he was seen by Dr Erik Jan, a physician. Dr Jan noted that Jeff had been hospitalized for depression and bizarre symptoms. A history of substance abuse was noted and, despite Jeff's denial, the drug screen was positive for opiates. His medication was as follows: Celexa, 20 mg hs (an antidepressant), Ativan 1 mg tid (an anti-anxiety) and Loxepac 25q 4 hprm (an antipsychotic).

A physical examination was undertaken, which was normal except for mood and mental stress. Dr Jan ordered physical exams, e.g., CAT, EGG, to rule out temporal lobe epilepsy or other underlying brain anomaly. These records indicated normal recordings.

Subsequently, Jeff continued to go in and out of hospital. In April, he was seen by Dr Albert Cook, who again noted that Jeff was feeling depressed and suicidal. While at home, he had made plans to hook the exhaust hose from a car into the vehicle and kill himself. Jeff was unable to relate the thought to any external stimulus, again describing the thought as spontaneous. The diagnosis was depression and Jeff was again admitted to hospital. Dr Smith saw Jeff and at follow-up. This in-and-out situation continued over the next few months; the records are redundant, reflecting, I believe, the concurring hopelessness and helplessness that Jeff—and his family—felt.

RAPPORT

And now a confession: I knew Jeff. He had been in the class of my eldest daughter, Lindsey—although they had seen each other rarely over the past few years. After grade 9 Jeff had isolated himself from his grade school friends (Jeff should now have been in grade 13, his last year of high school). He had developed a new set of friends, "a druggy group". Jeff had been our paperboy for some years in his youth, before high school. I knew about his depression and first suicide attempt in grade 9. After the attempt, my wife, Susanne Wenckstern, who works for the education system, and I did a prevention programme for the parents of students at his school, not only because of Jeff, but there had been three other suicidal events at that same school. We offered our assistance because it was our community, and our kids. After the programme, Jeff's mother spoke to me about Jeff and his needs. It was really the first time that I learned about the details of Jeff's pain.

Some four years after the school contact, on 4 July 2000, Jeff's mother contacted me, informing me about Jeff's suicide risk, current hospitalization and refusal at that time to speak to anyone. His latest suicide attempt had been intervened and Jeff was quite angry about this fact. He simply wanted out of the hospital. She asked me to see Jeff, so how could I refuse? Out of desperation, Jeff's mother had contacted a number of Jeff's friends' parents, including a minister and me. The intent was to set up a larger community support system. We both went to see Jeff—after all, as I have often stated, suicide prevention requires the combined effort of a community.

COMMUNITY APPROACH

Community action is a key—sometimes this approach is called a wraparound process (van den Berg & Grealish, 1996). The concept is not new. Many of us in the field have always seen the community approach as necessary. It was central to the counselling strategies at the beginning of the crisis centre movement, the Los Angeles Suicide Prevention Center (LASPC).

The LASPC, which began on 1 September 1958, employed a multi-people, multi-component approach. Disciplines included nursing, social work, psychiatry, psychology, and a large group of lay volunteers. The volunteers—trained in appropriate response—did the main work, answering the calls of people in distress. Many people provided the rescue. An active community referral source was established. The success of the LASPC was due to many people working together, intervening with the suicidal person. It was a community approach (Shneidman & Farberow, 1999) and this has become a basic to intervention with highly suicidal people.

Thus, a basic tenet of suicide prevention, since the LASPC, has been: Suicide prevention with highly lethal people is best done not alone. It takes a community approach (or to use a newer term, a wraparound process). Therefore, utilizing the TGSP, Jeff's historical protocols would resonate to item 33. Jeff had lost people and ideals (e.g., happiness). Suicidal people have often experienced a loss in some direct or indirect way (both evident in Jeff). Jeff, in fact, had become so isolated and alone since his very first attempt. He was estranged.

The main tactic with such a person is to increase that individual's psychological sense of possible choices and sense of being emotionally supported. A suicidal person cannot be or remain so isolated. He/she, in fact, needs not only the attachments, but also to tell his/her story. Relatives, friends, and colleagues should, after they have been determined to be on the side of life, be considered in the total support process. The person needs other objects (people) with whom to identify. Others can assist in establishing and/or re-establishing positive relations. Jeff needed his friends, family, and so on. This will help to build constructive tendencies, whether self-esteem, self-support, or some other life-enhancing processes. When so perturbed, individuals cannot simply give up even a negative part of their identity, nor can they often search out healthy objects on their own. They are simply in too much pain and too pessimistic to do so.

Jeff's attachments were increased. A community approach was undertaken to assist beyond his doctor, his therapist (and the ever-increasing hospitalizations)—this included family, relatives, friends, neighbours, a minister, and so on. Lindsey and many other (old) friends were called upon to be supportive—and they were. I was asked to be one more auxiliary ego. Indeed, with at-risk people like Jeff, suicide prevention, as we stated, is best not done alone. A combination of consultation, ancillary therapists, social networking, and use of all the interpersonal and community resources that one can involve, is, in general, the best way of proceeding. Of course, there are issues of boundaries in this case; yet, it was clear that my support was not as Jeff's primary therapist (he had Dr Smith and Dr Jones), but as one more supportive person (albeit I was a therapist). We all have to do what we can to save a life.

FIRST CONTACTS

We contacted Dr Smith and permission was given for me to see Jeff at the hospital. I met Jeff's mother on 6 July 2000 at the hospital—a 4-minute walk from my office. We talked about Jeff and she sent me a letter the next day, stating:

... please help Jeff open up and not want to take his own life but make a life for himself, to be able to cope. Jeff has become extremely and more depressed since we moved out of Windsor in October/99. I suppose it was something he just could not cope with, although it has been wonderful for the rest of the family.

He has always been a quiet person but now I feel he has closed himself off almost completely. He is sensitive and kind and compassionate, loves his family and is loved by his family. He is extremely artistic, musical, intelligent but only rarely plays his guitar anymore.

After my discussion with Jeff's mother, I met with the nursing staff, informed them who I was, and asked about Jeff's status. They were aware from Dr Smith about my visit. They reported that Jeff was very depressed and at a high suicide risk. He was under care and treatment with medication, but Jeff had for over a week refused to speak to anyone. Next, the staff located Jeff, who, upon seeing me, ran (one can readily score items 24 and 26 of the TGSP[1]). Only after some time, and the encouragement of his mother, did Jeff come to speak to me, but said that it was difficult for him because he knew me. Yet, I stated that his mother requested that I talk to him (I later learned that he had also seen the minister—the mother of another old friend—the day before). I stated, "How could I refuse?" I noted, if someone asked him to help my daughter, if she was in a similar state, what would he do? He then spoke: "I would help." He looked at me and said, "Okay, I understand." "Good," I remarked in my notes, "there is rapport." I then explained that I wanted to help him, to be one more person in his community to help.

Jeff reported that he was depressed; his moods were up and down, and he had been suicidal. He stated, however, that he was "not suicidal now" (dissembling?). His mood was depressed; he was agitated. He reported sleep disturbances. Jeff also stated that it was difficult for him to communicate. I accepted that statement and listened.

Jeff stated that he did not want help. He said that he saw Dr Smith, but Dr Smith was not helpful and added, "You won't." I responded by stating that I was not replacing Dr Smith or Dr Jones, but offering to be one more support person. I stated that we could give it a chance, again adding: What would he do if a friend were in such a situation? Reluctantly, I suspect, he stated that he would try—upon which I said, "I will try too." He discussed his background, most of that is described previously. I then again addressed the limit of my supportive role (not to replace Dr Smith or Dr Jones) and the issue of confidentiality due to suicide risk. I suggested that I would see him next week at the hospital, not wishing to be too intrusive in his care (Jeff was not my patient).

After our visit, I spoke to the staff and his mother. The mother reported that Jeff was angry with her for calling the minister, adding, and you "but I'm desperate". I stated that I understood and would see Jeff. At my office, I made some notes and completed the TGSP. Jeff's TGSP is shown in Appendix 14.1

A few days after my visit, Jeff's mother called. Jeff had become violent, tried to escape from the closed hospital ward and had been put in restraints. He was quite

---

[1] Explanations of all implications/items are given in Chapter 12.

angry. She had spoken to Dr Smith and he encouraged me to see Jeff (he was still refusing to talk to anyone).

I saw Jeff a few days later, first having spoken to the nursing staff. They reported that after Jeff's outburst he had become more sociable and talkative, even going to OT (Occupational Therapy). Once more, the extreme mood swings were evident.

When I met with Jeff, he was more open, despite stating that he was reluctant to express himself in words (Jeff was quite artistic, musical, and excellent in maths, but not languages). Jeff spoke about being depressed and feeling "lonely" more often. When I asked him what hurts, he said the "pain". "I feel so isolated," he said. Although he was positive about his family, a few years earlier his family had moved from the city of Windsor to the country and Jeff now saw the solution to his problem as returning to the city. He morbidly related to the fact that his new home was next to a cemetery. Outside his window, he saw the tombstones. He would obsess for hours, looking at one grave, imagining that he was in that grave. He would look and look, day in and day out. He so wanted to escape his malaise. Windsor became a "mecca". Jeff said that he wanted to see his friends again. Yet, when I asked if he wished to see his friends at the hospital, he said "no". He refused to allow me to tell my daughter (his friends learned anyway). As I listened to his story, it became obvious that Jeff was, indeed, a very isolated, depressed, deeply pained young man.

We discussed whether he would like to see me again; he agreed. I followed up with the staff and contacted Jeff's mother. We discussed Jeff's agreement to talk to me. The minister, friends, and others were also more frequently contacted—a supportive environment was available.

THE SUBSEQUENT VISITS

On 19 July Jeff was allowed to leave the hospital with his mother, on a short release, to see me at my office, a four-minute walk. Rapport was good. I noted in my notes, "He's accepting me," probably because of our established, but distant relationship (he had been the paperboy). (On a professional aside, I think, as professionals, we should still keep clinical notes, even if in supportive roles, in such cases.) Jeff talked. He talked about his cycles of depression and his feelings of hopelessness. He reported that when he gets in his depressed mood, "everything goes down". He stated, "I spiral down", feeling so hopeless and helpless that "only suicide is a solution".

He discussed his treatment, questioning his need for medication. I strongly supported the need and encouraged him to speak to Dr Smith, Dr Jones and others about his medications. (We know that he increased his contacts.) A number of other topics were discussed, notably his insomnia. I listened and discussed some ways to reduce that perturbation.

Jeff's pain was his enemy; he wanted relief from his intolerable inner anguish (item 1). For him, suicide had adjustive value. It abolished pain. It allowed him to escape.

Jeff wanted to go to a better life, devoid of his pain. Our—all members of the support system—task was to translate his belief that death was the solution into a wider adaptive belief: something more than stopping painful tension by death.

I began to attempt to redefine the trauma (his depression) to Jeff as painful but tolerable. I disagreed with his "I can't live with this". I asked something like, "When you say, Jeff, you can't live with this, what is the this?"... We then began to talk and learn how to block the exits (item 34).

Jeff was unwilling—did not want—to accept his painful moods. We focused on the "problem" that Jeff was trying to solve—the loss, the loneliness, etc. Again, Karl Menninger's dictum: The person is always right. It is our task, even as a supportive person, to discover, "how is he/she right?" Then, we needed to assist Jeff in developing alternative solutions to the alcohol, drugs, and suicide. People attempted to help, and Jeff needed to know that something was being done to help him through the pain—to block the final egression.

After the visit, Jeff agreed to see me (as well as other people in the community, e.g., the minister, other friends' parents), as an additional support to Dr Smith. By 10 August Jeff was released from the hospital.

I met Jeff on 10 August; Dr Smith had reported that Jeff was doing better. Jeff was not depressed and was alert. He was socializing and seeing his friends—more accurately, his old friends. I reinforced his social integration (item 2). To save a person's life, we need to develop attachment—with teenagers, this includes peers (not as therapists or counsellors, but as community adjuncts). Jeff's friends, including my daughter, offered support and encouragement.

Peer counselling—especially because teenagers prefer to talk to teenagers—is seen by some as the best mode of treatment for suicidal teens. This is a deadly error (Leenaars & Wenckstern, 1999). I am not suggesting that peer groups have no utility, only that they do not address the needs of truly suicidal people (King, 1997; Leenaars & Wenckstern, 1990). Peer counselling is not the same as psychotherapy. There is no research to suggest that peer counsellors can provide the therapeutic care that suicidal youth need. On the other hand, as with Jeff, a peer, minister, family doctor, and so on, may greatly assist in identification, referral, and support. Jeff's friends were essential supports—but he still needed to see Dr Smith. The fact that teenagers prefer to talk to teenagers is no justification for following their (often defensive) wishes (dissembling). This defence is an expression of the magnitude of their pain and their inability to cope with it, not health promoting.

Further community action may include putting information that the person is in trouble about "a thing" into the stream of communication, letting others know about it, breaking what could be a fatal secret, proffering help, and, if possible, showing interest and deep concern. All such efforts aim at increasing the person's attachments. This was done with Jeff.

When Jeff and I met, we began to explore the stimuli that resulted in his spiralling reaction, focusing on inner dynamics. He revealed that he had learned from his various therapists that as soon as he became "unhappy" about "anything" it would grow and grow. The pain would become deeper. He would be so obsessed about the "anything", become depressed and begin isolating himself. The spiral downwards would continue. In response, I asked, "What can you do as soon as the trigger, i.e., feeling unhappy, occurs?" I reinforced what he had learned about effectively coping with life's demands.

We talked about his resources, e.g., friends, Dr Smith, Dr Jones, the minister, me. He continued to see Dr Smith and had visits with Dr Jones. We also explored the possibility of some part-time work, something more to anchor him into the "real" world. Jeff had not worked or gone to school for some years.

The next week, Jeff came to see me. He was more agitated and tired, reporting increased sleep disturbances. He reported that he could not sleep, falling asleep at 2 or 3 a.m. He was restless and felt anxious. I noted in my notes, "I worry about a cycle. He gets so anxious, agitated. What is the impact?" I asked what helped before and he stated "Ativan"; after my appointment, Jeff was to see Dr Jones and he agreed to discuss his state and needs (which records show he did). When I asked if something else helped, he stated "meditation". We discussed this approach and I showed him some basics of relaxation techniques that I know. He was excited about such approaches, agreed to see me, and kept our next planned appointment, to provide additional community support (items 3 and 4).

Whether alone or in a community approach, all interveners can focus on any number of emotions with the suicidal person, notably the distressing (painful) feelings such as worthlessness, distress, or anxiety. The key with Jeff was to improve the external and internal situations, related to these emotions and other aspects of his suicidal mind, a JND (Just Noticeable Difference). This was attempted through a variety of methods: ventilation, medication, guidance, and support in the outside world. This implied, when working with a highly lethal person like Jeff, a heightened level of interaction during the period of heightened lethality. Jeff's parents, his doctor, the minister, his friends, and I, attempted to give Jeff transfusions of hope. We wanted his pain to subside enough, to reduce the lethality to a tolerable, life-permitting level.

The goal of everyone's assistance was to keep Jeff alive. The goal of our support was quite simple: It consisted almost by definition of lowering Jeff's lethality; in practice, decreasing or mollifying the level of perturbation did this. In short, we diffused the source of Jeff's constricted focus on suicide. We created familial/social (community) interest around him. We attempted to make Jeff's unbearable problems and/or injustices just sufficiently better to enable him to think, and reconsider, and try to see alternatives. Jeff needed to give himself time.

On 30 August Jeff came to see me for what was to be his last visit. Jeff had seen Dr Jones, was taking his medication and was reported to be "doing well". (Dissembling?) Despite Jeff's presentation, Dr Smith, Dr Jones, I, and others continued to see Jeff as a suicide risk, albeit lower than the month before. His risk fluctuated so. Jeff was, however, again questioning whether any of us could help. Typically, in an upswing, Jeff would be more independent, denying his problems and needs. We talked about whether I was helpful; he acknowledged the growing relationship, stating that he would try to work with Dr Smith, his friends, others and me.

THE DEATH

On 12 September Jeff was found dead; he hanged himself at an elementary school. He had left a note, scratched into the glass of a school window. His note read, "Take care of Joe [his nephew] and each other." I subsequently met with his family. They told me that Jeff was known to have been drinking excessively that day. Much later a further note was found and a copy given to me. The note read:

> Dear mom. I love you and could you buy a rose for Jill (a girlfriend) from me and all my friends and family.
>   I love you and
> I'm sorry

Jeff's family and friends mourned. There was a large funeral. The church was full of young people. There were the usual eulogies, but the family also asked me to speak at Jeff's funeral, highlighting not only Jeff's pain, but that help was available for suicidal people. They were concerned about his friends, who also might be suicidal and needed help. Here is what I said:

> This is not my usual platform and I apologize not only for my awkwardness, but also because I have been asked to do a eulogy, when many here knew Jeff better. Nevertheless, let me begin:
>   [In front of a picture of Jeff's favourite WWF pro-Wrestler, The Rock, with the caption, "The Great One".]
>   Jeff was The Great One. He was the best paper carrier I ever had. I first knew Jeff, with the rest of my daughter, Lindsey's, friends, from Central Elementary School. I met Jeff at school and at my home. Jeff had many skills, especially right brain ones. He was artistic, like Vincent van Gogh.
>   But like Vincent, Jeff suffered from Depression. Depression, in both Jeff and Vincent, was biologically based. There are Bipolar Disorders—the manic-depressive person, who goes up and down in moods. And, there are Unipolar Disorders—only the depression, the downs are felt. These disorders are often biological, just like ADHD (Attention Deficit/Hyperactivity Disorder). Jeff was depressed; he struggled with depression for years. We need to try to understand Jeff's depression, his pain. We need to try to understand, "Why did Jeff kill himself?"
>   Suicide is complex, more complex than most imagine. Suicide is not simply due to a stimulus—whether Jeff's school dropout or his move to Essex County. Suicide is more complex.
>   The stimulus for suicide is pain, unbearable pain. It is the pain of pain. It is anguish. What William Styron, the author of Sophie's Choice—who also struggled with depression—calls, "A howling tempest of the brain."
>   Research shows that about 90% of people who kill themselves had an identifiable mental disorder at the time of their death. Forty to sixty percent of suicides suffered from depression. It is difficult to understand suicide...but to answer the why, we need to understand the pain, PAIN.
>   And then there are our feelings, our pain about Jeff's death. His pain is now in our mind, we the survivors. We might feel sad, angry, numb, guilt, and so on. I feel guilt. I wonder if I could have done more...and my daughter, Lindsey—who said I could share her pain—feels guilty. Jeff had visited her a few evenings before his death, at

1:00 a.m.—he sometimes stopped by that late—and she spoke to him briefly, but now wonders, if she could have done more. We all have our guilt—and other feelings. These feelings and thoughts are normal. These are survivors' feelings. Don't listen to those who say, "You should not feel . . . guilty or sad, whatever." We all have feelings. Don't deny or avoid these reactions.

But, if these feelings get out of control, if they become unbearable, please get help. One of the reasons why Judy and Tom XX asked me to speak to you is to encourage you to get help if you are in pain and/or suicidal.

The XXs asked for help with Jeff. They asked his friends. They asked Wendy, our minister today, to help. They asked me. They persisted in trying to get help for Jeff. The XXs, and I, encourage you to get help, if you're suicidal.

People who are suicidal, need help. Often, people avoid getting help. There is a taboo about getting help for depression. But depression is like a heart condition. Would you not get help if you had a heart condition? It is the same. Depression and a heart condition are the same; they are both, among other things, biological problems.

There are all sorts of ways that we can help. Medication can help, e.g., antidepressants for depressed people, has been shown to be effective. Hospitalization can help. Psychotherapy can help. Each one of us can help. Our community can help.

There are things that do not help. Drugs and alcohol do not help. We know that Jeff was drinking a lot the day he died. These things do not help. There are, however, many things that can help suicidal people.

Jeff was blessed with many friends. He loved his parents and friends. His last note read, "Take care of Joe [his nephew] and each other." Jeff wanted people to take care of people.

Yet, Jeff himself was so isolated. He felt so pushed away. He felt that he was spiralling down. Sadly, Jeff found his solution—but there were others. Jeff, in his pain, was so mentally constricted. He was intoxicated with his pain.

We are now left with our feelings. We need to talk about our feelings. Next Saturday, those who want to talk . . . share about Jeff, are welcome to our home—Lindsey's home, for a sharing. And we will provide the lunch.

Thank you and goodbye Jeff.

CALCULATED RISK-TAKING

The question could be asked: Should Jeff have remained hospitalized? The problem here, of course, is that it would have been for months, if not years. He had been hospitalized for the first time four years earlier, and frequently after that first occasion. Patients may be discharged from inpatient care, especially if they are a chronic risk. Traditionally, these patients were hospitalized for years, some for all of their lives, and some involuntarily. Most hospitals around the world no longer support prolonged inpatient care—a decision that is related to commitment laws, health care costs and so on (Maltsberger, 1994). Sometimes the response to hospitalization is poor, if not iatrogenic (it was for Jeff), but calculated risks must be taken—which has no doubt raised, and will continue to raise, problems (see Chapter 21). The decision is complex and cannot be simply guided by costs *per se*, or any one other variable. A calculated choice was made with Jeff—a community network was sought, in addition to his therapist, psychiatrist. A reasonable decision was made, and perhaps in hindsight something more could have been done, but I am convinced that Jeff had decided to kill himself months before his death. His pain was too much to bear.

Maltsberger (1994, pp. 202–203) raises six important questions to ask in such cases. They are:

- Has the patient been afforded all reasonable treatment for the depressive and/or psychotic aspects of his illness (if there are any)?
- Is there a reasonable post-discharge treatment plan?
- Is the patient competent to give informed consent to the discharge and to the proposed post-hospital treatment, i.e., does he/she understand the calculated risk?
- Has the patient given consent to the treatment plan?
- Has full consultation been obtained in support of the discharge plan?
- Have those close to the patient been informed of and agreed to the plan?

Jeff's discharge was not foolhardy. As Maltsberger (1994) states, "when on balance the benefits of discharge outweigh the risks of continued inpatient confinement, it is both ethically and legally prudent to discharge patients suffering from chronic suicidal character problems" (p. 204). Risks have to be taken in care, whether in hospitalization, medication, psychotherapy, and so on; regrettably, there is no cookbook. We must make the best clinical judgements, and sometimes we will be wrong. Yet, in light of Jeff's death, I continue to espouse a community approach. The next case of Jennifer illustrates the life-saving value of such an approach.

WHAT HAVE WE LEARNED FROM THIS CASE?

David Lester, in his review of my manuscript, suggested that each case should have a conclusion/summary at the end indicating "What have we learned from this case?"; or, stated differently, "What are the essential features of or implications for treatment that prevented this suicide?" (or would have prevented this suicide). Although David does qualitative research, his strength is quantitative. I hereby, and in subsequent chapters, follow his advice.

The interventions with Jeff were sparse (items 24, 26, 1, 34, 2, 3, and 4). Our first intervention associates to item 24, attachments that were too unhealthy. We needed to establish a relationship, but, I believe, we were too late. Jeff had already decided to kill himself; he was only waiting for his opportunity. Establishing relationships would have been most critical; we needed to actively involve others. Jeff's parents tried, but even the community became impotent.

Of note, item 24 is also the single most frequent intervention. It was noted in all six cases, from Justin to Joe. What is the essential feature of treatment that would have prevented this suicide? The answer is attachments. I have no doubt about this fact!

It is also of note that, more than any patient that you will meet in this book, my focus with Jeff was on implications to reduce the unbearable pain. This is the *sine qua non* of treatment with people who are at the very centre of the suicidal storm— regardless of our role in the treatment. Implications 1, 2, 3, and 4 were invoked with Jeff; yet, his pain continued to howl.

Finally, I am also somewhat wary of the question posed; there is no such thing as *the* essential list of features or applications. At best, we can address the question in this case, not in general—although every theoretician is tempted. Thus, I will give way to Dr Lester's request and provide a section, "What have we learned from this case?" at the end of each case, as I have provided for Jeff. For the last case, Joe, I even provide a quantitative, arithmetical summary of what I did in all the cases—with a strong caution from me as a qualitative, idiographic researcher: We always need to treat the unique person.

CONCLUDING REMARKS

After Jeff's death, his family sought professional help and went to a survivor support group that is available in our community. I also mourned. I once wrote, "there will be casualties" when working with suicidal people, but I never anticipated that Jeff, who came to my home, delivered my paper, and so on, would be "a casualty". The pain (especially guilt) that some of our friends or patients leave us is deep. I became a survivor.

I continue to ask, "What could we have done to rescue Jeff?" David Lester, who read the entire manuscript (all of which added to the scholarly aspect), responded with the same consultation to this chapter. David asked: "Could Jeff have been saved in hindsight/retrospect?"; "What would you/Dr Jones/Dr Smith, etc., have done differently?" And, he asked the question that I had early in my involvement, "Would another medication have helped?" Would lithium, sometimes prescribed with difficult cases of mood disorders, have helped? Could we have improved the community support system? Would a long-term treatment centre, if such were available in Canada, have helped (i.e., long-term hospitalization)? Would greater consultation (i.e., communication) between all involved have helped? Which, as we will read in Chapter 19, medication(s), hospitalization(s), and environmental control(s), would have assisted? How could we all, including Jeff, have survived his tempest?

Appendix 14.1

THEMATIC GUIDE FOR SUICIDE PREDICTION

I CLIENT DATA

Date: 6 July 2000

Name: Jeff   Age: 18   Sex: M

Date of Birth: _____   Marital Status: _____

Education Status: _____grade 9_____   _____
                         (years)   (degrees)

Current Employment: NIL

II SUICIDAL EXPERIENCE

1. Has the patient ever seriously contemplated suicide? (If yes, note particulars)   Yes

2. Has the patient ever attempted suicide? (If yes, note particulars)   Yes

3. Does the patient know anyone who attempted suicide? (If yes, indicate family, acquaintance, etc.)   Yes

4. Does the patient know anyone who committed suicide? (If yes, indicate family, acquaintance, etc.)   Yes

III REFERRAL DATA

1. Purpose: To assess risk
2. What is the referral question? Can you help Jeff?
3. What is the presenting problem(s)? Hospitalization. Refused to talk.

IV INTERVIEW SITUATION

1. Observations: See note
2. Other procedures (e.g., tests, interviews)
   _____

V INTERPRETATIONS

	Low	Medium	High
1. Perturbation rating: scale equivalent	Low 1 2 3	Medium 4 5 6	High 7 8 9
2. Lethality rating: scale equivalent	Low 1 2 3	Medium 4 5 6	High 7 8 9

3. Guide summary:
   scores: I: 1, 2, 3, 4, 5, 6;   II: 7, 8, 9;   III: 10, 11, 12;
            IV: 13, 14, 15;   V: 16, 17, 18;   VI: 19, 20, 21, 22, 23, 24
            VII: 25, 26, 27, 28, 29, 30, 31, 32;   VIII: 33, 34, 35

Conclusions: Jeff presents a history of risk and ongoing risk.
Jeff had made a decision to kill himself.

VI REMARKS

See notes.
Jeff is being seen, provide support.

INSTRUCTIONS

Your task will be to verify whether the statements provided below correspond or compare to the contents of the patient's protocols (e.g., interview, written reports). The statements provided below are a classification of the possible content. You are to determine whether the contents in the patient's protocols are a particular or specific instance of the classification or not. Your comparison should be observable; however, the classification may be more abstract than the specific instances. Thus, you will have to make judgements about whether particular contents of a protocol are included in a given classification or not. Your task is to conclude, yes or no.

Intrapsychic

I *Unbearable Psychological Pain*

	Circle/Check
1. Suicide has adjustive value and is functional because it stops painful tension and provides relief from intolerable psychological pain. (P)[1]	Yes ✓ No
2. In suicide, the psychological and/or environmental traumas among many other factors may include: incurable disease, threat of senility, fear of becoming hopelessly dependent, feelings of inadequacy, humiliation. Although the solution of suicide is not caused by one thing, or motive, suicide is a flight from these spectres. (P & D)	Yes ✓ No
3. In the suicidal drama, certain emotional states are present, including pitiful forlornness, emotional deprivation, distress and/or grief. (P & D)	Yes ✓ No
4. S appears to have arrived at the end of an interest to endure and sees suicide as a solution for some urgent problem(s), and/or injustices of life. (P)	Yes ✓ No
5. There is a conflict between life's demands for adaptation and the S's inability or unwillingness to meet the challenge. (P)	Yes ✓ No
6. S is in a state of heightened disturbance (perturbation) and feels boxed in, harassed, especially hopeless and helpless. (P)	Yes ✓ No

---

[1] The letter P refers to a specific highly predictive variable, whereas the letter D refers to a specific differentiating variable of the suicidal mind.

II *Cognitive Constriction*

7. S reports a history of trauma (e.g., poor health, rejection by significant other, a competitive spouse). (P & D)   Yes ✓   No

8. Figuratively speaking, S appears to be "intoxicated" by over-powering emotions. Concomitantly, there is a constricted logic and perception. (D)   Yes ✓   No

9. There is poverty of thought, exhibited by focusing only on permutations and combinations of grief and grief-provoking topics. (D)   Yes   No ✓

III *Indirect Expressions*

10. S reports ambivalence; e.g., complications, concomitant contradictory feelings, attitudes and/or thrusts. (P & D)   Yes ✓   No

11. S's aggression has been turned inwards; for example, humility, submission and devotion, subordination, flagellation, masochism, are evident. (P)   Yes ✓   No

12. Unconscious dynamics can be concluded. There are likely more reasons to the suicide than the person is consciously aware. (D)   Yes ✓   No

IV *Inability to Adjust*

13. S considers him/herself too weak to overcome personal difficulties and, therefore, rejects everything, wanting to escape painful life events. (P)   Yes ✓   No

14. Although S passionately argues that there is no justification for living on, S's state of mind is incompatible with an accurate assessment/perception of what is going on. (P)   Yes   No ✓

15. S exhibits a serious disorder in adjustment. (P)   Yes ✓   No

   (a) S's reports are consistent with a manic-depressive disorder such as the down-phase; e.g., all-embracing negative statements, severe mood disturbances causing marked impairment.   Yes   No

   (b) S's reports are consistent with schizophrenia; e.g., delusional thought, paranoid ideation.   Yes   No

   (c) S's reports are consistent with anxiety disorder (such as obsessive-compulsive, post-traumatic stress); e.g., feeling of losing control; recurrent and persistent thoughts, impulses or images.   Yes   No

   (d) S's reports are consistent with antisocial personality (or conduct) disorder; e.g., deceitfulness, conning others.   Yes   No

   (e) S's reports are consistent with borderline personality; e.g., frantic efforts to avoid real or imagined abandonment, unstable relationships.   Yes   No

   (f) S's reports are consistent with depression; e.g., depressed mood, diminished interest, insomnia.   Yes ✓   No

   (g) S's reports are consistent with a disorder not otherwise specified. S is so paralysed by pain that life, future, etc. is colourless and unattractive.   Yes   No

V *Ego*

16. There is a relative weakness in S's capacity for developing constructive tendencies (e.g., attachment, love). (D)   Yes ✓   No

17. There are unresolved problems ("a complex" or weakened ego) in the individual; e.g., symptoms or ideas that are discordant, unassimilated, and/or antagonistic. (P)   Yes ✓ No

18. S reports that the suicide is related to a harsh conscience; i.e., a fulfilment of punishment (or self-punishment). (D)   Yes   No ✓

Interpersonal

VI   *Interpersonal Relations*

19. S's problem(s) appears to be determined by the individual's history and the present interpersonal situation. (P)   Yes ✓ No

20. S reports being weakened and/or defeated by unresolved problems in the interpersonal field (or some other ideal such as health, perfection). (P)   Yes ✓ No

21. S's suicide appears related to unsatisfied or frustrated needs; e.g., attachment, perfection, achievement, autonomy, control. (P)   Yes ✓ No

22. S's frustration in the interpersonal field is exceedingly stressful and persisting to a traumatic degree. (P)   Yes ✓ No

23. A positive development in the disturbed relationship was seen as the only possible way to go on living, but such development was seen as not forthcoming. (P)   Yes   No ✓

24. S's relationships (attachments) were too unhealthy and/or too intimate (regressive, "primitive"), keeping him/her under constant strain of stimulation and frustration
    (D)   Yes   No ✓

VII   *Rejection–Aggression*

25. S reports a traumatic event or hurt or injury (e.g., unmet love, a failing marriage, disgust with one's work). (P)   Yes   No ✓

26. S, whose personality (ego) is not adequately developed (weakened), appears to have suffered a narcissistic injury. (P & D)   Yes ✓ No

27. S is preoccupied with an event or injury, namely a person who has been lost or rejecting (i.e., abandonment). (D)   Yes   No ✓

28. S feels quite ambivalent, i.e., both affectionate and hostile towards the same (lost or rejecting) person. (D)   Yes   No ✓

29. S reports feelings and/or ideas of aggression and vengefulness towards him/herself although S appears to be actually angry at someone else. (D)   Yes ✓ No

30. S turns upon the self, murderous impulses that had previously been directed against someone else. (D)   Yes   No ✓

31. Although maybe not reported directly, S may have calculated the self-destructiveness to have a negative effect on someone else (e.g., a lost or rejecting person). (P)   Yes   No ✓

32. S's self-destructiveness appears to be an act of aggression, attack, and/or revenge towards someone else who has hurt or injured him/her. (P)   Yes   No ✓

VIII   *Identification–Egression*

33. S reports in some direct or indirect fashion an identification (i.e., attachment) with a lost or rejecting person (or with any lost ideal [e.g., health, freedom, employment, all A's]). (D)   Yes ✓ No

34. An unwillingness to accept the pain of losing an ideal (e.g., abandonment, sickness, old age), allows S to choose, even seek to escape from life and accept death. (D)   Yes ✓ No
35. S wants to egress (i.e., to escape, to depart, to flee, to be gone), to relieve the unbearable psychological pain. (P)   Yes ✓ No

Chapter 15

JENNIFER: A TEENAGER'S SUICIDE ATTEMPT

(And Then Her Mother Killed Herself)

Jennifer, a 14-year-old teenager, first arrived at my office in the beginning of spring. She was referred by a paediatrician; with the referral, the doctor provided the following case notes.

THE REFERRAL

Interview with Jennifer

Jennifer stated that she had a fight with her boyfriend over the phone. She remembered that her dad had pills in the home so she took the pills but she doesn't remember what she was thinking. Jennifer then called her mother because she panicked from what she did and she didn't want to die.

Jennifer stated that there is a person at school that has been harassing her and she even hit her boyfriend. Jennifer doesn't want to switch schools because she has already had to switch schools in grade school because of this same person.

Jennifer and her dad just moved to an apartment and she had to get rid of her dog that she had for seven years. Dad couldn't afford the house anymore.

Jennifer stated that she's glad that her parents are separated because they didn't get along.

Jennifer states that a few months ago she was suicidal by mutilating her wrists. She states that she was upset remembering her grandmother's death. Jennifer admits to skipping school a lot. Jennifer describes bad mood swings; she can be quite irritable. When she is down she cries a lot.

Mom is concerned that things are too permissive for Jennifer living at Dad's. Mom and Dad separated last May 1997. Jennifer chose to live with Dad because he is so permissive according to mother. Jennifer called mother that night while she was at work and told her that she had taken the pills. She said that she had broken up with her boyfriend.

Dad just told mother last night that Jennifer had attempted to cut her wrists a couple of months ago. Dad also informed mom that Jennifer had disclosed to him that she had been raped while she lived in Florida with Mom. Mom confronted Jennifer on this and she denied to mother that she had been raped, she just wanted to get Dad's attention.

According to Mom prior to parents separating they really did not have any serious problems. After parents split up, Jennifer was very angry with them. Dad was fighting custody. Jennifer was in the middle of parents' fight. Another student has threatened Jennifer at her school.

Jennifer had just made a suicide attempt. She was hospitalized, about to be released and her father, William, wanted Jennifer to see a psychotherapist. Jennifer's own reasons for accepting the referral to me were the following: "I am not speaking to my mother and I am drifting away from a lot of friends."

BACKGROUND

William was concerned about the impact of the family conflicts and divorce on Jennifer. Jennifer was especially estranged from her mother, Mary (something that proved to be circular); yet, the stated catalyst for the attempt was a problematic understanding with her boyfriend, Aaron. Jennifer and Aaron had been seeing each other for six months. They had met at school and quickly became sexually active (Jennifer's first sexual relationship, not Aaron's). The relationship was, however, conflictual (mirroring her parents) from the beginning. On the day of the attempt, Jennifer and Aaron had a fight. Aaron said "hurtful things", stating that he had had three affairs (although later he reported that that was a lie; I wonder). Jennifer became forlorn. Later, she said, "I felt such pain." The pain escalated and Jennifer saw suicide as a way out. Her father, being a pharmacist, had an accessible amount of medication; Jennifer managed to secure some and took an undisclosed amount of pills. At some level, wanting to be rescued, William discovered Jennifer, called the ambulance and Jennifer was hospitalized.

At a previous attempt to commit suicide, Jennifer had slashed her wrists. Her beloved grandmother had died. She felt overwhelmed with loss and sadness, wanting "to join my grandmother". "I wanted to escape," she said later. There were no other attempts at the time of my first interview, and she denied any intent, plans, and so on. Of importance, however, she reported that her mother had made a suicide attempt. Her mother, Mary, she reported, had a history of infidelity. At one time, she had a relationship with a "rich" boyfriend, who rejected her. Mary responded with a suicide attempt. Yet, even more significant, Mary had been diagnosed with a Bipolar Disorder, something that "ran in her family". The most painful stimulus for Jennifer was that her own relationship with her mother was chaotic, often Jennifer reported "I feel rejected. Sometimes she loves me and then she is gone," she added. Jennifer's latent reason for accepting the referral was, in fact, her relationship to her mother.

Jennifer's own behaviour was most consistent with a childhood Depressive Disorder (recurrent). She felt irritable most days (she said after the divorce). She had not attended school (failing all her grades); she reported that she could not concentrate. Jennifer was eating less (symptoms of bulimia were evident), and suffered from insomnia. She was often quite agitated; William, in fact, reported a history of mood swings in Jennifer for over two years. There is also, of course, a history of suicide ideation and attempts. Questions arose, given the positive familial history of a manic-depression, whether Jennifer may be developing a Bipolar Disorder.

Subsequently, a consultation with William (at this time, Mary refused to attend), and then with the paediatrician were undertaken. We especially addressed approaches to environment control; William pill-proofed the apartment (see Chapter 19). Issues of confidentiality were discussed, given the high risk, and a rescue plan was drawn up. Additional family members, especially an uncle Bob, were identified as added supports. As we have learned, intervention with high-risk people is best not done alone. A community approach was established (implication 2^1). In suicide, there are psychological and/or environmental traumas. Although there are many possible risks, interpersonal ones are figural; for example, rejection by a loved one. Thus, it implies that a community approach may be most useful; for example, it may include, in Jennifer's case, putting information that she is in trouble about her loss into the stream of communication, letting others know about it, breaking what could be a fatal secret, proferring help, and, if possible, showing interest and deep concern. One should have, at least, a provisional rescue approach with moderately lethal individuals, like Jennifer, and always an action plan with highly lethal individuals. Her TGSP scores are 1, 2, 3, 4, 5, 6, 7, 8, 9, 10, 12, 15(f) (a?), 16, 17, 19, 20, 21, 22, 23, 24, 25, 26, 27, 28, 31, 32, 33, 34, 35.

EARLY VISITS

26 March.   Jennifer arrived quite perturbed; William had set a rule about not seeing Aaron. Aaron was identified as "quite troubled" by many; indeed, one of Aaron's friends was on the local news the night before, having been arrested in his home for a series of break and enters. Aaron had been at his friend's home, when the police had arrived. William responded: "You can't go there." Jennifer hated rules of any kind, often being quite angry if any were imposed. Jennifer wanted to do what Jennifer wanted. Jennifer now reported that "I hate my father", suggesting today that her "good" parent was Mary.

At the end of the session, I invited William to join us (often therapeutic work with young teenagers is family therapy). Jennifer quickly changed her tone and behaviour; with William in the room, she focused on Aaron, stating that, "He cheated". Somehow this eased William's worry, but, as we learn, Jennifer was dissembling.

On the next visit, Jennifer continued to focus on Aaron. She reported that she had been quite upset at Aaron's sexual acting out. She reported, however, that she had met Aaron's best friend and had sex with him. "He (Aaron) got upset," she said, reporting that she felt good with her revenge (items 27, 28, and 32). Jennifer was, in fact, singly focused on one narcissistic injury; namely Aaron had been lost (i.e., abandonment). Jennifer was preoccupied with Aaron. I said, "Tell me what's happening. What hurts?" Jennifer talked and talked about her pain, mainly interpersonal. This implied that to help Jennifer, at times I went into her real world as an ombudsman, someone had to reduce the interpersonal distress.

---

[1] Explanations of all implications/items are given in Chapter 12.

Jennifer felt quite ambivalent. She was not only affectionate and hostile towards Aaron, but she was also ambivalent about life and death. I first worked with the life and death issue, putting my weight on the life side of the balance. I then worked with the affectionate feelings (protective factors) towards Aaron, William, and others.

Jennifer's self-destructiveness appeared to be an act of aggression, attack, and/or revenge towards Aaron (and her mother, and so on), that had hurt or injured her. Suicide is often a dyadic event (Shneidman, 1985). Jennifer often felt hurt, slighted and under attack. Revenge was frequently involved in her behaviour (as it was with others in her real world). As therapist, I created activity—something, of course, different from consciously or unconsciously attacking another person (e.g., Mary).

Jennifer, when talking about her own sexual behaviour, spontaneously associated to her mother's unfaithfulness. "I know my father's hurt," she said, "but, I did it too." We began to discuss her sexual acting out, beginning to attempt to get her to think before acting. She also reported that lots of boys in grade 11 and 12 were interested in her. She said, "They think that I am cool," lacking insight into an older boy's motivation. She did not grasp their wish to act out too. She did what she wanted, without reflection on the consequences (suggesting heightened impulsiveness).

During our early visits, I also began to associate her behaviour to her mother's suicide attempt. About three months before Jennifer's attempt, her mother had made an attempt. Mary had a fight with her then boyfriend. Jennifer had been upset at her mother's behaviour and had rejected her, until her mother's suicide attempt. Jennifer quickly attempted to heal the rift, but Mary was distant. "She always pushes me away," Jennifer said. I began to examine Mary's behaviour with Jennifer; for example, I asked if the only reason for her mother's attempt was the fight that day. Jennifer began to examine if suicide was something more than just a response to a situation, whether her or her mother's attempt was only due to a rejection. I attempted to get Jennifer to slow down and think (a common goal with adolescent patients).

CONSULTATION

Psychotherapists often wish they had consulted more; I was fortunate to have discussed Jennifer with Dr Shneidman. I recall his advice to me for Jennifer: "The trick in life is not to spoil and ruin it, no matter what happens." Obviously, we need to target acting out behaviour that was not only destructive, but at times highly suicidal. As is so often the case with young people, we "need to develop a larger view of life". Patients like Jennifer need to learn to cope with the frustrations of life, their thwarted needs, wants, wishes, and so on. They need to strengthen their ego.

Shneidman suggested that one has to accept the patient's view of life. With Jennifer, his statement would be, "This is the greatest trauma that you personally could suffer. Your mother had abandoned you...." Although, with some caution, one could add, "She's doing everything you are against." Shneidman would develop rapport with such patients; his psychotherapeutic goal with suicidal patients would be to act as the auxiliary ego and say, "I'm here to tell you that that's not what life is."

Jennifer's life, like many of our patients' lives, Shneidman noted, "is like a gyroscope. It spins. We need to find what will prevent the person from moving fast." You say to the patient, something like "Let's not go quickly, just slowly. Then, you decide." He suggested that, in a fatherly way, he would tell Jennifer something like "Believe me in this—listen to me. Don't do things impulsively. Have some restraint on your behalf." I strongly believe that Bronowski (1973), in his book *The Ascent of Man*, is correct when he said that what makes a person a person is the ability to wait, to think, to talk, before the act, and, I would add, before one kills oneself.

Shneidman noted that suicidal people "pour oil into troubled waters". A key task is, therefore, the following: "Calm things down!"

Characteristically Shneidman's consultations led to discussion of countertransference issues (he is an excellent teacher). Ed was never restrained in his insights. As we talked about Jennifer, he asked, "Are you overreacting yourself?" He asked: "Are you going too fast?" This is good advice with most suicidal patients. "Slow down", Shneidman advised, as I was preparing to help set the table for our frequent barbecues under his birch tree at his home on Kingsland Street, LA.

THE CONFUSIONS

28 March.   Unexpectedly, a call from Mary occurred. We discussed Jennifer's suicide attempt and our response; Mary reported that she wanted to be a support for Jennifer. I subsequently discussed matters of risk with both parents, although Mary rarely attended any visits with Jennifer.

31 March.   I received a call from a social worker; she reported that Aaron had made a suicide attempt. Aaron had been assessed as at high risk, was hospitalized, and placed in a youth treatment centre was planned. At our next visit, I evaluated Jennifer's risk; however, she appeared to show low perturbation and low lethality. She was less focused on Aaron, being more focused on the fact that "people blame me". She reported that Aaron had told people that he tried to kill himself because of her. Once more, we talked about suicide and I rejected the concept that she alone caused his attempt. Jennifer agreed; yet, we also explored people's possible perception, especially given the fact that even in the hospital Aaron reported, "I tried to kill myself because of Jennifer."

The stimuli from Aaron's report were that a grade 12 boy, Sam, had expressed interest in Jennifer, had dated her and engaged in sex with her. Aaron had been quite perturbed, feeling possessive. Jennifer now concluded that "Aaron loves me" and said, "I want to be with him." I attempted to slow her down, specifically suggesting that she allow Aaron time to heal, but Jennifer stated, "I do what

I want." Subsequently, with Jennifer's informed knowledge, discussions about the current risks with the paediatrician, William and others occurred.

Our next appointment with Jennifer was a "no show". I called William; Jennifer had gone to her mother's. I called and Mary informed me that Jennifer no longer wanted to see me. I once more discussed the heightened risk, but like Jennifer, Mary wanted to escape, minimizing the risk. She said that Jennifer and she did not need help (dissembling). Jennifer called back a few days later, saying that she wanted to see me.

The next appointment was kept with Jennifer, along with Mary. I first spoke to Mary (her first visit); my main goal was simply to communicate: "It is serious." I did not agree with "nothing" was wrong. I stated something like "I understand the wish to fly into happiness; but it is not true. Jennifer's suicide risk is serious." I again discussed the attempt, concluding: "It is serious." Mary reluctantly agreed (did she?). Upon questioning, Mary also gave the contretemps of the relationship to William a different read. She said, "William is the problem."

When I was alone with Jennifer, I asked, "What happened about our meeting?" It was clear that she had lied to her father and me; she had made plans to go out.

Jennifer reported that Aaron was "crazy", being still in the treatment centre. She also reported that Sam "played me. He's off with some rich girl." However, she reported that her brief liaison was positive because "older guys were now interested in me". She said, "I'm mature, like them. We're mature." I asked what she meant, so much related to her need for security (item 21). Jennifer's suicidal behaviours appeared to be related to unsatisfied or frustrated needs. Her pain related to the frustration. It should be the therapist's function to help the individual in relation to those thwarted needs. Even a little bit of improvement can save a life. The possible needs that are frustrated or blocked are expansive. Here is a partial list of Jennifer's needs, adopted from Henry A. Murray's *Explorations in Personality* (1938):

- *Aggression.* To overcome opposition forcefully; to fight; to attack or injure another; to oppose forcefully or punish other.
- *Autonomy.* To get free, shake off restraint; break out of social confinement; avoid or quit activities of domineering authorities; be independent and free.
- *Dominance.* To control other humans; influence or direct others by command, suggestion or persuasion; or to dissuade, restrain, or prohibit others.
- *Exhibition.* To make an impression; be seen and heard; to excite, amaze, fascinate, entertain, shock, intrigue, amuse, or entice others.
- *Rejection.* To exclude, abandon, expel, separate oneself or remain indifferent to a negatively seen person; to snub or jilt another.

Her esteem also needed building, something more nurturing than was achieved by acting out with the older boys. She so wanted to be loved (attachment).

As rapport is so essential in psychotherapy, I explored her commitment to therapy. At one point, she said, "I don't want to come back," yet, as she left, she agreed to return. Of course, non-compliance with treatment is a risk issue (Leenaars, 1997).

Our next visit was cancelled; Jennifer was sick. When she returned, we began to explore her relationship with boys. She was explicit about sex. "Some girls want it," she said, suggesting that there was nothing wrong. Of course, as we have learned, there is never any room for judgement, criticism and the like in therapy with suicidal people; rather, I continued to explore, "What will make you happy? What will add to your self-esteem?" and so on. Yet, I also explored the fact of safe sex. She, like many teenagers, was practising unsafe sex. I said something like, "If you are going to have sex, be safe." We also discussed birth control; Jennifer had refused such intervention from the paediatrician, who had earlier expressed her concern to Jennifer and her father. I referred Jennifer to a teenage medical centre, where she was able to obtain condoms and birth control pills. Jennifer complied with the referral. She also attended some educational sessions with a public health nurse, who became part of the community response team. Jennifer informed her father about her protective behaviour (not only to sexual disease, but to death).

Jennifer reported that she was "frustrated with Aaron". "He plays other girls," she said, "and then tells me." I asked, "Why might he do that?" She said "To make me jealous." Once more I encouraged her to slow down. We also discussed what was meant by "Aaron is crazy. Aaron is troubled." She needed to understand people better. Once more, she had a new boyfriend, Mike, and I again began to explore the trouble with acting out in life. Our next visits continued to focus on her impulsive behaviour; I suggested, "There is a need to think before you act" (remembering some of Shneidman's suggestions with Jennifer). We focused, for example, on her belief "I can do what I want", adding the conjunctive "if it is safe" (items 7 and 8).

Aaron, a Competitive Mother, and a Frequently Constricted Jennifer

It is imperative that the reader again be reminded that in working with suicidal people, the person defines the crisis. Jennifer needed to define her trauma, but a trauma is a perception. Jennifer was, figuratively speaking, "intoxicated" by her overpowering emotions and her constricted logic. I, thus, did not buy into her anguish. It is vital, in fact, to counter the suicidal person's constriction of thought by attempting to widen the mental blinders and increase the number of options. We did so on many practical items as we did on the traumatic ones. What is important is that it is possible to lower a patient's lethality by reducing his/her perturbation. We can widen the range of visible and realistic options. Suicide intervention is long-range problem-solving. We began to talk about boys; for example, Mike. Who is he? Is he like Aaron? What does he want? What are your needs? (Item 9).

There was poverty of thought in Jennifer, not only about suicidal states. She exhibited blinders on many topics. She often believed that something was either black or white. Something was either "A or not-A" and she knew what A and not-A were. It is not necessary to accept, as a therapist, the patient's view of the world as "A or not-A". To suggest such an "A or not-A" world is a limited and harsh view of life (e.g., either mom loves me or not, either Aaron loves me or not, either Mike is good or not). Thus, the task with Jennifer was to increase the permutations and combinations of her thoughts, to reframe her world. (See Wazlawick et al., 1967.)

School began to be discussed now as Jennifer was failing all her classes. Her marks had fallen since last year. Jennifer saw the failures as being the fault of her teachers. She said, "It (her marks) is justified. The teachers cause the trouble." Once more, we began to explore her denial, avoidance, projection and so on, often to a reluctant Jennifer ("My mother says it's the teacher's fault."). Despite Jennifer's statement the real motivation was boys. She skipped classes, did not do her homework, etc., to be with various boys. "Boys seem to be the only thing that interests you," I suggested. I also asked: "Will that get you to grade 12?"

14 May.   My notes read: "Mike is out. Daniel is in." Daniel was a grade 12 student at another high school. Aaron continued to be ignored; he, however, was angry, even getting some girls to beat Jennifer up. There was, in fact, an increase in female violence at Jennifer's school. Yet, Jennifer dismissed her own problem with aggression (items 29 and 30).

Once more, the principle was: Slow down. Think.

THINK BEFORE YOU ACT

Jennifer had many feelings and/or ideas of aggression and vengefulness towards herself and actually also towards other people (e.g., her mother and Aaron). One does not exacerbate the anger in the sense of making it more real for the person by talking about it. One should not buy into the taboo of "Don't talk about anger, suicide and death." Jennifer was already angry and hostile. Ventilation, lightening of angry feelings, adequacy of expression and need for contact, have a critical place in psychotherapy. Others need to know that the trauma is "real". One has to address the social taboo of talking about aggression, hate and rage, including suicidal and homicidal rage (even terrorism).

Jennifer had murderous impulses that had previously been directed against her mother, Aaron, and others. The focus with Jennifer was not immediately on "why" the aggression or "why" it had been turned inwards or "why" suicide had been chosen as the method of solving the problems, but these questions were addressed as therapy progressed. These are, in fact, best addressed once the lethality is reduced. Jennifer needed to learn ways of reducing her urgently felt impulses or wishes, which were central to the suicidal ending of her reveries. To address the impulses, including the aggressiveness, I addressed her unmet needs.

At the next visit, the relationship to Daniel had developed. Once more her relationships seemed to be primitive and immature (items 17 and 24). There were unresolved problems ("a complex", weakened ego) in Jennifer. One had to assess the discordant, unassimilated and antagonistic in Jennifer. I had to evaluate her complexes, anxiety, and other important aspects of her dynamics, psychopathology, and reaction patterns. Simply stated, I had to know Jennifer to treat her. Jennifer's relationships (attachments) were too unhealthy and too regressive, keeping her under constant strain of stimulation and frustration. Jennifer needed to have needs and wishes stimulated and inhibited to a healthier degree. Thus, I had to both increase and decrease her relationships, some of which were suicidogenic.

Daniel had first been reluctant in his relationship to Jennifer; "he said I was too young". They had met and had sex. Daniel now said, "It was not my age." Yet, importantly, Aaron "was back". She reported that she had been seeing Aaron again and "having sex". Once more, Jennifer had been dissembling. She reported, "I am excited with Aaron." She reported, for example, that she stole out of her apartment after 11:00 p.m., met Aaron, and had sex. When I began to explore her reason, she said, "I'm bored." She reported that only Aaron was stimulating. "I love him," she said. When I asked about Daniel, she saw no problem with several relationships at the same time. "Aaron does it" (of course, the association to her mother is obvious). I explored "Is it healthy?"; "Is it best?"; and so on. The issue of safe sex occurred again ("Aaron does not like condoms"). The motto that I again stressed, regardless of the specific self-destructive behaviour, was: "Be safe."

The contacts with the parents continued.

28 May.   The next visit, I asked about Aaron. She reported that she was quite upset at him. She reported that she heard that Aaron had said bad things about her. "He said, 'I am a slut'." I responded, "Your relationship with Aaron is up and down." She agreed and we discussed his mood disorder to which I added, "Is it like your mother?" Jennifer said, "yes" seeing the similarities (how they are alike and yet different).

Despite Aaron's lability, she said, "There is no one else. I only love Aaron." Mental constriction was pervasive; I responded with widening the blinders. And the ever present: Think before you act.

The next visit was kept with her father, William. Jennifer had reluctantly accepted a referral to a child psychiatrist, but she refused suggestions of an antidepressant ("I'm not crazy," she said). We began to explore then, and in subsequent joint visits, issues of rules and expectations (the usual issues over telephone, room cleanliness, etc.). Much of our conversation centred on responsibility. Jennifer saw herself as very responsible, unlike most other people; I began to explore with her what it meant to be responsible.

The next appointment was cancelled; William began to discuss concern about hard drug use. We all knew that Jennifer smoked marijuana, especially with Aaron—but the use of a "hard" drug was new. Later, when I explored her father's concerns, Jennifer admitted to marijuana use, but denied use of other drugs (dissembling?). She did, however, report that Aaron used multiple drugs. On the next visit, Jennifer was more open and said, "I used acid." When I asked about LSD, she said, "I used acid, not LSD." I suggested that these are the same; like many teenagers, she was uninformed about drugs. One teenager once reported, "I do acid, not marijuana. Marijuana is more dangerous." Drug education is often essential with suicidal teenagers (drug use is only one more face of self-destructiveness). Jennifer was willing to listen because, she said, "I had a bad experience." She reported visual hallucinations, paranoia, and panic after a recent use. She was quite uncharacteristically expressive of her fear, stating that "someone gave Aaron rat poison", reporting that she used it. Jennifer was upset and she cried for the first time. I used the occasion not only to teach her about drugs, but once more to slow the process. Once more, I explored the wisdom of thinking before doing (one often has to be redundant, concrete and explicit with suicidal teenagers).

Jennifer continued to see Daniel and, unknown to anyone, Aaron. They continued late night liaisons. Aaron continued to want to have sex, but Jennifer reported, "I said 'no'." Aaron had become quite angry about the refusal, raging at her and being verbally abusive ("You whore"). Jennifer began to question Aaron's motivation, asking, "Does he love me?" Her relationship to her mother also continued to be up and down, and again we associated Aaron and Mary's behaviour.

Jennifer had failed all but one course in school. I asked, "Is this what you want?" At school, too, the issue of violence continued (and we explored issues of school bullying, violence, and so on).

2 July.   The relationship to Aaron continued to be volatile. Aaron was discovered to be "dating" someone new; yet, despite Jennifer knowing this fact, she continued her own liaison. Aaron would call and Jennifer would sneak out of the apartment at night. "Why does he call?" I asked. Jennifer said, "sex". I noted a push–pull relationship; I suggested that he rejects her, tells her about dating, and so on, and then, because Jennifer feared the rejection, loss, and abandonment, he pulls her in. I showed the cyclical nature of the dynamic behaviour (Shneidman, 1985, called it more accurately, elliptical). I suggested that these patterns were dysfunctional and manipulative. She agreed and we associated the relationship to Aaron with her relationship to her mother, Mary. Both were habitual; I began to draw a habit cycle allowing Jennifer to see her cycle (e.g., triggers, relapse, reaction to relapse, pretend normal phase).

SUMMER HOLIDAYS

13 August.   William had called; he reported that Jennifer was doing better. "She is a better person," he said. Yet, I cautioned him about summer holidays, and to see how Jennifer does after school starts again in September. He agreed; yet, I reluctantly accepted the suggestion to reduce visits to every other week during the summer, because Jennifer did not want to come every week.

Jennifer herself also reported that she was doing better; in fact, her clothes even changed. She started wearing "prep clothes". Jennifer reported that she had developed new friends ("They don't do drugs. They are not boy crazy.").

Over the summer, she reported, "Aaron is out. Aaron still calls, but I don't see him often." She also stated "I don't have sex with him." She reported that with her new friends, she was meeting new boys ("They just don't want sex."). I encouraged her new better adjustment. She reported, in fact, "I feel better about myself." I continually reinforced her positive, protective behaviour (ego-strengthening).

During the summer, we also reflected on her past behaviour, especially being motivated by boys and not school. Specifically, about school, we explored: "How can we do better this year?" I was attempting once more to increase her thinking/planning behaviour.

20 August.   Jennifer arrived with her parents, William and Mary (our only joint meeting). Mary was manic; she was very talkative, flying from one ideation to the next. She had, in fact, called the meeting, reporting "a crisis".

Mary was blaming Jennifer for *all* the problems, from money to drugs. Mary had learned that Jennifer had been using drugs other than marijuana. She said "what if _____" and "what if _____". Mary was in a panic; she said, "Jennifer is suicidal." When I asked what she meant, she said, "Drugs are the same as pills. She's trying to kill herself." I shared some basics of suicide, especially regarding intent. Jennifer had denied intent; William did not see any risks. Yet, despite our efforts, Mary continued to worry about suicide risk. We discussed drug use, community support, etc. Our support in treatment that had been provided to Jennifer by this time was outlined, but Mary's own plan was different. "I have to stop the drug use," she said. Of note, William kept silent when Mary was racing in her talk from one topic to the next. I accepted that Jennifer had impulse control problems; yet, I suggested that simply telling Jennifer not to do drugs would fail. Mary left upset; I did not do what she wanted me to do (item 12).

There were no doubt unconscious dynamics in Jennifer (and Mary). There were many more reasons for Jennifer's behaviour than she was consciously aware of. The focus of action in therapy is on the individual in both his/her conscious and unconscious mind. The focus with Jennifer was on the person in her totality; not simply her stated conscious perception. This implied that I must see Jennifer with a decentred frame. There was much more to her destructive behaviours than just what Jennifer stated. The suicidal mind is deep, deeper than the conscious mind is aware of.

PROTECTIVE FACTORS

3 September.   Jennifer made plans to go to school. There had, however, been a further conflict with some girls the previous weekend. Jennifer had been threatened; and her solution was to escape. She said, "I want to go to another school"; yet, with encouragement, she returned to her old school. I used the occasion to discuss her quick decision to escape. Egression was a pervasive problem in Jennifer (and most suicidal people) (items 34 and 35).

Jennifer was often unwilling to accept her pain. She wanted to escape from her life. I needed to focus on the "problem" that Jennifer was trying to solve—the loss, the school failure. Again, repeating Karl Menninger's dictum: The patient is always right. It was my task to find out, "How was Jennifer right?" Then I needed to assist her in developing an alternative solution(s) to her life's problems.

Jennifer often wanted to flee, to be gone, to relieve uncomfortable feelings of pain. The suicidal person wants to escape. It followed that, where possible, the means of exit, not only suicide, needed to be blocked, especially since Mary and Aaron also exhibited such egression. Jennifer needed to develop better patterns of adjustment, protective factors to accept life, beyond those she had learned from her environment.

I associated her response to her patterns with her mother. If there was a conflict, Jennifer ran away. "Is this the best way to solve the problem?", we began to explore. (Of course, Mary herself used escape techniques.) Jennifer began to use words like "chaotic" and "intense" to understand the relationship to her mother, and how she had learned to cope with the chaos, by escaping. For example, Mary was now demanding that Jennifer see a new psychologist ("Someone who will tell you what to do," Mary said). We discussed that, by her age, Jennifer could decide whom she sees for treatment. I asked Jennifer: "What is in your best interest?" Jennifer decided to not see a new doctor, but continue with me, the paediatrician and the public health nurse (who continued to provide Jennifer with practical information and protective care). Mary, I learned, was quite upset!

From time to time, Jennifer and I discussed her mother's Bipolar Disorder. What it was. What it causes. How can it be treated? (Mary refused all medication and rarely saw any type of doctor for assistance.)

Jennifer's acting out continued; she started having body piercings, despite William's objections. It was of greater concern that Jennifer was drinking more. Her new friends did not do drugs, but they did drink. On one occasion, she reported that she drank 10 drinks of Vodka. "I got sick," she said. Once more, we began to explore her need to think, before acting. We explored: What is normal? What are the consequences? Can you learn from your mistakes? Jennifer was more able to reflect, think and plan (and the nurse provided Jennifer with educational information). Mary, however, was not.

Mary had called after the last visit; she was raging at me. She was angry with Jennifer and me; Mary said, "I was the victim." I, however, questioned her perception, suggesting that she and Jennifer were both causing problems in their relationship, not only Jennifer. Mary reported that Jennifer was disrespectful, did not do what Mary wanted, and said "hurtful things". Once more, I accepted that this might be true from her point of view and suggested that both had problems in their relationship. As Mary was suicidogenic, I attempted to provide more realistic perceptions, beyond the singleness of Mary's: "Jennifer is all the problem."

I encouraged Mary to come in and participate in Jennifer's treatment, not only in a crisis response. I suggested (as others and I had before) that she should see a counsellor too. I suggested that everyone needed to learn to cope better; regrettably, Mary never really participated in treatment, whereas William did. Mary also continued to refuse any intervention. Jennifer's relationships continued to be a focus in her therapy, as were her mood swings and how she could cope better. For example, we explored "how do you cope with your mother if you disagree?"; "how can you use time out (escape) effectively?"; and importantly, "how can you have a positive time with your mother?"

School was going well (she was passing all her subjects). There were fewer conflicts. Aaron was not being seen. And Jennifer got a part-time job.

30 October.   Jennifer reported that, overall, she was doing better. The new job, however, presented new challenges and we discussed how she could cope with these challenges. She found the job "chaotic". When we began to explore what she meant by "chaotic" (a frequent description of her family), she said that the job was not predictable. It was too unstructured ("I don't know what to do"), something that made Jennifer anxious. We explored the association with her history; Jennifer was now able to see how her history and current situation were enmeshed (item 19).

Jennifer's problems appeared to be determined by her history and present interpersonal situation. Jennifer's suicidal behaviour was not just determined by the present; it had a long history. Regrettably, the clues to her suicide risk and maladaptive patterns were usually not seen, heard, or even responded to before the attempt. Only if there was a suicidal crisis did the family acknowledge the risk. It followed, as a more general implication for psychotherapy, that a preventive approach to suicide, as all destructive behaviours, with our patients (and their families) is education about the risks, clues, what to do and so on. Much of my (and the public health nurse's) work with Jennifer's family was educational.

Jennifer, at first, responded that she did not want to return to her job ("I want to quit"). I accepted that "the job is difficult for you" and, I added, "You can do it. You can do other things too." (I had learned that her tasks were mainly simple clerical ones; e.g., filling shelves.) I reinforced her wellness (Jennifer got tears in her eyes). Jennifer had a need for nurture and reinforcement; fortunately, within the non-threatening context of psychotherapy, one can assist in addressing the needs and this often strengthens them. Jennifer had so little nurturance from Mary. Jennifer decided that she would continue the job and she went to work the next day.

12 November.   Jennifer had met a new boy, Andrew. She described him more realistically; she feared, however, being rejected. "I can't cope being rejected," she said; Jennifer verbalized such about Mary and Aaron. She asked, "Will it happen again?" "What if . . . ?" Of course, one cannot give her a false sense of reality; rather I reframed her worries as how to cope with life's demands (item 20).

Jennifer was weakened and defeated by unresolved problems in her interpersonal field. She appeared so preoccupied with the current unresolved problem that she was unaware of her developmental history, and of how she had previously adjusted to stressful events [a basic tenet in social learning theory (Bandura, 1977)]. She was fixated on the present. Yet, there was a history, her serial (sameness) way of coping with life's problems. She had suffered similar repeated defeats. This implied that I had to widen her protective processes including, but not limited to, helping Jennifer to understand her past learning. One has eventually to address history, with suicidal patients, to protect their future. And I added, "You can do it."

Jennifer continued to do well. She was getting B's (and "some A's") at school. She was motivated ("I don't want to fail twice.") Indeed, the very subjects that she had reported to hate were now her best. It was important that she should show herself that she could do it and, fortunately, many adults (her father, her teachers) were reinforcing her protective behaviour. Her relationships to others, especially females, also developed more positively.

The relationship to Andrew developed slowly. Jennifer did not become sexually active immediately; Andrew did not push ("I thought all guys were like Aaron"). The relationship, however, surfaced a deeper issue; i.e., trust. "After Aaron," she asked, "can I trust again?" I added the association with her parents' divorce. Jennifer was beginning to understand her more latent issues, dynamics and so on, in her life.

7 January.   Jennifer arrived upset; "Andrew cheated on me," she said. She reported that she was upset because the relationship was "different" ("we talked"). We explored "what should she do". Jennifer was learning how to slow down and think. She said, "I don't have to accept it" (like with Aaron, Mary, etc.) and I added, "You're too valuable to accept it." Jennifer especially associated to Aaron's past acting out; she said that she allowed it, but not now. She decided to break off the relationship with Andrew; "I'm going to decide," she concluded. She did make the decision and broke off with Andrew. Besides the events with Andrew, Jennifer's life was becoming less and less chaotic. She was doing well at school; she reported "I got a 98" (once more, I reinforced her abilities).

The relationship with Aaron, despite some distance, continued. "I love him," she said, but she realized that he had too many problems; e.g., mood swings, drugs. He also continued sexual relationships with several girls ("He can't commit"). We concluded: "You can love someone, but can't be with them." She developed a similar stance with her mother; this approach helped her with both relationships and other relationships.

On one occasion, she arrived suggesting that she wanted to move in with her mother. Her mother had asked, she added, "What should I do?" (she is thinking). I stated that given the past, what would most likely happen? Jennifer answered, "I'd be stressed." Although I often believe that it is in the patient's best interest to make his/her life's decisions, sometimes I am quite free in my advice about suicidogenic people. In this case I said, "I can't support it." I suggested "someone will get hurt again", providing a series of previous examples. I wondered whether Jennifer would do what she wanted—and had she learned to slow down.

Predictably, Jennifer never moved in with her mother, Mary. As Mary, in fact, had found a new boyfriend she no longer wanted Jennifer to move in, and said so ("I don't want you here"). This was one more rejection. Jennifer and I discussed her mother's decision: She does what she wants. It was one more opportunity to cognitively explore the belief "I do what I want". She stayed with her father and we continued therapy.

THE MOTHER'S SUICIDE

22 April.   Jennifer began to question her termination from psychotherapy. She said, "I don't need to be here." I responded by asking about her coping skills and suicide risk; she responded, "I'm happy to be alive." Jennifer, in fact, stated quite explicitly what she was happy about: her father, friends, and even school. She continued to love Aaron; yet she saw no future. She stated, "This makes me

unhappy," but again noting that other things did make her happy now ("Aaron is not the only thing that makes me happy now"). Her father, teachers, and the public health nurse all agreed about Jennifer's progress. We began the process of termination and some months later terminated mutually, always leaving the door open . . . and then her mother killed herself.

About three months after termination, I received a call from William. Mary had killed herself; the new boyfriend rejected her, she left a note and took an overdose. Jennifer called to see me; I agreed and we saw each other that day. I also saw William and her together. That same evening, I went to the funeral home to be supportive, if needed.

The funeral home was quite a sad event. There was a lot of pain. I met Jennifer's extended family, notably the oldest uncle, Bob (Mary's brother). I monitored Jennifer and, once we judged that she was coping with the sad events, I left the funeral home, after speaking to her father, her uncle and herself. Jennifer came to see me a few days later. Her main theme was: "I loved my mother. I miss her so." Jennifer came to see me a few times, talking about her mother. She never returned to psychotherapy, but she did talk about her loss for a few visits. Slowly, Jennifer needed to learn to cope the best that she could with the suicide of her mother. Jennifer had to learn to become a survivor. She and her father were referred to a support group and attended a series of meetings with other survivors, assisting in their healing.

Importantly, we also had a family meeting with her extended family; Bob served as the liaison. We discussed some basics in prevention, such as risk issues and how to respond if there was a suicidal risk. A family plan for prevention was established (a sort of wraparound net) and used to date on three occasions with three different extended family members (who suffered from depression and showed mild to moderate suicide risk). We all accepted: "It takes a family to prevent suicide."

WHAT HAVE WE LEARNED FROM THIS CASE?

The first focus of treatment with Jennifer was item 2: We had to help to stop the unbearable anguish. Much of Jennifer's treatment focused on implications under interpersonal relations (not only with her mother) and rejection–aggression. There was such aggression. It was key to her pain, namely, to do something about her troubled, primitive relationships. This needed intervention—this is what kept Jennifer alive. The specific implications were as follows: 2, 27, 28, 32, 21, 7, 8, 9, 29, 30, 17, 24, 12, 34, 35, 19, 20.

Chapter 16

SUSAN: A YOUNG ADULT'S ISOLATION
(And Then Her Father Killed Himself)

Susan was 13 when she made her first suicide attempt. Her father had also made a previous attempt. On the night of Susan's attempt, she came home a few minutes late. Her father, as typical, was drunk. He raged at Susan and she cowered away after the yelling stopped. She always froze when her father let out what she called "a red red roar". She went upstairs to the bathroom and swallowed "13 or so" aspirins. Susan was asthmatic and her body reacted. Fortunately, her mother heard Susan and called the emergancy services. Susan was hospitalized. She was referred to a counsellor, but said later to me, "we didn't connect." "I had to keep the secrets, dad had warned me," she added.

Susan is now 23, a young adult (see discussion on young adults in Chapter 9); she is an energetic person who arrived at my office quite distraught. She had an alcohol problem. "I binge at times," she said, "and then I get depressed and feel guilty." She feared the excessive use and had been thinking of killing herself. "Every time I drink, I say, now I have to kill myself" (the classical suicidological "therefore" conclusion).

Susan was depressed; her DSM symptoms included: depressed nearly every day, often being quite irritable and angry; lack of pleasure in almost everything; fluctuating sleep disturbances; fatigue; deep feelings of worthlessness and excessive (even suicidogenic) guilt; and frequent thoughts of suicide. Yet, Susan denied any plan: "I only want the pain to stop," she said.

I rated Susan's perturbation as 7 (high) on a 1 to 9 scale, where 1 is non-perturbent and 9 is the worst. Her lethality was a 4, maybe a 5 (mild–moderate). Her TGSP[1] scores were: 1, 2, 3, 5, 6, 7, 9, 10, 11, 12, 13, 15(f), 16, 17, 19, 20, 21, 22, 23, 24, 25, 26, 27, 28, 33, 35. Susan's Shneidman's Psychological Distress Questionnaire (PDQ) is presented in Appendix 16.1.

---

[1] Explanations of all implications/items are given in Chapter 12.

When asked, "What hurts?" Susan described her current problem as "alcoholism".

Susan stated that her relationship with her parents was "okay"; her father always drank and, in recent years, her mother—who had recently been hospitalized for depression—drank daily. The biological links are obvious. Susan herself, being a nurse, wondered about this fact. She often reacted to her problems, frustrations and so on, with depressive reactions. "It is so hopeless," she would often say.

After Susan's first suicide attempt, her then boyfriend, Dan (15), became more involved. They were sexual almost immediately after they met ("Dan wanted sex") and they dated for five years. Then, when Susan was 18, Dan died tragically in a motor vehicle accident (MVA) with two other girls in the car. It was a painful loss and Susan reported, "I never dealt with it." There were walls to her grief. At the funeral, she learned that Dan had been unfaithful, not only with one of the other victims of the MVA, but with a number of her best friends. She became numb, never talking to those friends again. "I became isolated," she said.

Susan was now in a new relation with Konrad ("the first since Dan"). Konrad was also 23, being employed as a youth counsellor at an agency. He had encouraged Susan to see me because of her occasional excessive drinking; when Susan drank she would become very angry. "Konrad can't stand my rages," she said. "I rage and rage" (the identification to her father was obvious, already at intake). "Konrad wants me to stop being angry," she said.

Work was positive; she enjoyed her work as a Registered Nurse (RN), but often felt bored. "I always wanted to be a doctor," she said. She denied that alcohol was a problem at work ("I binge on weekends").

In treatment, I began immediately to address the alcohol abuse. I began with the least intrusive intervention, and said something like: "Look, you and I both agree that the alcohol is a problem (no disagreement). You want to stop (nodding of her head). Let's begin by a verbal agreement that you will not drink." She said, "Yes." I do not mean to suggest that such verbal contracts should be the sole intervention with alcoholism or any habit. It is, however, a good first step; one can at least gauge the person's intent. Susan was motivated. I did suggest, however, that there were further steps that we could take, mentioning medication and hospitalization as two examples. I also suggested Alcoholics Anonymous (AA), but Susan refused such a referral. (I did suggest that we might need to rediscuss this option, if needed, and she agreed.)

Rapport was easily established. Susan wanted help. As an aside, Susan discussed a few dreams at her first visit. She reported: "I dream of vampires. They eat, devour everyone around me...but not me." She also reported a second dream: "I dream of Dan. I see him, but he does not see me. He is on a school bus. He sits beside someone else, holding hands."

THE NEXT VISITS

I began our second visit with, "We talked about a lot last day, what would you like to focus on today?" Susan suggested that we talk about her anger and alcoholism.

About the latter, Susan associated with her vampire dream; "I'm like them," she said.

She reported that she drank once since we met. She had had a frustrating day and had a drink. She was then even more frustrated and angry with herself. She said, "I can't control it." I reframed her thought that actually she did quite well. "You had a slip, but you did not slide." We began to negotiate what she could do in the future, if she felt an urge to drink. We were now arguing about an action plan (see Chapter 11 and item 16 of Chapter 12).

There is a relative weakness in almost all suicidal people's capacity for developing constructive tendencies, not only about attachment or love, but also about many aspects of their lives, drug and alcohol abuse being examples. The key to intermediate, and long-range, effectiveness with such people is to increase the options for action, something more constructive than, as in Susan's case, to drink. One widens the constriction beyond *the* solution, whether suicide or alcoholism or some other destructive (both self and other) behaviour. Keep in mind that the regressive act is an effort by the person to stop unbearable pain. The individual wants to do something to stop the psychache, one made out of weakness, not strength. Drinking was such an escape for Susan. Knowing this guided me as to what Susan's treatment needed to be: increase the constructive tendencies (or protective ones) and decrease the destructive one(s). Not drinking was a protective factor.

Susan never binged again, although from time to time, early in treatment, she would regress and have a beer or two (I have no information to suggest otherwise). Susan and I also discussed the need for medication, something she was more open to consider on the second visit. I suggested that the medication would make her pain easier. "You are using the alcohol to numb yourself. You want the pain to stop ('Yes'). You're using alcohol to medicate yourself but it does not work. It will make you worse (induction)." Susan agreed and, with the assistance of her general practitioner, she was prescribed an antidepressant, Zoloft (50 mg daily), with a good response.

Susan was well aware that the drinking was an acting out behaviour (she had taken a number of university courses in psychology, receiving all A's). She associated with Dan; "He always drank," she said. We began, as I do with all substance abuse cases, to understand her use cycle.

We also began to find alternative ways to cope with stress. She said that talking to me helped. She also decided to join a gym, something she did in high school, but not in the last two years. It made a JND. She also joined a volleyball team, excelling in the sport. (I often reminded myself to ask her how the games went.)

A therapeutic alliance had been developed, although this was in part due to her need for attachment. She was so lonely.

Susan cancelled the next appointment. At the next visit, she reported that she had a drink again, the night before our visit. She felt bad. (I assumed that there were deeper dynamic/transferences such as fear of my rejection, but I decided to address these later.)

Susan was, with some assistance, able to also see some gain in her wellness (a JND). She said, "I have more control now." I agreed. We continued our relapse work: What is the cycle? What are the stressors (triggers, buttons, whatever word the patients use)? What are the reactions? (Etc.) This work continued from time to time. Susan had a lot of resilience; her relapse work became a protective factor.

DAN

Susan and Konrad had had a fight. Susan said, "I raged. I don't want to rage. It hurts." She associated these feelings to Dan, when asked. She had never talked to anyone about Dan, but she began to break down the walls.

Susan said that Dan had used her and that he wore masks (dissembling). He was always sexual with her, she reported, "and with many others" she added. "How could he?" she asked. "He had sex with my best friends." She was so ambivalent, feeling love and hate (items 10 and 16). There were complications, concomitant contradicting feelings, attitudes and thrusts. Susan both loved and hated Dan— and many other people, as we will learn. She was deeply equivocal, sometimes even about living.

Intervention often took the form of changing one thing in Susan's life, such as the wish to love or be loved. In general, the therapist must address the ambivalence in suicidal people—with our energies on the life-directed aspects of the ambivalence. Susan and I, as we will see, needed to address her unconscious and many other indirect expressions in her mind to develop sound protective factors (ego strength).

Dan had also dissembled to his parents. They only knew Susan, and had accepted her as family. At the funeral, Dan's mother held her, and Susan went home with Dan's family that day. Yet, shortly after his death, Susan lost Dan's family too. "I only see them at the memorial services now," she said. "We don't talk. They learned about the other girls and blamed me."

Susan said, "I loved Dan so much. I still love him ... but I am so angry too." Susan needed to learn about ambivalence. She needed to accept that people can in the mind be both A and not-A. Often before, Susan would find the hate, rage and so on (all not-A for her) to be unacceptable and she would become suicidal. Once more we had to address Susan's ambivalence.

We continued to talk about Dan in Susan's psychotherapy.

Although Susan was quite volatile at times, she was most often avoidant. Her typical beliefs or thoughts were as follows: "I cannot tolerate unpleasant feelings." "If people get too close to me, they will discover my depression and reject me." "All men are critical, controlling, deceiving or rejecting." "I should avoid painful situations at all costs." "Unpleasant feelings will escalate and get out of control." "If I feel or think something unpleasant, I should try to stop it—for example, drink, or freeze or even plan my suicide." (See Beck et al., 1990.)

Throughout therapy, we would often address these automatic thoughts. Susan associated these patterns to Dan and, at a deeper level, as we will learn, to her father.

There were also real circumstances (the stage) to address. For example, Susan reported that she was going to see her family at a cottage, north of Toronto. She feared these occasions. "Everyone drinks," she said. "My grandmother comes and she drinks even more than my mother." "I don't want to go back to that," she concluded. We discussed the circumstances and what she could do on such occasions. Susan developed a plan of action.

During the next visit, she reported that she did not drink. We worked at strengthening her ego (items 17 and 18). There were unresolved problems ("a complex" or weakened ego) in Susan; for example, there were symptoms and ideas that were discordant, unassimilated, and/or antagonistic. While working with Susan, I realized that I should not attempt to cure all the complexes in her personality immediately. We first simply had to keep her alive. This is the *sine qua non* of responding to the would-be suicide. However, it is critical that I had to assess what was discordant, unassimilated, or antagonistic in Susan. I had to evaluate her complexes, anxiety, avoidance, and other important aspects of her dynamics, psychopathology, and reaction patterns. Her ego was weakened. Simply stated, I had to know Susan to treat her. It follows that I had to reinforce Susan, to strengthen her ego—and this, as we will see, was a constant.

Practically speaking, when working with suicidal people like Susan, we do what we can. We throw in our energies against death. We need to strengthen our patient's individuality and sense of reality, and that is often life saving.

KONRAD

Susan reported that she had another conflict with Konrad. She noted that now it was not alcohol (she did not drink), but her anxiety that was triggering conflicts. She began to describe deep feelings of irritability and worry. Susan had become angry because Konrad had failed to see her as promised. When they met the next day, Susan was angry, but Konrad dismissed her ("My father did that") and she "roared". Konrad left and said that he never wanted to see Susan again. Susan felt alone and abandoned. Her suicidal ideation increased, and her lethality was a 5 (on a 1 to 9 scale; i.e., moderate).

"I don't know how to handle my anger," she said. She associated to her family. She reported that as a child, her father would rage. Her mother and her sister, Kay, would rage back. "I just sat," she said. Susan would, in fact, sit at the kitchen table "for hours". At those times, she recalls she felt sad and "always thinking of killing myself". "I wanted it (the pain) to stop."

Susan continued to not drink. She was now three months into treatment and we continued to work on relapse prevention. Susan also often told about the stressors at work, often about "controlling, demanding doctors". "I cannot tolerate these type of people." She associated this reaction to her father.

20 July.   Susan had gone home again; Konrad (who had called Susan again) had joined her. All her family got drunk and she and Konrad left. "I felt so sad," she said. We began to discuss what she can and cannot control. I told her of a Zen story of a jackass tied with a rope to a pole. The jackass fights the rope, but only when he stops, can he be free. The jackass has to accept what she—I say "she" when the patient is female—cannot control. The secret for most suicidal patients is to accept what they cannot control (see Chapter 17 for more details of the Jackass story). Susan accepted that she could not control her father, mother, or sister (she was also often drunk). Susan decided that she could leave, but felt sad about that choice. I suggested to her: "Often in life, we have to choose between sad and sad, not happy and sad." I said, "At those times we have to decide which is the sadder and which is the least of two sad choices." She associated to feeling guilty if she leaves, but she learned to accept that leaving (time-out) was the better of the two sad possibilities.

Susan began to be more at ease, learning to accept her feelings and the situations at home. She reported to be doing better and appeared less anxious (a JND).

There were more familial issues, some new, some historical. Even last year, when she was 22 and still living at home, her father gave her a curfew while her younger sister, Kay, never accepted one. "He tries to control everything," said Kay. Susan, with her avoidant style at home, complied. She left home that year, moved to Windsor, some two hours away from her parents. The move had helped.

27 August.   Susan missed an appointment again. As now predictable, she had had a drink the night before our scheduled meeting. Susan was testing me. Would I reject her? We began to verbalize these patterns; how these reactions were a transference to me, Konrad, and others. She said, "I never understood that. But I can see what you say." (There is a benefit if a patient acts out several times during therapy. One incident can be dismissed, but not two.) I was developing Susan's need for understanding. As she did, she felt more control. She also began to understand how her past was haunting her present.

Susan felt so rejected. She was at home and then there had been Dan.

16 September.   Susan arrived for our visit. She said, "I'm stupid." I asked, "How are you stupid?" She often thought that she was "stupid"; her father had often said so and Konrad and Dan both did. I, however, would not accept the statement and she began to explore this automatic thought. Susan learned some basic thought-stopping techniques. There was, in fact, no evidence that she was stupid. She was a bright woman and I often said so.

23 September.   Susan was sad when she arrived. Konrad had walked out again, after a fight, and Susan began to cry in my office. When I asked, "What hurts so?" she said that she remembered sitting at the kitchen table as a child. A conflict would occur; afterwards, her father would throw the food across the room ("plates would fly"). Her sister, Kay (two years younger than Susan), would yell. Susan would sit "as if nothing was happening". She would dissociate (there is some evidence of derealization). "It was all I could do," she said. "At times, after it was all over, I'd go to my room and cry myself to sleep."

I agreed that that was maybe the best that she could do then, but she was not a child now and could learn to cope better—and I added that she was, in fact, coping better. I said, "You are talking here. That is better." She agreed. No one ever talked in Susan's home.

I told Susan about an Inuk (singular for Inuit) that I had met in the Arctic. Sexual abuse was not rare in the Arctic towards the Inuit by white men, even by the priests and ministers. Once, a woman came to speak to me. She said, "I was raped twice. This is not fair. I'm going to kill myself." If I had debated with her (about her "therefore"), I believe that she would be dead. Rather, I did not accept her major ("Life has to be fair") premise. I said, "The difference between you and I is that I don't accept that life has to be fair, often life is not and we have to learn to cope with it." The Inuk looked at me, somewhat surprised, but agreed. She was learning to cope with the intolerable.

As I told Susan the story, she listened and said, "Oh, like me." "Yes, like you. The Inuk learned to survive; after all, her people have survived in a barren land for thousands of years. She had strengths." Susan saw the identification. This is a type of resilience, a protective factor. In treatment I continually reinforced Susan's ego development.

DAN REVISITED

Susan began to talk more and more about Dan. She was learning to trust me. She said that after learning about Dan's infidelity, she could not trust any males. "I loved Dan. I trusted him. After that, I trusted no one" (a cognitive constriction). Susan did not trust Konrad. Susan also could not commit. I once suggested that she discuss this with Konrad, keeping in mind we were now six months into treatment.

7 October.   Susan reported that the conversation did not go well with Konrad. Susan had tried to talk to Konrad about their relationship, but he walked away. "He avoids more than me," she said. Konrad had said as he walked away, "You are thinking about Dan. Talk to Dr Leenaars about it."

I, on the other hand, encouraged Susan to talk here and elsewhere. I said, "Do you want what occurred in your childhood at the kitchen table again?" "No" was the emphatic answer. We, because Konrad was correct in some ways, began to talk more and more about Dan. I even verbalized partial agreements with Konrad, but, at the same time, I suggested that I also saw it differently from Konrad's view of encouraging avoidance/inhibition, not talking about it. Some of the problems were Konrad's.

I discussed briefly that Freud (1974m) had distinguished between positive and negative responses to life's traumatic events. Freud, I reported, saw remembering, repeating, and re-experiencing as positive, and forgetting, avoidance, phobia, and inhibition as negative. "The negative reactions", I said, "in your family are all too common. A typical response is simply to deny it." "Don't talk about it," I suggested, only exacerbated her problems, including those about Dan. She agreed. Yet, I also told her that to talk about painful events means that you risk making the feelings worse, especially the uncomfortable ones; the failure to talk, however, increases the pain even more. She agreed and so, years after Dan's death, we began some basic grief work.

She began: "It is difficult to let go. I cannot let go: No one remembers Dan." I suggested that she did not have to forget about Dan, but she did need to learn to say goodbye to him.

14 October.   Susan brought in some cards, letters and pictures. She had kept everything from Dan, even some of the clothes that he had left at her place. There were graduation pictures; there was a favourite sweater. All were held on to as treasures, but bittersweet ones.

Here is the text of a Christmas card:

> Listen Babe [*his pet name for Susan*], I know that lately I haven't been the greatest friend, I realize that and I am very sorry. You have to understand though that no matter what, you'll always be very important to me even if I don't always show it. I won't ever let anything or anyone come between us and I think you have learned that over the years. So, I hope you have a great Christmas and Happy New Year. I Love You Babe!

Dan, she had learned, had been having an affair at that time.

A card from Florida read:

> Dear Susan, I hope you had a great time in Collingwood [*a place north of Toronto*]. Florida is fun, we're meeting tons of people and I've scored a few times. I'll tell you about it when I get home Babe. I hope there's no hard feelings between us. I don't think anyone worth fighting over when it comes to you because you mean so much to me. We'll catch you later. Love Dan.

Susan said that Dan had "scored" with a number of girls in Florida for spring break. "The catch you later," she said, referred to having sex with her. There were many more letters like the ones above. All reflective, she had learned, of dissembling. "Dan had lied about everything," she concluded.

The sharing of the letters, pictures and so on were steps to her healing. We began to talk about Dan's affairs and she started to target her anger. Susan read the cards over and over and began to learn that it was okay to love and hate the same person.

I also began to explore Dan's death. I asked, "If Dan had not died in the accident and been alive, would you have continued to date him, after you learned about his lies?" Susan, waiting a few seconds, looked at me and said, "No!" I suggested that the problem is that he died.

30 October.   Susan arrived with Dan's sweater; she said, "I'm going to give it away." She had spoken to one of Dan's old friends; he had told her that there were "hundreds" of other girls. "How could he?" she asked. She was learning that Dan's behaviour was not acceptable, but her anger was. Susan was learning that it was acceptable to say goodbye. Their relationship was not one of intimacy, but one of identity diffusion for her and narcissism for Dan. Susan said, "I'm going to send the sweater to his friend. He wants it." We agreed that it was a good decision.

Susan also began to talk about Dan's risk-taking behaviour. He would drink and drive. On the night of the MVA, he and some female friends decided to go to Toronto. They had been drinking, having sex, and decided to go to Toronto, two hours away. Dan drove, travelling 140+ in a 100 km (60 miles/h) limit. They never made it. Susan was learning to accept the facts; Dan's behaviour had killed him. Accepting this fact somehow lessened the survivor guilt.

10 November.   Susan's sense of reality was more grounded. She was less stuck (glued) to Dan. The relationship was dysfunctional, even before Dan's death. Susan had seen the relationship as the only possible way to cope with her life and remained frustrated (TGSP's items 20, 21, 22, 23).

Susan's history and her current circumstances (the stage) determined her problems. She had been weakened and defeated by unresolved problems in her interpersonal field (the outer phenomenology). Suicidal people, like Susan, are often obsessively preoccupied with unresolvable dilemmas. The traumatic events in their history are persistently re-experienced. Susan, however, also characteristically persistently avoided any stimuli associated to her traumatic past. She was, in fact, initially almost amnesic to the events and how she had previously adjusted to her traumas—she just wanted to avoid all uncomfortable feelings, memories, etc. At a conscious level, she was fixated in the current pain. Yet, there was a history, a deeper pain.

Pain is deep. The worst ever pains are the unbearable energies that fuel a person's perturbation. Susan had suffered repeated defeats and was weakened. Denial, repression, avoidance, and so on had often resolved her problems. These defences, of course, are not only ineffective, but with suicidal people, they are suicidogenic. This implied that I had to widen Susan's adjustment processes including, but not limited to, helping Susan to understand the past, her past inhibitions, and how to cope better.

With Susan, as with all suicidal patients, we have eventually to address the history of unresolved problems and thwarted needs in the interpersonal field (or some other ideal). The frustrated needs—primarily, I believe, ones of attachment (affiliation)—must be addressed with all suicidal people. Susan's behaviour appeared to be related to the following unsatisfied or frustrated needs: attachment (affiliation), achievement, aggression, inviolacy, order, succorance, and understanding. Susan's pain related to the frustration or blocking of these important psychological needs; that is, needs deemed to be important by her. It was my function to help her in relation to those thwarted needs. Even a little bit of improvement helped and maybe saved her life. Susan needed some indication of the value of life, an affirmation of self—something she never got at home and, as she learned, never got from Dan. Often just the possibility of a small amount of gain in the satisfaction of needs gives a perturbed individual like Susan enough hope and comfort to divert his/her suicidal course. It provides an increase in resilience (e.g., self-esteem). As with suicidal people in general, the goal with Susan was to increase her psychological comfort by addressing her frustrated needs, especially the one of attachment (or what Erikson called "intimacy"). I needed to mollify all of Susan.

Susan's frustration in the interpersonal field was exceedingly stressful and persisting to a traumatic degree, probably since early childhood, but especially after the loss of Dan (not only an object, but also an ideal). The goal of her therapy was to reduce the traumatic aftershocks—the real-life pressures, the frustrated needs—which were driving up Susan's sense of perturbation. We needed to decrease the distress, at least, to just below the traumatic degree. I had to assist Susan in making the pain bearable, but also not to deny, repress, or deflect the pain, for this would serve as the energy for change. She was already undoing, a solution that added to her pain. Often, suicidal people's solution to their problems results in greater problems than they had originally. Susan needed to face her trauma, the loss of Dan. Suicidal behaviour, drinking, etc., were escapes—a way of avoiding the reality of Dan's deceitful behaviour and cruelty towards her, as well as his sudden death.

A positive development in the disturbed relationship was seen as the only possible way to go on living, but such a development would never be forthcoming. She always wished to have Dan back, "back" meaning not only alive but also innocent of his crimes. Dan could not be alive. Susan was stuck (with crazy glue, to use a euphemism) in her mind on Dan, the lost object. Somehow, I had to decrease Susan's interpersonal perturbation; Dan's death was fuelling her intolerable pain. I responded, "That is sad, what can you do now and stay alive?"

At the visit on 10 November, Susan said, "It is like a ton of bricks being lifted off my shoulders." We discussed that she only loved a dead man, not living on the side of life. She spontaneously added, "I know what Dan would have done, if I died. He would have f***** after my funeral." Susan's anger was less and less externalized. There were fewer rages and less fights with Konrad. Susan's pain was less; it became bearable.

The positive work continued around Dan, but also her father and Konrad. Denial was so prevalent in these relationships too. Alcohol was everydayness; Susan, however, continued her sobriety. I continued to reinforce her ego development, i.e., her individuality and sense of reality. Susan still needed to solve the adolescent's dialectic of identity vs identity diffusion. She was becoming more Susan.

Susan's relationship with Dan, of course, was associated to her family. Her family was dysfunctional. Susan's relationships had been constantly put under strain (item 24).

Susan's relationships (attachments) had been too unhealthy and too regressive, keeping her then and now under constant strain of stimulation and frustration. Therapeutically, I had to assist Susan to detach herself from a too highly cathected (and even suicidogenic) person—this was true not only about Dan, but also about her father. Susan needed to have her wishes and needs stimulated and inhibited to a healthier degree. She needed to develop intimacy. We had to increase and decrease her relationships; this was the main task in all her psychotherapy. And, as with most suicidal people, when one needs to increase the relationships, one may need to actively involve others in the individual's system (for example, with Susan, this meant at this time Konrad and members of her family). Not too infrequently suicidal behaviour, as in Susan, signals a system distress (Richman, 1986).

Susan's family drank, but Susan continued to be sober, and as I continued to reinforce her sobriety Susan became aware that the drinking was conditioned behaviour. She recalled Pavlov and his dog. "They are like Pavlov's dog," she said. "Something, anything happens and they drink. No one at home can tolerate unpleasant feelings:" Susan especially blamed her father: "He always drank."

GOODBYE TO KONRAD

14 January.   Christmas and New Year had gone well. Susan did not drink ("the first in years"); and again I reinforced her wellness. There had been, lately, little suicidal ideation. She had, however, met again with Dan's friend. "He's a jerk," Susan said about Dan. She was using her anger more constructively, letting go of the entanglement with Dan.

At the same time, the relationship with Konrad was fading. He was less and less attached, but not only to Susan. He quit his job and moved back home, some three hours away. Susan said, almost in relief, "Our relationship will soon end." Susan was not sad; and she displayed no suicidal thoughts over the loss. She concluded, "It is best."

Her job was going well; she had received a raise and promotion. "They say that I'm more friendly and helpful," she reported with a smile. Once more, I reinforced.

26 January.   Susan was becoming less passive; she continued on her medication. Yet, her anger cycle continued. Susan's anger had been, for example, very problematic at a volleyball game. She got overtly angry with a fellow player, which was a surprise to her friends. She was most often passive–aggressive and her friends expected such behaviour. (Susan had already begun to explore this dynamic; she said, "It is always the same, but why?")

Susan typically presented herself as the "sweet" Susan. It was only with Konrad that the rage was seen; yet, there were impulsive episodes. The volleyball game was one such event; her friend missed the ball and Susan yelled, "You're stupid." Everyone became silent. "I wanted to crawl away after," Susan said.

Susan accepted now that she could be "mean" ("I can be quite mean"). She had been "mean" with Konrad. Yet, she also accepted the view of the glass as half full (a useful tactic with most patients). Susan recognized her good self too.

She occasionally still saw Konrad, but he wanted to discuss nothing. Susan was frustrated, "but I can't talk to him about it." I suggested that I understood, but could not control whether Konrad listened or not, and that she could talk about her anger here. Aggression is a common emotion in suicidal young people, but eventually, in almost all cases, it has to be discussed. It was essential with Susan.

Sometimes Konrad would call or come to see her. They would have sex and he would leave. It was cyclical and Susan spontaneously began to see the pattern. "He only wants sex," recalling the same behaviour with Dan. It was elliptical. Susan concluded that Konrad needed help, but Konrad met any suggestion with, "You are the crazy one." Susan began to accept what she could not control. I advised her that the non-committal nature of the relationship was repetitive, and Susan reported, "Konrad said it was all me." Susan, however, began to learn that Konrad himself could not develop intimacy. "He'll never love me," she concluded. The relationship with Konrad faded even more. Susan stopped all sexual contact and Konrad did not call again. "He wants what he wants. He is like Dan." Susan began to explore her repetitive choices, losses, and rejections in her relationships (items 25, 26, and 27).

Susan reported repetitive traumatic hurts throughout her history (e.g., the unmet love, failing relationships). The most effective way to assist people like Susan is by mollifying the whole person, reducing the elevated perturbation. With Susan, I had to reduce her anguish, tension, and pain. Shneidman's rule is: Reduce the elevated perturbation and the lethality will come down with it.

Susan, whose personality (ego) was not adequately developed, appeared to have suffered a series of narcissistic injuries. Konrad was just one more. This implied at least two things: (1) the key to intermediate and long-range effectiveness with Susan included the following: to increase the options for action available to Susan, to increase awareness of adjustment processes, to widen the angle of the blindness, to address the irrational (spontaneous) beliefs and to increase objects available (beyond the narcissistic ones); and (2) the usual methods of psychotherapy had to be employed. One does not leave a patient, like Susan, with her "weak", "primitive" inadequately developed ego—she needed long-term, extensive therapeutic assistance (few truly suicidal people benefit sufficiently from short-term intervention).

Susan was persistently preoccupied with events or injuries, namely people who had abandoned her. This was the felt trauma, the disturbed relationships. Frequently, I said, "Tell me what's happening. Where does it hurt?" Susan, for example, told me about her loss, rejection, and abandonment—Dan, Konrad, and her father. This implied that to help Susan, one had at times to address her external world (the stage). She needed to find acceptance and affiliation from someone. She needed to develop intimacy. I needed to do all this without producing an unhealthy dependency. At the same time, I needed to recognize that I was a decisive element in this therapeutic process, not only in developing a healthy relationship, but also in developing Susan's positive identifications (a critical protective factor).

24 March.   The relationship with Konrad was now historical. Konrad continued to be quite upset and told Susan's friends that Susan's mental problems caused the break-up. Susan learned about the "gossip". In response, unlike her old self, Susan had called Konrad and demanded to speak to him. He refused and Susan told Konrad "it was over". She recognized that her termination needed to be said; she never could with Dan. Undoing can be a protective factor.

Konrad had pleaded with Susan on the telephone to try to make the relationship work; yet, he refused to talk about their problems. Susan kept to her decision. She also noted, "I need to work on my own ability at commitment. I need to sort out my choices, my relationships and whom I love."

Susan had been having problems with the occurrence of her menstruation, but her GP said that it was all anxiety. However, I questioned that simplistic view. Susan had been taking birth control pills; but without Konrad in her life, she stopped. Her moods shifted to the positive shortly afterwards. I encouraged Susan to ask her GP to refer her to a specialist, which she did. I stated to Susan, "I know you're anxious, but I don't believe that this is all anxiety. We are biopsychosocial beings." This was correct, of course. Susan had biological problems. She suffered from premenstrual syndrome (PMS) to which her rages were often associated. Of course, the Zoloft helped. Susan had said her final "goodbye" to Konrad.

Susan's treatment was now every other week. She had suggested the change and I have long learned that if the patient decides to have fewer sessions, then, provided they are well, it is almost always a good choice, a JND.

THE FATHER

21 April.   Susan began to raise a question: "Is it a pattern?" She was becoming more and more aware that her serial way of coping was problematic. Her solution had become an unbearable problem, and resulted in uncomfortable pain (items 33 and 34). Susan, in some direct or indirect fashion, had developed problematic identifications (i.e., attachments) with lost and rejecting people. Susan had lost someone, a highly cathected person (Dan), but there were more and deeper rejections (her father). The main point with Susan was to increase her psychological sense of possible choices in life, not only love of a deceased man or rejecting father. She needed a sense of being emotionally supported. With suicidal people, relatives, friends, and colleagues should, after they have been determined to be on the life side of the individual's ambivalence, be considered in the total treatment process. Konrad could not do this for Susan. Susan needed other objects (people with whom to identify).

Other people can assist our suicidal patient in establishing and/or re-establishing positive relations, and this was a priority with Susan: to learn to develop positive identifications (intimacy). This was undertaken to help build her constructive tendencies, whether self-esteem, self-support, or some other life enhancing processes. When so perturbed, Susan could not simply give up even a negative part of her identity (Dan). She was simply in too much pain and too pessimistic to do this. She needed assistance.

An unwillingness to accept the pain of losing Dan allowed Susan to choose, even seek to escape from life and accept death. She was suicidal to avoid her unresolvable pain. Centrally, I needed to focus on the "problem" that Susan was trying to solve—her intimacy. Karl Menninger has provided us with an important dictum that is worth remembering once more at this point: "The patient is always right." My task was to find out "how is Susan right?".

Susan associated how Dan and even Konrad were like her father. She asked, "What is the attraction?" We explored how her reactions were spontaneous. I suggested that we needed to understand her unconscious, however, better to answer her question, and she agreed. "I am not aware why I am doing it, even when I was; but, I know now when I am doing it."

Susan noted that "You can't trust the men that I choose. Why do I do that?" Susan began to associate to her father. "My mother says that you can't trust my father. He had affairs." Susan revealed, in fact, that her mother began to drink the day that she found out about her husband's "infidelity". "My mother", Susan added, "says you can't trust any men. They are all alike." I asked if she thought that was true. She thought and said, "No, I trust you." And I quickly added, "I believe that there are men and women who you can trust." Susan agreed.

The drinking at home got worse. Susan's mother, one day, announced that she was going to a treatment centre for addictions. She had noted, with pride, that Susan did not drink. "She actually praised me," said Susan. Susan supported her mother, who went into the treatment and stopped drinking. She attended AA and, with Susan's encouragement, started seeing a psychiatrist, who provided psychotherapy. Once she stopped, Susan's father, however, drank more.

Susan's father was getting worse. Not unusually, once one person gets better in a dysfunctional family, others may reveal their dysfunctions more. Mental disorders are often associated to family systems (Haley, 1971; Richman, 1986). The more Susan's father drank, the sicker he became. His blood pressure was very high. His eyes were bloody. He was often sick, vomiting, and having diarrhoea. Yet, despite efforts, Susan's father continued to drink and he raged mercilessly (Ahab was alive). Susan concluded: "He's an alcoholic." She was learning to accept that she could not control whether he drank or not. Susan's needs were frustrated. She was anxious. Susan was, however, not suicidal, and was beginning to accept the unacceptable.

Susan also explored further who Dan was and began to understand her history better. Suicide prevention often involves mollifying the whole person.

Work was going well, although Susan was confronted with a "sexual harassment" situation. A coworker had been very explicit about sexual wishes. Susan, unlike in her old passive style, was assertive; she said "no". The coworker got frustrated and angry; the harassment increased. When this occurred, Susan had flashbacks of sitting at the kitchen table again. She froze for a minute and then, "I imagined myself getting off the table and I said something." Susan told her boss and fortunately the coworker was warned about his behaviour (Susan did not want him to lose his job). This assertive action seemed to change Susan. "I can do it," she said proudly. "Yes, I know," I replied. She smiled.

BEN

30 June.   Ben, who was a 29-year-old doctor, was quite interested in Susan. He started talking to her and asked her for a date. They had "a wonderful time."

Susan continued to do well; yet, she continued to experience anxieties. We continued to explore this pain and I asked: "What can we do to lower the worries?" Shneidman's rule is: Reduce the perturbation.

The relationship with Ben grew. One day, Susan decided to tell Ben about her therapy. He reacted with surprise. "Why do you need therapy?" he asked. Susan attempted to explain. Ben said he "accepted" it. Did he understand it?

17 August.   Ben and Susan were dating each other exclusively. There were problems, however. On one occasion, Susan was to go out with Ben. She waited. She called his home and there was no answer. He finally arrived three hours late, stating that he had been out with a friend. Susan was understandably upset; yet, "the red, red roar" did not come out. At the same time she asked, "Is this a yellow light?" (I often use "the green, yellow and red light" metaphor with people who want to stop serial behaviour). Susan associated Ben's behaviour to Dan and Konrad; she also recalled how her father often promised Kay and her an outing, never keeping his promises.

Susan and I talked about Ben. She concluded that Ben's behaviour was not like Dan's. Yet, Susan was conscious of the events now. On one occasion, she said, "Will he just leave me too?"

Susan had been referred to a medical specialist, a gynaecologist, who had suggested that she, indeed, suffered from premenstrual syndrome (PMS). Susan agreed. This is only one possible sex difference that a therapist needs to know to treat women and men effectively. Susan and I talked about what helped with her PMS, such as no caffeine, exercise and so on. The association with depression is obvious. I also discussed with her something that I learned from John T. Maltsberger: antidepressants, such as Zoloft, help with PMS. Susan continued her medication.

SEX DIFFERENCES

Susan's case raises the question of gender differences; and let me here digress briefly. The main sex difference, as we read in Chapter 1, is that females complete suicide less than males, but attempt suicide more often than males (Lester, 1992). Suicide, however, is rare during pregnancy (Lewsi & Fay, 1981; Marzuk et al., 1997). The menstrual cycle may have a more positive association, but this is not a simple one. Ekeberg and colleagues (1986) found no association between suicidal attempts and the menstrual cycle. Targum et al., (1991) found no association. Fourestie and colleagues (1986) suggested, however, that there was an associated risk, but only on days 1–7 and 28+. Oral contraceptives in this study appeared to be a protective factor at these times; whereas Vessey et al. (1985) found the opposite (as well as for women using an IUD, but not diaphragms). The associations are not simple.

Lester (1990) carried out a meta-analysis of studies on attempted and completed suicides over the menstrual cycle and concluded that there was no association. Yet, although the link between the menstrual cycle may be very specific, if any link exists, research (e.g., Merikangas et al., 1993) has shown that females with menstrual problems—not simply the cycle *per se*—were more likely than females with no menstrual problems to have a major depressive disorder. They were also more likely to make suicide attempts. Thus, the association may be more related to individual pathological issues than to the menstrual cycle *per se*. Skutsch (1981a, 1981b) suggested that the associations are related to physiological differences. Oestrogen may inhibit the output of dopamine (which reduces the likelihood of depression). Thus, perhaps the risk issue is associated to the mediating factor of depression (and, thus, pain) in those women with menstrual problems, such as PMS. This was true for Susan; I suspect that the fluctuating levels of perturbation were associated to an underlying depression, which may well have heightened during times of physiological dysfunction. Of course, PMS is only one possible physiological risk factor. As we learned earlier, there is a wide array of physical and medical disorders or disabilities that render a person at high risk for suicide. Not all would be at risk; it is still the individual with PMS, diabetes, or some other disease that kills him/herself. Suicide is a multidimensional event and is not, for example, only due to PMS. I repeat, it is the individual who kills him/herself.

THE FATHER CONTINUED

1 September.   Susan's father continued to drink heavily. Ben had accompanied Susan on a home visit and found out about Susan's father's addiction. He was silent on the way home. "He didn't say anything," Susan said. "I know that he was upset, but he didn't say anything. Why?"

Susan was frustrated; yet, she was not overly angry. She recognized that the real anger was at her father. She recalled how, as a teenager, she never invited friends over, because she feared her father's drinking habits. "My father never cared about what my friends saw. I felt so embarrassed."

Despite a few negatives, Susan saw a greater balance on the positive side about Ben and continued the relationship.

At this meeting, Susan also reported a dream: "I see Dan. He is in a coma. I see him. His mother is there, crying. I begin to accept that he is dying. I woke up, crying." We again discussed her acceptance of Dan's death. I reminded her that grief takes a lifetime, even healthy grief.

30 September.   Susan was talking more to Ben; he was talking too. She said, "It is different than before." I listened and encouraged her in the relationship. Yet, she did note that Ben did not want to visit or talk about her family.

Her mother continued to go to AA and not drink. However, at home, it got worse. Her father was becoming more and more physically abusive. Her mother and sister, Kay, moved out. Her father raged even more. "He can't accept it," Susan said. "He wants what he wants. He can't cope with change." Susan and I freely associated to her past and current skills. I also cautioned her about enabling: "You can't rescue him. He does not want your help." Susan knew this and sadly accepted the feeling of impotence.

TERMINATION

19 October.   The relationship to Ben continued to go well. Susan continued to talk about Dan. One day, she arrived with a box full of old letters, notes and pictures.

We went through them, she chose a few, and left the rest in my office in the garbage pail. "I can let go of them now," she said. "I know that he's dead."

Susan started to talk about termination. I accepted her plan. She also planned to stop her medication and, with consultation with her GP, she did so. Susan did continue with the Zoloft for 10 days during the time of her PMS (a suggestion of Dr Maltsberger, who has often been my consultant on medication issues).

23 November.   Susan arrived and said, as she sat down, "I'm in love." She said that she was happy. "Ben says that he loves me." Susan reflected on Dan and Konrad. "It is so different," she observed. "Ben really loves me."

20 December.   Susan continued to plan to terminate; she decided to see me for one last visit in the new year.

26 January.   Susan arrived smiling. "Happy New Year, Dr Leenaars," she said. We discussed our history, her relationship to Ben and the things that were still painful, notably her father. "He drinks all the time now," she said. Yet, Susan had accepted that she could not control her father's drinking. He refused to stop.

We said goodbye, although, as always, I left the door open. I typically say something like, "Let me know how you're doing some time."

AND THEN HER FATHER KILLED HIMSELF

A few years after Susan terminated, she called and asked, "Can I see you?" We arranged to meet; Susan wanted to talk about Ben.

Susan's father had now become quite depressed. He often called Susan, sometimes speaking to Ben. Ben was upset about these conversations; and Susan's father was always drunk. Yet, Susan and Ben had planned to live together. Ben had accepted a new appointment in Boston, while Susan, following my encouragement, had applied to medical school in Boston and was accepted. They were both moving to Boston in a few months, and although Susan saw this as a new endeavour, Ben's preoccupation with her father was still an issue. He often refused to talk about this topic, saying simply that it made him uncomfortable. Ben often, Susan reported, avoided uncomfortable circumstances. "He avoids more than me," she said. I listened and suggested that she could not control Ben's avoidance. I acknowledged her frustration, but noted no suicidal ideation. Her pain, lethality, and so on were a 1 or 2 on a 1–9 scale. I have learned that patients prefer these simple subjective measures and they can also be useful to clinicians, even if researchers find it problematic empirically. It is one of Shneidman's simple measures of suicide risk: Ask the patient. These measures allow a patient and clinician a quantitative view of the patient's inner phenomenological world.

About Ben's avoidance, I suggested that Susan should try to speak to him, "Ask him, 'What is wrong?' 'Why do you avoid this problem?' 'Is there a reason why it hurts?'" (She knew little about Ben's past and I suspected that this was significant.) She said that she would, but did not call again until a few months later.

Susan arrived at an appointment with Ben. She wanted me to meet him, and I agreed (item 33). Shneidman has often reminded me that suicide prevention is best not done alone. A combination of consultation, ancillary therapists, social networking, and the use of all the interpersonal and community resources that one can involve is, in general, the best way to proceed. This was true with Susan. At this point, this meant seeing Susan with Ben (and later, with her mother).

Susan wanted to discuss what Ben wanted—whether he wanted a commitment or not. She wondered if he was avoiding. From our meeting, we did not learn an answer. Yet, he did avoid me, and offered only some surface talk. I suspected that he was fearful of a commitment, but uncertain as to why (dissembling?). I feared that the relationship would not last.

A few weeks later, on 20 June, Susan called. "My father died," she said. "Can I come to talk to you?" We agreed to meet the next day; Susan was two hours away at her father's home.

21 June.   Susan arrived, understandably upset. She said that she went home, found her father drunk "and then he killed himself". There have been few moments, as a psychotherapist, that I have felt overcome with deep sadness, but this was one. There have been others, and I still vividly recall the pain of such events. Shneidman tells me that, in his later years, the memories of such occasions in therapy get even sharper. These are issues for all psychotherapists. For example, some years ago a couple arrived at my office as an emergency. Their baby had just died the day before in a car accident. They were so sad; I quickly felt their pain, imagining the loss of my own child. This is loss!

As we have learned, countertransference comprises all of the therapist's reactions to the patient. These—as in this case—originate in our own history. They may not be only negative; indeed, they can be positive. Although it is the negative ones that result in the most problems (countertransference hate being the best example); the positive ones can also be problematic. I was emphatic; yet, I had developed a positive countertransference to Susan. It was not only my association to my parents (my father was dead), but to Susan herself. I felt her pain. She was so sad and I was sad. It was a loss!

I am not suggesting that therapists should always be a blank screen; in fact, this is often suicidogenic with truly suicidal patients. I am seldom a *tabula rasa* with suicidal patients. Indeed, on such sad occasions, by the very fact that we are human, we must feel, react, etc., to such pain. We have to be human, an I/Thou. It is acceptable to be sad on these occasions, and Dr Shneidman agrees. Yet, we also have to be conscious of our reactions to our patients. We have to know our own history, reactions, unconscious, and so on.

Susan cried. Susan talked. I listened. Her father had uncharacteristically asked her the day of his death, "Do you love me?" (Love is, I recall, a frequent word in suicidal notes.) Susan had said "yes" (she did). And a few hours later, she said, "I found him hanging in the garage! I stood there numb. I was that child again . . . but I knew that I had to call for a doctor." Susan did what she could. She did not sit at her kitchen table.

When her mother and Kay arrived later, they too were overwhelmed. Susan's sister began to drink, but both Susan and mother did not.

I listened and listened. Then Susan reported that Ben was not there. She had called, but he was not at home. She learned, in fact, that he had gone to Florida to a resort for a long weekend. She did not know; Susan called him; yet, he said that he could do nothing and never came home. Susan felt so alone. She talked and talked. I saw Susan for a few successive days, and then less frequently.

CONSULTATION

As fortune would have it, I had planned a visit to see Dr Shneidman; after all, it was Canada Day again (we almost always meet around the first of July).

As I told Shneidman about Susan and the recent events, he said "how sad". At the same time, however, he addressed my feelings of sadness. "Be careful," he said. "This countertransference can be dangerous. She needs you, not your overwhelming sadness." We talked often about our reactions to our patients; "They help keep the person alive, but be careful." Ed has always advocated that our attachments to our suicidal patients are critical, and so are their losses. We talked about my history, my losses. We talked about his losses (such as the death of Henry Murray). Later, after his wife Jeanne Keplinger Shneidman died, we talked about this loss. As therapists, we need to be conscious of our pain.

Dr Shneidman, during the consultation, also said something that proved to be true: "She won't see Ben again. He thinks that she has bad seeds. He'll leave."

Ben, in fact, did not see Susan again, after the death. Susan and I discussed Dr Shneidman's insight. Susan agreed that "Ben was always uncomfortable about the diseases in my family". "He takes a medical view of everything," she said. I suggested that, although life-saving in a medical crisis, this view does not allow one to cope with one's life. I suggested that his view is too limiting. We discussed Ben's avoidance. "He is too uncomfortable. He will run." He did, and Susan now had to cope with two losses.

Shneidman had also suggested that I tell Susan, "Don't make haste." Ben and Susan had planned to move to Boston. "Things are different now," I suggested. "Let's talk about your alternatives." Susan smiled; she had gone through this type of problem solving with me before. We reviewed her options. She accepted that there was no rush; yet, she ranked medical school first on her list. "Dr Leenaars," she said, "I always wanted to go. I don't want to lose this dream." "I understand," I replied. We then decided how we could have her therapeutic needs met in Boston. A few calls later, I referred Susan to a colleague. (A great benefit of having friends around the world is that I can refer almost anywhere to the best in the field. I have even referred someone to a friend in Tokyo.) We had a plan of action; we now focused on the here and now.

Susan now had to learn to live with her father's suicide, which is often a Herculean task.

SURVIVORSHIP

The pain of the suicide becomes the pain of the survivor. Anguish, guilt, anger, sadness, shame, and anxiety are a sample of the pains. Arnold Toynbee (1968) makes the point that death is a two-party event. He writes:

> The two-sidedness of death is a fundamental feature of death—not only of the premature death of the spirit, but of death at any age and in any form. There are always two parties to a death; the person who dies and the survivors who are bereaved ...
>
> The sting of death is less sharp for the person who dies than it is for the bereaved survivor.
>
> This, as I see it, is the capital fact about the relation between living and dying. There are two parties to the suffering that death inflicts; and in the apportionment of this suffering, the survivor takes the brunt. (pp. 327–332)

Toynbee here resonates to Saint Paul's question, "O death, where is thy sting?" As I see it, the brunt is even more for the survivors of suicide. The suffering is greater. The inflicting is more intentional. There are deep feelings of rejection, often perceived as the ultimate one (van der Wal, 1989–1990). There is frequently a belief that the sting was malicious (Clark & Goldney, 1995). Survivors ask, "Did he (or she) want me to hurt so?"

Suicide is a traumatic event. Shneidman (1972, p. 10) noted,

> I believe that the person who commits suicide puts his psychological skeletons in the survivor's emotional closet—he sentences the survivor—to deal with many negative feelings and, more, to become obsessed with thoughts regarding his own actual or possible role in having precipitated the suicidal act or having failed to abort it. It can be a heavy load.

The load is, indeed, a heavy burden; the skeletons live. Traditionally, survivors were burdened with the costs, and consequences of the intentional death, whether the suicide was seen as a crime or a sin (see Chapter 1). Even today, survivors of suicide experience more blame and attribution of mental disturbance than survivors of other deaths (Rudestam, 1992). Often, these survivors feel that they are blamed for the death (Silverman et al., 1994–1995). Today, survivors of suicide are not seen as sinners or criminals; they continue, however, to be often seen as mentally sick. There is a stigma. Whether the stigma is real or not, is still a question for research. (There is, in fact, much more to learn about survivors of suicide and all deaths.) Be that as it may, the pain is felt as real and endless. The survivors of suicide themselves, in fact, feel greater responsibility for the deaths (Bailley et al., 1999). The living suffer, sometimes unbearably! Suicide, in a few, becomes the choice. Greater focus on the skeletons in our patients is needed, when their father, mother, or other loved one has killed him/herself.

This was true with Susan. The aftershock for Susan was sharp, prolonged and could have been self-destructive if Susan's ego had not been strengthened. I believe that psychotherapy strengthens not only our suicidal patient, but also survivors of suicide. Sadly, most survivors of suicide remain in agony alone. The closet doors are closed (dissembling).

LEARNING TO LIVE AGAIN

3 July.   Susan talked about death. She talked about the general, "what is death?" Young adults are typically not close to death. Older adults, understandably, are closer. As we learn in later adulthood, acceptance of one's finite life is critical for wellness (integrity vs despair). Young adults are more focused on the dialectic of intimacy vs isolation.

Susan also talked about the specific—her father. She again discussed the conversation with her father, before his suicide. "He never asked me before, do I love him?" "I felt strange." We explored her thoughts and feelings more. As is so typical, she expressed survivor guilt. This is a common reaction in bereavement (even the DSM spells it out). Susan also felt, again, typical of suicide survivors, that it was her fault. "I should have known that he was going to kill himself. I should have known that when he asked me that question (about love), that he was going to kill himself." This is common. They believe that there is some "it" that predicted the death. Often survivors believe that they should have seen it, whatever the "it" was. One patient, I recall, discussed how his father's preoccupation with his furnace was a clue to suicide. I recall expressing that I was perplexed. I said something like, "I know something about suicide (*he nods*). In all my readings, I have never read that preoccupation with a furnace is a clue to suicide (*he looks*). Yet, I understand your feelings. It is common. Let's talk about your feelings of helplessness, lack of control and so on. Let's talk about your pain." (We did).

There are clues to suicide. Blocking suicide is best accomplished though prevention. Prevention is education. People—doctors, psychiatrists, psychologists, teachers, rabbis, ministers, crisis counsellors, and so on—must be educated. Such education is enormously complicated (item 19).

Susan's suicidal behaviour had a history. There were clues. Regrettably, the clues to suicide, depression and so on, are usually not seen, heard, or even responded to before the act. This was true with Susan—maybe because others in her stage also avoided "everything". It follows, as a more general implication for response with people like Susan, that the ultimate prevention of suicide is public education, which will make a major contribution to saving the lives of people like Susan, Jeff, Vincent, etc.

Postvention refers to those things done after the event occurred. Postvention deals with the after-effects in the survivors. Again, such an endeavour is complicated; it involves prevention, once the level of perturbation is low enough to bear it. Prevention is, however, not postvention. Yet, at our earliest meetings we can educate our patients about surviving. Survivor groups do this all the time (Shneidman, 1972). I did with Susan.

We talked about her father, his alcoholism, and his chronic suicidal career. "How could you have predicted it?" Did he say, "I'm going to kill myself?" ("No.") "Hindsight is always easier. You did not know. How can you say it was your fault? (*She looks.*) Let's talk about what hurts, your feelings and reactions." Susan did.

Later I also talked to Susan about the difficulties in prediction (see Chapter 5).

Susan and I also talked about the services that were available. We talked about a local survivor group. She accepted a referral and I called my friend, Anne Edmunds. Anne is a survivor and is one of Canada's leading advocates for survivors. Anne Edmunds met with Susan and Susan started to attend the group. Many assisted in Susan's healing. Later in Boston, she continued with a group there. One should not hesitate in referring one's patients to such services. I am indebted to a number of other leading survivors such as Iris Bolton, Karen Dunne-Maxim, and Ed Dunne in educating me about survivorship; they and many community-based people help to heal the skeletons that are in the mind of the survivors. We psychotherapists owe them a lot.

As Susan left, she asked if her mother could come and see me tomorrow for our next meeting. As has been, and will be, made clearer in subsequent case studies, suicide intervention often involves familial networking.

4 July.   Susan and her mother arrived. Her mother was somewhat dishevelled; yet she, when I asked, "How are you?" reported, "I cope." She stated that her husband had been quite ill, in pain and feeling hopeless. "He found a solution," she said accepting what she believed was inevitable. She also reported that there had been many suicides "for generations" in her late husband's family.

When asked why she came to see me, she said, "I worry about Susan. Susan as a young girl was so attached to her father. She was his favourite. She was daddy's girl." Susan's mother was also angry with Ben. "Why doesn't he talk to her?" she asked.

Susan listened quietly to our conversation; however, at the end, we talked about community supports and so on. Susan's mother had planned to join Susan at the survivor group that night and to attend one in her community. She also knew that the door, with Susan's permission, was open at my office, if she wanted to talk more. She agreed, but never returned. She came, I suspect, to make sure Susan was "okay". As she left, she said to Susan, "We loved you. Your dad loved you. He wanted you to be well. He just couldn't cope with his alcoholic pain." Susan teared.

I continued to see Susan, less as time went on, before she departed to Boston.

SAYING GOODBYE

11 July.   Susan arrived, stating, "I don't want to talk." This was her old pattern; unlike earlier, it was easier to get her to talk (the statement was an invitation to do so). "What hurts?" I asked.

Susan started to cry and she made the following statement: "It (father's death) can't be true"... "I don't believe it"... "I think about my dad at home and work all the time." Susan was less numb; she started to cope with the memories, thoughts, and flashbacks. The closet door was open. The skeletons were coming out. She was expressing common reactions to her tragic loss.

Susan cried; she trusted me to allow her sadness to be expressed. Despite her pain, she reported no suicidal ideation or self-destructive reactions. She did not drink. I reinforced her normality in her grief.

Susan, again common in survivors, began to share other feelings and reactions. She was angry. At work, some fellow workers did not speak to her ("People shut me out"). Yet, her main target, of course, was Ben. "He has gone to Hawaii on a vacation for 3 weeks," she said with a slight red roar. I allowed her to ventilate (a JND). Susan noted that he has not supported her ("he's done nothing"). We talked and, as I often do with patients who are left by a significant other during a difficult time, I began to explore his very ability to support her. We talked about relationships being in sickness and in health and in richness and in poorness and so on. I cognitively reframed his abandonment as his problem. I asked, "Could he help you in the future"? She reflected, "Will he always be like that?"

Susan was more and more accepting that the relationship with Ben was maybe not a bad loss. "It hurts but what would happen if I got sick? What would he do if I got depressed again? Would he just run away?"

Susan's mother was doing well, attending her survivor group weekly and sometimes with Susan in Windsor. Susan said, "We feel the support of these people. They help."

Susan continued to see me. Yet, as Susan would be leaving for medical school in a few months, our plan of a transfer became more concrete. I spoke to the receiving psychiatrist and Susan began the transfer mentally.

18 July.   Susan arrived, speaking about Ben. "He is dating someone else," she said. Once more, we rediscussed Dan and her relationships in general. The issues of trust re-arose. We also discussed our relationship and began more and more the process of saying goodbye.

25 July.   Susan walked into my office in tears. I asked the prototypical, "What hurts?" She said, "Did my dad love me?" We talked. Susan reported a dream, revealing the earlier dreams about Dan: "My father is in a coma. I try to talk to him. I try. I say, 'I love you.' He wakes up." We talked about his death and about death in general. We again talked about painful acceptance of our losses (she reported no suicidal thoughts). Susan also talked about her survivor group. She talked about listening to other survivors' losses. "We support each other," she said, adding, "it is so different from when I was a child at home." Susan had learned to be attached in "I/Thou" relationships, not "I/It".

We continued to talk about our relationships and how she anticipated that loss. At the same time, I reinforced the new relationship with her doctor in Boston. She had already visited once, while there to prepare for medical school. She reported that she liked him, "He listens to me, like you." She would visit the new therapist once more in August, before she moved to Boston. Healthy transferences are possible, but they require work.

Susan offered the following dream: "We were talking together. Someone else came into the room. You left. I left. You were pissed off with me." This transference needed work!

8 August.   Susan continued to talk about her father, Dan, Ben, etc. She often reflected on her own depressive states. She especially questioned about her irritability ("Dad was like that"). We talked about these concerns, but at the same time, I reframed the focus on her strengths. I said something like, "You have coped with a lot. You did as a child; you did the best that you could then. You are coping the best that you can now." Susan listened intently.

We continued to process her goodbye dream. She recognized that she was leaving. "I'm having a hard time saying goodbye." I shared, remembering Shneidman's advice that I too would miss our time; however, we both agreed that she was moving towards something important (see Chapter 3). She was attaching herself to an ideal: medical school.

GOODBYE

By mid-August, Susan was busy preparing to leave. She had stopped working and had started to say goodbye to her friends. "There are so many people calling me." I listened, nodding.

Susan was also preparing to say goodbye to her survivor group, although she planned to return on occasion, when she came to visit. Her mother continued with her group. Susan's sister, Kay, however, never attended. "Kay doesn't want to talk about Dad," she said, adding, "how sad".

We had two visits left. On our first, Susan focused on "all the changes." I talked about Shneidman's advice: "Don't make haste." Susan needed to reflect; I quickly divided the changes into positive and negative (it is easier to look at changes, once cognitively reframed). She continued to see Boston as positive; yet she said, "There are too many changes."

I directed our conversation to our change, our goodbye. We rediscussed her dream. Termination is always difficult. We spoke about choices, that her choice to go to Boston was in the service of the ego. I reinforced her choice. We talked again about what we can and cannot control, and having the wisdom to know the difference. I spoke about her resilience.

Despite an open discussion, I felt that I was not being as understood as I usually was by Susan. I discussed this fact and that maybe we were both feeling the sadness of our goodbye. She agreed and then verbalized her pain of losing our time together.

At our last visit, Susan again focused on accepting the unacceptable (a key protective factor). Susan spoke about her father's death and Dan's too. Susan had gone to the cemetery before our visit (I suspect intentionally). She spoke about talking to her father. "I said goodbye and told him that I would always love him. That I love him." I listened sadly. Susan just needed to tell her story. The suicide does in his/her note. Patients need to tell their narratives.

Susan and I also did the practical. We discussed her transfer to her new psychotherapist. She reported that she was pleased with "your friend" (an identification). We had planned a few follow-ups by phone. Once the practical issues were addressed, we said goodbye. "Goodbye Dr Leenaars," she said tearfully. "Goodbye, Susan."

WHAT HAVE WE LEARNED FROM THIS CASE?

Susan's first implication for treatment was item 16, to increase her constructive tendencies. This was a must with Susan. The specific implications were: 16, 10, 16, 17, 18, 20, 21, 22, 23, 24, 25, 26, 27, 33, 34, 33, 19. Most of the direct interventions with Susan fell under ego and interpersonal relationships. This is not surprising because her ego was so weakened by her painful attachments, current and historical. It is also of note that item 33 was repeated in her intervention. This related to the loss of a highly cathected person, Dan—and then her father. She so needed other people with whom to identify.

POSTSCRIPT

As a postscript, Susan called me a few times as arranged. She was well. She enjoyed medical school, standing near the top of her class (I was not surprised). And she met a new doctor, Wilhelm. She said, "He loves me. I know Wilhelm loves me." They married, had three children, and were happy together. Susan was no longer sitting at her kitchen table.

Appendix 16.1

SHNEIDMAN PSYCHOLOGICAL DISTRESS QUESTIONNAIRE (PDQ)

Copyright © 1993 by Edwin S. Shneidman

Name: _____ *Susan* _____ Age: ___23___ Sex: ___*F*___ Date: _____

Definition: Psychological pain is *not* bodily pain; it is how you feel as a person; how you feel in your mind (your joys or sadness, guilt or shame); how much you "hurt" as a human being, independent of your body. It is mental suffering; it is the opposite of "peace of mind".

1. My psychological pain relates mostly to my *feelings* of (check three):

( ) abandonment	( ) dread	( ) jealousy
( ) anger	( ) emptiness	(√) loneliness
( ) anguish	( ) fear	( ) powerlessness
( ) anxiety	(√) guilt	(√) rage
( ) bad conscience	( ) hopelessness	( ) shame
( ) confusion	( ) humiliation	( ) worry
( ) disgust	( ) inadequacy	( ) Other:

2. The *intensity* of my psychological pain is (circle one number below):

1	2	3	4	⑤	6	7	8	9
Little psycho- logical pain; almost non- existent	Mild	Moder- ate	Some- what bother- some	Present but manage- able between moder- ate and severe	Definitely hurtful	Harsh; rather severe	Definitely rather severe	Unbear- able; the worst discom- fort a person can ever experi- ence

3. My psychological pain is tied to my frustrated *needs* for (check three):

( ) *Achievement:* to accomplish the difficult; to master; to overcome.
(√) *Affiliation:* to affiliate with others; to remain a member of a group.
(√) *Aggression:* to overcome opposition; to oppose forcefully.
( ) *Autonomy:* to be free and independent of social confinement.
( ) *Counteraction:* to make up for failure by restriving; to overcome.
( ) *Defendence:* to defend or vindicate myself against others.
( ) *Dominance:* to control or influence others by persuasion or command.
( ) *Exhibition:* to make an impression; to entertain or shock or amuse.
( ) *Harmavoidance:* to avoid pain or injury or illness; out of harm's way.
(√) *Shame Avoidance:* to avoid humiliation or embarrassment or scorn.
( ) *Inviolacy:* to protect myself from others' interference; my own space.
( ) *Nurturance:* to gratify the needs of others; to help or console.
( ) *Order:* to put or keep things or ideas in good order; to be orderly.

( ) *Play:* to act for fun; to laugh or joke for its own sake.
( ) *Sentience:* to enjoy sensuous experiences and comforts of the senses.
( ) *Succorance:* to want to be helped or taken care of by others.
( ) *Understanding:* to want to know the answers; to ask questions; to speculate.

[From Henry A. Murray (1938). *Explorations in Personality.* New York: Oxford University Press. Reproduced with permission.]

Chapter 17

PETER: AN ADULT'S SUICIDAL PAIN

(I Now Understand the Words of My Brother's Suicide Note, "No One Loves Me")

Too little attention has been given to suicide in middle adulthood (Maris, 1987). The relative neglect of suicide during the midlife period appears concerning, especially since females have a high rate in their 40s in many countries (Lester, 1983). We will see the more general fact about the need for greater attention in the specific case of Peter.

MIDDLE ADULTHOOD

First, where does midlife fall? Common usage describes the term middle age as a period falling just before old age. For our purposes, midlife can be thought of as the period 40 plus or minus 15 years or, if you prefer, 25 to 55 (or 60) years, which correlates roughly to Erikson's (1968) stage of middle adulthood.

I thought it would be useful to consider some of the major writers who have studied this period before proceeding to our case study of Peter. Based on studies of biographies and autobiographies conducted in Vienna during the 1930s, Buhler (1968) described the 25- to 45-year period as a time when vitality is still high and self-direction and specification have replaced the shifting attitudes and uncertainties of youth. This period is often experienced subjectively as the culmination of life, one's generativity. She then observed that the transition to the 45- to 65-year period is often introduced by a crisis. The unfolding of one's individual powers comes to a standstill, and all that depends on physical abilities and needs enters a period of decline. Weighing against this biologic down slope are new and increasing interests in the results and productivity of life.

Kuhlen (1964), citing a number of studies, offered an even starker view of midlife events. He suggested that there is a shift from active direct efforts at gratification to indirect and vicarious methods. Moreover, the second half of life is marked by increases in the importance of anxiety and threat as sources of motivation.

Both Buhler and Kuhlen viewed life's midpoint as a marker for major stressful shifts, as we will see in Peter. Both regarded the relative success in making these shifts as crucial for subsequent adjustment.

Jung (1971) viewed the early part of midlife as a continuation of the "period of youth", which extends from puberty to age 35 to 40. He indicated that the major tasks during youth are giving up childhood dreams, dealing with sexual drives, and feelings of inferiority. This phase is characterized by a widening of the horizon of life. He believed that disturbances during this period are usually indications of attempts to continue the programme of childhood into the period of youth. He pointed out that the 35- to 40-year period calls for major changes in that "...we cannot live the afternoon of life according to the program of life's morning..." (p. 17). He maintained that it is "fatal" to look back and viewed neurotic disturbance during this period as a sign of attempts to cling to what was meaningful during youth. The major challenge is to find purpose for the latter half of life. Essential to this endeavour is the acceptance of death as a goal, which in turn is dependent on the discovery of meaning and wholeness in life through an inward turning of attention and self-exploration.

According to Kimmel (1974), the term "midlife crisis" was probably coined by Jacques (1965). He, like Buhler, studied biographical material. He chose for his subjects, 310 artists, who were painters, sculptors, composers, poets, and writers. Jacques reported a higher than expected death rate between 35 and 39, followed by a lower than expected death rate between 40 and 44. He also claimed a progression in their works from "lyrical and descriptive" in early adulthood to "tragic and philosophical" content during the crisis years to greater "serenity" in their productions after this period. He regarded a growing awareness of mortality as the main theme of the midlife crisis.

For Erikson, three principal conflicts or dialectics mark this period of adulthood; the one in question is called middle adulthood (the ages of 25–55). Before this period, there is young adulthood (before 25), as we saw with Rick. The opposing tendencies are between seeking intimate relationships as opposed to a sense of isolation. By intimacy, Erikson means mutually close and committed relationships, which may well involve feelings of fusion and self-abandonment. Only a person with a strong sense of personal identity (the healthy solution in the crisis for teenagers) can be secure enough to risk such closeness. Those still afflicted with confusion about their identities feel forced to stand well back from such intimacy and to endure a sense of profound isolation; their interpersonal relationships, sexual and otherwise, are problematic (e.g., promiscuous) in nature and their behaviour is role-like and stereotypic, as we saw in Rick. In the healthy course of events, this dialectic is ending as middle adulthood is beginning. The healthy solution is through compromise and synthesis, rather than by siding with either of the polarities. The enduring legacy of a successful synthesis is the virtue or ability to live in a committed way.

Early in middle adulthood the striving for intimacy and expressions of life are supplanted or perhaps expanded by a more general caring and striving for a sense of generativity, which is a wish to do and produce in ways that have enduring value. This can be expressed in child-rearing, but broader communal concerns and the world of ideas are certainly included as well. Failure at this stage results in a sense of stagnation, the feeling that one has and is going nowhere.

Towards the end of middle adulthood, as one approaches age 55 (or 60), increasing concern about the finitude of life and the approaching nearness of death lead into the next and final stage in Erikson's system. The crisis marking the close of life is one of integrity versus despair. The crucial task is the recollective one of evaluating and accepting one's own life as unique and meaningful. Such self-accepting individuals tend to be accepting of the behaviour (and lives) of others: even those that are widely discrepant from their own. On the other hand, those who are dissatisfied and sense that life is too short to begin again are subject to feelings of despair and self-disgust, as we will see in Joe. The virtue or strength that grows out of the integrity versus despair crisis is that of wisdom, which is characterized by a sense of wholeness and meaning. Such people are truly sage models that can be viewed as patterns to follow as well as representing successful solutions for the ending of midlife and the beginning of life's last end.

It is perhaps ironic that Erikson, who is so associated in popular thinking with the term midlife crisis, has not really described life's midpoint as a time particularly prone to crisis. In this, he stands in contrast to the other writers discussed in this chapter so far. Although he viewed a crisis as possible at any time, one is more likely to occur in his view at the boundaries of life-spans. Thus, in the case of midlife, one would expect more difficulty at about 25 to 30 years and again at 55 to 60 years. As we will read, Peter's life crisis, indeed, occurred in the latter part of his middle adulthood—and I would suggest that therapists should not dismiss the potential suicide risk of their patients during this developmental period.

PETER AND RITA: REVISITED

Peter, a 40-year-old male, as we learned in Chapter 11 on crisis intervention, came from a dysfunctional family (his only brother had killed himself two years earlier). He was married to Rita, someone who came from an even more dysfunctional family (her mother, like Rita, had a major affective disorder, Bipolar Disorder). They were first seen for marital therapy, an attempt at intervention that was very short term. On intake, Peter was quite perturbed (anxious) over Rita's infidelity. Rita had run off with David, a man 10 years younger; Peter presenting the problem, "My wife left me."

On the second visit (2 June), Rita had run off with David. Peter had denied suicide intent on that first meeting, but was highly perturbed and moderately lethal on the second visit. He refused a referral for medication or hospitalization. Instead, a perhaps not optimal plan of crisis intervention was started (see Chapter 11), including environmental control (i.e., removal of guns from the home), and then followed by psychotherapy. We will begin the process of psychotherapy after Peter's suicide attempt (which was detailed in Chapter 11). His TGSP[1] scores are: 1, 2, 3, 4, 5, 6, 7,

---

[1] Explanations of all implications/items are given in Chapter 12.

8, 9, 10, 12, 13, 15(f), 15(g), 16, 17, 18, 19, 20, 21, 22, 23, 24, 25, 26, 27, 28, 29, 30, 31, 32, 33, 34, 35.

Some six visits after intake, the work with Peter was more and more psychother-apeutic, not only crisis intervention. Yet, it is often more difficult to make such clinical distinctions than academic ones: When does therapy begin after a crisis response? On that visit, Peter announced that "the pain is unbearable", even using the word, "hopeless" to describe the pain. Peter stated, "It is hopeless"; he added, "I wish I did kill myself." He noted that death would relieve the pain, "like for my brother". Yet, he added a critical negation, "But I can't." When I explored the "can't", he associated to his children, noting that Rita had already abandoned their children, Peter Jr and Lianne.

Peter also began to discuss his need for punishment—self-punishment. He blamed himself for Rita's abandonment ("I am not man enough"). Peter obsessed about reading, among other things, Rita's diary, where he had read many "hurtful things". There was a pervasive need to be guilty. He reasoned something like: Rita is a good person; she left me; I must be a bad person; I must be guilty; it's all my fault (and at times he added the suicidological conclusion: "Therefore, I have to kill myself").

The loss was overwhelming and a deeply felt narcissistic injury. Peter stated, "She is my best friend." He suggested something that was obviously not true, "There is no one" (implications/items 14 and 26). Although Peter passionately argued that there was no justification for living on, his state of mind was incompatible with an accurate assessment/perception of what was going on. He was overwhelmed, perplexed, and confused. The only way to come back from this suicidal abyss is to develop relatively firm logic. In this regard, the statement "There is no one" was false. It was a constriction. Peter needed to perceive life as not just hard, bitter, unjustified, and hopeless. There were "someones".

Peter's personality (ego) was not adequately developed. He had suffered a nar-cissistic injury. This implied that, at least, a key to intermediate and long-range effectiveness with Peter was to increase the options for action, to increase aware-ness of adjustment (protective) processes, to widen the angle of the blindness, and to increase objects available—beyond the narcissistic ones. Peter needed help; for example, he needed psychotherapy. One doesn't leave the patient with his/her "weak", "primitive", inadequately developed ego after a crisis response. One must develop ego strength in the patient.

We began to explore who his friend was and who he could talk to, including his father, son, and daughter. Indeed, Peter Jr and Lianne were central to the treatment that often had a familial basis. Both were seen individually and together as needed, even after Peter's visit above, Lianne called me (the children have been an essential part of the treatment plan). Two days later, Peter was seen. He had explained the number of people to whom he spoke. In his self-defending style, he spoke to some of Rita's friends and they had confirmed Rita's belief "I am abusive". Obviously, not all people in the environment can or will help; some are suicidogenic (item 24).

Peter's relationships (attachments) were too unhealthy and/or too intimate (regres-sive, "primitive"), keeping him under constant strain of stimulation and frustration.

I had to assist Peter in detaching himself from a too highly cathected (or sometimes even suicidogenic) person, Rita. Peter needed to have his needs and wishes stimulated and inhibited to a healthier degree. Thus, I had to both increase and decrease relations. Not too infrequently suicidal behaviour signals a system distress (Richman, 1986).

PETER'S CHAOS

6 June.   Peter continued to see Rita; on 5 June, for example, Peter had seen Rita and she told him that she wanted to return home. Yet, her friends and her medical doctor advised "no". This ambivalence was short lived. On 6 June, when Peter was seen, he said that Rita had again suggested that the marriage was over. Peter started to question whether he was schizophrenic ("Am I crazy?", "Am I schizophrenic?"). Rita had suggested such a diagnosis (item 15).

About 90% of suicidal people exhibit a mental disorder, and some have symptoms that are consistent with schizophrenia; e.g., delusional thought, paranoid ideation. This, however, was not true for Peter, although he did exhibit symptoms consistent with an Axis I, DSM disorder of depression; e.g., depressed mood, diminished interest, insomnia. I deferred the decision whether there was a personality disorder at that time. There were symptoms consistent with item 15(g) of the TGSP. Peter was paralysed by pain so that his life, future, etc., were colourless and unattractive. He felt stagnant. Yet, Peter's suicidal behaviour is best understood by going beyond these nosological categorizations, although, I believe, such classification may assist in psychotherapy. Yet, in treatment, we constantly need to keep in mind that it is the individual who commits suicide, not some category. I needed to emphasize what was unique in Peter. At the same time, I had to look for what is ubiquitous regarding suicide, psychopathology, and personality functioning in general. I needed to understand Peter's mind.

Peter was informed that he was not schizophrenic, but that he did suffer from a depressive disorder and was in significant situational distress. Often, accurate information calms people's worries about their mental state, although one should never falsely minimize a suicidal person's true mental state. I have especially noted a number of people with a borderline personality who engaged in self-mutilating behaviour and had been told that this was only the result of their past history, such as sexual abuse. I believe that our patients do not need us to minimize, inhibit, etc., their mental health problems (nor maximize them). They need healthy, auxiliary egos.

10 June.   Peter continued to be obsessed and anxious about Rita, asking, "What will she do?" Peter wanted answers now—he could not tolerate the wait. He also expressed ongoing worry about the children, for example: "What will they do?; What will happen to them?" The next day, Rita called. Peter had made another suicide attempt (keep in mind that Peter had refused medication, hospitalization, referral to a psychiatrist, etc.). Rita was quite upset. Peter arrived the next day at the office, and I asked him what had occurred. He said in a calm fashion, "I found

a painless way." Peter had planned to take Rita's medication; yet, the attempt was stopped by Rita's unexpected appearance at the home. She had called the police, but the police did not take Peter to the hospital. They interviewed him and he assured them that he would see me today (obviously not an optimal response from the police—there is a need for prevention).

That visit lasted a few hours. We began with Peter's statement "Only suicide is a solution" and began to open the blinders (items 7, 8, and 9). Peter defined the trauma. He was, figuratively speaking, "intoxicated" by overpowering emotions and, concomitantly, with constricted logic and perception. I could not buy into his emotions and logic. I did not agree with his constriction. Peter's visit was not just for me to agree with his intoxication. There was poverty of thought. Peter's thinking was black and white. Thus, with Peter and other suicidal people, to presume that that suicidal individual either wants to kill him/herself or not is an extremely limited point of view. This is true, even if the person generates *only* such permutations and combinations in his or her thoughts, as Peter did at times. Thus, the task was to increase the permutations and combinations of Peter's thoughts, and this was critical in keeping Peter alive. Of note, it was especially his attachments to his children and his father, and his thoughts about these relationships (and ideals) that were so crucial in keeping Peter alive in those early months of treatment.

On 12 June, Peter was feeling better. We talked about his children; yet, he also spoke about Rita and David. He had spoken to David, stating that, "he is playing games". Somehow—although he was unclear—David had "given me hope". Somehow, which was again unclear, he dreamt that he would get Rita back.

On 13 June, Peter and Peter Jr were seen; Lianne did not show, as she was now siding with her mother. Peter Jr talked about the years of conflict and how, "they (parents) are angry all the time". Yet, he saw Peter, his father, as "okay", but his sister now disagreed. Peter himself continued to talk mainly about Rita. "She is against me," he said, "and now Lianne too." Lianne had often vacillated between her parents. Peter Jr confided that his mother was angry all the time; he said that the family was often "chaotic". This visit, once more, resulted in a call to the family doctor (suicide risk calls for careful consideration of the usual concerns of confidentiality). We discussed Peter and Rita's diagnoses, suicide risk issues, and plan of care. We agreed that Rita needed help, but she refused all suggested assistance from her doctor, as she had with others ("Peter was the problem").

On 14 June Peter was seen alone. Lianne had left with Rita the day before, but had called home four times since that departure. Rita had taken Lianne to her new apartment and then abruptly left to see David. Lianne wanted to come home. The "chaos" continued, for which Peter blamed David; he was, in fact, quite expressive of his anger towards David. Peter was so angry that he himself raised fears about his temper; yet, at the same time, he felt equally guilty about his rage. Telephone calls continued and Peter and Peter Jr were next seen on the 17 June. Lianne had stayed at her mother's apartment, but Rita never moved in—she lived with David. Peter responded by suggesting to Lianne that she should come home. Rita, in response, "blew". David got involved and the trauma escalated. Peter used words like "only"—"only Rita loved me", "only she will make me happy", "only if David leaves". In response, I asked, "Will Peter Jr make you happy?" "Does Lianne love you?" He responded with "yes"—his state of mind was too constricted to see even the obvious. His attachments to his children were so important.

We also began to explore—and predict—Rita's and David's behaviour. The unpredictable was predictable, and it was the predictability of the events that helped to reduce Peter's perturbation (a JND). Once life is more understandable (sameness), one is less anxious. It is in the range of expectations.

19 June.   Peter was feeling better, even though he had seen Rita, who announced, "I love David." Lianne had left her mother's place and, with Peter's help, had rented her own apartment. Rita and Peter had agreed to divide their assets (even then Peter believed that David was only after the money, "millions"). Peter reported that Rita was now calmer ("She is not panicking"). They were able to talk—my association was that this state had resulted in Peter's lethality being lower. There were no depressive mood swings. Yet, the next day, Peter called because Lianne had physically attacked her mother, Rita. Lianne had gone to see her father after the incident and they planned to see me the next day. Lianne's behaviour needed to be slowed down (and again, as in subsequent occurrences, a phone call was made to the family doctor).

Peter arrived on 21 June without Lianne. Peter, however, continued to be less perturbed and lethal (they were marked as "low" in the notes). We began to discuss expecting "worse"—what he can and cannot do, control and not control, and so on. Therapy often teaches the difference between what one can control or cannot control, and knowing the difference between them (an association to the Serenity Prayer is intended). Lianne was seen a few days later, and started being more involved in the treatment process at this time.

27 June.   Peter was seen (lethality was low); and he talked more and more about his hurt and anger (although he continued to deny the latter from time to time). He reported that Rita was "losing it" (something confirmed by the family doctor who suggested that she was quite manic at this time). Despite Peter's wishes, Rita had also begun to address the practical issues: she divided even the furniture as she wished. Peter unsuccessfully asked her not to rush, but this resulted in the opposite. Yet, Peter began to accept the unacceptable fact: Rita had left him. Regrettably, however, Peter also suggested that dating was a solution—he had already gone out with a new friend, Lisa. His family cautioned him—and so did I. I further suggested that this escape would also add to his problem (item 35).

Peter wanted to egress (i.e., to escape, to depart, to flee, to be gone), to relieve not only unbearable psychological pain, but any uncomfortable feeling. He attempted to escape from too many of life's problems. He needed better coping strategies. Explosive situations needed to be defused so that Peter no longer needed a suicidal weapon. I attempted to reinforce his constructive tendencies (protective factors)—talk about the hurt, need to escape, not act out (something Rita was increasingly doing).

CONSULTATION

30 June.   I am, as you have already learned, honoured to count Edwin Shneidman as one of my best consultants. As should be obvious to the reader by now, I believe that consultation with highly lethal patients is often good practice. Peter was an obvious case for consultation.

Shneidman's first rule was: Reduce Peter's perturbation. Shneidman asked: Why would he talk about Rita? What needs are frustrated? Etc.

Shneidman said that with Peter, as with so many perturbed (anxious) patients, we have to "play for time". For example, Peter's rash of choices, actions, disinhibitions, can be responded to with "It is not a good idea to make decisions now. You can wait with these decisions. Let us focus on what is a priority in your crisis." Therapists often have to pace their suicidal patients.

The obstacle to Peter's slowing down, "creating a monastic environment", was Rita. Peter loved Rita a lot, but not wisely. Rita was very seductive. She aroused Peter's heightened excitability. Rita, Shneidman concluded, "is like being introduced to a drug." (We saw the same in Scott.) How do you help an addict, whether alcohol, sex, aggression, whatever?

2 July.   Peter was seen; he reported that he was "okay", but despite our efforts to slow him down he continued to act out. He had gone out nightly, engaged in numerous sexual relationships and so on. He had approached Lisa sexually but she had declined his advances. (I remarked in my notes, "Good".) Despite this rejection, as Peter called it, he continued to see Lisa (and saw other women sexually). Rita became angry with him about Lisa (something Peter was positive about).

Overall, Peter was doing better; yet, he needed to continue to slow his pace. He was egressing; there was a growing tendency towards denial ("I'm all okay"). The lethality was, however, low. Thus, Peter and I now planned to see each other weekly, and more if needed.

On 9 July Peter focused on Rita's ongoing problem with Lianne; Rita was quite "upset"—and so was he. Indeed, his characteristic "racing" recurred ("My body is speeding"). He even saw that his relationship to Lisa was "too quick", asking "Am I using her?" (Peter's children continued to be seen.)

On 18 July Rita called, asking for the names of psychologists that she could see. I was positive to her about this request (not hopeful) and provided her with a few names. Rita, as predicted, never followed up. That same day, Peter was seen; his anger at Rita was heightened. He said "I am over her", "I don't care"—yet, another escape(?). Peter, however, also talked about his temper, especially towards Lisa, and towards himself—he clearly did have an anger management problem. Shneidman had noted, "Peter has to slow down his rage", associating to his favorite book, *Moby Dick*. In fact, on 18 July Peter said, "I do have a problem with anger." This was an important step (items 25, 26, 27, 28, 29, 30, 31, and 32).

REJECTION–AGGRESSION

Rejection–aggression was central to Peter's suicidal behaviour, and to much of his usual behaviour. A traumatic event or injury had occurred. Experience has taught us the important fact that it is neither possible nor practical to respond to an individual like Peter by the use of punishment, moral persuasion, confrontation, or the like. The most effective remedy was to mollify the felt trauma, reducing the elevated perturbation. It is the elevated perturbation that drives and fuels the elevated lethality; therefore, I tried to reduce Peter's anguish, tension, and pain. Shneidman's rule is: Reduce the elevated perturbation and the lethality will come down with it.

Peter's personality (ego) was not adequately developed. He had suffered a narcissistic injury (and many before). Peter needed psychotherapy and further intervention because he was too preoccupied with this injury. Peter was, in fact, often preoccupied with disturbed relationships. I frequently asked, "Tell me what's happening. Where does it hurt now?"

Peter was quite ambivalent. He expressed feelings and/or ideas of aggression and vengefulness towards himself, although he often appeared to be actually angry with someone else. Ventilation, lightening of angry feelings, adequacy of expression, and need for contacts had a critical place in his intervention, in regard to his ambivalence and anger. Peter's anger (or other feelings) needed to be heard (rather than introjected and especially not acted out). One had to address the taboo of talking about such issues.

Peter had turned upon the self, murderous impulses that had previously been directed against someone else. The focus with such highly angry and lethal people, like Peter, should not be immediately on "why" the aggression has been turned inwards or "why" homicide or suicide has been chosen as the method of solving the problems, but—and this is critical—once the lethality is lowered, the focus with people like Peter must be on those very questions (or problems). They need to understand and alter *this* process to stay alive. It is deadly.

To address Peter's aggressiveness, I addressed his unmet needs. I did so not only in the consultation room but also in his real world. Peter calculated the self-destructiveness to have a negative effect on Rita (and his mother, just as the suicide of his brother, Adrian, had been). Despite such Ahab-like rage, the therapist needs to constantly remind him/herself that Eros can work wonders against Thanatos. Or, similarly stated, with Peter, constructive goals worked wonders against destructive ones.

Finally (item 32), Peter's self-destructiveness appeared to be an act of aggression, attack, and/or revenge towards Rita (his mother, etc.) who had hurt and deeply injured him. Suicide, we should recall, is often a dyadic event. Peter often felt hurt, slighted, or under attack in his relationships. Revenge was a frequent motive. As his therapist, I created activity—something, of course, different from consciously or unconsciously attacking Peter. I was also constantly reminded, working with him, of a basic of intervention with such highly lethal individuals: Thinking is not a sufficient plan of action.

PETER'S HISTORY

22 July.   Peter reported that his relationship to Lisa was developing, but with Rita, there was more conflict—and his subsequent guilt. I suggested, noting the repetitive themes, that some of the thema were his personality—beyond simply a response to Rita. ("Some of this must be you.") He agreed. We then began to explore his anger, acting out, depression and so on—including biological, psychological, and sociological aspects.

Peter began to take greater responsibility—not simply the irrational guilt. He began to accept the belief, "Rita did not make me...". Responsibility is so critical in therapy with suicidal patients, and with responsibility comes freedom. Freedom allows you to be less mentally constricted on the *only* solution. Yet, this did not mean that Peter was well. For example, he reported on 29 July that he had asked Lisa to move in ("He's moving too fast," I wrote). Fortunately, Lisa said "no" and again I suggested going "slow!". Peter's worries became different. We, for example, learned that there had been questions about AIDS, etc., by the family doctor. Rita had been indiscriminate in her sexual behaviour before David. Fortunately, tests proved to be negative (both for Peter and Rita).

6 August.   As treatment developed, I began to ask Peter more about himself, his mother, his father, and his brother (what were the dynamics to his death?) On 6 August Peter, for example, shared a memory of his family at age 10. He had gone on a picnic with his grandparents at an amusement park, Boblo Island. He recalls seeing people squeezed into a transfer boat and having his first conscious anxiety attack. He associated to two images. In the first, his mother is scaring him during a storm. In the second, he recalls his mother, who weighed over 300 lbs, sitting on him, while his brother, Adrian, teased him (although often Adrian had been the target of "my mother's rage").

Memories about his brother, Adrian, were primarily horrific—survivor's memories. He recalls in morbid detail the suicide; his brother had shot himself and Peter had seen the "blood everywhere". Images of blood were frequent in Peter's memories and dreams. And, despite being in shock, Peter's family asked him to "do everything". His parents withdrew. His brother, still alive, was taken to hospital after shooting himself, but was kept on life support. There was no medical hope of recovery and, Peter said, "I had to pull the plug" at the hospital (guilt). He recalls having to identify the body, making the funeral arrangements, cleaning the blood, and so on. He talked about feeling "sad and angry"—"but having had to keep his feelings inside". "I was not allowed to weep," he said. "We were not allowed to talk about Adrian," he added. He noted that his father especially denied the event—"My father always denied everything, even mom's abuse." Peter added, "My father kept his head in the sand." Of course, by implication, we began to explore suicide as an escape.

Adrian, I learned, was also a very impulsive person, often resulting in problems with everyone, including the police. Adrian had been arrested for drunk driving, released, and was awaiting trial. He had threatened suicide at the time of the arrest; Peter recalled thinking at that time, "hope he is faking"—and then Adrian put a bullet through his head. Our discussions about Adrian and his death broadened, as can be seen in Chapter 11, especially about his mother and his brother's suicide note; "No one loves me. Mom hates me. I'm all alone. I have no reason to live." Peter at one point in treatment concluded, "I now understand the words of my brother's suicide note, 'No one loves me'."

12 August.   Peter reported more trauma. Rita had come unannounced to the house, when there was a party. She arrived "angry", "lost control" and "blew up" at Peter and other guests, including his parents. Peter was dismayed, questioning whether Rita was psychologically regressing. He told her that she needed help, yet she refused and continued to refuse help.

Peter's relationship to his father, Frank (and the father's personality) started to be more figural in the psychotherapy. At the party, Frank withdrew, being described as "rigid" and not showing himself (dissembling). After Rita arrived, Frank simply got up and left, leaving even his wife.

PETER'S NEEDS

Peter continued to worry about his children. On 19 August he spoke about Lianne. She continued to be depressed, but refused help. He wanted Lianne to get help now! Peter needed "to help", but his need for control was frustrated (item 21). The possible needs that were frustrated or blocked with Peter were expansive. Here is a partial list of needs, adopted from Henry A. Murray's *Explorations in Personality* (1938):

- *Aggression.* To overcome opposition forcefully; to fight; to attack or injure another; to oppose forcefully or punish other.
- *Autonomy.* To get free, shake off restraint; to break out of social confinement; to avoid or quit activities of domineering authorities; to be independent and free.
- *Counteraction.* To make up for failure by restriving; to overcome weakness or repress fear; to maintain self-respect and pride on a high level; to overcome.
- *Defendence.* To defend or vindicate the self against assault, criticism, blame; to conceal or justify a misdeed, failure, or humiliation.
- *Dominance.* To control other humans; to influence or direct others by command, suggestion, or persuasion; or to dissuade, restrain, or prohibit others.
- *Harmavoidance.* To avoid pain, physical injury, illness, and death; to escape from a dangerous situation; to take precautionary measures.
- *Rejection.* To exclude, abandon, expel, separate oneself, or remain indifferent to a negatively seen person; to snub or jilt another.
- *Sentience.* To seek and enjoy sensuous experience; to give an important place to creature comforts and satisfaction of the senses—taste, touch.

- *Succorance.* To have one's needs gratified by the sympathetic aid of another; to be supported, sustained, guided, consoled, taken care of, protected.

Although I listened to his concern about Lianne, I reframed the event by exploring his need for control (although he labelled it as "help"). Peter was impulsive, wanting quick solutions. We attempted to slow his pace. He would react quickly when things did not go as he wanted ("I like stability"). We began to explore alternatives to life's problems, learning to cope, even if one has no control. I told Peter about one of my favourite therapeutic stories (I do not recall the source). The Japanese Zen story goes something like this: "There is a jackass tied with a rope to a pole. The jackass, thinking like a jackass, pulls and pulls at the rope. The more he (or she) pulls, the tighter it gets. But, the Zen master says, 'If the jackass stops thinking like a jackass, it can sit here and there and, after a while, the rope will be loose and the jackass can be free. But, as long as the jackass thinks like a jackass, the tighter the rope becomes." The implications are multitudinal.

6 August.   Peter was doing well; yet he continued to worry. For example, he questioned his relationship to Lisa. He said, "I *only* want love"; yet, I again explored his needs for stability (sameness). Once more, I suggested that Peter "slow down". He continued to want to deny, deflect, and run away. He did not want to accept the unacceptable pain: Frustration.

16 September.   The relationship to Lisa continued to develop, but the relationship to his parents was up and down. He often reflected on his mother's "cruelty". As treatment continued, Peter also began to associate his impulsive acting out to his history (i.e., his social learning). He described it as a malaise for his brother too, but even worse. Peter began to drink early, and so did Adrian, but even more so. Adrian also abused drugs. The more conflicts in the home with their mother, the more they abused drugs and alcohol. Peter stated, "It was the best way to escape."

30 September.   "Lisa may be pregnant," Peter announced (something that proved not to be true). His children were upset, especially Lianne, who had only recently moved back home with Peter. Problems also continued with Rita; she was fighting the separation agreement and was demanding millions of dollars.

Yet, Peter also was looking forward to the next few weeks. Peter and Lisa were going on a cruise (a positive egression). One could see a genuine smile on Peter's face as he left the office. Egression in the service of the ego has always been healing.

21 October.   The cruise went well, but back home, Peter Jr and Lianne had been fighting. Peter Jr was angry that Lianne had moved back. For some time, he and his father shared the home. Lianne was seen as intrusive. Peter Jr demanded that Lianne leave. Eventually, Peter Jr left, but by November Lianne had also planned to move out. One can see that with weakened (fragile) egos, problems in adjustment are frequent.

28 October.   Civil court issues became figural. Rita was now accusing Peter of slander, and claimed that Peter called her a "F****** Bitch". Peter wondered what would happen; "What would she do?", he asked. I explored his belief, but also his suspiciousness. I learned that he first remembered being suspicious when young.

He was often tense, fearing when he would be hit next by his mother. He concluded, "Being suspicious was useful." As a child, and in his relationship with Rita, this process continued to be useful. He recalled, for example, a fire incident. Rita had accidentally started a fire in the kitchen. She called the emergency services, left the house, and closed the door. Peter was sleeping upstairs, only to be fortunately awakened by the smoke. Yet, we began exploring the belief, "I need to be suspicious all the time", to "some of the time" (a JND).

18 November.   Lisa moved in, and much of the following sessions related to this event and his children's reaction the change. It was also an opportunity for Peter to talk about change and his reaction to the same. He was less rigid, although more confused ("I am more confused") as we began to explore his fixed—sometimes delusional—beliefs. For example, at first, he could only see Rita's anger, not his own. Yet, in time he was more and more aware of his moods, including aggressive ones. By 9 December the court had settled the separation agreement, leading to divorce. The settlement was for much less than anticipated and the judge had been critical of Rita's lack of responsibility to the children. Peter concluded that the court went well from his view, whereas Rita went into "a rage" and "David broke". Peter was relieved.

16 December.   Peter and his family were planning for Christmas. His father had become more open and assertive. His despair was more often discussed with Peter now, especially about Adrian's death. Peter genuinely began to care about his father and his father openly returned the care. His father told him that he did not want to lose his last son. Peter reported that, "I'm his (father's) only sparkle." Peter was puzzled, but relieved with his father's attachment. Christmas went well for all (Rita was away).

THE MOTHER'S DEATH

18 January. Peter's mother died! Peter arrived quite upset, in a state of shock and grief. He showed the expected symptoms of bereavement, but especially guilt. He felt guilty about his anger towards his mother, his lack of love, and things he should have done for her. He stated, "I should have loved her." He concluded with "I'm the coldest of all." We began to explore his shoulds ("I should . . . "), associating to his harsh conscience (superego) (item 18).

Peter had a harsh conscience; i.e., his behaviour often included elements of fulfilment of punishment, not only about his mother's death. Self-punishment was a motive in his suicidal acts. This implied with Peter: Don't punish. Don't moralize. Don't preach. Don't pass judgement. Above all, I did not agree with Peter's major premises (e.g., "All bad boys deserve to be punished, to die," "I am bad," therefore, "I deserve to die").

Practically (when working with Peter), I did what I could. And—which is critical—I threw in my energies against punishment, and that was often life-saving. I questioned his belief, "I am bad" (something his mother often said, as well as "You F****** kid", "You bastard", etc.—all negative inductions). Attachment in psychotherapy is, in fact, often critical and in many ways life-saving. And, with assistance, Peter also associated to his history, concluding, "Mother didn't love me."

On 20 January Peter attended his mother's funeral. Rita was there; he said, "We were so cold." Rita had arrived at the funeral home, when "she blew up". Lianne was the target. When Peter attempted to interfere, Rita said "You F****** asshole." The police had to be called. Once more, we discussed Rita's own abusive history and her serial way of coping. Rita, obviously, showed borderline features, suggesting a possible Axis II of DSM diagnosis of Borderline Personality Disorder, comorbid with the more obvious Axis I diagnosis of Bipolar Disorder.

Yet, Peter also continued to focus on his more healthy relationships. With suicidal people, one must always continue to foster positive attachments in psychotherapy. The implication once more is as follows: Eros can work wonders over Thanatos.

Peter Jr had moved back to the home, and we explored the positive and negative of the frequent moves of his children. They, too, used escape. We began to investigate how Peter could respond to the demands of young adults in a healthy fashion. Lianne's problems were serious, and having been the primary target of Rita's rages she lacked ego strength. Lianne needed to develop mature coping strategies; "She acts like a child," Peter said. Psychotherapy was something Lianne needed now but was willing to accept only briefly. She rarely saw Rita, who had told her, "People who go to shrinks are crazy—look at your father."

RITA GOES ON AND ON

27 January.   Peter came in, with an unusual concern for Rita. Rita had made "a suicide attempt". "She's hurting herself," reported Peter. Rita had been cutting herself, and called Peter, who then called an ambulance. Rita was hospitalized, but she soon signed herself out. Peter now revealed years of suicidal behaviour in Rita. There had been attempts, threats, and self-abusive behaviour (parasuicide), often cutting herself. Peter began to understand Rita better. He said, "She goes on and on. It never stops." A common benefit of psychotherapy: Understanding people's behaviour, their serial way of coping, allows one to cope better. This is often a necessity with suicidal people. They not only do not understand themselves, they do not understand people, especially their closest attachments. The concern of Rita was, however, short-lived.

On 17 February Rita was accusing Peter of sexual abuse. The children immediately denied the allegations and authorities took no action. Rita raged more, accusing Peter of all sorts of behaviour. Once more, all Peter could do was understand Rita— we often spoke of her mental disorders, her poor abilities to cope with her pain, and so on.

Yet, other sex themes entered treatment. Sexual themes—like aggressive ones—are, of course, as we have read in this volume, not unusual in suicidal patients. On one occasion, a 21-year-old female, an employee of Peter, had approached Peter. He was excited, but fearful; yet, he acted out sexually. Hurt, rejection, and fear of closeness were continual themes in his treatment—and so was his acting out. He often set the stage.

Peter continued to grieve for his mother. On one occasion, to his total surprise, a cousin had said, "You were the apple of her (mother's) eye." Peter was bewildered; "how could I be an apple to her?", he asked. He puzzled. He wondered what it would have been like if his mother, if Rita, if someone, loved him?

15 March.   Peter reflected on his marital years. He now began to see himself as "harsh", not in the previous self-punishing ways. He, having explored his cognitive constriction and suicidal behaviour earlier, noted "my horse blinders affect me in many ways". He noted that, as a child, he learned to deny events (he often repeated to himself, "Nothing happened. Mom is good"). With Rita, "I turned a blind eye on things," adding, "just like my father did." He reported that talking about his mental constriction allowed him to see and perceive events better ("I know now how it affects me").

RELATIONSHIPS

22 March.   Peter was increasingly questioning his relation to Lisa. We began to explore his ambivalence—his love/hate, yes/no, was so characteristic. We associated to his ambivalent relationship to Rita. "It's like habit," he concluded. He wondered even, if Lisa acted like Rita, would it be easier ("Would it be easier if Lisa was not as kind?") (item 20).

Peter was weakened and defeated by unresolved problems in his interpersonal field (he was so before he met Rita). Peter was so preoccupied with current unresolved problems that he was often unaware of his history, how he had previously adjusted to trauma, whether interpersonal loss or otherwise. He was generally fixated in the present pain, forgetting his previous ones. Yet, there was a history, his serial way of coping with problems. His problems had often been resolved by, for example, denial, repression, projection. This implied that I had to widen the adjustment (protective) processes including, but not limited to, helping the person to understand the past, e.g., how his relationships to Lisa and Rita were different. This implied that I not only resonated to Peter's immediate unresolved problem, but also to his long-term needs. Indeed, Peter arrived at almost every session with a new trauma. His thinking was often catastrophic. I had to address his elliptical history of coping with unresolved problems in his interpersonal field.

Peter also continued to explore the prototype of his relationship, his mother. He noted that especially if one got close to her, she would rage. This often occurred with Adrian. "One never knew when she would attack—she especially was vicious to Adrian." He often wondered about his mother's role in Adrian's death. "No one did anything," he said. "She knew; he told her, but she just walked away," asking, "how could she?" He also began to see better his father's role: "He never did anything at any time." He concluded that his father was an "enabler" (reinforcer) and so was he with Rita.

By this time, trust was a core issue in treatment (as it had always been for Peter). Historically, there was no trust in his family. "With David, I lost my trust," he stated. We explored trust, whether he could trust people (e.g., "Can you trust me?"). He continued to associate to his mother. "How could you trust," he said, "she raged mercilessly." Once more, Adrian's death was discussed. He concluded, "we learned to be islands. We trusted no one, not even ourselves." I then explored how the mistrust affected him now. He asked, "Can we unravel it?" I answered, "Yes, but slowly, like peeling an onion."

Erik Erikson's developmental model first isolated "Basic trust vs mistrust" as the dialectic of the first stage of development (approximately to age 2). The role of the mother is crucial at this time in the child's life. If the mother is warm and responsive, the child develops trust; but, if not, the child develops a deep insecurity (Frager & Fadiman, 1984). Erikson (1963) wrote that basic trust "implies not only that one has learned to rely on the sameness and continuity of the outer providers, but also one may trust oneself and the capacities of one's own organs to cope with urges" (p. 248). Peter developed mistrust early as an infant and this affected his subsequent life. Early on, Peter developed a deep inner pain. According to Erikson (1963), this pain marks the child's first experience of evil. The virtue of hope is not developed; there is a lack of trust in self, mother, and the world.

Subsequently, people like Peter with a ground work of mistrust must, according to Erikson (1963), develop subsequent dialectics of autonomy vs shame or doubt (approximately 2–4 years), initiative vs guilt (4–6 years), industry vs inferiority (6–13 years) and then the subsequent development of young and middle adulthood. In Peter, one can see the mistrust, shame, doubt, guilt, and inferiority. He developed few virtues to cope with life's demands.

13 April.   Peter exhibited mild suicidality, but no risk. Lisa and Peter had had a conflict. He said, "I tried to push Lisa into a fight," recognizing that he had done the same with Rita—and that his mother had frequently done so. Again, we explored his habits, his serial way of responding. Projection was a common defence ("She is angry at me", not "I am angry"). I also wrote in my notes, "Even here he is testing me" and we explored these behaviours as they appeared as transferences in treatment (items 20, 22, 10, and 11).

Peter had been weakened and defeated by unresolved problems in his interpersonal field. He was overly fixated. He needed to learn to cope better on the interpersonal stage. His frustration in the interpersonal field was all too often exceedingly stressful and persisting to a traumatic degree. Everything was a trauma (a constriction). His needs were frustrated. A goal in treatment was to reduce these real-life pressures, the frustrated needs that were driving up his sense of perturbation. We had to reduce his pain. To do this, I assisted him to make the pain more bearable, but I did not deny, repress, project, or deflect the pain (this he did characteristically). The pain, in fact, served as the energy for his change. He needed to face his real trauma, whether interpersonal or otherwise. Suicide was an escape, a way of avoiding his life's problems. For example, he did not cope well with his own aggression, sometimes even turning it inwards. He was ambivalent almost all the time. Peter often exhibited complications, concomitant contradictory feelings, attitudes and/or thrusts. Even about his suicidal behaviour, he showed the deepest ambivalence between wanting (needing) to be dead and yearning for possible intervention or rescue. The rescue with Peter often took the form of improvement or change in one of the major details—one thing—in his world such as the wish to be loved, to have autonomy and so on—and this was a JND.

In general, I worked with the life-directed aspects of Peter's ambivalence without, of course, being timorous about touching upon the aggressive elements in Peter. Peter was, in fact, overly angry. His aggression, at times, was turned inwards; submission, subordination, and flagellation, were evident. But, a highly aggressive state, like the suicidal state, is characterized by its transient quality. The expression of intense aggression turned outwards or inwards is usually of brief duration. This was true for Peter—yet, the danger was that, in a few seconds, he could act out towards himself or others.

Peter, of course, never learned to cope with anger as a child. He associated to escaping, when, for example, his mother was angry. Once, he stated, "I stayed under the porch, hiding. My mother then started hitting me with the broom stick."

Problems with Rita continued. She had hired a new lawyer, asking for an appeal of the settlement. "I feel squeezed," he said (which we associated to his mother often setting on him). He noted insightfully, "She doesn't want my money, but punish me." "She wants me to rage like her," he added. We even concluded, probably accurately (see Chapter 10, on Scott), that if he does not react, she will rage even more. He associated this insight to an event as a child. His mother had been angry at him about a bath, but he did not react; so she filled the tub with ice-cubes and ice-cold water. Then Peter reacted—but she held him down in the water. "I thought I would die," he said.

Peter also now revealed a sexual abuse incident (later verified by his father, Frank). Peter had been sexually abused at age 5 by a maternal uncle (who had later killed himself, when confronted with his sexual abuse by a neighbour, some 10 years later). Peter's history was a series of events and trauma, beginning with his mother, that had undermined his adjustment abilities.

Peter's relationship to Lisa, on the other hand, was more positive. "I feel close to her," he said, stating that he found this satisfying, gratifying his need for nurturance.

UNDERSTANDING THE CHAOS

1 June.   Peter and I reviewed and understood more aspects of his chaotic life. We began to explore the aetiology of the chaos more. Biological (such as the basis for Bipolar Disorder); psychological, both conscious and unconscious; and even socio-logical/cultural (e.g., his Dutch ancestry) aspects were identified. We even began to unravel the unconscious dynamics, especially those related to love. Patients need to learn the multidetermined nature of behaviour, beyond a situational explanation

("Rita caused all the problems"). No single event accounts for behaviour such as suicide. One is reminded of the statement, somewhat misquoted: Those who don't know their history are bound to repeat it. (George Santayana: "Those who cannot remember the past are condemned to fulfil it.") To rephrase somewhat, I would state, "Those that know only one situation or event of their history to explain their suicidal behaviour are bound to repeat it and fulfil it." That is a common state of suicidal people.

8 June.   Peter began to report more dynamic material, much that is open to inter-pretation of the unconscious. He recalled the following three scenarios, almost in a dreamlike fashion, when he was about 8:

1. I'm walking in the country with my mother. There is a big black car. We get in . . . it feels weird.
2. I'm ready to go to school. All at once I get taken by mother on a 600-mile bus trip to see her father, she said. We stop, we meet a man. My mother looks happy and I'm surprised.
3. I'm by my house alone. I see a black car; my mother and a man are having sex. The man chases me.

He also recalls worrying about his mother, however. For example, he recalls walking with his mother and grandmother. His mother falls down a ditch and breaks her leg. He helps; she accepts his help. He concluded, "She loves me." Yet, most of his memories were more problematic, all centring around coping with one trauma after another. He, for example, asked, "Was my mother schizophrenic?"; "Was she abusive?"; and "Was I sexually abused?" About the latter, Peter began to recall more and more sexual abuse memories, and not only with his uncle. He recalled at around age 6, being in a bathtub with Adrian and both being molested by a much older female cousin. When 10 and so on, he recalled having "sexual play" with a much older male. Peter also recalled, around the age of 10 to 12, his mother talking about his "big penis" to his aunt in front of him. He remembered feeling mixed up, both pride and shame. He concluded that "a lot was disturbing". He began to ask about "what is normal?".

The sexual dysfunction continued with Rita. Peter associated to Rita's sexuality, wondering even more what was normal. Rita, he said, was sexually active, often excessively involved in pleasurable activities. They, as teenagers, had sex the first day they met. Often, she talked about wanting sex with other boys, suggesting that they go to sex parties. Peter said that Rita was often manic sexually. They often had sex, but Rita was rarely satisfied. Often the sex was pleasurable for Peter, but "sometimes painful". Yet, he did what Rita wanted, "otherwise she'd rage". Peter was often worried that she would have sex elsewhere (which he later learned that she frequently, indeed, had).

On this topic, it is of note that Rita from time to time accused Lisa of being "a hooker". The accusation had no factual basis. This too, however, resulted in Peter asking questions about sexual normality. He also recognized that his brother had problems sexually; when a teenager, he was charged for date rape but was found not guilty. Sexuality and aggression were serially problematic impulses for Peter and much of his family.

SUICIDE IN ALCOHOLISM

6 July.   Peter announced that he had been drunk on Saturday. After discussing the event, noting that the stimuli was "confusion" (Rita, Lisa, Lianne), Peter stated, "I need to escape." Yet, he denied suicidal thoughts. He revealed that alcohol had always been an escape, but "second on my list". As a digression, I will provide here a comment on the topic of alcoholism, based on a study of suicide notes in alcoholism (Leenaars et al., 1999b).

Alcoholism is associated with a vast number of suicides (Murphy & Robins, 1967; Murphy, 1992). The lifetime risk of suicide in alcoholics is about 2.5% (and 3.5% for those with a history of inpatient treatment). The most systematic study of suicide in alcoholism is the work of Eli Robins and George Murphy (Murphy, 1992). Their primary mode of study was the psychological autopsy. In the Murphy study of 50 cases (1992), 16 suicide notes are identified. The notes, until Leenaars et al. (1999b) had remained unanalysed.

Leenaars's (1988a, 1996) multidimensional model for the study of suicide was utilised to analyse the notes: unbearable pain, cognitive constriction, indirect expressions, inability to adjust, ego, interpersonal relations, rejection–aggression, and identification–egression. The purpose of the study was to assess whether the 16 suicide notes of alcoholics in the Murphy archive differ from matched suicide notes of non-alcoholics in the above dimensions (and the 35 specific protocol sentences that comprise these dimensions in the TGSP). The comparison sample was derived from a sample of over 2000 notes, matching for age and sex (see Leenaars, 1988a). The notes of alcoholics met a strict criterion for alcoholism (Murphy, 1992) and were by 11 men and 5 women whose mean age was 45.1 years (age range 32–57).

Comparisons of neither the eight clusters nor the 35 specified protocol sentences reached significance. The main conclusions about suicide in alcoholism are in support of the hypothesis that there may be more similarities than differences in suicide, regardless of whether one is an alcoholic or not.

Data from a descriptive point of view suggest that suicide in alcoholism is often associated with several factors: suicide in alcoholics is a response to unbearable pain, often the alcoholism itself. There is a history of trauma, e.g., a failing marriage, the inability to stop drinking, and the person is mentally constricted on these events. The alcoholic person is hurt, injured, and angry. Although there is much more to the death, the alcoholic person in the end wants to escape, finding the alcohol an insufficient egression. Of course, there are limitations to this study; yet, it is of methodological significance that the study of suicide notes yielded the same main conclusions as the more expensive psychological autopsy approach. Much more needs to be learned about the suicide of alcoholics and substance abusers through diverse methodologies; yet, clinically, the importance of alcoholism in our suicidal patients must be addressed at this time.

ACCEPTING THE UNACCEPTABLE

20 July.   Peter continued to be agitated, often feeling confused; he noted at least three anticipating anxiety-producing events: (1) 6 August was in court with Rita; (2) Lianne was moving back home on 1 August; (3) the relationship with Lisa was resulting in ongoing ambivalence about closeness (and, he added, "My need for a self"). Once more, we discussed the Jackass story, and Peter fighting the ropes. This is a common pattern in suicidal people. Often it means accepting the unacceptable. Shneidman (1996) tells of the story of the Japanese Emperor Hirohito to explicate the prevention statement of history. Shneidman (1996, p. 161) writes:

> In the rescript of capitulation on August 14, 1945, in which Emperor Hirohito, by unprecedented radio broadcast, almost none of his subjects had ever heard his voice before, ordered his loyal subjects to surrender, he touched on the two main antidotes to suicide: the sense of futurity; and the redefining of the key term, variously defined by the person as unbearable, unacceptable, intolerable, unendurable. With great presence, the Emperor commanded all members of his nation-family.
>
>   It is according to the dictates of time and fate that we have resolved to pave the way for a ground peace for all generations to come by enduring the unendurable as suffering what is insufferable. He ordered his people to live.

We continued to address his worry, making an imperative: Stop drinking; it was clear that alcohol was developing into a bigger problem. Despite reluctance, Peter did agree verbally to stop drinking and there were no known subsequent drinking episodes.

7 August.   Next, Peter focused primarily on Lisa; he stated, "I wish she was gone." This was a constant struggle, the ever-present approach/avoidance in his relationship. We also noted that his ambivalence was heightened when there was a move, and this time Lianne had moved back home. We began to explore his needs again. Shneidman (2001) recently made the following comment about the primacy of needs in psychotherapy with suicidal people:

> In general, the sources of elevated psychache are thwarted or frustrated psychological needs. These psychological needs—from Henry A. Murray (1938)—include the needs for abasement, achievement, affiliation, aggression, autonomy, counteraction, defendence, deference, dominance, exhibition, harm-avoidance, inviolacy, nurturance, order, play, rejection, sentience, shame-avoidance, succorance, and understanding...Two sets of needs can be distinguished: modal needs, the disposition of needs one ordinarily lives with, and vital needs, the needs that one would die for. That is what suicide revolves around. A basic aspect of the therapist's task is to understand the patient in terms of this template of blocked needs. There are many unnecessary deaths, but there is never a needless suicide. (pp. 181–182)

Peter struggled with his own commitment. On the weekend, he met a 19-year-old female, Sam, a friend of Peter Jr, and had sex. Lisa discovered the fact; Peter stated, "I can't stop". Once more, the can'ts, won'ts, should's, etc., became the focus of psychotherapy. For example, "When you say you can't stop it, what is the *it*?"; "when you say can't, what do you mean?", and so on. Of note, despite the sexual liaison with the younger woman, Lisa did not leave and, surprisingly, Frank, his father became more involved. They went fishing ("The first time ever"). His father began to talk about Peter's behaviour, saying, "You're acting like Adrian." He told

Peter that, at age 2, Adrian had already run away. Adrian had killed an animal and ran! Frank said, "Your sex with Sam is a running away. I know because that is what I did. You need to stop." Frank so feared the loss of Peter.

Sex, like much else, had been an escape. Rita had been very demanding, "When she was upset, she wanted sex." He recalls, for example, when her favourite grand-father died, she "only" wanted to have sex, even in the funeral home's parking lot. She often, in fact, engaged in sexual behaviours in public places, "wanting us to get caught". Sex was egression! Yet, we continued to explore how uncontrolled impulses, whether sexual or aggression, were unhealthy.

I provided him with a metaphor: Our impulses, wishes, needs, etc., I suggested are like the horses in front of a chariot. They are excellent horses, but they need the charioteer to guide and control them. The charioteer needs to hold onto the reins. "You need to hold the reins," I said. "If you throw them away, the horses will run wild and chaos, disaster will happen." It is a frequent story that I tell my patients, whether suicidal or not.

The pattern of sexual acting out, for example, was problematic for Lisa and now Peter. Lisa continued to be upset about Peter's liaison with the 19-year-old. Peter's conclusion was "It is Lisa"; I suggested an alternative, reframing it as his inner beliefs, conflicts, and so on. Yet, he continued to believe, "Getting Lisa to leave is the only solution." Of course, the risk factors for suicide are risk factors for other acts of destruction. I continued to focus on "Is the decision, emotional . . . constricted?" We explored rational reasons. I asked questions like, "Do you want to do this?", "How will this affect you?, Do you have the reins of the horses?", and so on. Peter reluctantly agreed to work at the relationship and went on a vacation with Lisa, but he returned with the statement, "I'm even more convinced that I want to leave." (Of course, I had questioned the relationship from the beginning; it was too fast.)

The dynamics in the relationship were of interest. Peter learned that Lisa vacillated between being passive/active. If he was passive, avoidant, etc., she became quite active in seeking out the relationship, but if he dominated, controlled, etc., she got very isolated and quiet. I began to question the dysfunction; even wondering if Lisa was stimulating Peter to reject her (a repeat of history).

Her reactions were, however, different from Rita's; Rita would rage at Peter's with-drawal. Yet, the process with Lisa was still problematic and circular. He also realized that he was acting like his father, when he isolated himself or did things to reject Lisa. His father was "self-absorbed"; he was "never there", adding "never was". Lisa, said Peter, was "never there". Peter's father was "hyper" and "a workaholic" (Peter escaped in work too). "It was part of my mother's rage and rejection. She rejected dad always." And I asked, "Are you trying to get Lisa to reject you?"; "Was the liaison such an attempt?"; and "Is it a way to escape?"

19 October.   Once more, Lianne had moved out and stayed at her mother's, but this was, as always, short-lived. A conflict occurred with David; a physical fight occurred with David and Lianne in the front yard. A neighbour called the police. Rita kicked Lianne out and she moved back to Peter's home. Peter said, "It was quite a mess." Peter Jr also continued his struggle. Peter was especially worried

about drug use by both children. He said Rita is associated with "losers" and all of them use drugs, suggesting that Rita was even supplying drugs to Lianne and Peter Jr. She often smoked marijuana with them. Peter suggested that Rita had a long history of multiple drug use, beginning as a teenager. He worried, but noted his lack of power ("it frustrates me"). "She will do what she wants," he said.

Lianne's drug use became more problematic, and frequent use of LSD occurred. This resonated to Adrian's problems; he too increased his drug use in the last year of his life. Peter noted that Lianne was also more unstable, upset, and angry. We began to explore options; e.g., medication, hospitalization; we had a case discussion on the same with the family doctor. We developed a plan for intervention. We found a treatment centre. Yet, Peter asked, "Will she go?"

Peter was overwhelmed with Lianne's problem, feeling hopeless and helpless (feelings associated to his earliest developments of trust vs mistrust and the associated virtue of hope). He said something like, "She will always use drugs. We can't do anything about it." He feared that Lianne was like Rita, questioning whether Lianne had a manic-depressive problem. Yet, despite her visits here from time to time for our family meetings, Lianne refused further treatment. This was regrettable, because she continued to race into problems.

INTROJECTS

9 November.   Peter arrived stating, "She is ugly." "Who?" I asked; "My mother often said that about Rita," he replied. He associated to the fact that his mother called all his (and Adrian's) girlfriends "ugly". He now noted that he hears his mother's voice in his mind saying, "She is ugly" about Lisa. After some discussion, I asked "That is the only reason for breaking off with her, your mother's voice?" "Is that rational?" I asked. Peter replied "no".

Peter and I began to discuss such voices (or introjects). I reminded him of another patient's story. A female patient in her 40s, suffering from a depressive disorder, had been preoccupied with a rejecting mother-in-law. Regardless of what she tried, the mother-in-law had not accepted her. This was most evident; if the mother-in-law was invited for supper, whatever my patient cooked it was "no good" ("It is not how I cook it," "My son likes it how I cook it"). We had discussed these dynamics in therapy, focusing on my patient's frustration of the need for acceptance, nurturance, and so on. At one point, the patient had recalled that her mother-in-law had been most favourable about some chili at a well-known restaurant. She purchased a take-out order, and served it as her own for supper, but the proverbial "This chili is no good" occurred. This stimulus allowed my patient to understand that the issue was not her cooking, but an intrapsychic problem of the mother-in-law. The interpersonal field had little to do with it. She had no control over the mother-in-law's dynamics. And I explored, "who had the problem?", suggesting your chili is okay.

He saw the meaning of that story. Next, I asked, "Why do you give your mother so much power?" He instantly said, "Because I would get beat." I noted his fast response and began to explore its applicability to his "here and now". Of course, we touched on the fact that his mother was dead, which placed the influence within a historical context (including his recent grief).

We also began to discuss how such statements developed into one's unconscious; for example, his harsh conscience. Habits are deep, deeper than the conscious mind is aware of. There are of course characteristics of identification with the aggressor. Basics in the cognitive approach were introduced; for example, the ineffective approach of "Don't..." as opposed to changing behaviour for a reinforcing reason (associating to the story of Adam and Eve, when God said "Don't eat the apple"). Once more, acceptance of the spontaneous beliefs/cognitions and at the same time development of new beliefs ("I can act rational") were suggested. Court issues continued. Rita continued to have her flare-ups. Lianne continued to have problems; for example, Lianne had assaulted a friend's boyfriend, with police needing to be called. Lianne's behaviour more and more sounded like borderline behaviour. In exploring the features with Peter, he agreed, worrying, but noting that he had learned to accept that he could not control Lianne. We continued to suggest intensive treatment for Lianne, but she continued to refuse, stating "I don't have a problem" (dissembling).

More insight into his mother, and by implication himself, occurred. He recalled whenever his mother was stressed, unhappy, whatever, she would act out against Adrian and himself. Sometimes they were locked in a dark room in a basement ("Everything was dark. I couldn't see anything"). Sometimes she sat on them. Sometimes she "clawed" them. "I got so anxious," he said. He noted that he felt impotent, much as at present with Lianne (and before, with Rita). "I feel trapped," he said. Once more, we needed to constantly widen the adjustment patterns.

4 January.   Peter, at his request, was now being seen every other week. Peter began to explore his new relationship with his father; Peter noted, "He is so different, with mother gone." His father, in fact, expressed uncharacteristically a "thank-you" for Peter's support, after his wife died ("You were there for me"). Yet, Peter, as typical in suicidal people, was perplexed; he did not see his father's movement towards him. The relationship was developing and they even began to speak about Adrian. For example, they talked about Adrian's struggle with life and his inability in the end to cope, and then how Peter could cope better.

18 January.   Court continued. On 18 January Peter reported that he was frustrated. "I want it to be over," he said. "It is causing stress," he added. Yet he, on his own, noted some relief in other frustrations (a JND). Lianne had finally seen the family doctor and had accepted a prescription of Zoloft, although this was short-lived. He continued to talk to his father. Peter Jr was fine. And although court continued, Peter reported that his rage was less. "I am controlling my behaviour," he said proudly, despite that much of his life continued to be problematic.

15 February.   Peter arrived all upset; Rita had called the police, reporting that Peter had abused her. The police arrived at his home at 1:00 a.m. unexpectedly and he was arrested. He claimed that she lied; stating that, after the police investigated

the facts, they accepted his story and he was released. They were, however, quite upset at Rita.

Lianne, too, had caused chaos again. She had wanted something to eat, but the bread was frozen. "She blew," Peter said. Lisa "flipped," while Lianne was breaking furniture, a TV, etc. Only with restraint was Lianne able to calm down. Peter, with me, continued to process the chaos, rather than feeling confused, hopeless, helpless—and suicidal. Yet, the event with Lianne, at least, resulted in her finally accepting to go to a drug treatment centre, as had been previously arranged. Her problem, however, continued to escalate; she was now formally charged with the assault of her friend's boyfriend.

Peter more and more explored how his past was controlling the present. He now recalled how his mother often placed ice-cubes in a bath, demanding that he (or his brother) learn not to react. If he or Adrian did, she would blow and then even more ice was added. It was "terror," he said. And now, whenever something is upsetting, he concluded, he blows (much like Lianne). He, for example, noted that the other day Peter Jr had put too many ice-cubes in his drink and he raged. "I have become my mother," he concluded; we began to explore this spontaneous cognition too.

More memories of terror arose. He recalled how his mother, while in the ice-tub on a number of occasions, tried to drown him. He was upset and she became even more so. She held his head down and "I only felt panic. She was going to kill me." Of course, child murder occurs (Lester, 1991b). Motivations range from psychosis, when a psychiatric person kills a child; spousal revenge, when the child is killed as a rage against the spouse; unwanted, when the child is not wanted (e.g., offspring of incest); altruistic, when the parent murders the child because the parent, often delusional, believes that the child will be better off dead; and accidental, when the child dies because of abuse (Resnick, 1969). Homicide–suicide also occurs all too frequently in troubled, disturbed patients.

"It was very real," he said. "She was going to kill me." "And," he added, "my father turned a blind eye." "My mother was crazy. Many people in her family were crazy. A number of them killed themselves."

Those were facts; one wonders, as we read in the chapter on Justin, how children cope with their trauma, their terror. How does a child cope with a homicidal or suicidal or homicidal–suicidal parent? Understandably, Peter had learned to panic—but now was learning new ways to cope.

THE LATTER VISITS

The relationship with Lisa, despite her up and downs, continued. Our relationship also developed. On 19 April we again discussed our treatment. Peter said, "I never trusted anyone." Once more, attachments are key (items 33, 16, 24, and 23). Peter directly and indirectly attached (i.e., identification) with lost and rejecting people (Rita, his mother, Lisa?). He had a relative weakness in his capacity for developing constructive tendencies (e.g., attachment, love). A key to his intermediate—and long-range—effective intervention was to increase constructive (protective) factors. Peter needed healthier relationships. Peter's relationships (attachments) were too "primitive" and too regressive, keeping him under constant strain of stimulation and frustration. I had to assist Peter in detaching himself from too highly-cathected, destructive (sometimes even suicidogenic) people. Peter needed to have his needs and wishes stimulated and inhibited to a healthier degree. Thus, I had to increase and decrease relationships. He also needed to develop his need for understanding, especially about dyadic events. I often spoke about the positive in relationships. How would such development be forthcoming? I often responded to him about his interpersonal events with: "That sounds bad. What can you do in the relationship to have more positive experiences—and stay alive?"

10 May.   Peter reported a dream: "There is a little girl in a nightgown to her knees. We play. She jumps from window to window. She's having fun. Then a roar. The girl is frightened and scared. I wake up (I was roaring while I slept)." When I asked about associations, he immediately saw himself as the child. The roar came from his mother.

This dream was also the stimulus where he began to better understand his mother. He knew that her father was "abusive" and "cruel". "He abused everyone," he had been told by his mother. Peter even wondered if his grandfather abused her sexually. He stated, "She often hinted about it, but never said so." One wonders what pain would have moulded his mother to become like her abusive father— one is here reminded of Ahab in *Moby Dick*. She never saw her behaviour as a repetition; fortunately, Peter did. He more and more was understanding of his parents, although he could not forgive her for the abuse. I suggested that was okay. It is acceptable that patients do not have to forgive the unforgivable. Peter found that healing; he no longer wanted to "be blind" (his mother's induction and father's common behaviour).

Of course, Peter's past raised many questions: What was the abuse? Who else abused him? I never believed the few incidents of sexual abuse. A different uncle, a minister, had once been visiting his home and was suddenly kicked out. "Something happened with me," Peter said, "but I don't remember what." He was never told. There were questions about his maternal grandfather. My notes read: "What all happened?"

11 June.   The judge finally made a decision; Rita was awarded 3 million dollars. He said, "This is a disaster," and planned to appeal (I advised against it). At such time, it was best to allow Peter to ventilate—and once he was calm to gently remind him that "life often is problematic". I reminded him that he had learned to cope with even larger problems (he was easily able to pay that sum of money).

12 July.   Peter continued to be more at ease. He was accepting of Rita's "win". We spoke about the process; namely, that he quickly gets very upset in response to an uncontrollable stimulus or event and then he calms down. This is not optimal, but before he would be suicidal, when perturbed. Now, he began to predict the cycle of his frustration of his needs, wishes, and so on and how to cope with his frustrations.

Once more stating Shneidman's rule: Lower the perturbation and then the lethality will come down.

The relationship with Lianne continued to be predictably problematic. She continued to rage ("I hate you"; "Give me money"). The relationships with Peter Jr and Frank continued to be more and more positive.

COPING WITH LIFE'S DEMANDS

26 July.   We focused on his life-long need to avoid; we noted that his father was even more so. For example, his mother once stabbed Peter with a rose clipper in front of his father. His father turned around and simply walked away, as Peter was bleeding and asking for help. Yet, the main avoidance, inhibition, denial, and so on in the family had been Adrian's suicide. Despite our talks, Peter struggled with the event—"It was extreme, even in our family," he said. It was a hallmark of Peter's life.

On 16 August Lisa finally moved out. Peter had pushed and pushed; the cycle was repetitive. They often argued; on one such recent occasion, while in his pool, Lisa, being frustrated with Peter, said, "Why don't you drown in the deep end." That statement triggered rage (= mother). Peter could only think about his mother drowning him, and he then asked Lisa to leave. I attempted to get Peter to understand his behaviour, but the deed was done. Lisa had left and never returned. As she left she said, "I have had enough abuse."

Peter began to cope without Lisa. Being alone was quite problematic. He especially encountered problems with sleeping (insomnia). "I need to touch," he said, adding, "I need closeness." I agreed that all people need attachment, but quickly discussed his ambivalent and conflicting behaviours. I also encouraged Peter to learn to tolerate being alone. We began to explore how his mother, Rita, and Lisa were alike, how they were different, and so on (a basic George Kelly approach to treatment, i.e., a personal construct). On the question of "alike" he concluded, "They all hurt me."

Lisa's life was now also revealed to have been abusive. Her family was dysfunctional. Her oldest brother, some eight years older, was especially problematic. He, like Adrian, had killed animals (once he killed the three family cats) and he sexually abused Lisa, from the age of 8, for six years. Peter wondered about her problems and could anything help her? He wondered if his choices were always unhealthy ones ("Why do I always associate to women who have abusive histories?").

Work continued around Rita, Lianne, and Peter Jr (school performance had become a problem for Peter Jr, despite an IQ of 142). He finally settled the divorce with Rita. Peter began to accept that psychotherapy did help; he even encouraged a referral for Lisa (and paid for her therapist), despite that they had separated.

13 December.   Peter associated to his childhood. He said, "it is a fog, maybe it didn't happen." Yet, I reminded him of the facts, even some physical scars (for example, from the rose clipper). And, of course, Adrian did kill himself. I blocked the blocking. Peter had learned enough about suicide to know that there was a

history to the suicide; it was not due to *a* situation. Suicide has a history. He could not be blind to that fact.

Peter became more aware of his ongoing tendency to deny a pattern that he learned at a very young age. Once Adrian and he were fighting, his father's response was to lock himself in the washroom, stating, "I don't want to see the monkeys." Yet, there was such abuse—"Rage was an everydayness." Adrian had even more problems; "he so acted out," said Peter. Adrian got hit more and got more ice baths. Peter withdrew, much like his father, but Adrian fought and then "mother raged even more." "It was useful to hide, to avoid." He understood his father's reaction to his mother's rage, but added, "My father watched it all." As was noted earlier, denial, avoidance, and inhibition are negative, but are sometimes the best that a young person can do. Our tendency in psychotherapy with suicidal people, like Peter, is to develop alternatives to lifetime negatives, sometimes destructive patterns—the patient needs to cope in the "here and now".

3 January.   There was a lot of pain. Peter explored how he was often called "a bastard". His mother was 15 when she became pregnant with Peter. Peter's father was 21. "She always blamed me," he said. "She said I ruined her life." "She would call me bastard" and rage about this and that. Pain is deep in the suicidal mind, much deeper than one first learns in psychotherapy. Imagine your mother calling you a bastard, because she was sexually acting out (dissembling).

The relationship with Lisa slowly disappeared, although Peter continued to pay for the psychotherapy. "I feel guilty," he said. Yet, he also began to develop a new relationship, Patti. Patti was 28; Peter was especially focused on her "nice body", stating, "I am excited." Attempts at slowing the relationship were rejected; Peter simply stated, "I want to have fun."

Peter's more positive relationship with his father, since his mother's death, continued. Peter even once spoke to his father about the abuse. Peter added, "Why didn't you do anything?" The father was unable to answer, but did not run. He only looked his son in the eyes, and then, they both cried.

Peter's relationship to Rita ended. With the settlement, Rita spent her money quickly—a new BMW, a new house, and so on. David was reported to be "happy". But, as one would predict, I learned that chaos continued (and continues today).

Peter Jr continued to do well (even his school performance improved and he eventually graduated with a business degree) while Lianne continued to struggle. Peter's need to control was strongest in response to Lianne, but he accepted that he could not control Lianne. "All I can do is offer to wait," he said, "she knows that I am here if she needs me."

His relationship with Patti (who did not come from an abusive past) continued slowly. Peter reported a more satisfying relationship, than before. "I love her," he said, "and she loves me."

21 February.   Peter spoke about going to horseraces with his father, with a few friends. A conflict occurred between two friends; his father simply left with the car alone. We again talked about accepting the unacceptable—his father's avoidance.

The psychotherapy was slowly ending, more by Peter's choice, than any specific reason. He came to see me once a month for four months. We talked about what we learned. His father continued to be a focus, and by implication, himself; e.g., black/white thinking, avoidance, impulsiveness. We explored how these family patterns resulted in problems, even suicide risk. Peter was able to better understand the complexity of suicide—and his life. Adrian's suicide was discussed over and over, not unusual for survivors of suicide. Peter himself, however, showed no suicide risk.

On 8 May Peter terminated, although the door, as in all suicidal cases, was left open. I usually end with something like "Let me know how you're doing." Peter has contacted me from time to time. Since our last visit, Peter has not been suicidal again.

WHAT HAVE WE LEARNED FROM THIS CASE?

Peter's treatment began—continued and ended—with addressing his inaccurate assessment of what was going on (item 14). We could listen to, but not accept his perception. This is not unusual with suicidal people. Cognitive constriction was a deadly state ("Only suicide is a solution"). It follows that it is vital to treatment (I highly encourage a good read of one of Aaron T. Beck's books). We had to address Peter's intoxications. Items 7, 8, and 9 were critical for Peter staying alive. The specific protocols that were addressed in his treatment were as follows: 14, 26, 24, 15, 7, 8, 9, 35, 25, 26, 27, 28, 29, 30, 31, 32, 32, 21, 18, 20, 20, 22, 10, 11, 33, 16, 24, 33. After constriction, implications under rejection–aggression were most important in Peter's therapy. He was often in a rage. Item 20, being unaware of his serial way of coping, and item 32, wanting to attach, were repeated over and over in his treatment. One had to stop, repetitiously, the rage. We needed to stop his murderous impulses.

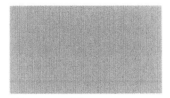

Chapter 18

JOE: AN OLDER ADULT'S SUICIDAL PAIN

(When My Wife Was Alive I Could Dance, Now I Can't Even Walk)

The elderly are at highest risk for death by suicide in many countries. Late adulthood is an obvious time-line in development (Frager & Fadiman, 1984; Kimmel, 1974). It is brought upon by one's increasing awareness of personal closeness to death (Kimmel, 1974), and it has its unique psychological issues. There is, however, a consistent controversy regarding what chronological age marks the beginning of this time-line. I tentatively supported the age of 55 (Kimmel, 1974; Neugarten et al., 1965). Utilizing the markers of 65 or 70 years makes less sense. These ages appear to be selected more for cultural reasons, such as age of expected retirement, than psychological (developmental) reasons. The age of 65 is also frequently selected in epidemiological studies, because the only available data, such as national statistics for suicide, often make comparisons on 10-year age groupings (i.e., 15–24, 25–34, etc.) (Lester, 1991a; McIntosh, 1991). Of course, no developmental period can be rigidly defined chronologically, and, at best, the marker of 55 approximates what can only be defined developmentally. Some people mature earlier, others later than the mean.

A DEVELOPMENTAL PERSPECTIVE OF LATE ADULTHOOD

It is important to note that this phase of development has been relatively well charted. It is the final time-line. Late adulthood is a stage marked by the development of a sense of integrity. The older adult continues to develop previous dialectics (such as identity vs identity confusion, intimacy vs isolation, and generativity vs stagnation); however, the crisis or dialectic of *integrity vs despair* becomes the central issue in the older person's life in Erikson's theoretical perspective.

Erikson (1963, 1968, 1980) was one of the first to pioneer the study of integrity (integrity vs despair) in late adulthood [although Butler's (1963) concept of life review includes many of the same issues and concerns]. By 55 or so, one becomes increasingly aware of the finitude of *one's own life*. Often this is triggered by changes in one's relations to the world, such as decline in health or loss of one's spouse. One begins (although the process might occur to a degree for many throughout the life-span) to evaluate one's life: Was my life meaningful? Has it always been unstable? What have I done? Was my life wasted? Was it unbearable? (etc.).

Erikson (1963, p. 268) wrote:

> It is the ego's accrued assurance of its proclivity for order and meaning. It is a post-narcissistic love of the human ego – not of the self – as an experience which conveys some world order and spiritual sense, no matter how dearly paid for. It is the acceptance of one's one and only life cycle as something that had to be and that, by necessity, permitted no substitution.

The acceptance of one's life, one's only life, becomes central. One's whole life is re-evaluated; indeed, one's *previous* development plays a crucial role. Has one's life been marked by instability? Have I been intimate? Have I generated something? One's accomplishments, especially one's physical (and mental) offspring are seen with new meaning. Even one's parents are seen differently. One not only evaluates whether life was meaningful, but whether it was bearable. A positive resolution results in acceptance. A negative resolution results in a deep sense of despair. As Melville noted in *Moby Dick*, those in despair live in "a damp, drizzly November in. . . (their). . . soul".

I do not wish to imply that one's concept of life and death does not develop after 55, only that 55—an arbitrary chronological number—marks the beginning. The person at age 55 or 60 does exhibit an awareness of one's closeness to death; however, such awareness may be different at 70 or 90. Peck (1956) has, in fact, attempted to define the issues of ageing more precisely by extending Erikson's insights into greater differentiation. (It would be of interest to study the suicide notes of those aged 55 to 70 and 70 and above—even more refined classifications. This, however, will be work for the future.)

What is *despair*? Erikson (1963, p. 269) wrote: "Despair expresses the feeling that the time is now short, too short to attempt to start another life, and to try out alternate roads to integrity." Elsewhere, Erikson (1968, p. 140) wrote:

> Such a despair is often hidden behind a show of disgust, a misanthropy or a chronic contemptuous displeasure with particular institutions and particular people – a disgust and a displeasure which, where not allied with the vision of a superior life, only signifies the individual's contempt of himself.

One's fate is not accepted. One's fellowship is lost, for example, by the death of the spouse. The person's life is meaningless. One's relations (e.g., self, spouse, child, job, book) are meaningless. The individual rejects everything. All was a waste. One plunges into despair. This despair is deep and getting deeper. One *is* despair. And this despair manifests itself in the non-resolution of death; for example, by the fear of death or, in a few, by the invitation to plunge oneself into death.

For most, however, there is a positive resolution and the person develops *wisdom*. Wisdom has many connotations for the older adult, for example, wit, accumulated knowledge, mature judgement, and inclusive understanding. Wisdom develops out of the dialectic of integrity and despair.

Not that each person can evolve wisdom for oneself; for most, the individual's tradition provides the essence. By the end of the life-span, those that positively resolve the encounter of integrity and despair develop a sense of wholeness and completeness. One is solid. One accepts oneself (identity) and one's relations (i.e., attachments). Helplessness is alleviated and so is dependence, both being feelings that often mark old age (Frager & Fadiman, 1984). Strength in the old, therefore, "takes the form of wisdom in all of its connotations". Erikson (1964, p. 133) wrote:

> Wisdom, then, is detached concern with life itself, in the face of death itself. It maintains and conveys the integrity of experience, in spite of decline of bodily and mental functions. It responds to the need of the on-coming generation for an integrated heritage and yet remains aware of the relativity of all knowledge.

JOE: AN INTRODUCTION

Next, we will learn about one elderly person, who felt such despair that suicide became a solution.

Joe was 65, a retired police officer. He first came to my office in May, some years ago now. Despite the time that has passed, I still remember Joe's statement, "When my wife was alive, I could dance, now I can't even walk." It is one of those statements that is aphoristic—it says it all, to use a colloquial expression.

Joe's wife had died in January. Joe was in bereavement. He had come to the clinical attention of his family doctor. As part of Joe's grieving reaction to his loss, he began to present symptoms of depression (e.g., feelings of sadness and associated symptoms such as insomnia, poor appetite, and isolation). Although Joe labelled the reaction as normal, he had sought relief from his pain. He wanted to escape from the mood, the insomnia, and so on. The duration of his grief was normal, but the expression of it, not so. Perhaps a diagnosis of Major Depression Disorder, single episode, was more appropriate as the symptom was present for some time and the expression of the severity was quite high. This, I believe, was associated to Joe's personality. Joe had had a high need for control. His career and life had been very structured and routine. Joe suffered little distress because much was inside the range of his predictability and control. Then, his wife, Stephanie, died. His world collapsed. Everything darkened. He became depressed. He withdrew. Thoughts of death occurred. Because of the pain, Joe went to see his doctor, more accurately, Stephanie's doctor, Dr Boring, as Joe had rarely seen a doctor in his life.

Joe saw Dr Boring, who had prescribed Prozac (an antidepressant), but Joe reacted poorly to the medication. He had stated, "It makes me feel out of control." He reacted similarly to other antidepressants, and thus, the physician referred Joe to a bereavement support group. Again, Joe felt uncomfortable, attended one meeting, and said that he could not talk in groups. Thus, Joe was referred to me for counselling.

FIRST VISIT

At our first visit, Joe was reluctant and anxious. He initially trembled and was sweating; yet, after a short time and a few calming inductions ("I understand; everyone is anxious when they first come to see me"), he became more at ease. After the usual intake information, I began with the usual question (item 1[1]): "What is wrong? Where do you hurt?" These questions with Joe seemed to be calming. Indeed, with many people, the very asking of such questions reduces the pain. I listened to "what" hurt Joe. I listened to his story of pain.

Joe began to talk about Stephanie. He said that he first met Stephanie in 1940 at a bus station. She had come to the city looking for work. He noticed her, as he was passing by and, as he stated, "I fell in love." Joe immediately went over to the unknown woman and said, "Hello." From that moment on, Joe never left Stephanie. They were married a few years later. He became a police officer and Stephanie stayed at home, raising three daughters and taking care of the home. All went well, except for the usual illnesses, problems, and so on. Then Stephanie developed bone cancer; she battled and they struggled together. "It was a horrible death," he said. She died and, to use a colloquial expression again, the rug was pulled out from under Joe's feet. First, bereavement and then depression set in.

At intake, Joe was clearly depressed. He exhibited a depressed mood every day. He had lost interest in everything; nothing gave him pleasure ("I can't be happy without her"). Joe also exhibited the following: weight gain, insomnia, agitation, fatigue, feeling worthless and guilty ("I should have been the one that died"), and had difficulty concentrating. He was having recurrent thoughts of death and suicide. When examining these thoughts, it became clear that some are commonly seen after the loss of a loved one; for example, wanting to be reunited and wanting to be in "heaven" together, but other thoughts were suicidal. He thought at times about taking his car, getting a hose, starting the engine and sitting, just waiting to die. Yet, there was no active intent. Joe dismissed the thoughts and wanted help. Risk was estimated to be low/medium (on a 1 to 9 scale, perturbation was 6; lethality was 4, although fluctuation would occur to a 6). Joe never wanted to die; he wanted the pain to stop. He somehow wanted his Stephanie back. The TGSP scores were: 3, 5, 7, 9, 13, 15(f), 17, 19, 21, 22, 21, 25, 26, 27, 33, 35.

JOE'S DESPAIR

At our first few meetings, Joe only talked about Stephanie. He felt so lonely. At the very first meeting, in fact, he stated the most revealing statement of his pain: "When Stephanie was alive I could dance, now I can't even walk." The pain was intolerable and Joe wanted it to stop. Suicide was one solution, but Joe also wanted to find other solutions. He reported that he could not think of "anything" (his cognitions were full of the "always", "everything", "nothing"). His trauma was the loss, having been dependent on Stephanie, despite an external dominant approach. The pain

---

[1] Explanations of all implications/items are given in Chapter 12.

of sadness and anxiety soared. "I was alone," he said. Emotional deprivation and guilt were figural emotional states. Joe, wanting to adjust, found himself—maybe for the first time in his life—unable to meet the challenge.

Joe's thoughts were only about Stephanie, in an obsessive neurotic style. He presented initially only permutations and combinations of grief and grief-provoking content. He was overwhelmed with the loss, feeling "weak" ("for the first time in my life"). Joe was figuratively intoxicated by the loss (items 7 and 8).

As a therapist, I needed to remember that Joe defined the trauma. A trauma is a perception. Yet, although Joe defined the situation, I did not buy into his overpowering emotion and constricted perception: His sadness, and generating only permutations of a grief-provoking content at the loss of Stephanie. Joe was grieving. It was, thus, vital that I countered his mental blinders, beyond the two options of either magically having Stephanie back alive or Joe being dead. I did not agree with his intoxication.

In all probability, Joe's bereavement, given the duration of symptoms, had become a depressive state (there was no medical record of a previous episode). In addition, it could be diagnostically noted that Joe had a weak ego. Individuals with a weak ego do not cope with life's traumas very well. Stephanie's death triggered a regression, resulting in discordant and antagonistic symptoms and ideas surfacing into Joe's consciousness.

Joe's ego was weakened (items 16 and 17). To develop ego strength is often an immediate goal in psychotherapy, but requires a long time to achieve. Joe had a relative weakness; he could not develop constructive tendencies without Stephanie. The key to intermediate—and long-range—effectiveness in suicide prevention with people like Joe is to increase the options for action, something more constructive than Joe's wish to unite with his wife. I needed to increase Joe's constructive tendencies and decrease the destructive one(s).

There were unresolved problems ("a complex" or weakened ego) in Joe. When working with such suicidal patients, one must not take on or attempt to cure all the complexes in the person's personality immediately. However, and this is critical, for one to respond to Joe effectively, I needed to assess if something discordant, unassimilated or antagonistic existed in him. One must be skilled in assessment and prediction with suicidal patients. We have to evaluate that person's complexes, anxiety, and other important aspects of their dynamics, psychopathology, and reaction patterns. Simply stated, to treat Joe, I had to know Joe (the person).

Despite the intrapsychic pain, Joe's main focus (or obsession) was with the interpersonal realm. There was a history and current situation: He lost Stephanie (items 19, 20, 21, and 22 of the TGSP). He was weakened. His needs for attachment and control, to name a few, were thwarted. His frustration in the interpersonal field persisted to a traumatic degree ("I'm lonely all the time"). Although Joe's primary frustrated need was attachment (affiliation) and control (dominance), the other Murray needs identified in Joe were: autonomy, counteraction, defendence, and harmavoidance.

In all probability, Joe's attachment to Stephanie—and hers to him, as she was de-scribed as "passive" and "always quiet"—was too intimate (i.e. dependent) result-ing in considerable strain, after the loss. Joe was hurt. The loss was a narcissistic injury ("She meant everything to me"). He felt so abandoned, but then he felt guilt about such feelings (of course, treatment allowed him to learn to accept such feel-ings). To put it simplistically, Joe was very attached (identification) to Stephanie. She died. Joe hurt. Joe wanted to escape from *the pain* (not life).

At the end of our first session, I asked Joe what he wanted from being here. He said, "I need a place to talk." He agreed to see me and, as his referring doctor was a regular referral source, exchange of information was undertaken with Dr Boring as needed. Joe never took any further medication.

CONSULTATION

After a few visits, I had occasion to consult with Edwin Shneidman about Joe (his wife Jeanne was there at times, passing by or joining in the conversation). We talked about ageing, understanding what it is like for Joe and themselves. Dr Shneidman shared his own life and his clinical bereavement cases, often supervising with his own rich personal life and clinical associations. We discussed our treatment plan: reduce the pain and the lethality, albeit low/medium, will come down. The way to do it, in this case, was to increase the attachment, the people—Joe had isolated himself, even from his children. I recall one more comment about the particular consultation; Jeanne Shneidman noted how important she felt it was for the therapist to understand the older person's world, especially if the therapist is young. Dr Shneidman and I had been talking about understanding Joe's (or any older person's) perception, not dominating, knowing, or controlling (after all, Joe would have escaped!).

THE SUBSEQUENT VISITS

After a few weeks, Joe came into my room in tears. I asked, "What is wrong?" Joe started to uncover a deeper bereavement. His father died when he was 3 (item 19), and thus, we had to address the history. He had a few memories, but mainly recalled the deep sadness in his home. "I believe", he said "my mother always stayed depressed." Joe became very attached to his mother, probably associated to her own separation anxiety or narcissistic need. Joe was shy and withdrawn as a child; yet, as a teenager, he struggled with this feeling and developed an external dominant appearance ("No one knew how I felt, except mom"). His mother died and he met Stephanie shortly afterwards. He described Stephanie as "lovely", expressing deep feelings for her—as he did towards his mother.

When I began to ask about his own daughters, he said that they were too busy. "I don't want to bother them," he said. He and his daughters had a number of "normal" conflicts over the years, usually when they did not do what Joe thought was the right or fair thing to do. Joe stated, however, that generally they got along.

Despite the usual conflicts interpersonally, he loved them and vice versa ("I've always loved them"). His daughters, Lindsey, Heather, and Kristen had all been supportive after Stephanie's death, but after a few months, Joe had told them that he was doing well (dissembling?). Only Heather continued to ask, questioning his appearance ("You look tired, Dad"). He would simply deny the problem, stating, "I get angry at her." I decided to increase Joe's sense of being emotionally supported (item 33). After they had been determined to be on the life side of Joe's ambivalence, his daughters, as well as some friends, were considered in the total treatment process. Joe needed other objects (people) with whom to identify, beyond his deceased wife. Others assisted in establishing and/or re-establishing positive relations, and all this helped Joe to build self-support. Given his level of perturbation, Joe could not simply give up even a dead part of his identity (Stephanie), nor could he search out objects on his own—his daughters. Joe was simply in too much pain and too pessimistic to do this.

Suicide prevention, as we learned, is best not done alone. Joe's daughters especially became part of Joe's community approach to treatment.

At the next visit Joe was restless; he was agitated. He again talked about Stephanie and his "mother", his losses. I listened. I also began to explore his anger, explaining that often depression is anger turned inwards. These dynamics are especially evident, I believe, in patients whose spouse has died from cancer or some other crippling death. They feel helpless and become angry, but anger at whom? When I asked Joe, he began to talk about his anger towards the health system, the decisions, operation and so on ("Everything, I am angry at everything") (items 25, 29, 31, and 32).

With suicidal patients, one must reduce the elevated perturbation and then the lethality will come down with it. With Joe, it was his anger that was heightened. Anger—in its many faces—is, in fact, a common emotion in suicidal people, as first noted by Wilhelm Stekel. I needed to reduce Joe's elevated anger.

One does not exacerbate the problem in the sense of making it more real for the person by talking about it. One should not buy into the taboo of "Don't talk about suicide and death", something that Joe was more than willing to do. Regrettably, people like Joe often create the silence. He did so with his daughters. Joe was already angry and hostile (and also hopeless and helpless). Ventilation, lightening of the angry feelings, adequacy of expression, and need for contacts had a critical place in his intervention. His daughters, too, needed to know that the trauma was "real" for Joe, even if they wished to defend against or deny the crisis. The suicidal person's anger (or other feelings) needs to be heard (rather than introjected and especially not acted out). I had to address the taboo of talking about death and suicide.

I am always reminded that constructive goals can work wonders against destructive ones (Eros over Thanatos). This became evident in Joe.

Shneidman, in my consultations, has often reminded me that suicide is a dyadic event. Joe felt hurt; he wanted to hurt someone—not Stephanie, but at times, he was angry at her—and then quickly felt deep guilt ("She abandoned me"; "How can I be angry at her, she is dead?"). As a therapist, I created activity—something of course, different from consciously or unconsciously attacking Stephanie. Death is, of course, often difficult to cope with—it arouses in all of us bewilderment and painful feelings, even aggression, attack, and/or revenge.

We also began to explore Joe's upswings, pleasures and so on. Joe loved the new Chrysler minivan and, while Stephanie was alive, had planned to buy one. He still wanted the vehicle, but felt that he should not be happy. We explored his belief (cognition) that he should not feel pleasure ("I can't be happy"). One often becomes concerned about practical items—retirement, medication, new home, new car, whatever (item 30)—with suicidal people. This was true about a new vehicle. With the usual psychotherapeutic induction, Joe decided to buy the van and expressed some real joy about the decision. Later he purchased the van, and said, "I bought the grey one, the one Stephanie liked. She would be happy." Joe was allowing himself to feel pleasure and was getting beyond his survivor guilt.

At the next session Joe was in one of what he called "valleys". He talked about boredom, stating that since Stephanie died he felt "bad easily", adding "even in our sessions". He wondered if he was getting worse; I discussed the cycling in grief (a term that was not completely accurate, but one that was healing Joe). We also discussed his guilt feelings about having bought the grey van; he expressed a deep ambivalence about being happy or not (item 28). Often the suicidal person, like Joe, is ambivalent—he is not only affectionate and hostile towards life, but he is also ambivalent about life and death. I worked first with the life and death issue, on the side of life. Then I worked with the positive feelings. Practically, however, I addressed both—siding with life, attachment (affection) is implied. Joe was—I suspect, a transference from his mother and wife—wanting my assurances, and fortunately, I could provide such transfusion. Joe became less ambivalent, wanting to live.

At the next visit Joe was, however, more irritable; he had gone to his cottage for the weekend. Stephanie and he owned a cottage along Lake Erie, one hour from the city. It was the first time Joe not only went to the cottage after Stephanie's death, but the first time ever alone. They always went together, he said. Subsequently with encouragement, however, he went often on weekends. Yet, the "boredom" (not so much "sadness"), but "boredom" (see Fenichel, 1953), lingered as an uncomfortable stimulus (item 3).

In psychotherapy, one can focus on any number of emotions. With Joe, we focused notably on the distressing (painful) feelings of deprivation, distress, and boredom. The latter was especially problematic. We attempted to improve the external and internal situations, related to these emotions and other aspects of his mind, a JND. This was accomplished through a variety of methods: ventilation, interpretation, instruction, and realistic manipulation in the outside world. I needed to give Joe some realistic transfusions of hope until the intensity of the boredom—in short— pain, subsided to a tolerable level.

Joe continued to question his need for therapy, despite reporting that the therapy helped. At the above meeting and the next, Joe especially needed someone to talk to him. "I don't talk to people," he said. It was a bind for Joe; his need to be in control was high. I began to address this need (item 21), basically what you can control and what you cannot control—and to paraphrase the AA (Alcoholic's Anonymous) Serenity Prayer, wisdom is knowing the difference (wisdom, of course, is Erikson's virtue of older age). I approached Joe about this need not only at a conscious cognitive level, but also at a somewhat insight-oriented level—he needed to learn to cope without Stephanie.

At the next meeting, now 17 July, Joe spontaneously began to talk about his "impatience", and how it affected him. He associated, for example, being overly upset at waiting for a plane. He labelled his behaviour as "overly", accepting the problem. He reported getting frustrated easily; yet, he began to cognitively realize "I can't control it." "I get upset at everything," he said, explaining his reaction in detail and learning to accept situations better, not only Stephanie's death.

Joe also freely associated to the first time that he recognized his impulsivity problem, when he was in his 50s. He had worked for the provincial police and had transferred to a local force. There he lost what he called "my freedom" having to "walk the beat". He became upset, adding, "I was probably depressed" (is the episode a recurrent one?). Joe concluded: "I don't cope with change well," associating to the loss of his mother, Stephanie, and so on. I supported him in his insight—and remarked about his viability, strength—I stated something like, "You've coped with a lot." In response Joe stated, "I'll make it" and I said, "I know you will", adding that it takes time (ego strengthening). He agreed.

THE LATTER VISITS

Joe was still not always "up", far from it. After a few visits in August, arriving uncharacteristically 10 minutes late, Joe was down. He again reported feeling depressed, having no meaning, no pleasure and so on (again, item 3). When I asked if anything had happened, he stated that he was planning on having his daughter, Lindsey, over with her family. The first visit to his home. He was anxious about the grandchildren, the noise, etc. I listened and accepted that he felt anxious, but, as I had actively sought the family's help, I encouraged the family event. He agreed that he wanted to, but was anxious. Once more, I encouraged attachments.

At the next meeting, Joe arrived happy. He actively reported that he had felt "enjoyment". During the visit, the kids made him happy. These visits continued and the family more and more actively sought out Joe's participation in familial events. This made a JND—a very significant JND.

On one occasion, Joe had to go to a wedding, which was an especially painful stimulus. He had recalled Stephanie, "I miss her so"; and I reminded him that it was only seven months and that "grief takes time—sometimes a life time".

We began to sort out the loss; "Is everything lost?" I asked (knowing that now he was actively socializing with his family, grandchildren, and even friends). He said, "No, not all." That is the important thing to do in psychotherapy with suicidal people: increase their attachments.

We began to sort out Joe's problems. Retirement had been one; after he left the police force, he had few interests or hobbies. Stephanie had been his only interest. Yet, earlier he had enjoyed the cottage, camping, and, fishing—and, with a few friends, playing cards. Joe started developing a plan of action; most importantly, he had decided to go camping the next summer in the Canadian Rockies. He and Stephanie went every summer. He missed this year, but decided he did not need to lose it next summer. One of his friends, also widowed, wanted to go too, and so his social world grew. By the beginning of September, Joe was active. He had been playing cards, was going to a fishing group, and started to attend church (he had stopped during Stephanie's illness; he was, like many, angry with God too). He had made definite plans for camping and fishing next summer. He often now came to the sessions accompanied by a daughter. The family, as in many of my cases, had been my best co-therapists.

This does not mean that Joe did not cycle. Once he arrived upset because a female friend had asked him out for a coffee at Wilber's, a local café. He liked the person and wanted to go, but felt guilt. He said, "Stephanie and I did that." We talked and explored, what would Stephanie want him to do or what would she do? "What would anyone do?" (I am now somewhat constricted, with my "anyone", "everyone"). He agreed that he could go. Joe often confused his emotions and thoughts; some were irrational ("If I go for coffee, I'll reject Stephanie"). Using basic cognitive strategies, I did not accept his basic premise (married people who see other women—even if the spouse is dead—are unfaithful). We addressed his thoughts and Joe opened his blinders more. Joe became less and less intoxicated with his grief and began to sort his beliefs out better. As therapy progressed, Joe's life improved. That is how we evaluate therapeutic success: Is the patient developing wellness? We need to look not only at the absence of pain, hopelessness, and so on, but the presence of protective factors, e.g., ego strength. Joe, for example, began to enjoy life. Eros can indeed work wonders over Thanatos.

By December of that year, Joe was feeling better. He was not depressed, had not felt suicidal for months, and was finding pleasure. His family and friends were involved in his life. His attachments had broadened and he was coping with his life's demands. Before Christmas, we decided to terminate. He thanked me and said as he left, "I'll always love Stephanie."

CONCLUDING REMARKS

When one is attempting to understand the suicide of adults, developmental age (time-line) is a significant variable to be accounted for in that perspective or model, as it was for Joe. The suicides of older adults are psychologically different from other adults, despite, I suspect, even greater commonalities.

As we have seen with our younger cases, a life-span developmental perspective is essential for understanding suicidal phenomena (Leenaars, 1991a), and no less so in the elderly, such as in Joe. To recapitulate the findings within Erikson's framework, the following can be tentatively concluded:

Finitude of one's life is obvious to most older adults. In our older years we evaluate our life. We evaluate its meaning. For example: Has my life been marked by insta- bility? Have I been intimate? Have I generated something? It would appear that the suicidal person, although not necessarily perturbed, despairs. He/she judges his/her life—his/her history—to have been too unstable. Without Stephanie, Joe's life was unstable and meaningless. He says that he cannot even walk. The damp, drizzly November in the soul of the older person is obvious to them. With the loss of Stephanie, Joe's life was drizzly. Older suicidal adults are direct and not ambivalent in their solution to the despair. They wish to die.

Older suicidal adults, as with Joe, see no alternatives. Indeed, there are few alterna- tives or contradictions in the suicide notes of older adults. They reject everything. All was a waste. As one reads their notes, one learns that the older adults' relations (e.g., spouse, child, job) are often now meaningless. Often in their notes, they do not even mention their interpersonal relationships. They are isolated. This latter observation is especially true for the males, as it was for Joe. Given his loss, there was no integrity for him and he despaired.

As a personal observation, after reading over 2000 suicide notes, I am struck by the lack of what Erikson calls wisdom in the notes of the elderly. I am not sug- gesting that this is surprising, only that developmentally there is a poverty of wit, knowledge, mature judgement, something that is obvious in most other writings of our elderly people. The notes are communications of despair. Although they wish to die, the suicidal older adult, by his/her plunge into death, does *not* accept death.

Erikson himself has not published much about suicide; the above are my specula- tions within his frame. However, in line with Erikson's position that death is "the most important overall aspect of life", he has made the following comment:

> All old people simply have to accept approaching death as a daily problem. They see it happen to their [*spouse*], relatives and friends and know that it is apt to suddenly come from somewhere when it was not expected. Their suicide, thus, is most of all *active* death: at least they have made the decision [*or suicidal behaviour*] and the choice of time and place. (Erikson, 1989, p. xii; words in brackets are mine).

This view is consistent with the wish to die. The suicide in late adulthood takes an active role in the demise. The older suicidal person sees suicide as a solution to pain and, according to Erikson (1989), this is an identity decision. Without Stephanie, Joe felt like a nothing (no "*I*"). Suicide is an identity. In this sense, the older suicidal person addresses previous dialectics. Suicide, Erikson (1989) states, "gives them an identity in life, even if it is an identity of one who brought about his own death" (p. xii).

As a more general comment, I wish to remind the reader that the current for- mulation about older adults should not be construed to mean that development is simply discontinuous. As we have seen in our cases from across the life-span, development is both *discontinuous* and *continuous* (Piaget, 1970). Development is dynamic, ongoing, and serial. The suicidal person does not respond anew to each crisis in his/her adult life, but one's reactions are consistent in many ways with that individual's previous reaction to loss, threat, impotence, etc. There is the eternal return of the same (sameness). As we discussed in Chapter 2, there is an *elliptical* nature to development (Shneidman, 1980, 1985). There is change and consistency. We saw this in Joe. Joe's reaction to Stephanie's death was continuous with his history; yet, with psychotherapy, Joe's life also showed a discontinuous flow. He learned to walk without Stephanie. Older suicidal adults can be successfully treated (De Leo & Scocco, 2001). Psychotherapy can be an avenue to wisdom.

WHAT HAVE WE LEARNED FROM THIS CASE?

Joe's treatment began with item 7, his history—the loss of his wife. Pivotal to his treatment was his interpersonal relations. All of the implications in this cluster could be invoked. We needed to increase his relationships; he needed to walk and

Table 18.1   Frequencies of each implication for treatment organized into meaningful clusters[a]

Intrapsychic	Interpersonal

I   Unbearable Psychological Pain
(1) 2   (4) 2
(2) 3   (5) 1
(3) 4   (6) 1
Total = 13
    $M = 2.16$
	VI Interpersonal Relations
	(19) 4 (22) 4
	(20) 5 (23) 3
	(21) 6 (24) 6
	Total = 28
	    $M = 4.66$

II   Cognitive Constriction
(7) 4
(8) 4
(9) 3
Total = 11
    $M = 3.66$
	VII Rejection–Aggression
	(25) 4 (28) 4 (31) 3
	(26) 5 (29) 3 (32) 4
	(27) 4 (30) 3
	Total = 30
	    $M = 3.75$

III   Indirect Expressions
(10) 3
(11) 2
(12) 2
Total = 7
    $M = 2.33$
	VIII Identification–Egression
	(33) 5
	(34) 3
	(35) 3
	Total = 11
	    $M = 3.66$

IV Inability to Adjust (13) 1 (14) 1 (15) 2 Total = 4 $M = 1.33$	
V Ego (16) 5 (17) 4 (18) 2 Total = 11 $M = 3.66$	

[a] Observations are based on 6 cases

even dance again. The specific implications in order of occurrence in the process of treatment were: 7, 8, 16, 17, 19, 20, 21, 22, 19, 33, 25, 29, 31, 32, 30, 28, 3, 21, 3. Item 19 was repeated frequently in this case; we had to educate his family. They needed to know Joe's pain and needs; Joe, like many men, would not tell them his story. He avoided doing so. We saw the extreme of dissembling in Rick. Masks are suicidal risks!

As a final remark on the question, What have we learned from this case?, I have been, as stated in Chapter 14, reluctant to do this task, but David Lester believes that it will assist the reader. I am reluctant because I do not want this to be seen as a cookbook (e.g., do items 1, 2, and 3 and no risk!). Dr Lester's question might suggest that there are primary ways to prevent suicide. This is not suicide prevention. Psychotherapy is a process, not a recipe. A recipe is just a wishful fancy.

Yet, as a researcher, I count numbers; thus, I will present some quantitative data (see Table 18.1). Item 24 (attachments) was the most frequent treatment technique, followed equally by items 16, 33, 20, 21, and 26 (5 out of 6 cases; Jeff did not give us time for psychotherapy). These relate to the following: to increase options or cognitions, to increase the individual's psychological sense of possible choices beyond death, to widen the adjustment processes (beyond the "same old, same old"), to address the frustrated needs, and to strengthen the person's ego. Arithmetically, these may well be keys—they are clinical keys.

Table 18.1 presents the frequencies of each implication observed in the six cases for treatment.

One final tally: the most frequent response was under Interpersonal Relations ($M = 4.66$), followed almost equally by Cognitive Constriction ($M = 3.66$), Ego ($M = 3.66$), Rejection–Aggression ($M = 3.75$), and Identification–Egression ($M = 3.66$). The least were: Indirect Expressions ($M = 2.33$), Unbearable Psychological Pain ($M = 2.16$), and Inability to Adjust ($M = 1.33$). The least invoked response, i.e., Inability to Adjust, is probably associated to my belief that it is essential to understand suicide from a psychosis, a neurosis, or a character disorder perspective, but it is not essential to treat the person. In psychotherapy, we treat the individual, not simply the disorder. It is the pain, anguish, and frustrated needs that we address, regardless of whether the person is depressed, or anxious, or whatever. We need to treat the pain, constriction, and so on, regardless of the mental disorder. This is essential to keep a person alive—treating the unique person.

Finally, I hope that the section, "What have we learned from this case?" at the end of each chapter has helped the reader. Quantitative and qualitative approaches are needed to study and understand psychotherapy with suicidal people.

Chapter 19

ADJUNCTS TO PSYCHOTHERAPY: MEDICATION, HOSPITALIZATION, AND ENVIRONMENTAL CONTROL

No psychotherapy with suicidal people can be an island unto itself. Often it requires adjuncts to treatment. Our treatment with suicidal people often has to be multicomponent. Medication, hospitalization, and direct environmental control may well be the most effective treatment. This is not to say that active out-reach and use of community resources (e.g., telephone crisis lines) are not. I however, view these approaches to be integral to psychotherapy with almost all suicidal people. My psychotherapy is a community approach. Dealing with a patient's reality and using community resources are a more direct, essential implication, based on what we have learned from suicidal people's own stories. There is a stage in the suicidal scenario. Medication, hospitalization, and more direct environmental control are different, but may be equally essential. They are protective factors and can be life-saving. The research, according to a World Health Organization (WHO) document, shows that these strategies may well be the most effective (Bertolote, 1993). I will briefly outline some thoughts on each topic, recognizing that the reader will need to learn more about each topic than is here presented.

On a point of consultation, as my knowledge on medication and hospitalization is limited, I was most fortunate to be able to consult with Dr John T. Maltsberger on medication and Dr Konrad Michel on hospitalization for this volume. My gratitude for these consultations is reflected in the following pages on these topics.

MEDICATION

Psychopharmacology does not work with suicidal people.

I thought that I would begin this section with a myth! I associate this fable with an equally absurd one. I here quote Stuart Montgomery (1997) in his paper, "Suicide and antidepressants". He writes, "One form of treatment that is known to be associated with the provocation of suicidal behavior is psychotherapy" (p. 332). The truth is that both psychotherapy and medication are effective and often necessary to prevent suicide (Möller, 2001; Slaby, 1994; Verkes & Cowen, 2000).

Psychopharmacological treatment is necessary for many suicidal patients. The same is true about psychotherapy. The combination of the two may be life-saving. Yet, like psychotherapy, there is no specific somatic treatment of suicidality (Möller, 2001). There is no antisuicide pill.

As in the development of psychotherapy, at this time, systems theory (von Bertalanffy, 1967) has taken precedence over linear models to explain the effectiveness of medication in the treatment of suicidal people. An essential prologue to psychotherapy is, in fact, an understanding of the basics in medication today (I highly recommend a read of Stahl's book, *Essential Psychopharmacology* (2000); I will borrow here extensively from that volume).

Psychopharmacology, to use a narrative metaphor, is the story of chemical neurotransmission. To understand the impact of, for example, a suicidal state on the brain (and vice versa), and the impact of drugs on the suicidal brain, it is absolutely essential that one knows the basics of chemical neurotransmission.

I cannot, of course, educate the reader fully in the field in this volume; Stahl (2000) does a matchless job to fill that need. As a student from the 1970s, I am struck by what has been learned in this field that is as dynamic as psychiatry and psychology are today. The topic is intricate. It is estimated, for example, that there are several thousand to millions of different brain chemicals. There are many unique chemicals (neurotransmitters), some similar to drugs we use. For example, the brain makes its own morphine-like drug (i.e., beta endorphin) and marijuana-like drug (i.e., anandamide). Stahl (2000) writes: "The brain may even make its own antidepressants, its own anxiolytics, and its own hallucinogens. Drugs often mimic the brain's natural neurotransmitters" (p. 18). Often the drugs are discovered prior to the neurotransmitter. This was true for morphine, but also, for example, the benzodiazepines diazepam (Valium) and alprazolam (Xanax) were known before the discovery of benzodiazepine receptors. The same is true with the antidepressants amitriptyline (Elavil) and fluoxetine (Prozac), which were known before the discovery of the serotonin transporter site. This is all more complicated than most readers need to know. Let it suffice to state that most drugs that act on the brain (i.e., the central nervous system) act in the process of neurotransmission and do so in a way that "mimics the action of the brain itself when the brain uses its own chemicals" (p. 19).

To understand this better, one must learn molecular neurobiology, again beyond the scope of this book (but is essential reading for any aspiring suicidologists). One has to know about the purpose of chemical neurotransmission. One needs to know how it alters postsynaptic target neurons; its long-term consequences on the postsynaptic neuron; and how it even regulates gene expression. This further means learning something about DNA and so on. It is a voluminous topic. On the critical relation to DNA, let me again quote Stahl (2000):

> The general function of the various gene elements within the brain's DNA is well known; namely, they contain all the information necessary to synthesise the proteins that build the structures that mediate the specialised functions of neurons. Thus, if chemical neurotransmission ultimately activates the appropriate genes, all sorts of changes can occur in the postsynaptic cell. Such changes include making,

strengthening, or destroying synapses: urging axons to sprout, and synthesising various proteins, enzymes, and receptors that regulate neurotransmissions in the target cell. (p. 21)

It is dynamic, not linear. This condensation overly simplifies the complexity. Let me, however, make one further jump in this story.

Chemical neurotransmissions regulate gene expression. Changes in genetic expressions lead to changes, for example, in the connection between the neurons in the brain and the functions of the connections. Thus, genes modify behaviour. The functions and, by implication, the behaviour derive from neuron functioning, and are controlled by the genes and the products that they produce (Stahl, 2000). This leads to two major and most relevant conclusions:

1. Genes exert significant control over mental processes and the associated behaviour, like suicidality, and may modify the behaviour.
2. Behaviour and perceptual experiences may alter gene expression. Stahl (2000) goes, in fact, so far as to ask, "(C)an behaviour modify genes?"

The latter question is debatable; Maltsberger (personal communication, 22 February 2002) suggested that the statement is "not correct". He believes that "Behavior and perceptual experience may alter gene expression." Stahl's view would be a paradigm shift (Kuhn, 1962). On the latter point, Stahl (2000) writes:

Learning as well as experiences from the environment can . . . alter which genes are expressed and thus can give rise to changes in neuronal connections. In this way, human experiences, education, *and even psychotherapy,* may change the expression of genes that alter the distribution and "strength" of specific connections. This, in turn, may produce long-term changes in behavior caused by the original experience and mediated by the genetic changes triggered by the original experience. Thus, genes modify behavior and behavior modifies genes. (pp. 21 and 23; my italics)

I prefer to believe Stahl, not Montgomery. To reduce it to psychopharmacology for dummies (and I include myself in this group), the brain and the mind are the same. There is no Cartesian dualism (except in the mind). Descartes led us astray. The mind is not in the foot. The suicidal mind is the suicidal brain. The suicidal brain is the suicidal mind. To focus on one, only neurotransmission, or only mentalism, is to regress to the days of the early 1900s. The simple fact is that psychotherapy modifies genes, drugs modify genes, and so do hospitalization and environmental control (and all vice versa). Treating one, whether the brain or the mind, is treating the other. Often the best practice with suicidal people is to do both. Each individual must be listened to about his or her unique needs (as we did with Susan, Peter, etc.).

Of course, there is much more in psychopharmacology. For example, one marvels at data such as that neuronal traffic speeds at up to 60 millionths of a metre per hour. Again, a good read of Stahl or some other similar text is essential. Let me note here however, one final fact. Learning, adjustment, cognitive strategies, the development of coping skills and so on are all related to neurotransmissions. Thus, it is imperative that people keep the brain healthy (a protective factor). The brain may be weakened in the presence of pain, depression, anxiety and so on. On the opposite side, mental stimulations, such as psychotherapy, strengthen the brain. A healthy brain (= mind) protects one against suicide. Often the brain does this automatically, but sometimes medication(s) is needed in some people. Medication for some suicidal people may be a key to healthy neurotransmissions, and thus, life. The most current selective drugs are, in fact, capable of interacting with different receptors; there are very selective keys to unlock specific unhealthy neurotransmissions. As in psychotherapy, it is often the selective key (the detail) that works better than a more global master key (the general).

These are some basics in the psychopharmacological approach to assist in the development of a healthy brain. It is assumed that effective treatment lessens the risk of suicide, although it has been difficult to demonstrate this (Verkes & Cowen, 2000). This echoes the problem in effective psychotherapy. What medication works? Which ones are effective? What medications are effective for which person? To address these questions, here is a brief shopping list of known current answers.

Answer 1

There are essential links between suicide and depression. Some 60% of suicidal people suffer from a mood disorder. There is strong support for the belief that suicides have a serotonin dysfunction (Maltsberger, 2002). The study by Asberg et al. (1976) left a pioneer's mark on suicidology, equal to Shneidman and Farberow's (1957a) book, *Clues to Suicide*. Asberg and her fellow researchers have subsequently produced a large body of work on brain research on the serotonin system. Indeed, Maltsberger concluded:

> We now have a general consensus that suicide victims have abnormal serotonin binding in the prefrontal cortex. Other research suggests that in a period immediately preceding suicide there is nonadrenergic brain overreactivity resulting in norepinephrine depletion (with compensatory increase in synthesis). This overactivity may be related to stress experiences (Mann & Arango, 1999). (Maltsberger, 2002, p. 86)

In depression, there is heightened perturbation. The pain or anguish, what Shneidman called psychache, is unbearable. Mental pain fuels the jump into the suicidal abyss. The pain is in the brain. It is an accepted fact that the behaviour of many suicidal people is related to serotonin dysfunction in the brain, associated to the depressed state. Thus, drugs that are specific serotonin re-uptake inhibitors can be most effective. Fluoxetine (Prozac), sertraline (Zoloft), and paroxetine (Paxil), are examples of the selective serotonin re-uptake inhibitors (SSRIs). They are specific keys. These drugs "have revolutionised the outpatient treatment of depression" (Maltsberger, 2002, p. 86). The use of SSRIs, in fact, in recent years has drastically increased. Isacsson (2000) has shown that in Sweden, suicide rates decreased in accordance with the increase in the prescription of antidepressants. Isacsson concluded that antidepressants might be one factor contributing to the decrease in suicide. There are a few such effective factors in suicide intervention; yet, Laukkala et al. (2001) have raised questions about the generalizability of Isacsson's findings. They noted that, in a Finnish sample, they found that the overwhelming majority of depressed people were not receiving antidepressants. There are still questions that are no different from those about the efficacy of psychotherapy. This is science.

Best practice would dictate that many—not all—depressed suicidal people could be effectively treated with the SSRIs. Yet, equally, good practice would dictate that this treatment be combined with psychotherapy. Maltsberger (2002) concluded:

> I continue to believe that psychotherapy in the treatment of suicidal patients remains extremely important, and that it often makes the difference between living and dying. The newer antidepressants, however, now are an essential part of the treatment of most depressions of any severity. Psychotherapy combined with antidepressant drugs is often the best treatment for the patients . . . (Maltsberger, 2002, p. 87)

Maltsberger's view is shared by many (for example, Hollon & Fawcett, 2001). Yet, there are cautions. "For a very small vulnerable subpopulation SSRI drugs may provoke suicidal states" (Maltsberger, 2002, p. 86).

Don Schell, a 60-year-old male, on the night of 12–13 February 1998, murdered his wife, Rita, his daughter, Deb, and his 9-month-old granddaughter, Alysa. Then he shot himself. Mr Schell had a long history of depression and had recently been prescribed Paxil (although he had a history of responding with somatic anxiety to another SSRI, Prozac). This homicides–suicide formed the basis of a wrongful death action against Smith Kline Beecham Pharmaceutical Co. in Wyoming Federal District Court. A June 2001 verdict—as reported in the *New York Times* on 8 June 2001—found against the company in favour of the surviving family members (J. Maltsberger, personal communications, 20 and 22 February 2002).

The defence had argued that no necessary (causal) connection between the homicides–suicide and a medical condition could be documented. There is no nomothetic data (e.g., double-blind randomized placebo-controlled trials). The surviving family's (plaintiff's) experts argued that in this case, Paxil, a SSRI antidepressant, triggered the violence. Dr Maltsberger was one such expert. He and the others argued for the idiographic approach, i.e., case study.

The case is detailed and let me here cite a few of Dr Maltsberger's main questions. Could causal inference be drawn from the individual case of Don Schell? This question is the same as those we have read by Gordon Allport, John Stuart Mill, Edwin Shneidman, and so on. In the Schell case, Dr Maltsberger's question is the following: In psychopharmacology, are there unique vulnerable individuals, who have reactions to otherwise comparatively innocuous drugs? Dr Maltsberger suggested a read of a quote by the late Paul Hoch (1972):

> Acute reactions can occur in certain persons following a single dose of one or more types of drugs or intoxicants. For example, the "pathological intoxication" occurring in alcoholism is often an acute organic reaction in predisposed individuals; such pathological intoxication, usually accompanied by an outburst of rage or fear mixed with disorientation and hallucinatory experiences, can occur after one dose of alcohol. . . . The same holds true for many other drugs; there are persons who develop acute delirious reactions after one dose of opium, or one dose of marijuana (*cannabis indica*), or one dose of a great many of the stimulants and intoxicants used all over the world. . . . So one must be aware that even a single dose, in predisposed individuals, is capable of occasionally provoking an acute organic reaction. (p. 160)

As we have learned, individual case reports tell us about the unique.

There are many more arguments, pro and con. There are also "politics"; we know, for example, that studies of SSRIs by the drug companies have shown negative side effects. Specific individuals were shown to have somatic anxiety, agitation, insomnia, and even suicidal behaviour and suicides. Dr Maltsberger (personal communication, 20 February 2002) used the term *Akathisia* to describe such states. Akathisia is a state of intense feelings of subjective anxiety and agitation as well as motor restlessness or agitation. It is a heightened state of perturbation; it fuels the lethality. In the Schell case, the Paxil heightened the suicide risk. Yet, for the vast majority, the SSRIs have been life-saving. Once more, whether in psychotherapy or medication, one has to treat the unique individual, not the general.

Dr Maltsberger's psychopharmacological advice is that patients who become agitated and anxious on SSRI drugs should be prescribed benzodiazepines or other sedatives. We need to treat each individual uniquely. In a recent Australian case (*R.* vs *Hawkins* [2001] NSWSC 420), the court ruled that a prisoner's culpability was greatly reduced after he killed his wife under the influence of sertraline (Zoloft). Thus, therapists are advised, especially if a medical doctor is the prescribing physician, to monitor all patients with caution (including during progressive withdrawal of medication) that are prescribed SSRIs or any medication. What is life-saving for many, may not be so for "John".

Yet, the fact remains that the new antidepressants help the vast majority of depressed suicidal people; they ease the psychache, the anguish. They are specific keys. Sertraline (Zoloft) and paroxetine (Paxil) are two such useful drugs. Venlafaxine (Effexor) is a different antidepressant as well as being an anxiolytic. Some patients that do not do well on the SSRIs, may do better on Effexor, especially if they show akathisia on the SSRIs. As antidepressants continue to be a major drug in the fight against suicide, it is worth remarking a little further on these medications:

- The use of antidepressants with selective neural reuptake blockade of serotonin generally has few side effects for most patients (Asberg et al., 1986), but not all.
- The dose depends on each patient's unique response; most may not show dangerous side effects—but, as we saw with Don Schell, some do.
- To quote Slaby (1994): "Not all depressions that may be predicted to be medication responsive respond to drugs, anymore than all cases of hypertension respond to antihypertension therapy. Stroke and heart attacks may still occur when a patient is on antihypertension medication, just as suicide occurs in some patients on antidepressants" (p. 145).
- Some patients experience associated panic or anxiety with the suicidal state; with these people benzodiazepines, as noted by Dr Maltsberger (see also below), may be effective in combination with antidepressants.
- One should be cautious with some antidepressants, such as MAO inhibitors or desipramine (Möller, 2001). These may actually increase drive [the same is true with some suicidal patients with ADHD, who are prescribed stimulants such as Ritalin and Dexedrine (Tanyo, 2001)].

- The immediate use of antidepressants is counterindicative in people who are intoxicated with psychotropic drugs (Möller, 2001).
- And finally, an old basic: One's clinical concern should be raised when any suicidal patient stops his/her antidepressant medication (or any drug) against advice. Often such people do not tolerate even minor side effects of medication, any more than they do their pain.

To conclude: Antidepressants help the vast majority of depressed suicidal people.

Answer 2

Lithium is the first choice in bipolar disorders, but it is also a good candidate (along with the antidepressants noted above) to prevent relapse in unipolar disorders. It may well be, in fact, the best choice in difficult cases of affective disorder (and even in some difficult personality disorders, e.g., borderline).

Lithium reduces suicidal behaviour—a fact that has been clearly demonstrated by Muller-Oerlinghausen (2001). A meta-analysis, for example, of 17,000 patients showed that the risk for suicide is 8.6-fold higher in patients without Lithium than in those with Lithium. Indeed, Lithium has probably been shown to be the most effective drug against suicide (Muller-Oerlinghausen, 2001).

There are further facts. Even if the patient does not benefit from Lithium in terms of episode reduction of the mood, it does reduce his/her suicidal behaviour and clinicians should think twice about stopping Lithium in suicidal patients, even if they continue to have depression/manic episodes. Muller-Oerlinghausen (2001) cautions very specifically about discontinuing or switching to another mood stabilizer in people at risk.

On a psychopharmacological note, "Lithium differs from other mood stabilizers and also most antidepressants by its marked serotonin-agonistic effects which are related predominantly to presynaptic functions" (Muller-Oerlinghausen, 2001, p. 88). It probably mimics chemicals in the brain; once more it relates to neurotransmitters. Lithium is an antiaggressive and antisuicidal treatment.

Answer 3

Benzodiazepine and some antidepressants work well with anxiety disorders, and states (e.g., anguish, psychache) both episodic and chronic. Lorazepam (Ativan) and alprazolam (Xanax) are two short-acting medications that work best for acute states of anxiety. Individuals who have chronic anxiety appear to respond better to clonozepam, a long-acting medication (Maltsberger, personal communication, 19 February 2000). Möller (2001) suggests that if a sleep disturbance predominates, the current non-benzodiazepine hypnotics may be recommended. Dr Maltsberger, my forever consultant on psychopharmacology, suggests that zolpidem (Ambien) is very good (it is a species of benzodiazepine). He also suggests trazadone (Trazadone); it is not a benzodiazepine, but works well with some suicidal people (although it makes some people feel hung over).

Answer 4

Suicidality in schizophrenics often requires medication. This is especially true during periods of anxiety or excitement. The standard treatment is low potency neuroleptics (e.g., Thioridazine, Levomepromazine). A different approach may be needed with schizophrenics who also show affective states (Möller, 2001). Clozaril (Clozapine) has also proved to reduce the rate of suicide in schizophrenia (Keck et al., 2000).

Answer 5

Personality disorders are frequently associated with suicide risk, often repetitively. Borderline patients and antisocial patients are especially at risk. Regrettably, the efficacy of drug treatment with these people is not well established.

Psychopharmacology is complex, certainly much more complex than presented here. Each individual needs to be treated separately as individual factors and drug factors may be critical in unique ways in each person. The Don Schell case dramatically illustrates this fact. For example, with impulsive, excited patients, the SSRI drugs can make the patient worse (Maltsberger, personal communication, 22 February 2002). I furthermore marvel how one suicidal person with depression reacts well to, say, Zoloft, while the next does not, but responds to Prozac. Indeed, some antidepressants in some individuals heighten suicidal risk; it is now established, evident by the labels themselves on these products, that caution is in order with some people. Once more, the Don Schell case illustrates this fact. Of course, specific adverse effects in specific individuals to all medication are a truism in the field.

As another example of the importance of the unique in psychopharmacology, age may be one factor in the individuality that needs to be taken into account. Psychopharmacology needs to be developmental psychopharmacology. It is not simply ageing that requires such a perspective, but, for example, diseases such as Alzheimer's and Parkinson's occur more frequently and these diseases are associated to depression. The same is true for people with strokes, congestive heart failure and so on. Antidepressants, in fact, can be very effective with these older people, as they are treated for their general medical condition at the same time. Yet, caution is warranted in using antidepressants as a treatment with suicidal older people, who also may be taking other drugs. One has to know about drug interactions. One does not want to open too many locks. Once more, psychopharmacology is all very complicated.

To conclude

Drugs can modify the brain. They can stop a suicidal death. Yet, best practice would probably call for the drug treatment to occur within the context of psychotherapy. It is best used as an adjunct to psychotherapy—a very effective one in some suicidal people. I would, in fact, alert anyone treating suicidal people *only* with drugs, whereas the treatment of suicidal people without drugs is common. Not all suicidal people need medication. It is, however, a necessary protective factor for some, and perhaps many.

HOSPITALIZATION

Shneidman (1980) on hospitalization writes:

> Hospitalization is always a complicating event in the treatment of a suicidal patient, but it should not, on those grounds, be eschewed. Obviously, the quality of care—from doctors, nurses and attendants is crucial. Stoller (1973), discussing one of his complex long-range cases says: "... there were several other factors without which the therapy might not have succeeded. First, the hospital. The patient's life could not have been saved if a hospital had not been immediately available *and a few of the personnel familiar with me and the patient.*" (p. 312)

Many patients can be saved only with hospitalization. Early treatment protocols (for, at least, the last few centuries) called for all suicidal patients to be hospitalized (Stone & Shein, 1968). This dogma is, however, no longer accepted. Indeed, as Shneidman noted, hospitalization for some suicidal people may be hurtful. Yet, other patients may readily accept the idea of hospitalization, but are equally fearful of being locked up. Hospitalization means different things to different people. For a few, it is perceived as the only hope to stop the unbearable pain, other than suicide. Even the offer of short-term care allows some patients to feel some control. Hospitalization, after all, is one of the oldest environmental control techniques used to prevent suicide. It often works!

The reason for hospitalization will always be, with few exemptions, to protect the patient (Goldblatt, 1994). Safety is foremost. Indeed, for some suicidal people, like William Styron (1990), hospitalization was the only thing that saved their lives. The decision to hospitalize a suicidal person is always complex. It is a decision about a unique individual. There are many issues involved, well beyond the space allotted here. Thus, I highlighted only a few associations to the word.

Hospitalization may be essential. However, the absence of facilities in some areas of the world, or the absence of effective hospitals in rural areas, may require alternative care or even transfer to a hospital with the means to treat the person. Regrettably, in some regions of the world, this is not even possible. Yet, even there, the establishment of a safe home with a caring trained person may be the only possible choice. At least this environmental control would be better than leaving the person in a suicidogenic place. Ultimately, it is the quality of care that the institute can provide that is critical. In most of the developed (and developing) world this remains the hospital. Yet, this is compromised and difficult today, especially with the era of decreasing health resources. Despite the cost, hospitalization for some suicidal patients is not only justified, but also a legal requirement. The development of high-quality hospital services, in fact, should be a major element in any national suicide prevention strategy (Hawton, 2000).

The first step to admission is assessment (see Chapters 5 and 6). Immediate assessment may be critical; appropriate procedures need to be in place in the hospital. This is not a time to reinvent the wheel. One needs an *a priori* guide.

Our understanding of the patient is a major factor in formulating a decision to hospitalize. Hospitalization during periods of acute perturbation and/or heightened lethality should be considered. For example, with patients who have a definite plan to commit suicide, hospitalization may be warranted, but sometimes not. One has to understand the person to develop a specific plan of action. Will psychotherapy be needed? Is it sufficient? Do we need medication? Is hospitalization needed? There are many questions. Ultimately, these can only be answered, if we understand Bill or Mary. Yet, as we saw with Peter (Chapter 17), even the best plan can be refused and we then need to consider the best response.

Different disorders or dysfunctions call for different response, regarding hospitalization. Depression may call for hospitalization, especially during periods of psychotic disintegration and/or a narcissistic injury (Goldblatt, 1994). Patients with Bipolar Disorders, especially if not treated with Lithium, may be especially in need of safety. Schizophrenia, especially during an acute psychotic episode, may need hospitalization. This is especially true if the patient reports that voices are telling him/her to commit suicide. Special attention needs to be given with paranoid schizophrenics. Hospitalization with patients with personality disorders is difficult and always problematic. This is especially true with borderline patients, since they are often preoccupied with suicidal and mutilating behaviours. Drug or alcohol abuse may be another risk factor, although sometimes short-term services for this group can be effectively provided in specialized drug treatment centres, rather than the hospital. Be that as it may, care should be given to each individual who abuses substances, as some require a secure psychiatric facility. The best guide to hospitalization is the cornerstone of this whole volume: Understanding the individual person. There is no general dogma today.

There are many more issues to consider. For example, a developmental perspective is necessary. The elderly, especially if isolated, should be routinely admitted during heightened lethality (Hawton, 2000). You cannot leave these people in their howling lonely despair.

There are further questions; for example, what if the patient refuses inpatient treatment? We will address this question and other ethical and legal issues in Chapter 21. These are an essential read for anyone working with suicidal people in an inpatient setting.

Hospitalization may have its negative consequences on psychotherapy (Goldblatt, 1994). If the therapist assumes the role of authority, the rapport and relationship may be strained. The attachment may regress. Furthermore, as Goldblatt (1994) notes:

> When the admission is against the patient's own judgement, the alliance may in fact break down. It is rare for a therapeutic alliance to survive when the admission is involuntary. The breakdown of the therapeutic alliance is frequently the price paid for forced hospitalization. (p. 154)

It is at times, however, a necessary calculated risk (Maltsberger, 1994).

Hospitalization, when available today, is also hampered by declining dollars for health care world wide. Funding is limited. Insurance companies, whether private or public, often refuse to authorize inpatient care. Hospitals are often crowded and waiting lists are too long. Sometimes the best decision then is not to hospitalize. There are risks and benefits to inpatient care (Goldblatt, 1994; Hawton, 2000). To quote Shneidman again, "the quality of care from doctors, nurses and attendants is crucial."

Research supports Shneidman's caution. Hospitalization often does little to inspire confidence in our patients (Michel et al., 2002). All too often, the staff is rejecting—a further blow to the suicidal mind. Studies have shown that hospital staff often have unfavourable attitudes towards suicidal patients (Ramson et al., 1975; Reimer & Arantewicz, 1986). Staff are often seen as not only unhelpful, but disapproving (Hawton & Blackstock, 1976). Treolar and Pinfold (1993), furthermore, have found that suicidal patients often consider medical staff to be unhelpful. Nurses and social workers are often seen as more helpful. Even more alarming is the finding by Barnes (1986) that the negative attitude is especially evident towards patients who repeat attempts. The greater the number of attempts, the greater the negative attitudes. This is not quality care. Our attitudes can be life-enhancing, but also death-promoting. Michel and his colleagues (2003) suggest that it is "a significant relationship" that allows a suicidal patient to be helped. It is our care. This is as true in the hospital as in our psychotherapy room. Dr Shneidman's wisdom should guide us in both places, "quality care".

There are numerous matters in managing suicidal inpatients (Sederer, 1994). As this is beyond the scope of this volume, I will here, by way of illustration, note only a few. All hospitals must have written and regularly updated policies and proce- dures. There are environmental precautions; for example, is the facility equipped for safety? Two examples of environmental control in a hospital are that windows need to be secured, and that toxic substances must be locked up (see more details below). What works with outpatients works with inpatients—i.e., environmental control.

There are also patient-specific interventions (Sederer, 1994). Have, for example, pa- tients' belongings been searched? During heightened risk, plans for observation need to be in place. One to one observations may be needed initially, followed by varying increments of time. Checks must be recorded. Some patients may re- quire direct supervision, whether in the protected facility and/or public settings. The use of seclusion with or without restraints, presents difficult challenges to care. There are numerous factors to consider in managing suicidal inpatients. There are no golden standards. One must rely on the same standards as in psychotherapy and community practice (see Chapter 21).

There are risks to hospitalization. While some suggest that suicides in hospital are rare, suicides do occur in hospitals, both general and psychiatric (White et al., 1995). In fact, Dr Konrad Michel (personal communication, 15 March 2002) believes that such events are not rare. Observations in Switzerland, he suggests, support this view. I agree; I believe that suicides occur much more frequently in hospital than our current data suggest. I know that this is at least as true in Canada as in Switzerland. My friends in the field around the world suggest the same. Jumping from windows, balconies, and internal open spaces (e.g., stairwells) are the most common methods of suicide in hospitals.

My own first experience of a patient's suicide occurred, in fact, in a hospitalized patient. He—I will call him John—was a 20-year-old person who suffered from paranoid schizophrenia. He had presented himself with his mother to an outpatient clinic at a large general hospital in a major Canadian city. I was then an intern and was asked to do the intake assessment; I immediately evaluated heightened risk (the mother had planned to go to the Caribbean with a man the next day). John had a definite plan; equally, he was actively psychotic. John feared that the police would get him. I contacted the supervising psychiatrist who supported my assessment. John was then taken to the hospital emergency, with our evaluations, but released by the psychiatrist on call. John was put on the waiting list for outpatient follow-up.

That same night, John's mother called the police (she still was going south) and reported that her son planned to burn down the apartment building. The police responded and John was arrested and taken to the same general hospital. He was hospitalized immediately (a crisis often precipitates action), and was put in an intensive psychiatric care unit. Observation procedures were put in place, etc. Yet, John killed himself a most unusual way. (I will keep that confidential. If published here, it may provide a method for a suicidal reader.) That night, he must have been determined. For him, the dreaded police captured him (and now his abandoning mother could go to the Caribbean). This case raises ethical and legal issues (see Chapter 21). There are regrettably casualties, even if we hospitalize.

Schizophrenia is a disabling disorder that, it is believed, afflicts some 20 million people. It has an early onset and is life-shortening, not only by suicide, but also by premature death (including homicide). It is estimated that about 5% of schizophrenics will kill themselves (Palmer & Bostwick, 2002). The risk is highest at the beginning of onset; indeed, the timing of many deaths by suicide is consistent with John's, i.e., early. Risk is heightened especially if there have been previous attempts (Bostwick & Palmer, 2002). There are further risk factors, as in John; hospitalization is a most pervasive one, especially shortly after discharge (van Heeringen & Apter, 2002). According to a systematic review by Sutton et al. (2002), other common risk factors are as follows: male, living alone, not living with family, recent loss, depression, motor restlessness, hopelessness, worthlessness/low self-esteem, impulsivity, drug abuse/dependence (but not necessarily alcoholism), and—very important—fear of mental desensitization. Indeed, insight into the problem may heighten risk (van Heeringen & Apter, 2002)—which has obvious implications for what we do in treatment. It is of note that some symptoms of schizophrenia, such as delusions and non-command hallucinations, are not risk factors (Sutton, et al., 2002). One should be especially cautious with schizophrenics who are suicide attempt repeaters and/or are depressed; mood factors continue to be a risk factor, also with schizophrenics. Protective factors include being married—attachments, of course, are so critical for all of us. John, I learned much later, was not unusual—he had almost all of the markers.

There are many more topics on hospitalization. Upon discharge from the hospital, after care is most important (Hawton, 2000), and psychotherapists must be part of any plan in the after care. Transitions are particularly critical and risky times. (Further issues in care are addressed in Chapter 21.)

Finally, one should be aware that hospitalization may affect the psychotherapist too (Goldblatt, 1994). The therapist's own experiences, feelings, etc. may play a role in the decision to hospitalize or to do the after care. These are matters of countertransference (see Chapter 11). The therapist's own countertransferences are as relevant to medication and hospitalization as they are to assessment and therapy. Rejections, even if only perceived, may be iatrogenic. Transference hate and countertransference hate may especially add great difficulties to treatment of suicidal people (Maltsberger & Buie, 1974). Therapists who have lost a patient to suicide need to be aware how this pain may affect subsequent care. Some therapists, for example, do not treat suicidal people again, while others may hospitalize sooner, sometimes too soon (Goldblatt, 1994). Consultation at such times is critical (Maltsberger, 1984–1985).

Hospitalization is complex, all treatment of suicidal people is complex. Many issues are involved. The topic is so vast that it calls for an urgently needed book itself, *Hospitalization of Suicidal People*.

To summarize the main point: Hospitalization should never be eschewed, if needed. It probably works best, however, in not only a multimethod approach, but also a multidisciplinary one (Leenaars et al., 1994b; van Heeringen, 2000). Hospitalization alone is not enough.

ENVIRONMENTAL CONTROL

The two main traditional solutions for preventing suicide in the last century have been the clinical treatment of suicidal people (i.e., psychotherapy, medication, and hospitalization) and the establishment of suicide prevention centres and community programmes (e.g., schools). However, a third approach to suicide prevention, which is one of the oldest methods of prevention, is known as controlling the environment. Removing the sword from the defeated soldier in battle, for example, is an ancient act of prevention. Yet, this prevention tactic has been infrequently discussed until recently. Presumably because most of the work with regard to the prevention and intervention of suicidal behaviour has remained within the realm of clinical settings, this neglect may be understandable, although given current research, too limiting.

Erwin Stengel (1964) was one of the first in this century to propose controlling the environment as a means for decreasing the incidence of suicide, noting, for example, that the detoxification of domestic gas (from coal gas with high carbon monoxide content to natural gas) might have reduced the suicide rate in nations where the switch had taken place. Subsequent research on the detoxification of domestic gas in England supported Stengel's proposal (Kreitman, 1976). More recently, a review of the research by Clarke and Lester (1989) and an international examination by Leenaars and experts (2000b) from 12 nations validated the approach in treatment.

This perspective on prevention is consistent with a report on suicide prevention of the World Health Organization (WHO). After careful analysis of all measures by an international team of researchers, headed by Bertolote (1993), a series of tactics to prevent suicide that had support in the scientific literature were proposed. The team provided six basic steps for the prevention of suicide. All but one, the treatment of psychiatric patients, are consistent with controlling the environment: gun possession control, detoxification of domestic gas, detoxification of car emission, control of toxic substance availability, and toning down reports in the press. They also offered further measures under the rubric of "other measures". These too are consistent with environmental approaches, such as fencing high buildings and bridges. Although there is no definitive evidence for the effectiveness of the "other measures", the research strongly supports the five measures that call for controlling the environment as effective means of reducing suicide.

Gun control is often cited as the prototypical example of controlling the environment to prevent suicide. Although countries differ in the most frequent method for suicide, firearms are a preferred method in many countries. An opportunity for studying the effects of legislative means restriction, e.g., gun control laws, on their use for suicide is provided by Canada's Criminal Law Amendment Act of 1977 (Bill C-51), enforced since 1978. This Act requires acquisition certification for all firearms, restricts the availability of some types of firearms to certain types of individuals, establishes procedures for handling and storing firearms, requires permits for those selling firearms, and increases the sentences for firearm offences. Early commentators on the impact of this Act found little impact of the Act on firearm suicide in Canada, but presented only simple charts, with no statistical analysis of the trends. Lester and Leenaars (1993) remedied this omission and reported a comprehensive study on the preventive effect on suicide of the Act in Canada. Their study suggested that strict firearm control laws might have reduced the use of firearms for suicide. Further, individuals did not switch to other methods. Subsequently, Leenaars and Lester (1998) showed that the gun control law was most effective with females and younger people (and, vice versa, least with people over 65). Furthermore, Leenaars et al. (2003) reported that even if one controls for social and economic variables, the impact of gun control is still evident. Environmental control works. Results on related phenomena on homicide and accidental deaths hold equal promise.

The tactic of controlling the environment is, however, more complex than gun control, although it is a prototypical example. Referring to gun control as a means for suicide prevention in Canada and in the USA probably makes sense because it is the main method of suicide in those countries. However, in other countries, guns are not a frequent means. Cantor and Baume (1998), for example, noted that in Australia there has been a modest decline in firearm suicide, but a major rise in hanging. Obviously, availability is only one factor; Cantor and Baume suggest that "acceptability" may be equally relevant to understanding the impact of the environment on suicide. Acceptability is consistent with the environmental view. Bowles (1995), for example, showed that drinking poisonous herbicides was, at one point in time, the most available and acceptable means of suicide in Western Samoa. Firearms may not be available in some countries. For example, in Cuba, firearms are not readily available and are the least frequent means for committing suicide in this nation. This is also true in Japan. As reported by Takahashi et al. (1998), the firearm control law in Japan is one of the strictest in the world. Only about 0.2% of suicides yearly are committed by guns; yet, the use of other acceptable means is frequent. For example, in the 1980s, Paraquat, a highly lethal herbicide, was often reported in the media as a lethal means. A series of suicides by this method, thus, occurred. Paraquat was readily available in every garden store and, according to Takahashi et al., it became a very accepted means—much like in Western Samoa and other regions of the world. Only after environmental controls were implemented did the use decline. Paraquat only became available upon a detailed buyer check, much like the implementation of gun-checks in some countries. The commercial concentration was reduced. An offensive odour and emissions were added. A massive educational programme was undertaken, and so on. Takahashi et al. have concluded that these environmental control measures resulted in a decrease in the use of Paraquat ingestion. Thus, one can see great variation in means in various regions and, although gun control may make little sense in some regions, the tactic of controlling the environment may still have applicability, as suggested in the WHO report. There may be, however, a need for culture-specific control of the environment (Takahashi et al., 1998).

Controlling the environment goes beyond issues of the method. The WHO noted, for example, that there was strong support in research for toning down reports in the press. The effect of the media has, in fact, been reported for centuries. For example, Goethe's (1774) novel, *The Sorrows of Young Werther*—the story of unrequited love, resulting in suicide (see Chapter 2)—had a reported contagion effect. Philips (1974) was one of the first in the last century to document the impact of the media on suicide rate. Several subsequent suicidological reports have indicated that there is an association between media reporting about suicides and suicidal behaviour in a society. A field experiment concerning mass media and suicide has been reported by Sonneck et al. (1994). In Vienna, after the implementation of the subway system in 1978, it became a common means of suicide. Mass media reported about these events in dramatic ways and subways became a readily available and acceptable means of suicide. Subsequently, efforts were made, under Gernot Sonneck and Elmar Etzersdorfer (see Etzersdorfer & Sonneck, 1998) to provide guidelines for media to report suicides. Reports in the media changed and the number of subway suicides and attempts dropped more than 80%, remaining at low levels since. Although available, it became less acceptable. Thus, once more, the principle of controlling the environment, in this case toning down media reporting, appears to have utility.

Controlling the environment is, in fact, not foreign to practising psychiatrists. Control of the availability of medicines is a common practice, and is one of the five steps for prevention found to be effective in the prevention of suicide by the WHO.

In 1972, Oliver and Hetzel (1972) first called attention to the adverse effects of the availability of medication. There are variations in mortality rates associated with overdoses of medicines (e.g., antidepressants, sedatives). Common practice calls for prescribing medications that are safe or in small amounts with high-risk patients. According to the WHO, this action is consistent with controlling the environment to prevent suicide. The WHO even suggested that the pharmaceutical industry could contribute by providing appropriate dosage units and packages. The approach of controlling the environment is much broader than control of toxic substance availability. Examining steps such as gun control and fencing bridges may broaden the understanding of the complex solutions needed to prevent suicide. Not only may this approach impact on direct service, but it may also be an occasion to reflect on the support of public health action. The detoxification of domestic gas, for example, was supported by the medical research of Kreitman (1976) in the 1970s, and has been estimated to have saved uncountable lives.

Although further research is needed, means restriction and the more general approach of controlling the environment may be a viable strategy to prevent suicide in all regions of the world. Yet, despite the recommendations of the WHO and the research, there has been a lack of impact on clinical practice globally. The lack of education about means restriction is a clear illustration. The study by Wislar and his colleagues (1998), for example, exemplifies this absence.. They conducted a chart review of youth receiving mental health evaluation, with 40% being suicide related, in an emergency department of a hospital. Chart reviews provided no evidence that means restriction education was provided. Although further prospective research is needed on the topic, Wisler et al.'s study, and other studies with similar findings, call for greater attention to controlling the environment in the treatment of suicidal patients. The lack of means restriction education may be a failure in care and applies not only to guns but to other means (e.g., availability of medicines). Consultations on a difficult case where there is imminent risk, especially with lethal means, are not only helpful (e.g., have we adequately controlled environmental factors?; has the gun been secured?), but are sound practice. There are broad global implications of this research, I believe, in the care and failure in care of suicidal persons.

To conclude, as noted elsewhere in this book, suicide and suicidal behaviours are multifaceted events. This complexity of causation indicates the necessity of a parallel complexity of solutions. Prevention of suicide or suicidal behaviours can be understood as being any action that contributes to a decrease in the frequency of the event. The approach known as controlling the environment has been shown to be the most effective. This third solution to prevention departs from the approaches of traditional treatment, such as psychotherapy, and suicide prevention centres or programmes; however, in light of research, this tactic cannot be ignored in clinical practice.

Finally, I will quote Clarke and Lester's (1989) most significant book on the topic, *Suicide: Closing the Exits*:

> There is no doubt, however, that there is a full agenda of policy work to be undertaken to reduce the availability of a variety of lethal agents. The discouraging history of gun

control in the criminal justice arena shows how much there is to be done about this lethal agent alone, though greater progress may follow from treating the widespread availability of firearms as a broader problem of public health. Much also needs to be done in the United States to institute more effective controls on a variety of medications. In other countries, controls are needed not only on guns and medicines, but also on pesticides, exhaust gases, and toxic domestic gas. Efforts to impose these controls will lead to a demand for new kinds of research to identify the most cost-effective and acceptable solutions. In other words, for public health professionals and researchers alike, there is a full program for the foreseeable future to close more of the exits to suicide. (p. 111)

CONCLUDING REMARKS

Medication, hospitalization and direct environmental control may well be necessary and very effective with suicidal people. Psychotherapy may not be enough for some very suicidal people. Our treatment calls for a multimodal approach. I endorse medication, hospitalization, environmental control—all methods that act as an anodyne. They are "medicines" that ease pain.

Part IV

IMPLICATIONS

Heraclitus, the pre-Socratic philosopher (around 500 BC) had taught that, "You can't step twice into the same river." All things are in process. Like the river, the suicidal patient is—and suicidal patients are—always changing. He or she is always in flux. Psychotherapists, thus, must constantly alter, change, reframe and so on, their understanding of each unique patient to prevent his/her suicide. Suicidologists must constantly learn. A permanent existing idea or *Vorstellung* is a mythical entity in psychology. As William James noted, our theories, whether of suicide or otherwise, need to be flowing, not static.

Heraclitus, however, also taught that, "In the same river, we both step and do not step, we are and we are not." Heraclitus, like Shneidman and myself, tries to comprehend and understand the underlying coherence of things—we are and we are not. Heraclitus called it, Logos (see Freeman, 1971, and Kirk & Raven, 1971). It is the "sameness", or the common. To understand, here is Heraclitus's guidance: "Therefore one must follow . . . that which is common." This, we attempt to do throughout this book; yet, even our order (theory) can be in flux. The waters flow ("Those who step into the same river have different waters flowing upon them").

I have learned that: You have to enduringly understand the person to treat him/her. Our psychotherapy has to be person-centred (or patient-centred). This is true of Jennifer, Susan, Peter, Joe, and anyone that we meet in our therapy room. We have to listen constantly and understand their story.

Although a marvel in 1682, we all now, like Newton then, could predict the observation of Halley's Comet in that year, waiting some 80 years to confirm its predicted return in 1759. However, if Halley's Comet had instead exploded in 1739, could Newton have predicted its explosion or, even more important, have prevented it? That is the task of the psychotherapist. This volume, to this point, has presented the thesis; the first chapter in this section, however, is antithetical in mood. It takes a second look at our theory and argues instead, echoing Heraclitus, that there are no *Vorstellungen*. It questions the notion that my schema, i.e., unbearable pain, cognitive constriction, and so on, is *the* golden road to the understanding of all suicide. Alternative schemata are needed and one is provided, showing that we must not expect too much of our theories. Of course, that is the challenge: Understanding each person as an individual and as a general and then to treat him/her effectively as an individual.

The second chapter in Part IV does the same as the first, but raises the whole spectre of ethical and legal issues. Ethical and legal issues are complex; to understand these issues, for example, from the predominant American writings, is too myopic. That is why this chapter is written with eleven colleagues: C. Cantor (Australia), J. Connolly (Ireland), M. EchoHawk (Turtle Island, renamed North America), D. Gailiene (Lithuania), Z. X. He (China), N. Kokorina and A. Lopatin (Russia), D. Lester (United States), M. Rodriguez (Cuba), L. Schlebusch (South Africa), Y. Takahashi (Japan), and L. Vijayakumar (India). I present the perspective from The Netherlands. I know that this has resulted in Chapter 21 being better than from one viewpoint alone, including mine. I am once more indebted to these people for allowing me to accommodate my formal operational level of understanding.

In Chapter 22 are some final musings on Edvard Munch, Fyodor Dostoevsky, Vincent van Gogh, and a little bit of Herman Melville. These come at the topic of this book from a somewhat different light, showing that understanding suicide is still the best step before the next one, psychotherapy. It concludes with, "Suicide can be prevented."

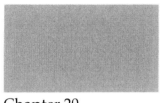

Chapter 20

THIS IS WHAT I HAVE LEARNED

What I have learned is that suicide is a multidimensional event. There are biologi-cal, psychological, logical, conscious and unconscious, interpersonal, sociological, cultural, and philosophical/existential elements in the event. The complexity of the event calls for a diverse set of strategies for prevention, and psychotherapy has been proposed as one possible strategy (Shneidman, 1985). Any intervention, however, must be based on sound understanding. This is as true in psychology as it is in biology.

Any element of the diverse event is a legitimate avenue to understand suicide. This volume is within the psychological tradition—the "trunk" of Shneidman's arboreal metaphor. Years ago, Allport (1942) and, later, Shneidman and Farberow (1957a), suggested that personal documents have a significant place in social sci-ence research, despite ongoing debate (Runyan, 1982a). Allport argued that those personal documents—e.g., poems, suicide notes, psychotherapy records—aid in the very aims of science: understanding, prediction, and control. There has, in fact, been a strong tradition of utilizing personal documents in the field of suicidology (Shneidman & Farberow, 1957a). Recently, an international task force of the Inter-national Academy for Suicide Research (IASR) echoed Allport's and Shneidman's conclusion that personal document "approaches should be utilized in the science of suicidology" (Leenaars et al., 1997, p. 141). This volume is in this tradition.

Regardless of the data source, Hempel (1966) has argued that the sciences have achieved their "deepest and most far-reaching insights" through theory, "below the level of familiar empirical phenomena" (p. 77). William James (1890) noted that only theory (a schema, classifications) in psychology will allow us to sort out the booming buzzing mess of experience. Leenaars et al. (1997) have made a similar argument in suicidology, stating that "there is no substitute for theory in research". Yet, despite early beginnings in the first half of the twentieth century, significant theoretical development has been lacking in suicidology (Lester, 1992). As therapists, however, we must bring order to the mess. We need to understand the patient because the patient needs to be understood. We, as therapists, are in the special position to assist in sorting out the person's "buzzing mess". This volume has been one attempt at theory building, by wedding personal documents to theory (there are few marriages of this kind in psychology). Shneidman (1988) once stated about my work that I was "doing the marvellous thing of scientising our field by the use of its most dramatic documents" (p. 10). These endeavours resulted in, to quote Shneidman further, "insightful clinical implications". It is empirically based intervention at its best.

To restate what we have learned, suicide notes are the ultra personal documents (Leenaars, 1988a; Shneidman, 1980). They are the unsolicited productions of the suicidal person, usually written minutes before the suicidal death. They are one of the best windows (or snapshots) to the suicidal mind—a window that is similar to the actual protocols that one hears in a therapeutic hour. The patient's words, like suicide poems, suicide notes, and so on, allow us to explore and understand the suicidal person's (conscious and unconscious) commonalities (Beck, 1976; Shneidman, 1985).

A theoretical–conceptual analysis, since the first formal study of suicide notes (Shneidman & Farberow, 1957a), has been seen as offering the richest potential to understand suicide. In response to this challenge, I developed a logical, empirical approach to study suicide notes (Leenaars, 1989a, 1989b, 1990, 1992a, 1996; Leenaars & Balance, 1984a), which not only presented a method for the theoretical analysis of suicide notes, but was also calculated to augment the effectiveness of previous controls. Essentially, Carnap's logical and empirical procedures (1959) have been used for the investigations. These studies, I believe, have given us not only snapshots, but full-length movies by which to understand the suicidal person.

A number of models of suicide have been subjected to analysis (see Leenaars, 1988a). These, to recapitulate, include the ideas of Adler, Binswanger, Freud, Jung, Menninger, Kelly, Murray, Shneidman, Sullivan, and Zilboorg. Using these theorists, the following empirically based multidimensional schema or template for understanding suicide was derived (Leenaars, 1998a): Unbearable pain, cognitive constriction, indirect expressions, inability to adjust, ego, interpersonal relations, rejection–aggression, and identification–egression. As we have seen in this volume, the model is not only useful for understanding suicide, but also for identifying specific strategies for intervention. Yet, this fact begets the core questions that I raised three decades ago: What classification or model best fits the empirical data? What schema best allows us to understand our patients? These are the central questions, when approached by each unique, suicidal patient in our therapy rooms. The purpose of this chapter is to give a critical examination of the multidimensional schema presented in this volume and, by implication, any frame that is accepted as a closed system (Shneidman, 1985); are there really only the 8 or 10 commonalities (like the 10 Commandments)?

As a final caveat to theory in science, psychology has a long-standing belief that people must make formulations about things to understand them (Benjafield, 1991; Goffman, 1974; Husserl, 1973; Kuhn, 1962). We have to have templates. IASR's task force recognized that this development is critical if suicidology is to advance into the twenty-first century, but is often neglected. In summary, the present study, like the 1989 study (Leenaars, 1989a), uses personal documents, i.e., suicide notes, to answer the question: What are the best fitting empirical groupings or classifications of the data?

A NEW STUDY

The method called for independent judges to verify whether the protocol sentences (see Chapter 5) did, in fact, occur in 140 suicide notes. These notes had been analysed for previous studies (such as age, gender, and so on, but only American notes) and used as a composite sample here. The number of notes constitutes the largest sample of suicide notes to be analysed in one study to date.

A series of studies, spanning four decades, have shown that clinical judges (i.e., psychologists, psychiatrists, and graduate students/interns in both disciplines) can be trained to produce reliable judgements. Independent researchers (O'Connor et al., 1999) have demonstrated substantial reliability with the method; thus allowing us to conclude that reliability has been well established for the method. Coefficients of concordance (Siegel, 1956) of 0.76 or greater in the various samples have indicated substantial inter-rater reliability ($p < 0.05$). Further efforts, such as the use of reconciled scores, have been used for the data in this comprehensive sample analysis. Validity studies have also been reported.

For the current study, a cluster analysis (Varaclus procedure, oblique principle component; SAS Institute, 1995) was undertaken to reduce the protocol sentences as scored in the 140 notes to a meaningful empirical schema. Our analysis produced a classification of eight discrete clusters (when an eigenvalue of 1:00 was used as the criterion). This number of clusters accounted for 55% of the variance (the same as the initial solution). The eight new clusters identified by a word or short phrase are as follows: I. Unbearable Psychological Pain; II. Cognitive Constriction; III. Disorders in Adjustment; IV. Suicide as Solution; V. Interpersonal Relations: Unresolved; VI. Identification–Ambivalence; VII. Vengefulness–Aggression; and VIII. Identification–Egression.

To compare the original (1989) cluster solution with the current one, the Rand (0.8504) and Morey and Agresti Adjust Rand (0.4308) were measured (SAS Institute, 1995). As can be seen, although there were some similarities, generally there are differences between the current and the original solution—as used throughout this volume. There is, as Heraclitus predicted, both sameness and flux.

The specific protocols in this new cluster solution are provided below, with both the current numerical scheme and the original number (in brackets), in the TGSP utilizing the Intrapsychic and Interpersonal schema:

Intrapsychic

I *Unbearable Psychological Pain*
1 (1) Suicide has adjustive value and is functional because it stops painful tension and provides relief from intolerable psychological pain.
2 (2) In suicide, the psychological and/or environmental traumas among many other factors may include: incurable disease, threat of senility, fear of becoming hopelessly dependent, feelings of inadequacy, humiliation.

Although the solution of suicide is not caused by one thing, or motive, suicide is a flight from these spectres.

3   (3)   In the suicidal drama, certain emotional states are present, including pitiful forlornness, emotional deprivation, distress and/or grief.

4   (6)   S is in a state of heightened disturbance (perturbation) and feels boxed in, harassed, especially hopeless and helpless.

5   (21)   S's suicide appears related to unsatisfied or frustrated needs; e.g., attachment, perfection, achievement, autonomy, control.

II   Cognitive Constriction

6   (8)   Figuratively speaking, S appears to be "intoxicated" by overpowering emotions. Concomitantly, there is a constricted logic and perception.

7   (9)   There is poverty of thought, exhibited by focusing only on permutations and combinations of grief and grief-provoking topics.

8   (11)   S's aggression has been turned inwards; e.g. humility, submission and devotion, subordination, flagellation, masochism, are evident.

9   (34)   An unwillingness to accept the pain of losing an ideal (e.g., abandonment, sickness, old age), allows S to choose, even seek to escape from life and accept death.

III   Disorders in Adjustment

10   (15)   S exhibits a serious disorder in adjustment.

    (a) S's reports are consistent with a manic-depressive disorder such as the down-phase; e.g., all-embracing negative statements, severe mood disturbances causing marked impairment.

    (b) S's reports are consistent with schizophrenia; e.g., delusional thought, paranoid ideation.

    (c) S's reports are consistent with anxiety disorder (such as obsessive-compulsive, post-traumatic stress); e.g., feeling of losing control; recurrent and persistent thoughts, impulses or images.

    (d) S's reports are consistent with antisocial personality (or conduct) disorder; e.g., deceitfulness, conning others.

    (e) S's reports are consistent with borderline personality; e.g., frantic efforts to avoid real or imagined abandonment, unstable relationships.

    (f) S's reports are consistent with depression; e.g., depressed mood, diminished interest, insomnia.

    (g) S's reports are consistent with a disorder (or dysfunction) not otherwise specified. S is so paralysed by pain that life, future, etc., is colourless and unattractive.

11   (18)   S reports that the suicide is related to a harsh conscience; i.e., a fulfilment of punishment (or self-punishment).

IV   Suicide as Solution

12   (4)   S appears to have arrived at the end of an interest to endure and sees suicide as a solution for some urgent problem(s), and/or injustices of life.

13 (5)   There is a conflict between life's demands for adaptation and the S's inability or unwillingness to meet the challenge.

14 (13) S considers him/herself too weak to overcome personal difficulties and, therefore, rejects everything, wanting to escape painful life events.

15 (14) Although S passionately argues that there is no justification for living on, S's state of mind is incompatible with an accurate assessment/perception of what is going on.

Interpersonal

V   Interpersonal Relations: Unresolved

16 (17) There are unresolved problems ("a complex" or weakened ego) in the individual; e.g., symptoms or ideas that are discordant, unassimilated, and/or antagonistic.

17 (20) S reports being weakened and/or defeated by unresolved problems in the interpersonal field (or some other ideal such as health, perfection).

18 (22) S's frustration in the interpersonal field is exceedingly stressful and persisting to a traumatic degree.

19 (16) There is a relative weakness in S's capacity for developing constructive tendencies (e.g., attachment, love).

20 (23) A positive development in the disturbed relationship was seen as the only possible way to go on living, but such development was seen as not forthcoming.

VI   Identification–Ambivalence

21 (26) S, whose personality (ego) is not adequately developed (weakened), appears to have suffered a narcissistic injury.

22 (24) S's relationships (attachments) were too unhealthy and/or too intimate (regressive, "primitive"), keeping him/her under constant strain of stimulation and frustration.

23 (10) S reports ambivalence; e.g., complications, concomitant contradictory feelings, attitudes and/or thrusts.

24 (28) S feels quite ambivalent, i.e., both affectionate and hostile towards the same (lost or rejecting) person.

VII   Vengefulness–Aggression

25 (19) S's problem(s) appears to be determined by the individual's history and the present interpersonal situation.

26 (29) S reports feelings and/or ideas of aggression and vengefulness toward him/herself although S appears to be actually angry at someone else.

27 (30) S turns upon the self, murderous impulses that had previously been directed against someone else.

28 (31) Although maybe not reported directly, S may have calculated the self-destructiveness to have a negative effect on someone else (e.g., a lost or rejecting person).

29 (32)   S's self-destructiveness appears to be an act of aggression, attack, and/or revenge towards someone else who has hurt or injured him/her.

30 (12)   Unconscious dynamics can be concluded. There are likely more reasons to the suicide than the person is consciously aware.

VIII   *Identification–Egression*

31 (25)   S reports a traumatic event or hurt or injury (e.g., unmet love, a failing marriage, disgust with one's work).

32 (7)   S reports a history of trauma (e.g., health, rejection by significant other, a competitive spouse).

33 (33)   S reports in some direct or indirect fashion an identification (i.e., attachment) with a lost or rejecting person (or with any lost ideal [e.g., health, freedom, employment, all A's]).

34 (27)   S is preoccupied with an event or injury, namely a person who has been lost or rejecting (i.e., abandonment).

35 (35)   S wants to egress (i.e., to escape, to depart, to flee, to be gone), to relieve the unbearable psychological pain.

Appendix 20.1 presents the TGSP-2, which I encourage the clinician to use as alternative constructs or schema—the same and different—to understand the patient.

A DISCUSSION: WHAT WE LEARN FROM THIS STUDY

Our discussion will focus primarily on the main topic: The failure to replicate our schema and its implication for theory development, and the applications for psychotherapy. After reading this chapter one may ask, "Why include this chapter? It invalidates the schema that you used throughout the book." I would reply, "It validates and invalidates the schema, but that is the most central clinical point of the book." Our understanding of a patient is like the river—it is both the same and different. Our commonalities or templates or unity thema or seals or whatever we wish to call them, should be process, not static. There is both the general and the unique. System models are more useful. This is the main insight that I have gained over the years of treating suicidal people: They are what I use to save a suicidal person.

To address the question from a pure quantitative view, the current results suggest that not only were the constructs of Leenaars (1989a) not validated, they were generally a different fit with the current data, despite similarities. Yet, if one reconciles and merges the qualitative with the quantitative methods of research, a different view emerges. There were both flux and similarities in the results. The current classifications, in fact, offer an alternative perspective on suicidal events. At this time, it can be concluded from the results that there are at least two and, by implication, more models to define suicide. There is more than one template, to use a nautical example, to build a ship. Of course, this is an everyday necessity in clinical practice, where the interventionist must constantly be mindful of his/her theory to fit the uniqueness of each person (the singular). This is *the* single most important fact that our patients teach us, not necessarily arithmetical research.

The current result was anticipated on the basis of the initial study (Leenaars, 1989a). It was noted then that there was some tentativeness to the results. There were methodological problems. For example, it was deemed that larger samples were needed, which is one purpose of this study. Questions were also raised about the statistical method, i.e., clustering. Cluster Analysis is a method of classification. Clustering methods are designed to create groups of entities and different clustering methods can and do generate different solutions (Aldenderfer & Blashfield, 1984). Clustering is classification seeking, although it actually imposes the structure. This is true, of course, for all approaches to mathematical groupings, e.g., Factor Analysis. Besides, the data do not have pure psychometric properties. One could even get more specific. The specific solutions are orthogonal, so things shift, etc. Put more simply, we are imposing order on the mess, when, in fact, it is a mess. Aldenderfer and Blashfield (1984) in their classical text on the topic, *Cluster Analysis*, in fact, state that clustering is "heuristic". In considering the present results as opposed to the previous one, we can say that both solutions are slightly different perspectives, one is no more valid than the other. Finally, if we continue to sample, to analyse, etc., we could get to a better fit of the multidimensional malaise in suicide, but never the thing itself (Husserl, 1973).

At a deeper theoretical level, there is a need to seek empirical uniformities. The Newton system, for example, sought to account for physical particulars. The theories of Freud, Murray, Shneidman, and the other seven suicidologists studied, offer an understanding of suicidal patients. Yet, our science still needs to bridge its theory to data—a necessary step in all sciences (Hempel, 1966). This is the challenge in suicidology. Yet, all psychology must remain open-ended (Heidbreder, 1933), by the very nature of its subject matter. A permanent existing idea or *Vorstellung* is, in fact, a mythological entity in psychology (James, 1890). Theories of suicide need to be flowing, not static. It was never intended in 1989 (Leenaars, 1989a) to propose that there are only eight possible classifications of suicide. There were no eight commandments. The model was a probable construction of suicide, like all theories of suicide. This is true of Freud's, Shneidman's, Beck's, or anyone's theory. Indeed, we must continue to define suicide, both the general and the unique, and, according to Shneidman (1985), this will remain the main task of suicidologists in the future. This endeavour is like a river; we need further theory building.

The current schema, based on the general framework of the new eight-cluster solution, with the Intrapsychic/Interpersonal frame, can be accounted for as follows:

Intrapsychic

I *Unbearable Psychological Pain*
The common stimulus in suicide is unbearable pain, an inner turmoil of deep anguish. The suicidal person is deeply perturbed and feels especially hopeless and

helpless. The psychological pain is driven, created by and sustained by frustrated needs. Suicide is a solution; it stops the intolerable frustrating, blocking or thwarting flow of the mind.

II   Cognitive Constriction
The common cognitive (or perceptual) state in suicide is constriction. There are mental blinders. There is a single-mindedness, often about one thing (or ideal). Figuratively, the person is "intoxicated" by constricted emotions, logic, and perception—a dissociated state. The person, in fact, exhibits subordination and submission to his/her constricted belief ("There is only one thing to do").

III   Disorders in Adjustment
It is helpful to understand suicide from a psychopathological perspective. The suicidal person—in almost 90% of cases—exhibits a mental disorder, with mood disorders being the most common. A psychosis, a neurosis or a character disorder is not unusual in a suicidal person; it is not a mere transient state. On one further point, as Freud (1974g) first documented in his paper, "Mourning and melancholia", the psychopathology of the suicidal person is often associated to a very harsh conscience, especially self-criticism, guilt, and shame.

IV   Suicide as Solution
There are urgent problems, injustices and/or unmet demands. The suicidal person is too weak to overcome his/her life's realities. The only solution is suicide, the person simply does not believe in a justification to live. The common belief is, "There is no reason to live."

Interpersonal

V   Interpersonal Relations: Unresolved
Unresolved problems in interpersonal relationships (or to some other ideal such as health, employment, public self) are the common field (or stage) in suicide. The person is frustrated and weakened interpersonally. The suicidal person lacks in the capacity to develop constructive interpersonal tendencies.

VI   Identification–Ambivalence
There is a narcissistic injury, a trauma. The person was deeply attached, but cannot cope with the perceived loss, rejection, and so on, of the object (person or other ideals). The attitude becomes one of ambivalence. There are ambivalences, complications, contradictions, and so on towards "punitive" relationships. There is both love and hate and there is both the wish to be dead and to be rescued.

VII   Vengefulness–Aggression
Aggression is a common emotion in suicide. There is both a current situation and a history to the aggression. Rage, and even vengefulness, not only towards others, but to oneself is omnipresent. Often, unconscious elements are associated to the

anguish of Thanatos. The aggression is, indeed, deep, deeper than the mind is aware of.

VIII *Identification–Egression*

Suicide is not random. There is a perception of a never-ending trauma or hurt or injury. The common need of attachment is frustrated, often experienced as abandonment. The real puzzle for the suicidal person is, "how to get out of it?" The common solution is escape, an egression. The purpose of suicide is to seek a solution, to be gone, to be elsewhere, to be dead.

SUMMARY

This volume has presented strong support for a multidimensional approach to understanding suicide and its treatment. Yet, the current schema did not replicate fully a previous one (Leenaars, 1989a). However, this is to be expected (and even anticipated) because theories are constructions, even empirically based models. We are not at the stage in the science of suicidology when we can make definite predictions, whether from psychology, biology, or sociology. We need to accept the limits of our theories. If they have become too rigid ("dogma"), then we will get stuck (functionally fixed) with a patient. Rather, we must continually understand the uniqueness of each individual. We have to remember Heraclitus. Theoretical understanding is a process, not a thing. Be that as it may, classification into meaningful sets is important in suicidology. There is, in fact, no substitute for theory building in science (Hempel, 1966), despite the limitations in the science of suicidology (Benjafield, 1991). We only have constructions (ideas), not the thing itself (Heidegger, 1962; Husserl, 1973). We do not have an observation like Halley's Comet in 1682, waiting some 80 years, to predict its return in 1759. However, if Halley's comet had instead exploded in 1739, could Newton have predicted its destruction and, even more important, explained why the comet exploded? And, most important, could Newton have prevented the destruction? Our data, i.e., suicides, remain elusive (Maris, 1981); yet, we must continue the development of theory in our field. Suicidology cannot be atheoretical. We must, however, acknowledge the complexities and issues in theory building in science (Hempel, 1966) and its application to psychotherapy and other treatments. But, then, this is true of all science, even for Albert Einstein's theory of relativity. Despite these facts, psychotherapists must constantly alter, change, reframe, and so on, their understanding of each unique patient to prevent suicide. The river is both the same and different. We, as humans, in fact, can do no better. What I have learned is: You must always understand the person if you are to treat him/her. This is true for Vincent, Rick, Sylvia, Jeff, Joe, and all suicidal people.

Appendix 20.1

THEMATIC GUIDE FOR SUICIDE PREDICTION: FORM 2

Copyright © 2001 by Antoon A. Leenaars, PhD, CPsych

I PATIENT DATA

Date: _____

Name: _____ Age: _____ Sex: _____

Date of Birth: _____ Marital Status: _____

Education Status: _____
(years)

_____
(degrees)

Current Employment: _____

II SUICIDAL EXPERIENCE

1. Has the patient ever seriously contemplated suicide? (If yes, note particulars)

   _____

2. Has the patient ever attempted suicide? (If yes, note particulars)

   _____

3. Does the patient know anyone who attempted suicide? (If yes, indicate family, acquaintance, etc.)

   _____

4. Does the patient know anyone who committed suicide? (If yes, indicate family, acquaintance, etc.)

   _____

III REFERRAL DATA

1. Purpose _____

2. What is the referral question? _____

   _____

3. What is the presenting problem(s)? _____

   _____

   _____

IV   INTERVIEW SITUATION

1. Observations _____

_____

_____

2. Other procedures (e.g., tests, interviews) _____

_____

V   INTERPRETATIONS

1. Perturbation rating:	Low	Medium	High
scale equivalent	1 2 3	4 5 6	7 8 9
2. Lethality rating:	Low	Medium	High
scale equivalent	1 2 3	4 5 6	7 8 9

3. Guide summary:
scores: I: 1, 2, 3, 4, 5;   II: 6, 7, 8, 9;   III: 10, 11;
          IV: 12 13, 14, 15;   V: 16, 17, 18, 19, 20;   VI: 21, 22, 23, 24;
          VII: 25, 26, 27, 28, 29, 30;   VIII: 31, 32, 33, 34, 35

Conclusions: _____

_____

_____

VI   REMARKS

_____

_____

_____

_____

_____

_____

_____

_____

_____

_____

_____

_____

_____

_____

_____

_____

Include on back any other relevant data.

INSTRUCTIONS

Your task will be to verify whether the statements provided below correspond or compare to the contents of the patient's protocols (e.g., interview, written reports). The statements provided below are a classification of the possible content. You are to determine whether the contents in the patient's protocols are a particular or specific instance of the classification or not. Your comparison should be observable; however, the classification may be more abstract than the specific instances. Thus, you will have to make judgements about whether particular contents of a protocol are included in a given classification or not. Your task is to conclude, yes or no.

INTRAPSYCHIC

I   *Unbearable Psychological Pain*

Circle/Check

1. Suicide has adjustive value and is functional because it stops painful tension and provides relief from intolerable psychological pain. (P)   Yes   No

2. In suicide, the psychological and/or environmental traumas among many other factors may include: incurable disease, threat of senility, fear of becoming hopelessly dependent, feelings of inadequacy, humiliation. Although the solution of suicide is not caused by one thing, or motive, suicide is a flight from these spectres. (P & D)   Yes   No

3. In the suicidal drama, certain emotional states are present, including pitiful forlornness, emotional deprivation, distress and/or grief. (P & D)   Yes   No

4. S is in a state of heightened disturbance (perturbation) and feels boxed in, harassed, especially hopeless and helpless. (P)   Yes   No

5. S's suicide appears related to unsatisfied or frustrated needs; e.g., attachment, perfection, achievement, autonomy, control. (P)   Yes   No

II   *Cognitive Constriction*

6. Figuratively speaking, S appears to be "intoxicated" by over-powering emotions. Concomitantly, there is a constricted logic and perception. (D)   Yes   No

7. There is poverty of thought, exhibited by focusing only on permutations and combinations of grief and grief-provoking topics. (D)   Yes   No

8. S's aggression has been turned inwards; e.g., humility, submission and devotion, subordination, flagellation, masochism, are evident. (P)   Yes   No

9. An unwillingness to accept the pain of losing an ideal (e.g., abandonment, sickness, old age), allows S to choose, even seek to escape from life and accept death. (D)   Yes   No

III *Disorders in Adjustment*
10. S exhibits a serious disorder in adjustment. (P)   Yes No
   (a) S's reports are consistent with a manic-depressive disorder such as the down-phase; e.g., all-embracing negative statements, severe mood disturbances causing marked impairment.   Yes No
   (b) S's reports are consistent with schizophrenia; eg., delusional thought, paranoid ideation.   Yes No
   (c) S's reports are consistent with anxiety disorder (such as obsessive-compulsive, post-traumatic stress); feeling of losing control; recurrent and persistent thoughts, impulses or images.   Yes No
   (d) S's reports are consistent with antisocial personality (or conduct) disorder; e.g., deceitfulness, conning others.   Yes No
   (e) S's reports are consistent with borderline personality; e.g., frantic efforts to avoid real or imagined abandonment, unstable relationships.   Yes No
   (f) S's reports are consistent with depression; e.g., depressed mood, diminished interest, insomnia.   Yes No
   (g) S's reports are consistent with a disorder (or dysfunction) not otherwise specified. S is so paralysed by pain that life, future, etc. is colourless and unattractive.   Yes No
11. S reports that the suicide is related to a harsh conscience; i.e., a fulfilment of punishment (or self-punishment). (D)   Yes No

IV *Suicide as Solution*
12. S appears to have arrived at the end of an interest to endure and sees suicide as a solution for some urgent problem(s), and/or injustices of life. (P)   Yes No
13. There is a conflict between life's demands for adaptation and the S's inability or unwillingness to meet the challenge. (P)   Yes No
14. S considers him/herself too weak to overcome personal difficulties and, therefore, rejects everything, wanting to escape painful life events. (P)   Yes No
15. Although S passionately argues that there is no justification for living on, S's state of mind is incompatible with an accurate assessment/perception of what is going on. (P)   Yes No

Interpersonal

V *Interpersonal Relations: Unresolved*
16. There are unresolved problems ("a complex" or weakened ego) in the individual; e.g., symptoms or ideas that are discordant, unassimilated, and/or antagonistic. (P)   Yes No

17. S reports being weakened and/or defeated by unresolved problems in the interpersonal field (or some other ideal such as health, perfection). (P) Yes No

18. S's frustration in the interpersonal field is exceedingly stressful and persisting to a traumatic degree. (P) Yes No

19. There is a relative weakness in S's capacity for developing constructive tendencies (e.g., attachment, love). (D) Yes No

20. A positive development in the disturbed relationship was seen as the only possible way to go on living, but such development was seen as not forthcoming. (P) Yes No

VI Identification–Ambivalence

21. S, whose personality (ego) is not adequately developed (weakened), appears to have suffered a narcissistic injury. (P & D) Yes No

22. S's relationships (attachments) were too unhealthy and/or too intimate (regressive, "primitive"), keeping him/her under constant strain of stimulation and frustration. (D) Yes No

23. S reports ambivalence; e.g., complications, concomitant contradictory feelings, attitudes and/or thrusts. (P & D) Yes No

24. S feels quite ambivalent, i.e., both affectionate and hostile towards the same (lost or rejecting) person. (D) Yes No

VII Vengefulness–Aggression

25. S's problem(s) appears to be determined by the individual's history and the present interpersonal situation. (P) Yes No

26. S reports feelings and/or ideas of aggression and vengefulness towards him/herself although S appears to be actually angry at someone else. (D) Yes No

27. S turns upon the self, murderous impulses that had previously been directed against someone else. (D) Yes No

28. Although maybe not reported directly, S may have calculated the self-destructiveness to have a negative effect on someone else (e.g., a lost or rejecting person). (P) Yes No

29. S's self-destructiveness appears to be an act of aggression, attack, and/or revenge towards someone else who has hurt or injured him/her. (P) Yes No

30. Unconscious dynamics can be concluded. There are likely more reasons to the suicide than the person is consciously aware. (D) Yes No

VIII Identification–Egression

31. S reports a traumatic event or hurt or injury (e.g., unmet love, a failing marriage, disgust with one's work). (P) Yes No

32. S reports a history of trauma (e.g., poor health, rejection by significant other, a competitive spouse). (P & D)   Yes   No
33. S reports in some direct or indirect fashion an identification (i.e., attachment) with a lost or rejecting person (or with any lost ideal [e.g., health, freedom, employment, all A's]). (D)   Yes   No
34. S is preoccupied with an event or injury, namely a person who has been lost or rejecting (i.e., abandonment). (D)   Yes   No
35. S wants to egress (i.e., to escape, to depart, to flee, to be gone), to relieve the unbearable psychological pain. (P)   Yes   No

Chapter 21

ETHICAL AND LEGAL ISSUES

Ethical and Legal Issues: Antoon Leenaars with Chris Cantor, John Connolly, Marlene EchoHawk, Danute Gailiene, Zhao Xiong He, Natalia Kokorina, David Lester, Andrew Lopatin, Mario Rodriguez, Lourens Schlebusch, Yoshitomo Takahashi, and Lakshmi Vijayakumar

Ethical and legal issues are complex, more complex than one person can be consciously aware of. This is true for a book on psychotherapy. One can write a book on psychotherapy for the world, but not the ethical and legal context for all nations. Thus, when I decided to write this book, a project by the International Working Group on Ethical and Legal Issues in Suicidology seemed to have a natural home. This chapter is the complete project of the group, although a number of papers have been published by the group (Leenaars, et al., 2000a, 2000b, 2001a, 2002a). This then constitutes the full report—and allows us to place the patient's psychotherapy within his/her historical–cultural–ethical context.

There is a rich history of thought about the ethical and legal issues in suicidology. We could begin our discussion with Plato or Confucius or Kant or Pemulway or Buddha or Lucien Taparti or Laotze or Hume, or any one of our global array of wise people. We have chosen here to begin with a story from Black Elk (Neihardt, 1932). Black Elk is one of the most sacred Elders of Turtle Island of the last century. Here, somewhat condensed, is one of his stories:

> A very long time ago, two scouts were out hunting for bison; and when they were on top of a mountain and looking north, they saw something coming towards them. "It is a woman," one said. They recognized that it was a sacred, young and beautiful woman and the one said, "Throw all bad thoughts away." Yet, the other looked and had foolish thoughts and a cloud came over them, and the foolish one turned into a skeleton.
> Then the woman told the wise one that she would come to his people. The people were to build a teepee in the centre of the village and she would bring a sacred gift. And the man told his people; they built the teepee; and the woman came to the teepee and said:
> With visible breath I am walking
>
> > *A voice I am sending as I walk*
>
> In a sacred manner I am walking
> With visible tracks I am walking
> In a sacred manner I walk.

And as she sang, she gave the chief a pipe, with a bison carved on one side to mean the earth that gives us birth and nourishes and with twelve eagle feathers to mean the sky and twelve moons. She said "With this you shall multiply and be a good nation. Nothing but good shall come from it." The people sang and the woman left the teepee, transforming into a white bison galloping away.

People of Turtle Island tell this story when people must think about issues of the good, the just, the moral, and so on. These are the concerns presented here, and thus, we light the pipe . . .

Of course, no one can light the pipe alone. Thus, when I wanted to light the pipe on ethical and legal issues for an international audience, I realized my limitations (i.e., a Canadian–Dutchman) and decided to invite a group of international experts to join me. I invited the following people with their culture/ nation identified in brackets: C. Cantor (Australia), J. Connolly (Ireland), M. EchoHawk (Turtle Island, renamed North America), D. Gailiene (Lithuania), Z. X. He (China), N. Kokorina and A. Lopatin (Russia), D. Lester (United States), M. Rodriguez (Cuba), L. Schlebusch (South Africa), Y. Takahashi (Japan), L.Vijayakumar (India), and myself (The Netherlands). We recognize that we do not represent the world or our own nation. We too have our limitations. Yet, we hope that our perspectives will cast a wider net over these issues than one view in isolation. One perspective on ethical and legal issues would be myopic, and this myopia has been a problem to date on the topic. No one person, or nation or culture can know the *"good"*, whether defined by Black Elk, Plato, Buddha, and so forth. To discuss such issues, say from the American view, which is the most prolific view on the topic, would be foolish. Thus, we hope that, with our diverse perspectives, we can come to a closer approximation to smoking the pipe.

An *a priori* step in our discussion is definition. What do we mean by "ethical" and "legal"? These terms are difficult to define; the whole chapter, in fact, is about definition. Yet, we begin with a definition from *The Oxford English Dictionary* (OED, 1993), the arbiter of the English Language, keeping in mind that we could equally use a Cuban dictionary, a Lithuanian one, and so forth. Thus, we read:

> *Ethical*—Of or pertaining to morality or the science of ethics; pertaining to morals. Dealing with the science of ethics or questions connected with it. In accordance with the principles of ethics; morally correct, honourable; conforming to the ethics of a profession, etc.

The word *Ethic* is defined as: A set of moral principles, esp. those of a specified religion, school of thought, etc.

> *Legal*—Of or pertaining to law; falling within the province of law. Belonging to or characteristic of the profession of the law. Required or appointed by law; founded on or deriving authority from law. Allowed by or in accordance with a particular set of rules; permissible.

The word *Law* is defined as: The body of rules, whether formally enacted or customary, which a particular State or community recognizes as governing the

actions of its subjects or members and which it may enforce by imposing penalties.

Ethical and legal issues are multifarious. This is as true in the area of suicidology as it is in any area. To narrow the possible topics, we chose to address the
list below, knowing full well that many issues would not be addressed. We felt
that the key ethical and legal issues are verily represented by the following topics:
suicide and attempted suicide; assisted suicide and euthanasia; standards of reasonable and prudent care; responsibility for care; failure to diagnose properly;
failure in care; liability and malpractice; means restriction; and postvention. And
further, the selections could be organized into three superordinate categories:
(1) Laws on Suicide, Assisted Suicide and Euthanasia (with the first two topics);
(2) Standards of Care and Liability (with the next five topics); and (3) Further Ethical and Professional Concerns (with the final two topics). We will discuss the ethics
and laws on each selection. We recognize that the list itself may be too narrow, and
perhaps too Western. There are, of course, special ethical and legal issues facing
each region of the world (which will need work in the future). Further, each case
in each region is unique; thus, individual (idiographic) issues are not necessarily
the same as general (nomothetic) ones. The nomothetic, however, are hopefully
applicable to the idiographic.

Of course, legal issues are complex across the globe and often not even uniform
within a country. For example, in the United States of America (US), legal issues
are complicated by at least two facts. First, the US comprises 50 states, and each
state has a certain degree of autonomy in setting its own legal rules and requirements. On occasion, local laws and rulings may be appealed to higher courts at the
federal level, the results of which modify the ruling of the lower court. However,
even here, the country is divided into several federal districts, each of which may
rule differently. Only when the United States Supreme Court rules on an issue does
some means of unity develop.

A second factor in the US is that civil suits play a major role in determining the
standards for the nation, but again, these suits begin at the local level and, only if
and when they are reviewed at the federal level, does a uniform standard develop.
Of course, from a global perspective each country/culture has its own standards.
We only give the US as an example of the complexity of the issues addressed
here.

We should also note that in some countries, such as Cuba, there are difficulties
in obtaining information. Furthermore, within Cuba, it is difficult to access the
information, even if it exists. Although there is a growing interest in ethical and
legal issues, the topics have rarely been addressed. Cuba is given here only as
an example because other countries from our group equally experienced problems in gathering information. And if some topics were discussed, others, such as
those related to care, liability and so on, were not. Lithuania is an example of the
latter.

Finally, we saw our report to be one opportunity for a global approach to suicide
and its prevention.

LAWS ON SUICIDE, ASSISTED SUICIDE AND EUTHANASIA

Suicide and Attempted Suicide

Suicide constitutes a serious public and mental health problem world wide. In many countries suicide ranks among the top 10 causes of death. Some of the countries represented here have some of the world's highest rates; e.g., Lithuania. The rates of suicide in a nation are also not static. A century ago, Russia, for example, had one of the lowest suicide rates (3 per 100 000). By the last decades of the Soviet Union's existence, the rates of suicide in the USSR had increased significantly from 17.1 in 1965 to 29.6 in 1984. However, this public health problem was persistently glossed over during that time. For example, the State Statistics Department of the USSR had not reported the statistical data on this issue before the mid-1980s. Thus, it is difficult to know what the numbers and actual rates may have been. We do know that, in 1996, the rate in Russia was 53.0 (per 100 000). Of course, people in other regions, such as Turtle Island, also have great variation within the region. The WHO estimated that in the not too distant future almost one million people would commit suicide yearly. In addition, at least 10 times as many persons engage in suicidal behaviour (i.e., attempted suicide, parasuicide or deliberate self-harm). The sheer number makes suicide and suicidal behaviour a public health and mental health problem of prime importance. This importance was as true historically as it is today.

Suicide has been viewed differently historically in various regions. Confucianism and Taoism in China, which are reflected in the Chinese traditional medical classic *Huang Di Nei Jing* valued life as more precious than to be measured by gold. The Chinese classic *Yi Jing* (The Book of Changes) stated "It is a delightful matter if a hopeless illness can be treated with no drug." And *Yi Zhuan* (500 BC) (The Annotation of Yi Jing) explained this concept as "The hopeless drug never be prescribed."

The *Old Testament* of the West does not directly forbid suicide, but in Jewish law suicide is wrong. During the early Christian years, there was excessive martyrdom, i.e., suicide, resulting in considerable concern on the part of the Church Fathers. St Augustine (354–430 AD) categorically rejected suicide. Suicide was considered a sin because it violated the Fifth Commandment, "Thou shalt not kill." By 693, the Church of the Council of Toledo proclaimed that individuals who attempted suicide should be excommunicated. St Thomas Aquinas (1225–1274 AD) declared suicide to be a grave mortal sin. The notion of suicide as sin took firm hold in the West for hundreds of years. Only during the Renaissance and the Reformation did a different view emerge.

The *Dharmashastras* (book on the codes of living in ancient India) are explicit in their condemnation of suicide. For instance, Yama Smriti (600 BC) says that the body of those who die by suicide should be defiled. If a person survived an attempt, he/she should pay a fine and if the person killed him/herself, the sons or friends should pay the fine (Thakur, 1963). Although suicide was condemned in the *Dharmashastras*, there is also a chapter on allowed suicides. Scriptures, such as by Manu and Kautilya, were against suicide. These sentiments were echoed for ages in India. Even today, attempted suicide is a crime under the Indian Penal Code though even the neighbouring country of Sri Lanka has removed attempted suicide as a punishable offence. Assisting and abetment of suicide is also a punishable offence under the Code.

In the US, only part of Turtle Island, there are over 500 federally recognized tribes and each tribe has its own culture and traditions. Yet, despite the diversity, it would be safe to say that suicide is viewed as a taboo.

The Native people of Turtle Island view life as a precious gift, which is to be cherished and protected. There is also the philosophy that to fully enjoy the "gift of life" one must live in balance in terms of the mental, physical, social, and spiritual aspects of the whole person. When there is a person who is "out of balance" or "out of harmony", then negative events can happen, such as suicide.

Historically, there were exceptions to the rules and laws in various nations. For example, in India, the *Dharmashastras* allowed some suicides. A person, for example, was allowed to commit suicide to expiate for sins like incest; hermits and ascetics suffering from incurable diseases and unable to perform their duties could embark on Mahaprasthana (Great Journey of Life; i.e., To walk in the north easterly direction subsisting on water and air, till death). Yet, as in the early Christian era, there was a tendency towards suicide as a mode of accepted religious practice and some actions were taken. Suicide by drowning at holy places like Varanasi and Prayag were supposed to relieve the soul from the never-ending cycle of birth and death. In 1802, legislation had to be formed to prevent people from drowning themselves before the Temple Car of Puri Jagannath.

Today there is a wide array of perceptions on suicide and attempted suicide. In the US, completed suicide is not against the law in any of the states (Victoroff, 1983). However, there are some local variations; six states have current penalties for attempting suicide. Both suicide and attempted suicide are not illegal at present in Japan. Throughout the history of Japan, there has been no period when suicide was prohibited by law, except in the early eighteenth century when a cluster of lover suicide pacts (Joshi) was triggered by Chikamatsu Monzaemon's dramas (Takahashi, 1997). In the Netherlands, the principle that all punishment for crime ends upon the individual's death was introduced in 1809 and was applied to suicide and attempted suicide. In the former Soviet Union, "suicide" was omitted from medical and legal discussion because it was dictated that such a problem could not possibly exist in socialist society. No laws were needed because the problem did not exist, except in mental derangements. Yet, by the mid-1980s, the problem was beginning to be acknowledged and addressed from a medical–legal view. Suicide and attempted suicide are not illegal in Australia. In South Africa, suicide is not a crime, although it is considered to be against public policy. There are also no laws in Cuba and Lithuania against suicide. Ireland was the last European country to decriminalize suicide in 1993 by the Criminal Law (Suicide) Act, where we read, "Suicide shall cease to be a crime." It is, thus, easy to conclude that not only in the past and present but also in the future, there will be great diversity about the laws governing suicide and attempted suicide. There is no *one* law.

Euthanasia and Assisted Suicide

The right to die concept is one of the most controversial and elusive issues facing the legal and ethical issues of suicidology around the world. The increased control that we have gained over biological life because of progress in medical treatment, especially with the terminally ill, will force a confrontation with the subject (Diekstra, 1992). More and more often, the question will be posed whether life or death is the humane choice in the terminally ill. This situation will have a profound impact on legal and ethical issues world wide. It will not only be about life and death, but also about the very definition of what is a suicide and what is not (Leenaars & Diekstra, 1997). Our very definitions will change.

Before we address the perspectives, we need to clarify our terms, mainly because there is considerable confusion about the terms, euthanasia, and assisted suicide. Euthanasia literally means an easy or good death. It refers to the practice of allowing the person to die with assistance, often by a medical doctor. Another person does not perform assisted suicide; rather, the means are provided by which the person can end his/her own life. These distinctions are critical, especially if one looks at the diversity of global views.

To illustrate the right to die debate, we will begin with the Netherlands. The Netherlands is chosen because euthanasia in the Netherlands is *gedogen* (gudoogun; a Dutch word having no good English translation, although tolerance may be the best (NRC Handelsblad, 1998)), probably more so than any area of the world. On 28 November 2000, the Lower House of the Dutch Parliament approved a bill for the "Review of Cases of Termination of Life on Request and Assistance with Suicide." The bill passed the Upper House on 10 April 2001 and became law on 1 April 2002. Euthanasia and assisted suicide are now treated as a legal act in the Netherlands, the first nation to do so, if carried out by a physician and certain criteria are followed. The law does not, however, decriminalize other forms of euthanasia and assisted suicide. The press release, including English text, of the Department of Justice can be obtained at the website http://www.minjust.nl—see Kerkhof and Connolly (2001) for the text. Yet, the Northern Territory Government of Australia had historically earlier legalized assisted suicide. There had been, however, numerous appeals and counter appeals in the Territory, with such practices being illegal at this time.

For those familiar with the right to die debate, the Dutch case of Nico Speijer is important (Leenaars & Diekstra, 1997). Nico Speijer was the Netherlands' leading suicidologist; Dr Speijer completed assisted suicide, after suffering from incurable terminal illness. He did so, after he wrote, with René Diekstra (Speijer & Diekstra, 1980), the rules and regulations for assisted death, entitled *Assisted Suicide: A Study of the Problems Related to Self-Chosen Death*. In this book, which was the first to address exclusively the issue of assisted death from ethical, legal, and professional perspectives, the authors outlined a set of criteria for assisting with self-chosen death by health care professionals in cases of unbearable physical illness without reasonable prospects for improvement or for recovery of an acceptable quality of life.

The criteria and rules of conduct for assisted "suicide" are formulated in the following:

1. Request made voluntarily and directly by actor
2. Actor *compos mentis* (mentally competent) at time of request
3. Wish to end life is longstanding
4. Presence of unbearable suffering (Subject)
5. No reasonable prospect of improvement (Object)
6. Remaining treatment alternatives uncertain/only palliative (offered but rejected)
7. Helper is acknowledged professional
8. Helper has used intercollegial consultation (1–6) (Actor has been seen/examined by colleague(s))
9. Avoidance of preventable harm/damage to others
10. Decision-making process and steps taken documented for professional and legal evaluation.

The book initially received little attention but the death of Speijer brought a drastic change in this respect. Speijer, in fact, had followed the rules of conduct in the book for his own demise. Three months after the event, in December 1981, the Court of the City of Rotterdam convicted a female lay volunteer who had helped an elderly chronic terminally ill patient to die by feeding her at her request a chocolate pudding in which barbiturates had been mixed. The court sentenced the volunteer to a suspended imprisonment stating that in providing assistance at the request of the deceased she had not (as she could not have because of the simple fact that she was a volunteer) acted carefully, which was then operationalized by reference to the rules of conduct as formulated in *Assisted Suicide*. By implication, the court asserted that had the assistance been carried out in accordance with those rules, the volunteer might have gone unpunished.

Jurisprudence throughout the country ever since has complied with the verdict of the Rotterdam Court. No health care professional that has been known to have assisted with death, and who carefully observed the rules of conduct, has been prosecuted or put on trial. This, in spite of the fact that assistance with death was punishable by law in the formal sense. It was a practice of *gedogen*, until the law of 10 April 2001 came into effect. For example, in the Assen case, a psychiatrist assisted a depressed 50-year-old female with her suicide after the death of her son, arguing that her pain was understandable and untreatable. In another case, a gynaecologist was charged for killing a 3-year-old girl born with multiple physical and mental handicaps. The new law includes regulation regarding minors. Youths of 16 or 17 can, in principle, make their own decisions, whereas children aged 12 to 16 need parental approval. These cases, and the inclusion of children in the new Act, raise the issue of the slippery slope (Lester & Leenaars, 1996). Other issues warrant caution; yet, some people, such as Herbert Hendin (1997), have attacked the Dutch position, based on his own *a priori* perspective, a foreign psychoanalytic one, rather than on the "objective" facts (Conwell, 1998). Hendin's perspective is at least one of forcing the data of another culture into one's own. This is not to say that there are no problems in the Netherlands, there are—problems of reporting, following the guidelines, issues of consent have all been raised (van der Maas et al., 1992). There are issues, for example, of how "unbearable suffering" is defined. Does it refer to terminal illness, depression, etc.? Regardless of one's view, the development of the Netherlands has sparked considerable debate and this debate, even with the new law, continues and it would be wrong to say that euthanasia and assisted suicide are no longer punishable under the law. The law only spells out that a physician must practice due care, as discussed earlier and as set out in a separate law—The Termination of Life on Request and Assisted Suicide (Review) Act, and he/she must report the cause of death to the coroner in accordance with the Burial and Cremation Act.

The rules of conduct are basically consistent with the previous guidelines. The due-care requests mentioned in the Criminal Code Article 293, para. 2, stipulate that the medical doctor:

(a) must be convinced that the patient has made a voluntary and well-considered request to die;
(b) must be convinced that the patient is facing interminable and unendurable suffering;
(c) has informed the patient about his or her situation and prospects;
(d) together with the patient, must be convinced that there is no other reasonable solution;
(e) has consulted at least one other independent doctor of the patient;
(f) has seen and given a written assessment of the due-care requirements as referred to in points (a) to (d);
(g) has helped the patient to die with due medical care.

Regional Review Committees exist to review if the due-care requests have been followed. Yet, debate and issues had occurred and continue to occur.

One should, of course, be cautious about transposing the Dutch perspective to other cultures (Lester & Leenaars, 1996). The views in the Netherlands itself are not uniform, nor are they across the world.

No legislation on euthanasia exists in China. Historically, under the condition of low production times and non-appearance of surplus products, people abandoned the old and sick when they moved to another habitat, as in almost all regions of the world historically. As late as in the seventh century, the famous Chinese monk named Xuan Zang (602–664 AD) witnessed a seeing-off ceremony that drowned a person in the Ganges River. The people on both sides of the river bid farewell to the euthanasic with drum and gong. A recent study of doctors (as well as of teachers and students) by Wang Hezhou (1989) found that 90–95% approve of euthanasia in China. Yet, there is an opposition to such practice without careful rules of consideration. In India, drowning occurred in the holy Ganges because of religious belief. There is a place called Sangamam, where three rivers unite and the belief is that if one dies there one can escape the cycle of births and deaths. Today, there are still no specific laws to deal with assisted suicide and euthanasia. The available medical facilities are inadequate for the population in India. A study of medical students, however, shows a much lower acceptance of such practice in India (about 50%) than in China (Etzersdorfer et al., 1997).

In Japan, assisted suicide and euthanasia are illegal under the penal code but there are some cases of assisted suicide and euthanasia that are well known, such as the famous Yamanouchi case in 1960 (Japanese Association for Dignified Death, 1990). In that case, a son killed his father suffering from apoplexy upon the latter's request by giving him milk in which pesticide was mixed. The Nagoya High Court's judgement on the Yamanouchi case in 1961 has often been cited. According to this judgement, euthanasia should be permitted under strict conditions, which meet the following six criteria:

1. The patient is suffering from incurable illness with the most up-to-date medical knowledge and technology, and the death is impending in the near future.
2. His/her agony is so severe that no one can see him suffering.
3. The purpose of terminating the patient's life is to palliate his/her agony.
4. In the situation that the patient's consciousness is so clear that he/she can state his/her wish, he/she should state his/her wish clearly that someone else should terminate his/her life.
5. The physician should terminate the patient's life. If someone else terminates the patient's life, there should be most reasonable circumstances for the act.
6. The method of terminating the patient's life should be something ethically acceptable (for example, the use of medical drugs instead of pesticide).

Any act fulfilling all the above six criteria can be considered as euthanasia, and can be acquitted under Japan's penal code (therefore, a vast majority of cases do not fully meet the criteria). The defendant of the Yamanouchi case was judged that he did not meet criteria (5) and (6). He was found guilty of murder at the victim's request and sentenced to one-year imprisonment with three years suspension of sentence.

In Russia, euthanasia is considered to be a medical issue. It strongly denies even the possibility of legalizing assisted suicide and euthanasia. The argument is that a Russian physician must fight for the life of his patient and must not put either "active" or "passive" euthanasia into practice to bring the patient's death closer. This is supported by the principles of national medicine. Medical personnel are not allowed to assist in death.

At the same time, a number of supporters of euthanasia have appeared recently in Russia. In the 1990s one of the most well-known supporters of euthanasia was the late Professor Sergey Dolsky, who supported the idea of a "merciful" death. However, judging by the publications in the Russian press, there is little support. The main argument against assisted suicide and euthanasia is the following: a doctor is called upon to keep the life, but not to destroy it. Legally, euthanasia is prohibited by the legislation of the Russian Federation. It means that medical personnel are never allowed to put euthanasia into practice, at a patient's request, to hasten his/her death. A person who promotes a patient's death is subject to criminal responsibility.

In Ireland, euthanasia and assisted suicide are illegal. In recent years, as much of the rest of the world, these topics have been given a great deal of public airing. The celebrated case of Dr Paddy Leahy is well known. Dr Leahy had publicly admitted to euthanasia with no legal prosecution. He, being terminally ill himself, had promoted the idea of assisted suicide for the terminally ill. Yet, there is little support for Dr Leahy's ideas; a survey of doctors found only 21% of doctors in favour of physician assisted suicide (Cusack, 1997), which is quite different from the surveys in China. Indeed, surveys across the world show considerable variation among medical doctors and the general population, reflecting each region's views.

The Medical Council of Ireland's Guide to Ethical Conduct (1994) explicitly states that euthanasia is professional misconduct. However, the Irish Supreme Court in re Ward of Court has allowed practice such as withdrawal of life sustaining treatment, with a decision in 1995. Withdrawal and refusal of treatment are now seen as quite separate from euthanasia and assisted suicide world wide, although debate continues on such issues. In the US, the landmark case on withdrawal was that of 21-year-old Karen Ann Quinlan. Yet, there are still questions here: Who decides when treatment is withdrawn? Is this action really different from (passive) euthanasia? Is the act of providing pain-reducing medication that will speed death, different from euthanasia, regardless of the physician's stated intent?

In the US, assisted suicide has received wide and varied attention, from Jack Kevorkian's practice advocating no debate ["...all of these (issues) have been well debated in the past and there is nothing new to learn" (Kevorkian, 1988, p. 2)] to Derek Humphry's 1991 book, *Final Exit*, that reached the best-seller list in the *New York Times* to Herbert Hendin's (1997) extreme opposite perspective in *Seduced by Death*. This is not to say that Humphry's or Hendin's books are not useful; they provide us with the extremes. In 1997, the United States Supreme Court decided that there was no constitutional right for physician-assisted suicide (that is, the American Constitution did not address the issue), leaving the matter of legislating physician-assisted suicide to each individual state. Despite the debate, at the present time, only Oregon has passed a law, the Death with Dignity Act, permitting physician-assisted suicide, when certified. The Oregon Act, as amended in 1998, permits a physician to prescribe a lethal medication to a patient who is terminally ill (that is, will die within six months) only if the patient is not suffering from a psychiatric or psychological disorder or depression causing impaired judgement. If the patient is suspected of suffering from such disorders, then psychiatric/psychological evaluation must be carried out to ascertain whether or not the patient has such a disorder. There are also requirements concerning such issues as the form of request, family notification, waiting periods, residency, reporting, etc. The full Act can be found at the following website: www.ohd.hr.state.or.us/chs/pas/ors.htm. However, there were and are considerable lawsuits to block the Oregon initiative, and the federal government, congress, and the courts, have all expressed reservations. Euthanasia and assisted suicide continue to be deeply controversial in Oregon and the rest of the US.

Murder, of course, is no more tolerated in the US, than in the other 11 regions. For example, Jack Kevorkian, on 26 March 1999, was found guilty of homicide in the death of Thomas Youk, a 52-year-old male with Lou Gehrig's disease. Kevorkian was also found guilty of illegally delivering a controlled substance. Some laws, such as those about murder, are universal.

Euthanasia is not often considered an issue at this time for the Native American population on Turtle Island. The most vulnerable time for suicide for Native people is youth and most attention is directed to this phenomenon (EchoHawk, 1997), a situation that has also been observed since 1994 in black South Africans, especially the young in post-apartheid South Africa. There are, of course, laws against causing death among Native people on Turtle Island that have application to the issues of euthanasia and assisted suicide. The Zuni tribe of New Mexico, for example, has a tribal code regarding "Causing a Suicide". There are strong sanctions against such practices.

In Cuba, there exists an article of the Penal Code, "The one who brings help or induces another to suicide, incurs a sanction of prevention of liberty for two to five years." Support among the health professions (e.g., doctors, nurses) is very low in Cuba; 34.5% in a survey supported euthanasia and then only in specific terminal cases (Vergara et al., 1998). Euthanasia and assisted suicide are forbidden in South Africa (although there is growing debate), Australia (except for a few months in the Northern Territory), India and Lithuania. Despite the differences in our regions, we believe that debate about these issues will be essential in the future, as we move towards a global world.

STANDARDS OF CARE AND LIABILITY

Standards of Reasonable and Prudent Care

Care for the suicidal person should be reasonable and prudent. Yet, what is "reasonable" and "prudent"? The community typically defines the yardstick. What is the standard in the community? Given the diversity of views here, there is no *one* standard. Yet, it is about the standards that most commentaries emanate from the US. We should keep in mind that we all have different communities, and thus, standards in one may not be accepted in other countries/communities. The writings of Thomas Gutheil (e.g., 1992), an American and one of the most prolific authors on this topic, espouses the community-based perspective. Gutheil (1992; Gutheil et al., 1983) described the elements in more detail in terms of community, court, and practitioner standards. The community standard—that of suicidologists—refers to what reasonable similarly qualified practitioners would have done. In some countries, such as the US, external circumstances (e.g., available resources) may be taken into account. This would be equally true in such countries as Lithuania, India, Cuba, and so on, especially since these countries lack resources. However, in some countries, such as Australia, the lack of resources does not itself offer protection, if standards are not practised (Cantor & McDermott, 1994).

In Japan, the community also sets the standards of reasonable and prudent care. In addition, the level of medical care, which was offered to a patient in controversy, is often taken into consideration to judge the reasonable standard of care. For example, a psychiatrist working at a medical college hospital is expected to know more about the most accurate and newest information on the side effects of some neuroleptic drugs published in the latest academic journals, than a general practitioner working in a remote rural area. Ireland, the Netherlands, Turtle Island, and South Africa also follow the rules of standards of care. In Cuba, the yardstick is probably applied; but that country is less clear about definition. At a community level, a national suicide prevention programme in Cuba has begun to establish definitions of what constitutes reasonable and prudent care for health professionals—e.g., psychologists, social workers—although practice still dictates that the primary responsibility falls on the family doctor. India and China follow the rule; yet, the overall lack of services is immense owing to the large populations in these nations.

In the former Soviet Union, despite official denial of the public health problem of suicide, the All-Union Scientific Suicidological Centre was established at the Moscow Institute of Psychiatry by Professor Aina Ambrumova at the beginning of the 1970s. It became the first medical institution of studies and treatment of suicide in Russia and became the standard for care in the region. The aim of the establishment was to address, which was unusual for that time, problems of medical care: the discovery of suicidal risk states among healthy people; working out new methods of aid to suicidal people to replace expensive psychiatric hospitalization which fails to adapt them; and, finally, prevention of re-attempts, often observed in the post-suicidal period.

In the 1990s, the rate of completed suicides in Russia exceeded 40 per 100 000. The Ministry of Health of the Russian Federation acknowledged this situation and in May 1998 issued the normative act "On specialized aid to citizens with crisis states and suicidal behaviour". This act sums up more than 20 years' experience of the Federal Suicidological Centre (Moscow) and the experience of some suicidological services in different regions of Russia. It shows the expediency of organizing complex structural departments of similar services; for example, based on crisis telephone service, socio-psychological aid consulting rooms, crisis states departments. The act also determines the staff standards for medical and other personnel of suicidological service departments; and confirms the improvement courses syllabus for suicidologists.

Lithuania offers an interesting point of observation because a reform in the health care system is in progress. In 1995, the Parliament of the Republic of Lithuania adopted the Law of Mental Health Care, creating mental health centres in municipalities. Special postgraduate training is offered to family physicians. Yet, there are few psychiatric care services for special populations. Mental health care for children and teenagers is almost non-existent, except in the largest cities.

People who attempt suicide in Lithuania receive emergency care, but only the immediate somatic condition is assessed and treated. Most attempters leave the hospital immediately after the emergency care, except for those suffering from serious mental illness. Eight psychiatric hospitals provide psychiatric care; but although qualified psychological and psychotherapeutic care is rare, it is developing in larger cities. In smaller communities, where twice as many suicides occur than in the cities, mental health care is lacking. The very first special crisis centres are being founded and telephone crisis services are now available in all cities, but the changes are gradual. The economic situation is still unstable and the reforms in the health service system proceed very slowly, but they are proceeding. Thus, the standards of care are changing and what the community labels as the "standards" is evolving.

Standards of reasonable and prudent care are developing; some are changing; and some are well defined. In conclusion, the standards in each community continue to define what is meant by the "good".

Responsibility of Care

Suicide, as we have learned, has been seen differently historically and currently across the globe. As nations moved away from legislating suicide and suicide attempts as illegal, a mental health perspective was adopted (see Shneidman & Farberow, 1957a), and responsibility for the care was moved to the health professional. Yet, there is no universal perspective on responsibility. The basic guide is reasonable and prudent care. Robert Litman (1988, 1994) and Bruce Bongar (1991; Bongar & Greaney, 1994) have written extensively on the topic. Their work offers major areas of reflection, albeit American.

Litman (1994), for example, offers the hospital setting as a prime example of care. Hospitals, in all countries represented here, are at the forefront of care with suicidal people. Litman asks, "How do we evaluate care?" Patients in hospitals have a right to receive "reasonable care"; yet, as Litman notes, the standards are unclear. Once more, the prevailing standard in the community should be our guide.

The responsibility for care, in all nations/cultures, is with the primary caregivers. This means that the medical doctor, psychiatrist, psychologist, nurse, social worker, crisis workers, and so on are the caregivers, depending on the resources available. Yet, in some traditions such as Turtle Island, responsibility is with the person, the traditional healer, and the community. The truth, of course, is that we need all sources of caregiving—Elders, priests, monks, parents, family members, and so on; in fact, anyone who is on the side of life.

Some regions of the world have set laws. In Japan, for example, according to Japan's Mental Health and Welfare Law, at least two psychiatrists with qualified mental health examiner's licenses should interview a patient, and if they agree that the patient is suffering from mental illness and imminent danger to others or self, the patient should be admitted to treatment, even if it's against the patient's wishes (Takahashi, 1992). In less severe cases, if a psychiatrist recognizes a patient's imminent suicidal risk while treating him at an outpatient clinic, and evaluates that the patient needs hospitalization, the psychiatrist is obliged to explain his/her evaluation to both the patient and the family and refer the patient to a hospital. The psychiatrist should be responsible until the patient is safely hospitalized. The responsibility of other service providers such as psychologists, social workers, and nurses in such situations, however, remains obscure.

In Lithuania, according to the 27 and 28 articles of the Law of Mental Health Care, if in the psychiatrist's opinion, the patient is suffering from mental illness and is in imminent danger to others or self, the psychiatrist may hospitalize a patient at risk for 72 hours. The Mental Health Commission of Municipality should accept the decision. If, within the span of 72 hours, the consent is not given, the involuntary hospitalization and treatment must cease. The responsibility of hospitals and medical personnel is regulated according to the Law on Patients' Rights and Compensation for Damage to Their Health, adopted in October 1996.

In Russia, the doctor–patient relation in the legal system is in an early stage of development due to the following factors: for decades national public health has not been supported by strong progressive legislation; the legislative base in the sphere of health protection has been imperfect; and the monopoly of state property, lack of effective (not declarative) mechanisms to provide the rights of the patients affected it greatly.

To some extent, "The principles of the legislation of the Russian Federation on the health protection of citizens" adopted in 1993 changed the situation for the better. For instance, there is a section, "Responsibility for damage to the health of the citizens", which underlines some general points of this problem. A new criminal Code of Russia adopted in 1997 also deals partly with the questions of responsibility (e.g., failure to help the patient, improper performing of the professional duties by medical personnel). It is quite obvious, however, that the aspects of responsibility, as far as suicidology is concerned, are missing in the above-mentioned laws. They do not appear in the latest law, "On psychiatric aid and guarantees of rights of the citizens who are rendered it" (1993). In this connection, the questions of the responsibility of both hospitals and medical personnel are still solved in accordance with the principles of medical practice.

In other regions, such as Cuba, it is difficult to establish responsibility of care. Institutions, hospitals, specific services/professionals, at different levels of the community, are often responsible. The Mental Health Law, specifically article 20, requires particular care, stipulating hospitalization for those patients at imminent risk. In those cases, two psychiatrists may involuntarily hospitalize a patient at risk; nevertheless, the person has a right to appeal to Revision Court (Ethical Medical Court) if considered competent. However, hospitalization against a person's consent is basically a theoretical stipulation in Cuba because practice dictates against hospitalization if the patient refuses, even in high-risk cases. Finally, there seems to exist the belief in Cuba that when a person kills him/herself, he/she only is responsible for the death.

The person him/herself is central in responsibility on Turtle Island. Traditionally, the main person responsible for one's life after reaching puberty is that person him/herself. Others are not allowed to interfere with what a person is experiencing, and unless that person requests help, or communicates in some way with another person or a traditional healer, the individual will probably be left alone. This, of course, leads to poor communication in the current era when traditions are lost and a person may be experiencing disharmony. This would be especially painful for Native youth not understanding their own traditions. They could translate respect for their privacy as "not caring" and/or not wanting to be "bothered".

The history of the destruction of the cultures and traditions of Native tribes will not be discussed here, but it is important to point out that Native tribes are experiencing the repercussions of lost cultures and traditions (EchoHawk, 1997). Native people are now forced to address issues of death, related to the disproportionately high rates of suicide among the youth. The suicide rate for Native Americans is different from that of non-Native Americans in that the highest rate of suicide for Native people is among the youth, while for non-Native Americans, the highest rate of suicide is among the elderly. However, it should also be noted that suicide rates vary from tribe to tribe. Some tribes have a much lower suicide rate than the general US population, while other tribes have a much higher rate than the general US population. The tribes with the strongest cultures and traditions appear to have the lowest rates.

Native tribes are considered to be sovereign nations and are responsible for developing their own laws to govern their tribes. While no universal standards of reasonable and prudent care have been developed by Native tribes, some tribes have presented serious concerns to Congress which have ultimately ended in legislation at the federal level. One of those laws is Public Law (PL) 99–570, the "Anti-Drug Abuse Act of 1986". This law recognizes the magnitude of the problem of alcoholism and alcohol abuse, which is highly correlated with completed suicides and suicide attempts among Native tribes. Of course, this is true across the world. For example, rates of suicide in Russia have been highly correlated with alcohol consumption.

The (American) Indian Health Service is the main federal health care provider and health advocate for Native people (US Department of Health and Human Services, 1996). Tribes have an option to take over the operation of the Indian Health Services facilities under the authority of a PL 93–638 self-determination contract (Title I) or a PL 93–638 self-governance contract (Title III) (US Department of Health and Human Services, 1996). It is not within the scope of this discussion to make a distinction between the two types of contract. The point to be made is that either the federal or tribal health programmes have the responsibility for care of Native tribes regarding suicide and suicide attempts.

One issue about responsibility of care generally, that we wish to note, is informed consent. Patients have legal and ethical rights to be informed about and participate in measures to prevent their suicide. Their self-destructive state does not obviate this responsibility. Such dialogue, even if the therapist elects to override the patient's ideas, not only fulfils their right but lessens paternalism and regression.

Responsibility for care varies; yet, from a global view, we wish to note that there may be global issues that apply to all (see Cantor & McDermott, 1994). The United Nations Working Group on the Principles for the Protection of Persons with Mental Illness and for the Improvement of Mental Health Care (United Nations, 1991) has, for example, offered some "good" principles. Its first principle on basic rights has as its second clause: "2. All persons with mental illness, or who are being treated as such persons, shall be treated with humanity and respect for the inherent dignity of the human person." Responsibility for care implies humanity and respect in care, otherwise it is not responsibility.

The UN report describes standards of care: "1. Every patient shall have the right to receive such health and social care as appropriate to his or her health needs . . . " and "2. Every patient shall be protected from harm including unjustified medication, abuse by other patients, staff or others, or other acts causing mental distress or physical discomfort." These are issues, we believe, of "the good" in our responsibility (see Cantor & McDermott, 1994).

Failure to Diagnose Properly

Once a mental health worker takes a person into care (even on Turtle Island, if a person has asked a traditional healer for help), he or she must assess the risk of that person being suicidal (Bongar & Greaney, 1994). Many of the care issues in the US, for example, are based on claims of misdiagnosis or failure to diagnose. The issue of diagnosis is universal; indeed, the very first question in care should be: Was the mental health worker's evaluation sufficiently thorough to assess suicidality?

An American case, *Bell* vs *New York City Health and Hospital Corporation* (1982) illustrates this view. In that case, a psychiatrist was found liable for premature release of an inpatient who committed suicide because the psychiatrist's examination of the patient prior to release was judged to be inadequate. He failed, for example, to request prior treatment records or to enquire about the patient's psychotic symptoms. Thus, he failed in assessment.

Yet, there are problems in prediction and assessment. In the Western countries in the 1960s and 1970s, there was a focus on prediction; however, it was soon realized that the statistical rarity of suicide and the imperfection of the prediction instruments led to so many false positives that the instruments had little utility (Beck et al., 1974a). In the 1980s, the focus shifted to assessment; i.e., rather than predicting the future occurrence of suicide in people, the intent was to assess potentially suicidal people in a more general sense, taking into account a multidimensional perspective. Difficulties continued, and in the US, the National Institute of Mental Health (NIMH) organized a think tank on assessment of suicidal behaviour and concluded that few tests, if any, were useful (Lewinsohn et al., 1989). Another overview, by leading suicidologists (Maris et al., 1992), came to the same conclusion. Thus, we are left with the clinician's own skills—which may include tests—to evaluate risk, a task that is enormously complex (Leenaars, 1995). The mental health worker is obliged to assess the risk, despite the problems and imprecisions (Cantor & McDermott, 1994). One sound recommendation with complex situations is a case consultation or conference with all staff and individuals beyond the mental health worker, especially in the community standard area, based on such beliefs. Such a case consultation will assist in diagnosis and may be necessary if a proper assessment is to be made (Takahashi, 1997).

There are more complicated issues, if one goes beyond the Euro–American–Australian view. For example, although there may be greater difficulties in assessing risk in youth than in other ages, a particular problem in assessment occurs with Native youth. Tests have not been normed for Native people, and even clinical cues that are used by psychiatrists and psychologists may not apply. Therefore, greater problems and biases occur with such tools. This will be equally true in applying, for example, American tests or perspectives (even Shneidman's 1985 definition of suicide begins: "In the Western world ... ") to other countries such as Lithuania, Cuba, China, and so forth. Not only are instruments, cues, etc., problematic in our clinical cases, but they may be even more so in their global application.

Failure in Care

There are issues in failure of care beyond assessment. These issues vary from India, with its limited services, to Lithuania, with its developing services, to the US, with its extensive services. Gutheil (1992) and Bongar (1991; Bongar & Greaney, 1994) have written extensively on the topic, although their perspectives are limited to the US and may not apply to even close countries like the Netherlands. Once more, the community defines "failure". The most common American failure issues identified are as follows: (1) failure to predict or diagnose the suicide; (2) failure to control, supervise, or restrain; (3) failure to take proper tests and evaluations of the patient to establish suicidal intent; (4) failure to medicate properly; (5) failure to observe the patient continuously (24 hours) or on a frequent enough basis (e.g., every 15 minutes); (6) failure to take an adequate history; (7) inadequate supervision and failure to remove belts or other dangerous objects; and (8) failure to place the patient in a secure room (see Robertson, 1988, pp. 198–199).

Although various proposals have been advanced for the above failures, typically the results of civil law suits in the US determine the final version of the standard. In *Bell* vs *New York City Health and Hospital Corporation* (1982), the psychiatrist was found to have failed in his care. In contrast, in *Dillman* vs *Hellman* (1973), the psychiatrist was cleared after a psychiatric inpatient jumped to her death when transferred to a less secure ward because the psychiatrist had based his decision on a well-documented and clear assessment. The court ruled that psychiatrists cannot ensure results or cannot be held liable for honest errors of judgement. Negligence on the part of staff, however, provides clear grounds for liability, and is an issue beyond failure. For example, in *Wilson* vs *State* (1961), an attendant forgot to lock a laundry chute, and a psychiatric inpatient jumped through it to her death. The attendant was clearly negligent in his supervision. We will address these issues in more detail below.

Failures in care are issues in all nations. In Japan, the judicial circle now has a consensus that even suicidal patients should be treated in an open atmosphere as long as the treating staffs record the patient's conditions in detail, evaluate suicidal risk repeatedly according to change of the clinical course, and often discuss risk–benefit analysis about the patient's condition and treatment. If the above-stated matters are considered but suicide happens, it is often considered that suicide was unpredictable. Otherwise the treating staff are judged to fail in their proper care of the patient. In Russia, failure in care is not believed to exist. Medical training is based on the following principle: a doctor must be trained in how to cure properly, and this is considered a guarantee from any possible mistakes. Thus, both in medicine and in suicidology, failure in care is rarely reflected and analysed in textbooks and manuals for medical students. As a rule, these issues are only discussed at a practical level, e.g., hospital rounds. However, change is occurring on these and other issues in the medical community of Russia today. In other nations with limited resources (e.g., India, Cuba) or developing resources (e.g., Lithuania), these issues have no consensus and are less clear. In Cuba, for example, problems in the health system, such as lack of qualified personnel, result in internal Ethical Medical Courts—which determine any failure in care—considering whether or not the suicide was unpredictable. Be that as it may, negligence, such as failure to diagnose, may result in sanctions; even suspension from practice, according to the Work Code and to Judicial Decree. Yet, issues such as calculated risk-taking, adequate protection measures, early release, failure to commit, or abandonment as (identified by Bongar and Greaney, 1994), will probably be confronted in Cuba and globally in the future, if not now.

Calculated risk-taking (see Maltsberger, 1994) is an essential element of care today, even in the US with the recent move to limited "managed" care, but it should be calculated, and not flippant or dictated by economics (e.g., insurance coverage). Calculated risk must be taken about hospitalization, discharge, and so on. Hospitalization, especially long-term hospitalization, often promotes regression. Fostering patient improvement commonly entails taking potentially life-threatening risks (Cantor & McDermott, 1994). Adequate prevention means, especially in hospital settings, that one must take reasonable care to safeguard the patient's environment. The abandonment issue is one that is frequently discussed; tersely stated, to abandon a patient is not consistent with Black Elk's "good". It is clear that there is a duty of care to a patient, and if for some reason or another one needs to transfer a patient, the therapist should take full responsibility for ensuring that the transition to another therapist is successful. In the US, further, it is failure in care to abandon a patient if his/her insurance fees run out. Failure to commit and early release are some other issues facing care.

We would be remiss if we did not note one final issue on failure in care. Native people on Turtle Island, and also in Australia, are overly represented in jail. Jail suicide, especially in youth, is a frequent occurrence, and most of these cases involve intoxication. There is a concern that this situation needs to be corrected in order to ensure the safety of the incarcerated person. Careful monitoring of the intoxicated person would be essential until detoxification had taken place. Yet, further safeguards would be needed; in fact, in Australia, Recommendations of the Royal Commission on Aboriginal Death in Custody (Johnston, 1991) made explicit the need for such care. It is likely that other regions and cultures would have their own special issues in care and failure in care.

Liability and Malpractice

What constitutes wrongdoing? What is "foolish"? What is malpractice? When are mental health workers liable? Gutheil (1992) suggested that there are fundamentals of malpractice, related to the following: the existing clinician–patient relationship;

negligence or the breach of duty (although negligence itself does not necessarily equate with liability); the negligence results in specific danger or harm; and the fact that the clinician was negligent resulting in the patient committing suicide (if the element of causation can be determined). Demonstrating causation is often difficult; and Gutheil offers a metaphoric example that best illustrates the issue:

> Consider a camel with serious osteoporosis of the spine, whose back is laden with straw. A final piece of straw (the proverbial "last straw") is placed on the back, and the camel's back breaks. In utilizing a clinical analysis of the situation, the clinician would consider the pre-existing condition of the camel and its back, the burden posed by the pre-existing straw, and the final straw leading to the condition of clinical compensation. (Gutheil, 1992, p. 150)

The legal viewpoint, at least in the US, focuses on the last straw, which is called the "proximate cause". The question is a "but for", and we quote Gutheil again, "But for this last straw, the camel's back would not have been broken" (p. 150). In suicide, the relation is more perplexing; yet, the metaphor applies. The question is, did the (failure in care) (negligence) cause the suicide? The answer lies in the statement "Dereliction of a duty directly causing dangers" (Gutheil, 1992, p. 150). Dereliction has application to in-hospital suicide, outpatient suicide, suicide after release; especially, misuse or non-use of medication, and so on. In all of these situations, are we acting like the hunter in Black Elk's story who acted in a negligent way, causing probable damage to the woman, or are we acting like the good hunter?

Malpractice and liability issues across the world are diverse, and even if they resemble those in the US, such as in Australia, Ireland, and the Netherlands, there are differences. For example, in the US, negligence, as defined by the American Learned Hand rule of 1947, refers to failure to invest resources up to a level commensurate with anticipated saving in dangers (Gutheil et al., 1983). This differs from Australia's approach regarding negligence as a breach of duty of care, and not some cost–benefit analysis (Cantor & McDermott, 1994). Thus, even if the laws appear to be the same, there are differences. Once more, caution is in order when comparing one country/culture with another. US laws cover staff working with Native people in America; yet, even here, there are traditional tribal practices that may result in complexities in malpractice issues.

Most countries/cultures have laws against causing suicide. These issues were somewhat addressed earlier, under Euthanasia and Assisted Suicide; yet, we will provide a few further examples here. In Cuba, there are two groups of sanctions that apply to medical and mental health workers. These sanctions are gathered in the Work Code and in a Judicial Decree. Negligence (affecting the life of a person) constitutes one of the most severely sanctioned behaviours. According to Judicial Decree a person "Acting with manifest negligence or indolence in the fulfilment of his/her work, contents and orders, implying serious alteration of health services due to the production of heavy irreversible lesions or death due to the patient" may be removed from the National Health System. There are less severe sanctions for other behaviours such as "the unfulfilment of medical indications or the delegation of a technical function to an unauthorised personnel" or "the unfulfilment of the obligation established for the performance of his/her function, or of the internal disposition of the Centre". In these cases the person may be moved from his/her place of work temporarily or definitely or may be separated from his/her centre. Yet, it is difficult to establish responsibility in many cases and there is a belief in Cuba that when the suicidal person had died, he/she is the only person responsible for the death. To date, there have been no reported malpractice suits due to suicide. The same is generally true in most regions. In Japan, for example, although attention is gradually being paid to malpractice suits for a patient's suicide, the number of malpractice suits due to suicide is still much fewer than those of malpractice suits due to improper treatments or operations for other physical illnesses.

Let us return, in conclusion, to the advice of Gutheil (1992), which may be globally applicable in some fashion to all. He suggests that the approach to liability prevention should involve responsible and prudent assessment, responsible and prudent intervention, and durable documentation and consultation. Regardless of one's culture/nation, maintaining the "good" standard of care prevails.

FURTHER ETHICAL AND PROFESSIONAL CONCERNS

Means Restriction

The two main traditional solutions for preventing suicide have been the clinical treatment of suicidal people (e.g., traditional healing, medication, psychotherapy, and hospitalization) and the establishment of suicide prevention centres and community programmes (e.g., schools). However, there is a third approach, which is called controlling the environment. A report from the WHO (Bertolote, 1993) provided six basic steps to prevention. All but one, the treatment of psychiatric inpatients, are consistent with controlling the environment: gun possession control, detoxification of domestic gas, detoxification of car emissions, control of toxic substance availability, and toning down reports in the press. All these measures could be applied to all the regions discussed here. Means restriction is especially important. Means restriction would include several of these approaches (e.g., gun control, control of toxic substance availability). Guns are a frequent means of suicide, especially in the US, and research on gun control (see Leenaars et al., 1998a) shows that this may be a useful tactic to prevent suicide.

In Russia, the rate of firearm suicides has dramatically increased from the beginning of the 1990s, and this is also true for attempted suicide. For example, in the Kemerovo region, attempted suicide by firearms has increased by 30% over the past few years. This increase stems from the availability of guns, which became possible for the following reasons: Firstly, in post-Soviet Russia, the system of selling firearms has changed greatly. It means that, nowadays, any citizen who has no previous convictions and is not registered with a psychiatrist can easily obtain a firearm from a specialized store. Secondly, the USSR disintegration gave rise to the black market sales of firearms with quite reasonable prices (for instance, an up-to-date model of an automatic Kalashnikov costs only a few thousand US dollars). Thirdly, continuous local conflicts, which occur in the territory of the former Soviet Union (Tadjikistan, Georgia, Chechnya, etc.), have become a source of unregistered firearms. Finally, regional peculiarities of some territories of the country may be the reason for the cases of suicides by explosives. These kinds of suicides take place in the Kemerovo region (the largest coal-mining basin of the country) where miners commit suicide by self-explosion. It is thus easy to conclude that the availability of lethal means may be related to the increase in suicide and attempted suicide.

Most countries have strict gun laws, but not the US. The Netherlands has strict gun laws and recent changes in 1986 made them even more controlled, addressing such global issues as international trade in guns and ammunition. The laws about gun ownership in Ireland are very strict. In Cuba, it is prohibited to sell, buy, or carry firearms, and only authorized personnel (e.g., police and army) may possess them. Gun control is in place in almost all the nations presented, except the USA.

Legal issues have had some impact on efforts to prevent suicide by restricting access to lethal means for suicide in the US. The sale of any medication must first be approved by the Food and Drug Administration (FDA) which also monitors adverse effects, including accidental and suicidal overdoses. However, so far, the FDA has not restricted the sale of antidepressants on the basis of their subsequent mortality rate. Gun control is even more problematic. Gun control laws in the US can be passed at federal, state, and local levels. Guns have been restricted on occasion primarily in an effort to decrease their use in criminal acts. The fact that restricting access to guns may reduce their use for suicide (Leenaars & Lester, 1998) has been a byproduct of the legislation. Finally, civil suits to recover damages for loss of life have been the primary impetus for some jurisdictions to also address other means of suicide, namely the fencing in of bridges (and high buildings), which have become popular venues for suicide. One bridge in Washington, DC, is now fenced in, and protective barriers have recently been installed on the Golden Gate Bridge in San Francisco. Of course, one could attempt to control the environment in different ways. In South Africa, for example, the world's first installation of 24-hour emergency telephones, manned by trained personnel on the Van Staden's River Bridge in Eastern Cape, was implemented. The bridge is one of the highest bridges in the country and was known in the community as "Suicide Bridge".

Referring to gun control as a means of suicide prevention in the US probably makes sense because it is that country's main method of suicide. However, in other countries, guns are not used so frequently. For example, in Cuba, firearms are the least frequent means of committing suicide in the nation. Meanwhile, hanging is the most common for men and fire the most frequent for women. The main method in Lithuania is hanging. In India, the common methods are poisoning by insecticides/pesticides and hanging. Hanging and drowning are the most popular in Ireland. Thus, one can see great variation in means and, although gun control may make little sense in some regions, the tactic of controlling the environment may still have applicability.

Japan, for example, has a very strict gun control law, only 0.3% of suicide victims use guns (National Police Agency, 1997). The vast majority of people who used guns were policemen, soldiers, and criminals. One recent example of restricting the means of suicide however, involves a reduction in the availability of poisonous Paraquat. The number of deaths by Paraquat in Japan increased dramatically from 594 in 1984 to 1021 in 1985. Among the 1021 deaths in 1985, 96.5% were suicides (National Police Agency, 1986). One of the most serious reasons for this sharp increase was that there were a series of indiscriminate killings using Paraquat. Victims got, from vending machines, soft drinks that were contaminated by Paraquat. Similar crimes happened all over Japan by drinking soft drinks contaminated by Paraquat, which in 1985 killed a total of 17 innocent people. Since the mass media reported this criminal act sensationally, Paraquat has become widely known to be extremely lethal.

Paraquat, which used to be purchased easily at gardening shops in Japan, is now only available upon production of detailed documentation by the buyer. In addition, vivid coloration, an offensive odour and emetics have been added to the chemical to make it unpalatable for anyone considering suicide. In addition, its commercial concentration has been reduced to make it less lethal (the Asahi Shimbun, 1985; Poisonous Substance Control Act, Revised, 1986). The National Police Agency conducted the Poisonous Substance Control Campaign in February 1986 and cooperated with related agencies to control Paraquat and other poisonous substances in an attempt to prevent crime using these substances. The number of suicides employing this herbicide has greatly decreased since that time.

Thus, although further research is needed (Leenaars et al., 1998a) means restriction and the more general approach of controlling the environment, may be a viable strategy to prevent suicide in all regions. Yet, despite the research and the recommendations of the WHO, there has been little impact on clinical practice globally. The lack of education about means restriction is a clear example. The study by Wislar et al. (1998), for example, exemplifies this absence. They conducted a chart review of youth receiving mental health evaluation, with 40% being suicide related, in an emergency department of a hospital. Chart reviews provided no evidence that means restriction education was provided. This is a failure in care and this applies not only to guns but to other means. There are broad implications globally in the care and failure in care of suicidal persons.

Postvention

Postvention, a term introduced by Shneidman (1975), refers to those things done after the event has occurred. Postvention deals with the traumatic after-effects in the survivors of a person who has committed suicide (or in those close to someone who has attempted suicide). It involves offering mental health services to the bereaved survivors.

Postvention services vary. They are almost non-existent in some countries (e.g., Cuba, India, Russia) and are only developing in some; for example, Lithuania recently developed its first programme in schools following the suicide of a student. Other countries, such as Ireland, have recently identified a gap in this area of care. The National Task Force in Ireland on suicide, in fact, recently identified postvention in all aspects being a major goal for future development in care. While the Samaritans have been a presence for many years in the support of the bereaved by suicide, in the past few years there has been a proliferation of support groups set up by voluntary organizations and health boards. As yet, however, no guidelines or standards of training for mental health workers in this field have been established and this is now a matter of urgency in Ireland.

Hopefully, in the wake of the publication of Ireland's Task Force report suitable structures and procedures will be put in place to address all of these issues. Already the health boards responsible for the administration of the health services in Ireland have set up local task forces to examine the recommendations of the National Task Force and find appropriate ways of adapting them and implementing them appropriately to local conditions and needs.

There continues to be a reluctance to develop postvention strategies. Japan illustrates the reluctance in such services. There is still a strong stigma towards suicide in Japan. When suicide unfortunately happens, Japanese people behave as if nothing took place. They believe that only time would heal the wound of the survivors and nobody outside the family needs to care for them. Survivors themselves feel that suicide is a shame for the family, who wish to be left alone and do not seek help from outsiders. In this atmosphere of the society, few efforts have been made for postvention in Japan. At present there are no self-help groups for the survivors of suicide in Japan, although there are numerous groups for those who lose significant others by accidents or physical illnesses. When suicide happens at school, at present there are almost no efforts of postvention by mental health professionals.

Other regions, such as Australia, the Netherlands, the US, have greater developed programmes; in fact, in the US survivors have taken a leadership role in not only providing postvention but also in preventing suicide. We believe that these directions are important because postvention is one of the best measures for legal self-defence, as well as being humane (the "good").

Gutheil (1992) and Bongar (1991; Bongar & Greaney, 1994) strongly advocate for postvention when a patient has committed suicide. Gutheil (1992) provides it as the fifth item in his list of approaches to liability prevention. Such approaches range from attending the funeral to outreach towards the survivors. Outreach, at times, may be ethically necessary and clinically crucial (Gutheil, 1992). Further, Bongar and Greaney (1994) suggest that malpractice action is often taken because of bad feelings, and if the clinician reaches out, feelings of abandonment are immediately addressed. Survivors informed about the context of the suicide are often relieved. As Gutheil (1992) notes, postvention is one of the best antidotes towards potential litigation. Yet, of course, confidentiality continues after death (Cantor & McDermott, 1994), although the content can be discussed in general terms, such as publicly known facts about depression, hospitalization, the death, without infringing on the confidentiality of the deceased. Postvention may also be a vehicle to providing information about survivor services in that community, if needed. Clinicians themselves may be in need of postvention. We too are at risk for the aftershocks world wide.

CONCLUDING REMARKS

The ethical and legal issues discussed have applicability globally. Yet, regions and cultures also have their own unique issues that go beyond the scope of our current project. Each nation needs its own study.

In the current project, we began our discussion about ethics and laws with Black Elk's guiding story advocating the "good". We could have equally begun with Plato's analogy of the cave (Hamilton & Cairns, 1961). In the analogy, people are depicted as fettered in their mind, seeing only shadows. One person becomes free of the illusions and sees the truth and travels further out of the cave to see the sun— the "good", the "just". In Black Elk's story and Plato's analogy, we are presented with the ethical and legal realities of everyday practical work with our suicidal patients. We constantly must decide to smoke the pipe—the "good".

We do not wish to suggest that we know the "good", or have smoked Black Elk's pipe or have seen Plato's sun. We only have our perspectives. These constructions are, we hope, better than one view alone. Indeed, we hope that our discussion will bring all of us somewhat closer to the good, the just, and so forth in suicidology world wide. Finally, we encourage our communities to respond to our dialogue on these difficult and complex issues as we embark on this millennium.

Chapter 22

MUNCH, DOSTOEVSKY, VAN GOGH, AND A LITTLE BIT OF MELVILLE

Many of us associate Edvard Munch's "The Scream" with suicide. It is a motif of the suicidal PAIN. Those of us who have seen "The Scream" resonate to its base expression of the inner turmoil of deep anguish, a window to Munch's mind—and the suicidal mind.

Edvard Munch's mother died when he was 2 years old and his beloved sister when he was 13, immortalized in his paintings, "The Dead Mother and Child," and "The Sick Child", respectively. Munch's family had a history of depression. He struggled all his life with attachment, despair, anxiety, jealousy, rejection, and so on, most strongly expressed in the "accidental" (?) shooting of his hand, when his female friend Tulla Larsen abandoned him (the association to Vincent Van Gogh's cutting off of his ear is obvious).

"The Scream" occurred on a trip to Ekebergsåsen. In his diary, Munch wrote:

> I was walking along a path with two friends
> the sun was setting
> I felt a breath of melancholy
> Suddenly the sky turned blood-red
> I stopped and leant against the railing,
> deathly tired
> looking out across flaming clouds that hung
> like—blood and a sword over the
> deep blue fjord and town
> My friends walked on—I stood
> there trem-
> bling with anxiety
> and I felt a great, infinite scream pass
> through nature.

Munch's paintings and life are worthy of extensive study. This is the role of research. Munch himself lived to be 88 years old, surviving years of unbearable pain. About one of his equally famous paintings, "Anxiety", Munch wrote:

> I saw all the people behind their masks—smiling, phlegmatic—composed faces—I saw through them and there was suffering—in them all—pale corpses—who without rest ran around—along a twisted road—at the end of which was the grave.

This is the suicidal mind. This is the suicidal brain.

Research helps us to understand the mask, the complexity—biological, psycho-logical, sociological, cultural, and so on—which lead some people to the suicidal abyss. Yet, research needs to do more; it should lead to effective intervention. In my day-to-day life, I see patients and I want to know what works. We need to know better how to reach through the suicidal mask.

The suicidal mind is, indeed, a mask. How can we understand this scream? As we have learned, like patients' stories, suicide notes are windows to the mind; they are a way through the looking glass. Here are a few more suicide notes:

> Dear Papa, I am twenty-three years old and I still have accomplished nothing. I am certain that I will never amount to anything, so I have decided to end my life . . .

Another person, N.N., ended his long suicide note with the suicidal "therefore", as follows:

> Therefore, in my uncontrovertible capacity as plaintiff and defendant, judge and ac-cused, I condemn this Nature, which has so brazenly and unceremoniously inflicted this suffering, to annihilation along with me . . . Since I am unable to destroy Nature, I am destroying only myself, solely out of the weariness of enduring a tyranny in which there is no guilty party.
> N.N.

These notes are a few of a large trove of notes collected by a researcher of the mind. He came across the notes accidentally when a clerk of a judicial system revealed that he had been keeping them for years. The researcher was Fyodor Dostoevsky.

Dostoevsky's collection (Dostoevsky, 1994) of suicide notes was written in the 1870s; they are a unique window to suicidal people of those times (and of all times).

Dostoevsky's study (as we had seen about Goethe's) suggests that he was a su-perb suicidologist. Dostoevsky battled against his own deep anguish; he is known to have made two suicide attempts (Orbach, 2003). As these are only endnotes, I will be brief and leave it to the reader to read Dostoevsky's insights into the suicidal mind—and suicidal mask. Dostoevsky and Shneidman (1985) both write about pain, "morbid anxiety", mental constriction, dissembling, escape, and so on. Dostoevsky puzzled in his diaries on the ever-present suicidal person, who leaves no clues, much like Shneidman and me. About N.N., the person who wrote one of the above notes, Dostoevsky mused:

> The man I told you about who committed suicide is indeed a passionate exponent of his idea—that is, the necessity of suicide—and not an indifferent or "cast-iron" sort of person. He is truly tormented and suffering, and I think I conveyed that clearly enough. It is all too clear to him that he cannot go on living, and he is utterly convinced that he is correct and cannot be refuted. He cannot escape confronting the highest and most fundamental questions: "What is the point of living when he is already aware that it is disgusting, abnormal, and inadequate for a human to live like an animal? And what is there to keep him living on earth in such a case?" He can find no answers to these questions and he knows it, for although he has realized that there exists, as he expresses it, "a harmony of the whole", still, he says, "I don't understand it and I never will be able to understand it. That I will never be able to share in that harmony is

the necessary and inevitable conclusion." And it was this sort of clear-cut conclusion that led him to his end. (pp. 734–735)

Fyodor Dostoevsky, author of such insightful novels as, *Notes from the Underground* (a favourite of mine in my late adolescence), concluded from his study that people kill themselves "precisely because their suffering has become unbearable". I echo this view. To know the mask, you have to know the person. You have to resonate to his or her pain, a psychache. To reach through the mask, you have to ask, "Please tell me who you are and where do you hurt?"

Not only Edvard Munch's paintings, but also Vincent van Gogh's paintings are associated to suicide. "Cornfield and Crows"—my favourite painting—is an obvious example. I will illustrate my view on psychotherapy with suicidal people with this last case study of Vincent van Gogh.

Vincent van Gogh was born in Zundert, the Netherlands on 30 March 1853. He was born to the village pastor, Theodorus, and his wife, Anna. As an aside, Zundert is a village next to my own village, Ulvenhout. As a child, I often heard about a famous painter from Zundert, but how crazy he was. I recall visits to the church and, later, a wonderful large statue of Vincent and his brother, Theo, holding each other for eternity. Only later did I learn how famous he really was and how he probably suffered from a manic-depressive disorder as others probably did in his family (Jamieson, 1993).

Vincent was born exactly one year to the day after the death of a brother, also named Vincent (see Honour, 1967; Jamieson, 1993, 1995; Lester, 2000; and Roskill, 2000, for details of this narrative). Vincent had the same number for a birth certificate. Anna, his mother, never recovered from her loss. She did not like Vincent; she wanted the first Vincent. No trust ever developed.

Theodorus and Anna had five other children after Vincent (in birth order): Anna, Theo, Elizabeth, Wilhelmina, and Cornelius. Like our Justin, all these children lived in a depressed household and suffered deeply throughout their lives. Every Sunday, for example, Anna would take the children to the cemetery to be with her beloved first Vincent. Vincent, like his siblings, grew up feeling unloved and rejected. Vincent van Gogh was often reminded that his mother wanted the real Vincent.

There is, of course, much more to Vincent's life. He struggled endlessly with his painting, but he never sold a painting during his life, only a few drawings. And even sadder, Vincent never developed a loving attachment. He had loved Ursula Loyer, the daughter of his landlord, while he held a short post as a preacher in London before he started his painting career. (Vincent, early on, tried careers as an art dealer, preacher, and teacher, all with little success.) Ursula never knew about Vincent's love. A similar unrequited love occurred when Vincent fell in love with a cousin, Kee Vos, who was widowed. When Kee learned of Vincent's love, she was horrified and rejected him. Kee had told Vincent, "No, never, never." In a letter to Theo, dated 3 November 1881, Vincent wrote, "Should I accept her 'no, never, never', or considering the question as not completed and decided, should I keep some hope and not give up?" Vincent kept his pursuit, but his love, like Werther's for Lotte, was unrequited. Vincent's logic was problematic (somewhat akin to Dr Shneidman's analysis of Natalie's logic). Vincent wrote:

> Then I thought: I should like to be with a woman, I cannot live without love, without a woman. I would not set any value on life, if there were not something infinite, something deep, something real. But then I said to myself: you said "she and no other", and you would go to another woman now, that is unreasonable, that is against all logic. And my answer to that was: who is the master, the logic or I, is the logic there for me or am I there for the logic, and is there no reason and no sense in my unreasonableness and lack of sense? And whether I do right or wrong, I cannot act otherwise, that damned wall is too cold for me, I need a woman, I cannot, I may not, I will not live without love. I am but a man, and a man with passions, I must go to a woman, otherwise I freeze or turn to stone, or in short am stunned. (Roskill, 2000, p. 138)

Yet, there was a great battle within Vincent. He suffered deeply from what he called "melancholy". Vincent, in fact, exhibited an incident of self-mutilation in his aftershocks, well before the well-known ear incident. Kee Vos had to go to Amsterdam; she and her parents refused to see Vincent when he pursued her there. Upon the refusal, he burned his hand in an oil lamp. He felt totally (narcissistically) rejected and struggled with his rage.

After Kee, in 1882, Vincent moved to The Hague, and met a vagrant, Christine. She too soon abandoned him. In 1884, Vincent had returned to his parents' home. The neighbour had a daughter, Margot, two years Vincent's senior. She was shy. Vincent fell in love with her and she requited his love, but when Vincent asked to marry her, Margot's father refused. Vincent again was rejected. Margot, once she learned of the refusal, attempted suicide; yet, Margot's parents continued the refusal. Vincent's parents offered no support, and once more his mother rejected him. Shortly after his father died in 1885, Vincent was told to leave the village. He felt rejected by everyone.

After the death of his father, Vincent feared a breakdown. In 1886, he moved to Paris to live with his brother and main life-support, Theo. It is known that at this point, Vincent bought a revolver. He continued to struggle, and began to drink more. He quarrelled with everyone and moved to Arles, wanting to start a school for artists (a dream never realized). We all know the story of the visit by Paul Gauguin in October of 1888. The relationship was deeply problematic and ambivalent. Van Gogh so wanted the relationship (attachment) to work; he wanted Gauguin's acceptance ("I have done two canvasses of falling leaves, which Gauguin liked, I think"). The relationship was, however, "terribly electric". Gauguin claimed that Vincent even tried to kill him. Gauguin alleged to have woken up twice, while in van Gogh's home, to find van Gogh moving towards him. Gauguin decided to leave. About 23 December 1888, Vincent wrote to Theo:

> I think myself that Gauguin was a little out of sorts with the good town of Arles, the little yellow house where we work, and especially with me.
>   As a matter of fact there are bound to be for him as for me further grave difficulties to overcome here.
>   But these difficulties are rather within us than outside.
>   Altogether I think that either he will definitely go, or else definitely stay.
>   Before doing anything I told him to think it over and reckon things up again.

> Gauguin is very powerful, strongly creative, but just because of that he must have peace.
> Will he find it anywhere if he does not find it here?
> I am waiting for him to make a decision with absolute serenity.
>
> (Roskill, 2000, p. 303)

The arguments continued; reports suggest that on 24 December Vincent was in "a state of terrible excitement and high fever". Gauguin was out on the street, and Vincent came at him, holding a razor. Vincent fled to his study, where he cut off his right ear. He tied a scarf around his head, put the severed ear in an envelope and gave it to a familiar girl, a prostitute, on the street. Vincent was hospitalized.

After hospitalization, Vincent van Gogh was exhausted. He felt such pain, describing his suffering as "anguish" and "emptiness". He continued to describe his mood in his letters as one of "melancholia", a term at the time for depression. He often thought of suicide and wrote about the topic ("suicide") to Theo. He once wrote to Theo, "I can understand why people drown themselves." Vincent saw only pain and "'no luck' in the future", only more anguish. He felt fearful and "cowardly". He was "paralysed". Vincent continued to not only struggle with the current situation, but also his history haunted him. This was most noteworthy about his parents. On 23 January 1889, Vincent wrote to Theo:

> Whatever I think on other points, our father and mother were exemplary as married people.
> And I shall never forget Mother at Father's death, when she only said one small word: it made me begin to love dear old Mother more than before. In fact as married people our parents were exemplary, like Roulin and his wife, to cite another instance.
> Well, go straight ahead along that road. During my illness I saw again every room of the house at Zundert, every path, every plant in the garden, the views from the fields round about, the neighbours, the graveyard, the church, our kitchen garden behind—down to the magpie's nest in a tall acacia in the graveyard.
> It's because I still have earlier recollections of those first days than any of the rest of you. There is no one left who remembers all this but Mother and me.
> I say no more about it, since it is better that I should not try to recall all that passed through my head then. (Roskill, 2000, p. 308)

Vincent regressed and in May 1889 he moved into an asylum in Saint-Remy. Here he learned to accept his illness, calling it "a fracture of the brain" and "a disease". Despite his seeming acceptance of his illness and feeling comfortable with the insanity of the other patients, Vincent's suffering was for him endless, having made several suicide attempts while at the asylum. Most likely these cyclical but acute troubling episodes were associated to manic (mood) attacks. He cycled often at these times, lacking in receiving modern-day, effective treatment, such as medication (Lithium) and psychotherapy.

While in Saint-Remy, he continued to paint. Indeed, his doctors encouraged him to paint. Van Gogh himself wrote to Theo, how his painting expressed his pain, "sadness", "loneliness". It was van Gogh's most effective anodyne. In April 1890, he went back to Paris. Theo had arranged for lodgings in a nearby town of Auvers with a doctor named Gachet. Yet, van Gogh began to fight with Gachet, almost immediately. Vincent thought that Dr Gachet was sicker than he was.

"Dr Gachet", remarked van Gogh in his letters, "hated it all." At these times, Vincent also continued to think about his pain. To Theo, in his penultimate letter, Vincent wrote, "I beg you, tell Mother and our sister that I think of them very often, also I had a letter from them this morning and will reply soon." This attachment was iatrogenic, repeated elliptically in his relationships, the final one with Dr Gachet. After one quarrel with the doctor, Vincent pulled out the revolver, but did not fire it. Vincent went back to his room and wrote a letter, his penultimate act. He felt that he was a nobody at this time, as he had been almost all of his life. After writing the letter, which was found on van Gogh's body, Vincent walked out to the countryside and shot himself. It was the 27th of July. Vincent once wrote, "One should learn to go on living, even if one is suffering." In the end, van Gogh, however, could not bear his suffering, and suicide became the only solution.

Vincent van Gogh had shot himself in the abdomen and was able to return to his room. Theo arrived the next day. Vincent died the next morning, 29 July 1890, at the age of 37. Theo himself never recovered, and had a mental breakdown. In a letter home, Theo wrote about Vincent's death and said, "Life was such a burden to him." The pain had become unbearable. Vincent's skeletons became Theo's. Theo van Gogh could not survive the suicide of his beloved Vincent and died on 25 January 1891.

Vincent van Gogh was not only a great painter; he, if you read his letters, was a prolific writer (Roskill, 2000). There are extensive collections of his letters, which, as we learned, allow us an intimate understanding of Vincent's life and suicide. They allow us to truly understand this individual, like the other people we met in this book. Here is van Gogh's suicide letter, addressed to Theo:

> My dear brother,
>   Thanks for your kind letter and for the 50 fr. Note it contained . . . Since the thing that matters most is going well, why should I say more about things of less importance; my word, *before we have chance of talking business more collectedly, there is likely to be a long way to go. . .*
>   The other painters, whatever they think of it, instinctively keep themselves at a distance from discussions about actual trade.
>   Well, the truth is, we can only make our pictures speak. But still, my dear brother, there is this that I have always told you, and I repeat it once more with all the earnestness that can be imparted by an effort of a mind diligently fixed on trying to do as well as one can—I tell you again that I shall always consider that you are something other than a simple dealer in Corot, that through my mediation you have your part in the actual production of some canvases, which even in the cataclysm retain their quietude.
>   For this is what we have got to, and this is all or at least the chief thing that I can have to tell you at a moment of comparative crisis. At a moment when things are very strained between dealers in pictures by dead artists, and living artists.
>   Well, my own work, I am risking my life for it and my reason has half-foundered owing to it—that's all right—but you are not among the dealers in men so far as I know, and you can choose your side, I think, acting with true humanity, but what's the use?

How can we understand van Gogh? The TGSP for his last note is as follows: 1, 2, 3, 4, 5, 6, 7, 10, 12, 13, 16, 17, 19, 20, 21, 23, 24, 25, 26, 31 (the dealers), 33, 34, 35. On the TGSP-2, the transposed scores are as follows: 1, 2, 3, 4, 5, 9, 12, 13, 14, 16, 17, 19, 20,

21, 22, 23, 25, 28, 30, 31, 32, 33, 35. Each is a different perspective on Vincent's last letter. Of course, like all stories, they are open to further Carnapian points of view.

Van Gogh was in PAIN, "a moment of comparative crisis." He called it a "cataclysm". All was not well, as one can read in an earlier letter, at the home of Dr Gachet, but there was a deeper pain. Vincent writes, "Things are very strained between dealers in pictures by dead artists, and living artists." Vincent was not selling his paintings—his generativity was not seen. He was forlorn and distressed. He did not see a solution. Were dead artists' paintings selling better? His own paintings did after his death. Was he hopeless about his paintings, mental state, and even Theo? Theo had married, had a child and was focused on his own affairs. This upset Vincent. What does Vincent really mean in his letter to Theo? Does he dissemble? One can read the ambivalence. There was such a deep history to his pain and his family's pain. Several siblings suffered like Vincent from depression. Theo struggled with his moods. His youngest sister, Wilhelmina, is known to have suffered a mental collapse and was hospitalized for decades. His youngest brother, Cornelius, is also believed to have killed himself at the age of 33. What all happened in their history? What were the biological markers? What were the essential elements of his intrapsychic drama? What were the critical aspects of the interpersonal stage? What were the unconscious processes in the van Gogh family and in Vincent's mind?

Vincent could not cope; he finds himself at the end exhausted and weak. He says that he cannot develop constructive relationships with dealers and others. He feels isolated. One can read, as in his paintings from this period, the unresolved problems. Vincent was defeated. His needs, especially attachment (affiliation), achievement, exhibition, and defendence, were frustrated and thwarted. His life had become exceedingly stressful to a "cataclysmic" degree. He wanted a way to go on living, but did not see it forthcoming ("no luck"). He suffered too many narcissistic injuries. He was intimately identified with his paintings, but he sold none. He felt so rejected and wanted to escape. He wrote, "Well, my own work, I am risking my life for it." He concluded to Theo—what is the latent meaning—as follows: "... you are not among the dealers in men so far as I know, and you can choose your side, I think, acting with true humanity, but what's the use?" The "what's the use?" is a concludifying, what Shneidman has called a lethal (suicidal) syllogistic conclusion. Dostoevsky's N.N. and Vincent came to the same "therefore." Vincent intended to kill himself—he says so in his penultimate act, his letter, a window to his mind and the suicidal mind.

What could we have done to help? Could Vincent's suicide have been stopped? Would psychotherapy have helped? There was so much pain and anguish, a psychache in his life. What would have worked to prevent his death? And why did Munch survive his pain, and van Gogh not? What were Munch's protective factors? Why did Jeff die and Susan survive? These are the most important idiographic (individual) questions. These are some of the questions one asks in person-centred psychotherapy. Did the attachments that Edvard Munch received help him to await the suicidal abyss? Why did Vincent and Rick jump into death? And, what could we have done to prevent these needless deaths?

In Herman Melville's—who was an equally troubled soul—monumental study of people's anguish and suicide, *Moby Dick*, Chapter 36, "The Quarter Deck", Captain Ahab—a personification of "The Scream"—speaks:

> Hark ye yet again—the little lower layer. All visible objects, man, are but as pasteboard masks. But in each event—in the living act, the undoubted deed—there some unknown but still reasoning thing puts forth the mouldings of its features from behind the unreasoning mask. If man will strike, strike through the mask! How can the prisoner reach outside except by thrusting through the wall.

We—researchers, clinicians, survivors, and so on—must understand and reach through the suicidal mask. There are research-based practices. Suicide can be prevented.

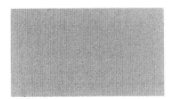

REFERENCES

Aaron, D. (Ed.) (1985). *The Inman diary: A public and private confession* (2 vols). Cambridge: Harvard University Press.

Abbey, S., Hood, E., Young, L. & Malcolmson, S. (1993). Psychiatric consultation in the eastern Canadian Arctic: III. Mental health issues in Inuit women in the eastern Arctic. *Canadian Journal of Psychiatry, 38,* 32–35.

Albom, M. (1997). *Tuesdays with Morrie.* New York: Doubleday.

Achenbach, T. (1974). *Developmental psychopathology.* New York: Ronald.

Adler, A. (1967). Contributions to discussions of Vienna Psychoanalytic Society—1910. In P. Friedman (Ed.), *On Suicide.* New York: International Universities Press. (Original work published 1910.)

Aldenderfer, M. & Blashfield, R. (1984). *Cluster analysis.* Beverly Hills: Sage.

Allport, G. (1942). *The use of personal documents in psychological science.* New York: Social Science Research Council.

Allport, G. (1962). The general and the unique in psychological science. *Journal of Personality, 30,* 405–422.

American Psychiatric Association (1987). *Diagnostic and statistical manual of mental disorders* (3rd edn, rev.) (DSM-III-R). Washington, DC: Author.

American Psychiatric Association (1994). *Diagnostic and statistical manual of mental disorders* (4th edn) (DSM-IV). Washington, DC: Author.

Anastasi, A. (1982). *Psychological testing,* (5th edn). New York: Macmillan.

Arbeit, S. & Blatt, S. (1983). Differentiation of simulated and genuine suicide notes. *Psychological Reports, 33,* 283–293.

Asberg, M., Nordstrom, P. & Traskman-Bendz, L. (1986). Biological factors in suicide. In A. Roy (Ed.), *Suicide* (pp. 47–71). Baltimore: Williams & Wilkins.

Asberg, M., Traskman, L. & Thorien, P. (1976). 5-H1AA in cerebrospinal fluid: A biochemical suicide prediction? *Archives of General Psychiatry, 33,* 1193–1197.

Axline, U. (1947). *Play therapy.* New York: Random House.

Ayer, A. (Ed.) (1959). *Logical positivism.* New York: Free Press.

Bailley, S., Kral, M. & Dunham, K. (1999). Survivors of suicide do grieve differently: Empirical support for a common sense proposition. *Suicide and Life-Threatening Behavior, 29,* 256–271.

Balance, W. & Leenaars, A. (1991). Suicide in middle adulthood. In A. Leenaars (Ed.), *Life span perspectives of suicide* (pp. 137–151). New York: Plenum.

Bandura, A. (1977). *Social learning theory.* Englewood Cliffs: Prentice-Hall.

Barnes, R. (1986). The recurrent self-harm patient. *Suicide and Life-Threatening Behavior, 16,* 399–408.

Barraclough, B. (1986). Illness and suicide. In J. Morgan (Ed.), *Suicide: Helping those at risk* (pp. 61–65). London: King's College.

Barter, J. & Weist, K. (1970). *Historical and contemporary patterns of northern Cheyenne suicide.* Unpublished manuscript.

Battegay, R. (1990). Suicide notes: Predictive clues and patterns [Review of *Suicide Notes*]. *Crisis, 11*, 74–75.

Battin, M. (1993). Suicidology and the right to die. In A. Leenaars (Ed.), *Suicidology: Essays in honor of Edwin Shneidman* (pp. 377–398). Northvale, NJ: Aronson.

Beck, A. (1963). Thinking and depression I. Idiosyncratic content and cognitive distortions. *Archives of General Psychiatry, 9*, 324–335.

Beck, A. (1967). *Depression: Clinical, experimental and theoretical aspects.* New York: Hoeber.

Beck, A. (1976). *Cognitive therapy and the emotional disorders.* New York: International Universities Press.

Beck, A. & Beamesderfer, A. (1974). Assessment of depression. The depression inventory. In P. Pichot (Ed.), *Physiological measures of psychopharmacology: Vol. 7, Modern problems in pharmacopsychiatry* (pp. 151–169). Basel: Kerger.

Beck, A. & Greenberg, R. (1971). The nosology of suicidal phenomena: Past and future perspectives. *Bulletin of Suicidology, 8*, 10–17.

Beck, A. & Rush, A. (1978). Cognitive approaches to depression and suicide. In G. Serban (Ed.), *Cognitive defects in the development of mental illness* (pp. 235–257). New York: Burnner/Mazel.

Beck, A., Beck, R. & Kovacs, M. (1975a). Classification of suicidal behaviors: 1 Quantifying intent and medical lethality. *American Journal of Psychiatry, 132*, 285–287.

Beck, A., Freeman, A. & Associates (1990). *Cognitive therapy of personality disorders.* New York: Guilford.

Beck, A., Kovacs, M. & Weissman, A. (1975b). Hopelessness and suicidal behavior: An overview. *Journal of the American Medical Association, 234*, 1146–49.

Beck, A., Kovacs, M. & Weissman, A. (1979a). Assessment of suicide intention: The scale of suicide ideation. *Journal of Consulting & Clinical Psychology, 47*, 343–352.

Beck, A., Resnick, H. & Lettieri, D. (Eds) (1974a). *The prediction of suicide.* Bowie, MD: Charles Press.

Beck, A., Rush, A., Shaw, B. & Emery, C. (1979b). *Cognitive therapy of depression.* New York: Guilford.

Beck, A., Schuyler, D. & Herman, I. (1974b). Development of suicidal intent scale. In A. Beck, H. Resnik & D. Lettieri (Eds), *The prediction of suicide* (pp. 45–56). Bowie, MA: Charles Press.

Beck, A., Weissman, A., Lester, D. & Trexler, L. (1974c). The measurement of pessimism: The hopelessness scale. *Journal of Consulting and Clinical Psychology, 42*, 861–865.

Bell vs *New York City Health and Hospital Corporation* (1982) 90. A.D. 2nd 270, 456 N.Y.S. 2d 787.

Bemporad, J. (Ed.) (1980). *Child development in normality and psychopathology.* New York: Brunner/Mazel.

Benjafield, J. (1991). The end of development. In A. Leenaars (Ed.), *Life span perspectives of suicide* (pp. 3–15). New York: Plenum.

Benjafield, J. (2002). Research methods: A history of some important strands. *Archives of Suicide Research, 6*, 5–14.

Berman, A. (1986, April). *Suicidal youth.* Paper presented at the conference of American Association of Suicidology, Atlanta, GA.

Berman, A. (Ed.) (1990). *Suicide prevention. Case consultation.* New York: Springer.

Berman, A. & Jobes, D. (1991). *Adolescent suicide: Assessment and intervention.* Washington, DC: American Psychological Association Press.

Berman, A., Leenaars, A. & Schutz, B. (1991). David: A case consultation. *Suicide and Life-Threatening Behavior, 21*, 299–306.

Bertolote, J. (1993). *Guidelines for the primary prevention of mental, neurological, and psychosocial disorders: Suicide.* Geneva: World Health Organization.

Bjerg, K. (1967). The suicidal life space: Attempts at reconstruction from suicide notes. In E. Shneidman (Ed.), *Essays in self-destruction* (pp. 475–493). New York: Science House, Inc.

Boismont, B., de (1856). *Du suicide et la folie suicide.* Paris: Germer Bailliere.

Bolton, N. (1972). *The psychology of thinking.* Edinburgh: T. & A. Constable Ltd.

Bongar, B. (1991). *The suicidal patient: Clinical and legal standards of care.* Washington, DC: American Psychological Association.

Bongar, B. & Greaney, S. (1994). Essential clinical and legal issues when working with the suicidal patient. In A. Leenaars, J. Maltsberger & R. Neimeyer (Eds), *Treatment of suicidal people* (pp. 179–194). Washington, DC: Taylor & Francis.

Bostwick, J. (2000). Affective disorders and suicide risk: A re-examination. *American Journal of Psychiatry, 157,* 1925–1932.

Bostwick, J. & Palmer, B. (2002, Sept.). The Novartis workshop on schizophrenia. Workshop presented at the 9th European Symposium on Suicide and Suicidal Behaviour, University of Warwick, England.

Bowers, K. & Meichenbaum, D. (Eds.) (1984). *The unconscious reconsidered.* New York: John Wiley & Sons.

Bowles, J. (1995). Suicide in Western Samoa: An example of a suicide prevention program in a developing country. In R. Diekstra, W. Gulbinat, D. De Leo & I. Kienhorst (Eds), *Preventive strategies on suicide* (pp. 173–206). Leiden: Brill.

Brenner, M. (1988, April). *Economic and behavioral risk factors. Accounting for suicide over the life cycle.* Paper presented at the conference of the American Association of Suicidology, Washington, DC.

Brent, D. (1992, April). *Psychiatric effects of exposure to suicide among friends and acquaintances.* Paper presented at the conference of the American Association of Suicidology, Chicago, IL.

Bronowski, J. (1973). *The ascent of man.* Boston: Little, Brown & Co.

Brown, L. (Ed.). *Oxford English Dictionary* (1993). New York: Oxford University Press Inc.

Buber, M. (1970). *I & thou.* (W. Kaufman, Trans.) New York: Charles Scribner's Sons.

Buhler, C. (1968). The developmental structure of goal setting in group and individual studies. In C. Buhler & F. Massarick (Eds), *The course of human life* (pp. 92–102). New York: Springer.

Busch, K., Clark, D., Fawcett, J. & Kravitz, H. (1993). Clinical features of inpatient suicides. *Psychiatric Annals, 23,* 256–262.

Butscher, E. (1976). *Sylvia Plath.* New York: Seaburg.

Butler, R. (1963). The life review: An interpretation of reminiscence in the aged. *Psychiatry, 26,* 65–76.

Cameron, N. (1963). *Personality development and psychopathology: A dynamic approach.* Boston: Houghton Mifflin Co.

Camus, A. (1955). *The myth of Sisyphus.* (J. O'Brien, Trans). New York: Vintage Book.

Canetto, S. (1994). Gender issues in the treatment of suicidal individuals. In A. Leenaars, J. Maltsberger & R. Neimeyer (Eds), *Treatment of suicidal people* (pp. 115–126). Washington, DC: Taylor & Francis.

Canetto, S. & Lester, D. (Eds) (1995). *Women and suicidal behavior.* New York: Springer.

Cantor, P. (1991). Developmental perspective on prevention and treatment of suicidal youth. In A. Leenaars (Ed.), *Life-span perspectives of suicide* (pp. 283–294). New York: Plenum.

Cantor, C. & Baume, P. (1998). Changing methods of suicide by young Australians, 1974–1994. *Archives of Suicide Research, 4,* 41–50.

Cantor, C. & McDermott, P. (1994). Suicide litigation: From legal to clinical wisdom. *Australia and New Zealand Journal of Psychiatry, 28,* 431–437.

Caplan, F. & Caplan, T. (1974). *The power of play.* Garden City, NY: Anchor.

Caplan, G. (1964). *Principles of preventive psychiatry.* New York: Basic Books.

Capstick, A. (1960). Recognition of emotional disturbance and the prevention of suicide. *British Medical Journal, 1,* 1179–1182.

Carnap, R. (1959). Psychology in physical language. In A. Ayer (Ed.), *Logical positivism* (pp. 165–197). New York: Free Press. (Original work published 1931.)

Clark, S. & Goldney, R. (1995). Grief reactions and recovery in a support group for people bereaved by suicide. *Crisis, 16,* 27–33.

Clarke, R. & Lester, D. (1989). *Suicide: Closing the exits.* New York: Springer.

Cohen, S. & Fiedler, J. (1974). Content analysis of multiple messages in suicide notes. *Suicide and Life-Threatening Behavior, 4,* 75–95.

Colarusso, C. & Nemiroff, R. (1981). *Adult development.* New York: Plenum.

Connors, E. (1995). The healing path: Suicide and self destructive behavior in North American native people. In A. Leenaars & D. Lester (Eds), *Suicide and the unconscious* (pp. 259–269). Northvale, NJ: Aronson.

Conwell, Y. (1998). Seduced by death. [Review of H. Hendin's *Seduced by death.*] *Suicide and Life-Threatening Behavior, 28*, 234–237.

Coppen, A. (1994). Depression as a lethal disease: Prevention strategies. *Journal of Clinical Psychiatry, 55*, 4 (Suppl.), 37–45.

Corder, B. & Haizlip, T. (1984). Environmental and personality similarities in case histories of suicide and self-poisoning in children under ten. *Suicide and Life-Threatening Behavior, 14*, 59–66.

Corder, B., Parker, P. & Corder, R. (1974). Parental history, family communication, and interaction patterns in adolescent suicide. *Family Therapy, 3*, 185–190.

Cusack, D. (1997). Physician-assisted suicide: Killing or compassion (Editorial). *Medical–Legal Journal of Ireland, 3*, 42.

Daly, M., Conway, M. & Kelleher, M. (1986). Social determinants of self-poisoning. *British Journal of Psychiatry, 146*, 406–413.

Daubert vs Merril Dow Pharmaceuticals, Inc. N092-102 (US 06/28/1993).

Darbonne, A. (1969a). Suicide and age: A suicide note analysis. *Journal of Consulting and Clinical Psychology, 33*, 46–50.

Darbonne, A. (1969b). Study of psychological content in the communications of suicidal individuals. *Journal of Consulting and Clinical Psychology, 33*, 590–596.

Davis, F. (1967). The relationship between suicide and attempted suicide. *Psychiatric Quarterly, 41*, 752–765.

De Leo, D. & Scocco, P. (2001). Treatment and prevention of suicidal behaviour in the elderly. In K. Hawton & K. van Heeringen (Eds), *The international hand book of suicide and attempted suicide* (pp. 555–570). London: John Wiley & Sons.

Descartes, R. (1972). *The philosophical works of Descartes*, Vols 1 & 2 (Trans. & Ed. by E. Haldace & G. Ross). London: Cambridge University Press.

Diamond, G., More, D., Hawkins, A. & Soucar, E. (1995). Comment on Black's (1993) article "Comparing genuine and simulated suicide notes: A new perspective". *Journal of Consulting and Clinical Psychology, 63*, 46–48.

Dickens, C. (1966). *Oliver Twist* (K. Tillotson, Ed.). Oxford: Oxford University Press.

Diekstra, R. (1992). Suicide and euthanasia. *Giornale Italiano Di Suicidologia, 2*, 71–78.

Diekstra, R. (1996). The epidemiology of suicide and parasuicide, *Archives of Suicide Research, 2*, 1–29.

Diekstra, R. (1997). Parasuicide: Is it a distinct phenomenon? In A. Botsis, C. Soldatos & C. Stefanis (Eds). *Suicide: Biopsychosocial approaches* (pp. 177–186). Amsterdam: Elsevier.

Diekstra, R. & Van der Loo, K. (1978). Attitudes toward suicide and incidence of suicidal behavior in a generalized population. In H. Winnick & L. Miller (Eds), *Aspects of suicide in modern civilization* (pp. 79–85). Jerusalem: Jerusalem Academic Press.

Diggory, J. (1974). Predicting suicide: Will-o-the-wisp or reasonable challenge? In A. Beck, H. Resnik & D. Lettieri (Eds), *The prediction of suicide* (pp. 59–70). Bowie, MA: Charles Press.

Dillman vs Hellman (1973) 283 So 2d 388 (Fla. Dist. Cf. App).

Dostoevsky, F. (1994). *A writer's diary. Fyodor Dostoevsky*, Vols 1 & 2 (K. Lantz, Trans. & Annot.). Evanston, IL: Northwestern University Press.

Douglas, J. (1967). *The social meaning of suicide*. Princeton, NJ: Princeton University Press.

Durkheim, E. (1951). *Suicide* (J. Spaulding & G. Simpson, Trans). Glencoe, IL: The Free Press. (Original work published 1897.)

Durocher, J., Leenaars, A. & Balance, W. (1989). Knowledge about suicide as a function of experience. *Perceptual and Motor Skills, 68*, 26.

Dyck, R., Joyce, A. & Azim, H. (1984). Treatment compliance as a function of therapist attributes and social support. *Canadian Journal of Psychiatry, 29*, 212–216.

Eagle, M. (1987). Revisioning the unconscious. *Canadian Psychology, 28*, 113–116.

EchoHawk, M. (1997). Suicide: The scourge of Native American people. In A. Leenaars, R. Maris & Y. Takahashi (Eds), *Suicide: Individual, cultural, international perspectives* (pp. 60–67). New York: Guilford.

Edelman, A. & Renshaw, S. (1982). Genuine versus simulated suicide notes. An issue revisited through discourse analysis. *Suicide and Life-Threatening Behavior, 12,* 103–113.

Eissler, R., Freud, A., Kris, M. & Solnet, A. (1977) *Psychoanalytic assessment: The diagnostic profile.* London: Yale Universities Press.

Ekeberg, O., Jacobsen, D., Sorum, Y. & Aass, G. (1986). Self-poisoning and the menstrual cycle. *Acta Psychiatrica Scandinavica, 73,* 239–241.

Eliot, T. (1944). *Four quartets.* London: Faber & Faber.

Ellenberger, H. (1970). *The discovery of the unconscious.* New York: Basic Books.

Epstein, S. (1994). Integration of the cognitive and psychodynamic unconscious. *American Psychologist, 49,* 709–724.

Erikson, E. (1963). *Childhood and society* (2nd edn). New York: Norton.

Erikson, E. (1964). *Insight and responsibility.* New York: Norton.

Erikson, E. (1968). *Identity: Youth and crisis.* New York: Norton.

Erikson, E. (1980). *Identity and the life cycle.* New York: W.W. Norton.

Erikson, E. (1989). Foreword. In D. Jacobs & H. Brown (Eds), *Suicide: Understanding and responding* (pp. xi–xiv). Madison, CT: International Universities Press.

Etkind, M. (1997). *. . . Or not to be: A collection of suicide notes.* New York: Riverhead Books.

Etzersdorfer, E. & Sonneck, G. (1998). Preventing suicide by influencing mass-media reporting. The Viennese experience 1980–1996. *Archives of Suicide Research, 4,* 67–74.

Etzersdorfer, E., Vijayakumar, S., Grausgruber, A. & Sonneck, G. (1997). Attitudes towards suicide among medical students—comparison between Madras (India) and Vienna (Austria). *Social Psychiatry and Psychiatric Epidemiology, 33,* 104–110.

Exner, J. (1986). *The Rorschach: A comprehensive system*, Vol. 1 (2nd edn). New York: John Wiley & Sons.

Eyman, J. (1991). Countertransference when counselling suicidal school-aged youth. In A. Leenaars & S. Wenckstern (Eds), *Suicide prevention in schools* (pp. 147–157). Washington, DC: Hemisphere.

Eyman, J. & Eyman, S. (1992). Personality assessment in suicide prediction. In R. Maris, A. Berman, J. Maltsberger & R. Yufit (Eds), *Assessment and prediction of suicide* (pp. 183–201). New York: Guilford.

Farberow, N. (1972). Cultural history of suicide. In J. Waldenstorm, T. Larsson & N. Ljeingstedt (Eds), *Suicide and attempted suicide* (pp. 30–44). Stockholm: Nordiska, Bokhanlelus, Forlag.

Farberow, N. (Ed.) (1980). *The many faces of suicide.* New York: McGraw-Hill.

Farberow, N. & Shneidman, E. (1957). Suicide and age. In E. Shneidman & N. Farberow (Eds), *Clues to suicide* (pp. 41–59). New York: McGraw-Hill.

Farberow, N., MacKinnon, L. & Nelson, F. (1977). Suicide. *Public Health Reports, 92,* 223–232.

Fawcett, J. (1997). The detection and consequences of anxiety in clinical depression. *Journal of Clinical Psychiatry, 58* (suppl. 8), 35–40.

Fenichel, O. (1953). On the psychology of boredom. In H. Fenichel & D. Rapaports (Eds), *The collected papers of Otto Fenichel. First series* (pp. 292–302). New York: W.W. Norton. (Original work published 1934.)

Fenichel, O. (1954). *The psychoanalytic theory of neurosis.* New York: W.W. Norton.

Fishbain, D., D'Achille, L., Barsky, S. & Aldrich, T. (1984). A controlled study of suicide pacts. *Journal of Clinical Psychiatry, 45,* 154–157.

Fishbain, D., Fletcher, J., Aldrich, T. & Davis, J. (1987). Relationship between Russian roulette deaths and risk-taking behavior: A controlled study. *American Journal of Psychiatry, 144,* 564–567.

Fourestie, V., de Lignieres, B., Roudot-Thoraval, R., Fulloi-Lemaire, I., Cremniter, D., Nahoul, K., Fournier, S. & Lejonc, J. (1986). Suicide attempts in hypo-oestrogenic phases of the menstrual cycle. *Lancet, 2,* 1357–1360.

Foulkes, D. (1978). *A grammar of dreams.* New York: Basic Books, Inc.

Fraiberg, S. (Ed.) (1980). *Clinical studies in infant health.* New York: Basic Books.

Frager, R. & Fadiman, J. (1984). *Personality and personal growth* (2nd edn). New York: Harper & Row.

Freeman, K. (1971). *Ancilla to the pre-Socratic philosophers.* Oxford: Basil Blackwell.

Freud, A. (1965). *Normality and pathology in childhood: Assessments of development.* New York: International Universities Press.

Freud, A. (1966). *The ego and the mechanisms of defense.* New York: International Universities Press.

Freud, S. (1974a). Psychopathology of everyday life. In J. Strachey (Ed. & Trans.), *The standard edition of the complete psychological works of Sigmund Freud, Vol. VI* (pp. 1–310). London: Hogarth Press. (Original work published 1901.)

Freud, S. (1974b). A case of obsessional neurosis. In J. Strachey (Ed. & Trans.), *The standard edition of the complete psychological works of Sigmund Freud, Vol. X* (pp. 153–318). London: Hogarth Press. (Original work published 1909.)

Freud, S. (1974c). The case of little Hans. In J. Strachey (Ed. & Trans.), *The standard edition of the complete psychological works of Sigmund Freud, Vol. X* (pp. 101–147). London: Hogarth Press. (Original work published 1909.)

Freud, S. (1974d). The future prospects of psycho-analytic therapy. In J. Strachey (Ed. & Trans.), *The standard edition of the complete psychological works of Sigmund Freud, Vol. XI* (pp. 139–151). London: Hogarth Press. (Original work published 1910.)

Freud, S. (1974e). The unconscious. In J. Strachey (Ed. & Trans.), *The standard edition of the complete psychological works of Sigmund Freud, Vol. XIV* (pp. 159–215). London: Hogarth Press. (Original work published 1915.)

Freud, S. (1974f). Dreams. In J. Strachey (Ed. & Trans.), *The standard edition of the complete psychological works of Sigmund Freud, Vol. XV* (pp. 83–228). London: Hogarth Press. (Original work published 1916.)

Freud, S. (1974g). Mourning and melancholia. In J. Strachey (Ed.), *The standard edition of the complete psychological works of Sigmund Freud, Vol. XIV* (pp. 239–260). London: Hogarth Press. (Original work published 1917.)

Freud, S. (1974h). General theory of neurosis. In J. Strachey (Ed. & Trans.), *The standard edition of the complete psychological works of Sigmund Freud, Vol. XVI* (pp. 243–483). London: Hogarth Press. (Original work published 1917.)

Freud, S. (1974i). A case of homosexuality in a woman. In J. Strachey (Ed. & Trans.), *The standard edition of the complete psychological works of Sigmund Freud, Vol. XVIII* (pp. 147–172). London: Hogarth Press. (Original work published 1920.)

Freud, S. (1974j). Group psychology and the analysis of the ego. In J. Strachey (Ed. & Trans.), *The standard edition of the complete psychological works of Sigmund Freud, Vol. XVIII* (pp. 67–147). London: Hogarth Press. (Original work published 1921.)

Freud, S. (1974k). The ego and the id. In J. Strachey (Ed. & Trans.), *The standard edition of the complete psychological works of Sigmund Freud, Vol. XXI* (pp. 3–66). London: Hogarth Press. (Original work published 1923.)

Freud, S. (1974l). New introductory lectures. In J. Strachey (Ed. & Trans.), *The standard edition of the complete psychological works of Sigmund Freud, Vol. XXII* (pp. 3–182). London: Hogarth Press. (Original work published 1933.)

Freud, S. (1974m). Moses and monotheism. In J. Strachey (Ed. & Trans.), *The standard edition of the complete psychological works of Sigmund Freud, Vol. XXIII* (pp. 3–37). London: Hogarth Press. (Original work published 1939.)

Freud, S. (1974n). An outline of psycho-analysis. In J. Strachey (Ed. & Trans.), *The standard edition of the complete psychological works of Sigmund Freud, Vol. XXIII* (pp. 137–207). London: Hogarth Press. (Original work published 1940.)

Friedman, P. (Ed.) (1967). *On suicide.* New York: International Universities Press. (Original work published 1910.)

Fryer, J. (1986). AIDS and suicide. In J. Morgan (Ed.), *Suicide: Helping those at risk.* (pp. 193–200). London: King's College.

Furth, H. (1966). *Thinking without language.* New York: The Free Press.

Garrison, C., Lewinsohn, P., Marsteller, F., Langhinrichsen, J. & Lann, I. (1991). The assessment of suicidal behavior in adolescents. *Suicide and Life-Threatening Behavior, 21,* 217–230.

Gergen, K. (1977). Stability, change and chance in understanding human development. In N. Daton & H. Reese (Eds), *Life span developmental psychology: Dialectical perspectives on experimental research.* New York: Academic Press.

Ginsberg, H. & Opper, S. (1969). *Piaget's theory of intellectual development.* Englewood Cliffs, NJ: Prentice-Hall.

Goethe, J. (1951). *Die leiden des junger Werther. Goethes Werke, Vol. 6.* Hamburg: Christian Wegner Jerlag. (Original work published 1774).

Goffman, E. (1974). *Frame analysis.* New York: Harper Colophon.

Goldney, R. & Spence, N. (1987). Is suicide predictable? *Australian and New Zealand Journal of Psychiatry, 21,* 3–4.

Goldney, R., Winefield, A., Tiggemann, M., Winefield, H. & Smith, S. (1989). Suicidal ideation in a young adult population. *Acta Psychiatrica Scandinavica, 79,* 481–489.

Goldblatt, M. (1992). *Richard Cory suicides: Diagnostic questions.* Paper presented at the annual conference of the American Association of Suicidology, Chicago, Il, April.

Goldblatt, M. (1994). Hospitalization of the suicidal patient. In A. Leenaars, J. Maltsberger & R. Neimeyer (Eds), *Treatment of suicidal people.* (pp. 153–165). London: Taylor & Francis.

Grad, O. (Ed.). (2001). *Suicide risk and protective factors in the new millennium.* Ljubljana, Slovenia: Cankarjev dom.

Greenglass, E. (1982). *A world of difference.* New York: John Wiley & Sons.

Greenwald, A. (1975). Consequences of prejudice against the null hypothesis. *Psychological Bulletin, 82,* 1–20.

Gulbinat, W. (1996). The epidemiology of suicide in old age. *Archives of Suicide Research, 2,* 31–42.

Gunnel, D. & Frankel, S. (1994). Prevention of suicide: aspirations and evidence. *British Medical Journal, 308,* 1227–1233.

Gutheil, T. (1992). Suicide and suit: Liability after self-destruction. In D. Jacobs (Ed.), *Suicide and clinical practice* (pp. 147–167). Washington: American Psychiatric Press.

Gutheil, T., Bursztajn, H., Hamm, R. & Brodsky, A. (1983). Subjective data and suicide assessment in light of recent legal developments. Part 1: Malpractice prevention and the use of subjective data. *International Journal of Law and Psychiatry, 6,* 317–329.

Haley, J. (Ed.) (1971). *Changing families.* New York: Greene & Stratton.

Hamilton, E. & Cairns, H. (Eds) (1961). *The collected dialogues of Plato.* Princeton: Princeton University Press.

Hartmann, H. (1939). *Ego psychology and the problem of adaptation.* New York: International Universities Press.

Hattem, J. (1964). Precipitating role of discordant interpersonal relationships in suicidal behavior. *Dissertation Abstracts, 25,* 1335–1336.

Hawton, K. (2000). General hospital management of suicide attempters. In K. Hawton & K. van Heeringen (Eds), *The international handbook of suicide and attempted suicide* (pp. 519–537). London: John Wiley & Sons.

Hawton, K. & Blackstock, E. (1976). General practice aspects of self-poisoning & self-injury. *Psychological Medicine, 6,* 571–575.

Hawton, K. & van Heeringen, C. (Eds) (2000). *The international handbook of suicide and attempted suicide.* London: John Wiley & Sons.

Hayakawa, S. (1957). Suicide as a communicative act. *ETC, 15,* 46–51.

Heidbreder, E. (1933). *Seven psychologies.* New York: Appleton-Century-Crofts.

Heidegger, M. (1962). *Being and time* (J. Macquairie & E. Robinson, Trans). New York: Harper & Row.

Heimann, P. (1950). On countertransference. *International Journal of Psycho-Analysis, 14,* 181–184.

Hempel, C. (1966). *Philosophy of natural sciences.* Englewood Cliffs, NJ: Prentice-Hall, Inc.

Hendin, H. (1997). *Seduced by death: Doctors, patients and the Dutch cure.* New York: Norton.

Hendin, H. (2001, Aug.). *AFSP—Suicide Data Bank—Recognizing and responding to a suicide crisis.* Paper presented at "Suicidality, Psychoanalysis" International Congress, Hamburg, Germany.

Hendin, H., Maltsberger, J., Lipschitz, A., Haas, A. & Kyle, J. (2001). Recognizing and responding to a suicide crisis. *Suicide and Life-Threatening Behavior, 31,* 115–128.

Henken, V. (1976). Banality reinvestigated: A computer-based content analysis of suicidal and forced death documents. *Suicide and Life-Threatening Behavior, 6,* 36–43.

Henry, A. & Short, J. (1954). *Suicide and homicide.* New York: Free Press.

Hoch, P. (1972). *Differential diagnosis in clinical psychiatry: The lectures of Paul H. Hoch, M.D.* (M. Strahl & N. Lewis, Eds). New York: Science House.

Hoff, L. (1984). *People in crisis.* Menlo Park, CA: Addison-Wesley.

Hollon, S. & Fawcett, J. (2001). Combined medication and psychotherapy. In G. Gabbard (Ed.), *Treatments of psychiatric disorders, Vol. 2* (pp. 1247–1266). Washington, DC: American Psychiatric Publication, Inc.

Honour, A. (1967). *Tormented genius.* New York: Morrow.

Horney, K. (1950). *Neurosis and human growth.* New York: Norton.

Hughes, S. & Neimeyer, R. (1990). A cognitive model of suicidal behavior. In D. Lester (Ed.), *Current concepts of suicide* (pp. 1–28). Philadelphia: The Charles Press.

Humphry, D. (1991). *Final exit.* Eugene, OR: The Hemlock Society.

Humphry, D. (1992). Rational suicide among the elderly. In A. Leenaars, R. Maris, J. McIntosh & J. Richman (Eds), *Suicide and the older adult* (pp. 125–129). New York: Guilford.

Humphry, D. (1993). Letter to the editor (Letter). *Suicide and Life-Threatening Behavior, 23,* 281.

Husserl, E. (1973). *The idea of phenomenology* (W. Alston & G. Nokhnikian, Trans), The Hague: Martinus Nijhoff. (Original work published 1907.)

Iga, M. (1993). Japanese suicide. In A. Leenaars (Ed.), *Suicidology: Essays in honor of Edwin Shneidman* (pp. 301–323). Northvale, NJ: Jason Aronson.

Isacsson, G. (2000). Suicide prevention—a medical break through? *Acta Psychiatrica Scandinavica, 102,* 113–117.

Isacsson, G., Bergman, U. & Rich, C. (1996). Epidemiological data which suggests anti-depressants reduce suicide risk among depressives. *Journal of Affective Disorders, 41,* 1–8.

Jacobs, J. (1971). A phenomenological study of suicide notes. In A. Geddens (Ed.), *The sociology of suicide* (pp. 332–348). London: Frank Cass & Co., Ltd.

Jacobs, D. & Brown, H. (1989). *Suicide: Understanding and responding.* Madison, CN: International Universities Press.

Jacobs, D. & Klein, M. (1993). The expanding role of psychological autopsies. In A. Leenaars (Ed.), *Suicidology* (pp. 209–247). Northvale, NS: Aronson.

Jacques, E. (1965). Death and the mid-life crisis. *International Journal of Psychoanalysis, 46,* 502–514.

James, W. (1890). *The principles of psychology.* New York: Henry Holt & Co.

Jamieson, K. (1993). *Touched by fire.* New York: Free Press.

Jamieson, K. (1995). *To paint the stars: The life and mind of Vincent van Gogh* [Video]. Georgetown: Georgetown Television Production, Inc.

Japanese Association for Dignified Death (Ed.) (1990). *Dignified Death.* Tokyo: Kodansha.

Jobes, D., Berman, A. & Josselsen, A. (1987). The impact of psychological autopsies on medical examiners' determination of manner of death. *Journal of Forensic Sciences, 31,* 177–189.

Jobes, D. & Maltsberger, J. (1995). The hazards of treating suicidal patients. In M. Sussman (Ed.), *A perilous calling: The hazards of psychotherapy practice* (pp. 200–214). New York: Wiley.

Johnston, E. (1991). *Royal Commission into Aboriginal deaths in custody. National report: Overview and recommendations.* Canberra: Australian Government Publishing Science.

Jones, E. (1953–1957). *The life and work of Sigmund Freud.* New York: Basic Books.

Jung, C. (1971). The stages of life (R. Hull, Trans.). In J. Campbell (Ed.), *The portable Jung* (pp. 3–22). New York: Viking. (Original work published 1933.)

Jung, C. (1974). Psychological types. In H. Read, M. Fordan & G. Adler (Eds), *The collected works of C.G. Jung, Vol. VI.* London: Routledge & Kegan Paul. (Original work published 1921.)

Kahne, M. (1966). Suicide research. *International Journal of Psychiatry, 12,* 177–186.

Keats, J. (1970). *You might as well live.* New York: Simon & Schuster.

Keck, P., Strakowski, S. & McElroy, S. (2000). The efficacy of atypical antipsychotics in the treatment of depressive symptoms, hostility, and suicidality in patients with schizophrenia. *Journal of Clinical Psychiatry, 61,* Suppl. 3, 4–9.

Kelleher, M. (1996). *Suicide and the Irish.* Cork: Mercier Press.

Kelleher, M., Corcoran, P., Keeley, H., Dennehy, J. & O'Donnell, I. (1996). Improving procedures for recording suicide statistics. *Irish Medical Journal, 89,* 16–17.

Kelly, G. (1955). *The psychology of personal constructs* (Vols 1 & 2). New York: Norton.

Kerkhof, A. & Connolly, J. (2001). Euthanasia and assisted suicide in The Netherlands. *Crisis, 22*, 1–2.

Kerkhof, A., Schmidtke, A., Bille-Brahe, U., De Leo, D. & Lonnqvist, J. (Eds) (1994). *Attempted suicide in Europe*. Leiden: DSWO Press.

Kerlinger, F. (1964). *Foundations of behavioral research*. New York: Holt, Rinehart & Winston.

Kevorkian, J. (1988). The least fearsome taboo: Medical aspects of planned death. *Medicine & Law, 7*, 1–14.

Kimmel, D. (1974). *Adulthood and aging*. New York: John Wiley & Sons.

King, C. (1997). Suicidal behavior in adolescence. In R. Maris, M. Silverman·& S. Canetto (Eds), *Review of suicidology, 1997* (pp. 61–95). New York: Guilford.

Kirk, G. & Raven, J. (1971). *The presocratic philosophers*. London: Cambridge University Press.

Kral, M. & Johnson, E. (1996). Suicide, self-deception of the cognitive unconscious. In A. Leenaars & D. Lester (Eds), *Suicide and the unconscious* (pp. 67–89). Northvale, NJ: Jason Aronson, Inc.

Kral, M. & Sakinofsky, I. (1994). Assessment of suicidal people for treatment. In A. Leenaars, R. Neimeyer & J. Maltsberger (Eds), *Treatment of suicidal people* (pp. 19–31). London: Taylor & Francis.

Kreitman, N. (1976). The coal gas story. *British Journal of Preventive and Social Medicine, 30*, 86–93.

Kreitman, N. (1977). *Parasuicide*. London: John Wiley & Sons.

Kreitman, N., Philip, A., Greer, S. & Bagley, C. (1969). Parasuicide. *British Journal of Psychiatry, 115*, 746–747.

Klerman, G. (Ed.) (1986). *Suicide and depression among adolescents and young adults*. Washington, DC: American Psychiatric Press.

Kuhlen, R. (1964). Developmental changes in motivation during the adult years. In J. Birren (Ed.), *Relations of development and aging*. Springfield, IL: Charles C. Thomas.

Kuhn, T. (1962). *The structure of scientific revolutions*. Chicago: The University of Chicago Press.

Laukkala, T., Isometsä, E., Hämäläinen, J., Heikkinen, M., Lindeman, S. & Aro, H. (2001). Antidepressant treatment of depression in the Finnish general population. *American Journal of Psychiatry, 158*, 2077–2079.

Leenaars, A. (1979). *A Study of the Manifest Content of Suicide Notes from Three Different Theoretical Perspectives: L. Binswanger, S. Freud, and G. Kelly*. Unpublished PhD Dissertation. University of Windsor, Canada.

Leenaars, A. (1985). Freud's and Shneidman's formulations of suicide investigated through suicide notes. In E. Shneidman (Chair), *Suicide notes and other personal documents in psychological science*. Symposium conducted at the meeting of the American Psychological Association, Los Angeles, CA, August.

Leenaars, A. (1986). A brief note on the latent content in suicide notes. *Psychological Reports, 59*, 640–642.

Leenaars, A. (1987). An empirical investigation of Shneidman's formulations regarding suicide: Age and sex. *Suicide and Life-Threatening Behavior, 17*, 233–250.

Leenaars, A. (1988a). *Suicide Notes*. New York: Human Sciences Press.

Leenaars, A. (1988b). Preventing youth suicide: Education is the key. *Dimensions in Health Services*, Oct.: 22–24.

Leenaars, A. (1988c). Are women's suicides really different from men's? *Women and Health, 14*, 17–33.

Leenaars, A. (1988d). The suicide notes of women. In D. Lester (Ed.), *Why women kill themselves* (pp. 53–71). Springfield, IL: C.C. Thomas.

Leenaars, A. (1989a). Suicide across the adult life-span: An archival study. *Crisis, 10*, 132–151.

Leenaars, A. (1989b). Are Young Adults' suicides psychologically different from those of other adults? (The Shneidman Lecture). *Suicide and Life-Threatening Behavior, 19*, 249–263.

Leenaars, A. (1990). Do the psychological characteristics of the suicidal individual make a difference in the method chosen for suicide? *Canadian Journal of Behavioural Science, 22*, 385–392.

Leenaars, A. (Ed.) (1991a). *Life-span perspectives of suicide*. New York: Plenum.

Leenaars, A. (1991b). Suicide in the young adult. In A. Leenaars (Ed.), *Life-span perspectives of suicide* (pp. 121–136). New York: Plenum.

Leenaars, A. (1991c). Suicide notes and their implications for intervention. *Crisis, 12*, 1–20.

Leenaars, A. (1992a). Suicide notes from Canada and the United States. *Perceptual and Motor Skills, 74*, 278.

Leenaars, A. (1992b). Suicide notes, communication and ideation. In R. Maris, A. Berman, J. Maltsberger & R. Yufit (Eds), *Assessment and prediction of suicide* (pp. 337–361). New York: Guilford.

Leenaars, A. (Ed.) (1993a). *Suicidology: Essays in honor of Edwin S. Shneidman*. Northvale, NJ: Jason Aronson.

Leenaars, A. (1993b). Unconscious processes. In A. Leenaars (Ed.), *Suicidology: Essays in honor of Edwin Shneidman* (pp. 127–147). Northvale, NJ: Jason Aronson.

Leenaars, A. (1994). Crisis intervention with highly lethal suicidal people. In A. Leenaars, J. Maltsberger & R. Neimeyer (Eds), *Treatment of suicidal people* (pp. 45–59). Washington, DC: Taylor & Francis.

Leenaars, A. (1995). Clinical evaluation of suicide risk. *Psychiatry and Clinical Neurosciences, 49*, Suppl. 1, 561–568.

Leenaars, A. (1996). Suicide: A multidimensional malaise. *Suicide and Life-Threatening Behavior, 26*, 221–236.

Leenaars, A. (1997). Rick: A suicide of a young adult. *Suicide and Life-Threatening Behavior, 27*, 15–27.

Leenaars, A. (Ed.) (1999a). *Lives and deaths: Selections from the works of Edwin S. Shneidman*. Philadelphia, PA: Brunner/Mazel.

Leenaars, A. (1999b). Suicide notes in the courtroom. *Journal of Clinical Forensic Medicine, 6*, 39–48.

Leenaars, A. (2002). In defense of the idiographic approach: Studies of suicide notes and personal documents. *Archives of Suicide Research, 6*, 19–30.

Leenaars, A. & Balance, W. (1981). A predictive approach to the study of manifest content in suicide notes. *Journal of Clinical Psychology, 37*, 50–52.

Leenaars, A. & Balance, W. (1984a). A logical empirical approach to the study of suicide notes. *Canadian Journal of Behavioural Science, 16*, 248–256.

Leenaars, A. & Balance, W. (1984b). A predictive approach to Freud's formulations regarding suicide. *Suicide and Life-Threatening Behavior, 14*, 275–283.

Leenaars, A. & Balance, W. (1984c). A predictive approach to suicide notes of young and older people from Freud's formulations regarding suicide. *Journal of Clinical Psychology, 40*, 1362–1364.

Leenaars, A. & Diekstra, R. (1997). The will to die: An international perspective. In A. Botsis, C. Soldatos & C. Stefanis (Eds), *Suicide: Biopsychosocial approaches* (pp. 241–256). Amsterdam: Elsevier Science.

Leenaars, A. & Lester, D. (1988–89). The significance of the method chosen for suicide in understanding the psychodynamics of the suicidal individual. *Omega, 19*, 311–314.

Leenaars, A. & Lester, D. (1990). What characteristics of suicide notes are salient for people to allow perception of a suicide note as genuine? *Death Studies, 14*, 25–30.

Leenaars, A. & Lester, D. (1991). Myths about suicide notes. *Death Studies, 15*, 303–308.

Leenaars, A. & Lester, D. (1992). A comparison of rates and patterns of suicide for Canada and the United States, 1960–1988. *Death Studies, 16*, 433–440.

Leenaars, A. & Lester, D. (1994). Assessment and prediction of suicide risk in adolescents. In J. Zimmerman & G. Annis (Eds), *Treatment approaches with suicidal adolescents* (pp. 47–70). New York: John Wiley & Sons.

Leenaars, A. & Lester, D. (Eds) (1996). *Suicide and the unconscious*. Northvale, NJ: Aronson.

Leenaars, A. & Lester, (1998). The impact of gun control on suicide: Studies from Canada. *Archives of Suicide Research, 4*, 25–40.

Leenaars, A. & McLister, B. (1989). *An empirical investigation of the latent content in suicide notes*. Paper presented at the American Association of Suicidology Conference, San Diego, CA, April.

Leenaars, A. & Maltsberger, J. (1994). The Inman diary: Some reflections on treatments. In A. Leenaars, J. Maltsberger & R. Neimeyer (Eds), *Treatment of suicidal people* (pp. 227–236). Washington, DC.: Taylor & Francis.

Leenaars, A. & Wenckstern, S. (Eds) (1990). *Suicide prevention in schools.* Washington, DC: Hemisphere.

Leenaars, A. & Wenckstern, S. (1991). Suicide in the school-age child and adolescent. In A. Leenaars (Ed.), *Life span perspectives of suicide* (pp. 95–107). New York: Plenum.

Leenaars, A. & Wenckstern, S. (1994). Helping lethal suicidal adolescents. In D. Adams & E. Deveau (Eds), *Threat to life, dying, death and bereavement: The child's perspective* (pp. 131–150). Amityville, NY: Baywood.

Leenaars, A. & Wenckstern, S. (1999). Suicide prevention in schools: The art, issues and pitfalls. *Crisis, 20,* 132–142.

Leenaars, A., Anawak, J., Brown, C., Hill-Keddie, T. & Taparti, L. (1999). Genocide and suicide among indigenous people: The north meets the south. *The Canadian Journal of Native Studies, 19,* 337–363.

Leenaars, A., Balance, W., Pellarin, S., Aversano, G., Magli, A. & Wenckstern, S. (1988). Facts and myths of suicide in Canada. *Death Studies, 12,* 191–210.

Leenaars, A., Balance, W., Wenckstern, S. & Rudzinski, D. (1985). An empirical investigation of Shneidman's formulations regarding suicide. *Suicide and Life-Threatening Behavior, 15,* 184–195.

Leenaars, A., Cantor, C., Connolly, J., EchoHawk, M., Gailiene, D., He, Z., Kokorina, N., Lester, D., Lopatin, A., Rodriguez, M., Schlebusch, L., Takahashi, Y. & Vijayakumar, L. (2000a). Legal and ethical issues. In K. Hawton & K. van Heeringen (Eds), *International handbook of suicide and attempted suicide* (pp. 421–435). London: John Wiley & Sons.

Leenaars, A., Cantor, C., Connolly, J., EchoHawk, M., Gailiene, D., He, Z., Kokorina, N., Lester, D., Lopatin, A., Rodriguez, M., Schlesbusch, D., Takahashi, Y. & Vijayakumar, L. (2002a). Ethical and legal issues in suicidology: International perspectives. *Archives of Suicide Research, 6,* 185–197.

Leenaars, A., Cantor, C., Connolly, J., EchoHawk, M., Gailiene, D., He, Z., Kokorina, N., Lester, D., Lopatin, A., Rodriguez, M., Schlebusch, L., Takahashi, Y., Vijayakumar, L. & Wenckstern, S. (2000b). Controlling the environment to prevent suicide: International perspectives. *Canadian Journal of Psychiatry. 45,* 639–644.

Leenaars, A., Connolly, J., Cantor, C., EchoHawk, M., Gailiene, D., He, Z., Kokorina, N., Lester, D., Lopatin, A., Rodriguez, M., Schlebusch, L., Takahashi, Y. & Vijayakumar, L. (2001a). Suicide, assisted suicide and euthanasia: International perspectives. *The Irish Journal of Psychological Medicine. 18,* 33–37.

Leenaars, A., De Leo, D., Diekstra, R., Goldney, R., Kelleher, M., Lester, D. & Nordstrom, P. (1997). Consultations for research in suicidology. *Archives of Suicide Research, 3,* 139–151.

Leenaars, A., De Leo, D., Goldney, R., Gulbinat, W. & Wallace, D. (Eds) (1998a). The prevention of suicide: Controlling the environment. Special issue, *Archives of Suicide Research, 4,* 1–107.

Leenaars, A., De Wilde, E., Wenckstern, S. & Kral, M. (2001b). Suicide notes of adolescents: A life span comparison. *Canadian Journal of Behavioural Science, 33,* 47–57.

Leenaars, A., Fekete, S., Wenckstern, S. & Osvath, P. (1998b). Suicide notes from Hungary and the United States. *Psychiatrica Hungarica, 13,* 147–159.

Leenaars. A., Girdhar, S., Dogra, T. & Wenckstern, S. (In progress). Suicide notes from India and the United States. (*Research in progress*).

Leenaars, A., Haines, J., Wenckstern, S., Williams, C. & Lester, D. (2003). Suicide notes from Australia and the United States. *Perceptual and Motor Skills, 92,* 1281–1282.

Leenaars, A., Lester, D. & Goldney, R. (Eds) (2002). Qualitative versus quantitative studies in suicidology. *Archives of Suicide Research, 6,* 1–73.

Leenaars, A., Lester, D., Lopatin, A., Schustov, D. & Wenckstern, S. (2002). Suicide notes from Russia and the United States. *Social and General Psychiatry, 12–3,* 22–28. (In Russian.)

Leenaars, A., Lester, D. & Wenckstern, S. (1999). Suicide notes in alcoholism. *Psychological Reports, 85,* 363–364.

Leenaars, A., Lester, D., Wenckstern, S. & Heim, N. (1994a). Suizid-abschiedsbriefe—Ein vergleich deutscher und amerikawischer abschiedbriefe von suizidenten. *Suizidprophylaxe*, *3*, 99–101.

Leenaars, A., Lester, D., Wenckstern, S., McMullin, C., Rudzinski, D. & Brevard, A. (1992). A comparison of suicide notes and parasuicide notes. *Death Studies*, *16*, 331–342.

Leenaars, A., Maltsberger, J. & Neimeyer, R. (Eds) (1994b). *Treatment of suicidal people*. London: Taylor & Francis.

Leenaars, A., Moksony, F., Lester, D. & Wenckstern, S. (2003). The impact of gun control (Bill C51) on suicide in Canada. *Death Studies*, *27*, 103–124.

Leenaars, A., Saunders, M., Balance, W., Wenckstern, S. & Galgan, R. (1991). Knowledge about facts and myths of suicide in the elderly. *Gerontology and Geriatrics Education*, *12*, 61–68.

Lester, D. (1969). Resentment and dependency in the suicidal individual. *Journal of General Psychology*, *81*, 137–145.

Lester, D. (1970a). Personality correlates associated with choice of method of committing suicide. *Personality*, *1*, 261–264.

Lester, D. (1970b). Factors affecting choice of method of suicide. *Journal of Clinical Psychology*, *26*, 437.

Lester, D. (1970c). Relation between attempted suicide and completed suicide. *Psychological Reports*, *27*, 719–722.

Lester, D. (1971). Choice of method for suicide and personality: A study of suicide notes. *Omega*, *2*, 76–80.

Lester, D. (1974). Demographic versus clinical prediction of suicidal behaviors. In A. Beck, H. Resnik & D. Lettieri (Eds), *The prediction of suicide* (pp. 71–84). Bowie, MD: Charles Press.

Lester, D. (1983). *Why people kill themselves* (2nd edn). Springfield, IL: C.C. Thomas.

Lester, D. (1987). *Suicide as a learned behavior*. Springfield, IL: C.C. Thomas.

Lester, D. (Ed.) (1988a). *Why women kill themselves*. Springfield, IL: C.C. Thomas.

Lester, D. (1988b). The perception of different methods of suicide. *Journal of General Psychology*, *115*, 215–217.

Lester, D. (1990). Suicide and the menstrual cycle. *Medical Hypotheses*, *31*, 197–199.

Lester, D. (1991a). Suicide across the life span: A look at international trends. In A. Leenaars (Ed.), *Life span perspectives of suicide* (pp. 71–80). New York: Plenum.

Lester, D. (1991b). *Questions and answers about murder*. Philadelphia: The Charles Press.

Lester, D. (1992). *Why people kill themselves* (3rd edn). Springfield, IL: C.C. Thomas.

Lester, D. (1993). *Suicide in creative women*. Commack, NY: Nova Science Publ., Inc.

Lester, D. (1994). A comparison of fifteen theories of suicide. *Suicide and Life-Threatening Behavior*, *24*, 80–88.

Lester, D. (1996). *Sylvia Plath*. Unpublished manuscript.

Lester, D. (1997). Suicide in an international perspective. *Suicide and Life-Threatening Behavior*, *27*, 104–111.

Lester, D. (2000). *By their own hand*. Chichester, UK: Aeneas Press.

Lester, D. & Hummel, H. (1980). Motives for suicide in elderly people. *Psychological Reports*, *47*, 870.

Lester, D. & Leenaars, A. (1993). Suicide rates in Canada before and after tightening firearm control laws. *Psychological Reports*, *72*, 789–790.

Lester, D. & Leenaars, A. (1996). The ethics of suicide and suicide prevention. *Death Studies*, *20*, 162–184.

Lester, D. & Murrell, M. (1980). The influence of gun control laws on suicidal behavior. *American Journal of Psychiatry*, *137*, 121–122.

Lester, D. & Reeve, C. (1982). The suicide notes of young and old people. *Psychological Reports*, *50*, 334.

Lester, D. & Wright, T. (1973). Suicide and over control. *Psychological Reports*, *32*, 1278.

Lester, D., Agarwal, K. & Natarajam, M. (1999). Suicide in India. *Archives of Suicide Research*, *5*, 91–96.

Lester, D., Beck, A. & Trexler, L. (1975). Extrapolation from attempted suicide to completed suicide. *Journal of Abnormal Psychology*, *84*, 563–566.

Levinson, D. (1986). Development in the novice phase of early development. In G. Klerman (Ed.), *Suicide and depression among adolescents and young adults* (pp. 1–15). Washington, DC: American Psychiatric Press.

Lewinsohn, P., Garrison, C., Langhinrichsen, J. & Marsteller, F. (1989). *The assessment of suicidal behavior in adolescents: A review of scales suitable for epidemiological clinical research*. Rockville, MD: National Institute of Mental Health.

Lewis, G. & Fay, R. (1981). Suicide in pregnancy. *British Journal of Clinical Practice, 35*, 51–53.

Lichter, D. (1981). Diagnosing the dead: The admissibility of the psychiatric autopsy. *American Criminal Law Review, 18*, 617–635.

Litman, R. (1967). Sigmund Freud on suicide. In E. Shneidman (Ed.). *Essays in self-destruction* (pp. 324–344). New York: Jason Aronson.

Litman, R. (1984). Psychological autopsies in court. *Suicide and Life-Threatening Behavior, 14*, 1988–1995.

Litman, R. (1988). Psychological autopsies, mental illness and intention of suicide. In J. Nolan (Ed.). *The suicide case: Investigation and trial of insurance claims* (pp. 69–82). Chicago: American Bar Association.

Litman, R. (1994). Responsibility and liability for suicide. In E. Shneidman, N. Farberow & R. Litman (Eds), *The psychology of suicide* (pp. 187–199). Northvale, NJ: Aronson.

Litman, R. (1995). *Suicide without a clue*. Paper presented at the annual conference of the American Association of Suicidology, Phoenix, AZ, May.

Loranger, A., Sartorius, N., Andreoli, A., Berger, P., Buchheim, P., Channabasavanna, S., Coid, B., Dahl, A., Diekstra, R. & Regier, D. (1994). The International Personality Disorder Examination, IPDE. The WHO/ADAMHA international pilot study of personality disorders. *Archives of General Psychiatry, 51*, 215–224.

Luborsky, L., McLellan, A., Woody, G., O'Brien, C. & Auerbach, A. (1985). Therapist success and its determinants. *Archives of General Psychiatry, 42*, 602–611.

Lukianowicz, N. (1974). Suicidal behavior. *Psychiatrica Clinica, 7*, 159–171.

Mackinnon, R. & Michels, R. (1971). *The psychiatric interview in clinical practice*. Philadelphia, PA: W.B. Saunders.

Mahler, M. (1968). *On human symbiosis and the vicissitudes of individuation*. New York: International Universities Press.

Mallon, T. (1984). *A book of one's own: People and their diaries*. New York: Ticknor & Fields.

Maltsberger, J. (1984–1985). Consultation in a suicidal impasse. *International Journal of Psychoanalytic Psychotherapy, 10*, 131–158.

Maltsberger, J. (1986). *Suicide risk: The formulation of clinical judgment*. New York: New York University Press.

Maltsberger, J. (1990). The prevention of suicide in adults. In A. Leenaars (Ed.), *Life-span perspectives of suicide* (pp. 295–307). New York: Plenum.

Maltsberger, J. (1994). Calculated risk-taking in the treatment of suicidal patients: Ethical and legal problems. In A. Leenaars, J. Maltsberger & R. Neimeyer (Eds), *Treatment of suicidal people* (pp. 195–205). Washington, DC: Taylor & Francis.

Maltsberger, J. (2000). Letters across the Pacific. *Crisis, 21*, 154–155.

Maltsberger, J. (2002). Letters across the Pacific. *Crisis, 23*, 86–88.

Maltsberger, J. & Buie, D. (1974). Countertransference hate in the treatment of suicidal patients. *Archives of General Psychiatry, 30*, 625–633.

Mann, J. (1996, April). Neurobiological regulation of the threshold for suicidal behavior. Dublin Award paper presented at the conference of the American Association of Suicidology, St. Louis, MI.

Mann, J. & Arango, V. (1999). The neurobiology of suicidal behavior. In D. Jacobs (Ed.), *The Harvard Medical School guide to suicide assessment and intervention* (pp. 98–114). San Francisco: Jossey-Bass.

Maris, R. (1981). *Pathways to suicide*. Baltimore, MD: Johns Hopkins University Press.

Maris, R. (1985). The adolescent suicide problem. *Suicide and Life-Threatening Behavior, 15*, 91–109.

Maris, R. (1987, April). *Mid-life male suicides*. Paper presented at the American Association of Suicidology conference, San Francisco, CA.

Maris, R. (1991). The developmental perspective of suicide. In A. Leenaars (Ed.), *Life-span perspectives of suicide* (pp. 25–38). New York: Plenum.

Maris, R. (1993). The evolution of suicidology as a professional discipline. In A. Leenaars (Ed.), *Suicidology: Essays in honor of Edwin Shneidman* (pp. 3–21). Northvale, NJ: Jason Aronson.

Maris, R., Berman, A., Maltsberger, J. & Yufit, R. (Eds) (1992). *Assessment and prediction of suicide.* New York: Guilford.

Maris, R., Berman, A. & Silverman, M. (2000). *Textbook of suicidology.* New York: Guilford.

Martin, G. (1998). Media influence to suicide: The search for solutions. *Archives of Suicide Research, 4,* 51–66.

Marzuk, P. (1989, April). *AIDS-related suicides.* Paper presented at the American Association of Suicidology Conference, San Diego, CA.

Marzuk, P. (1994). Suicide and terminal illness. In A. Leenaars, J. Maltsberger & R. Neimeyer (Eds), *Treatment of suicidal people* (pp. 127–138). Hampshire, UK: Taylor & Francis.

Marzuk, P., Tardiff, K., Leon, A., Hirsch, C., Portera, L., Hartwell, N. & Iqbal, M. (1997). Lower risk of suicide during pregancy. *American Journal of Psychiatry, 154,* 122–123.

Maslow, A. (1966). *The psychology of science.* New York: Harper & Row.

McBride, H. & Siegel, L. (1997). Learning disabilities and adolescent suicide. *Journal of Learning Disabilities, 30,* 652–659.

McLeavey, B., Daly, R., Ludgate, J. & Murray, C. (1944). Interpersonal solving skills training in the treatment of self-poisoning patients. *Suicide and Life-Threatening Behavior, 24,* 382–394.

McIntosh, J. (1991). Epidemiology of suicide in the United States. In A. Leenaars (Ed.), *Life span perspectives of suicide* (pp. 55–69). New York: Plenum.

McIntosh, J., Hubbard, R. & Santos, J. (1983, April). *Suicide facts and myths: A compilation and study of prevalence.* Paper presented at the American Association of Suicidology Conference, Dallas, TX.

McLister, B. (1985). *Content analysis of genuine and simulated suicide notes using Foulkes' Scoring System of Latent Structure.* Unpublished PhD dissertation, Windsor, Canada.

McLister, B. & Leenaars, A. (1988). An empirical investigation of the latent content of suicide notes. *Psychological Reports, 63,* 238.

Meehl, P. & Rosen, A. (1955). Antecedent probability and the efficiency of psychometric signs, patterns, or cutting scores. *Psychological Bulletin, 52,* 194–216.

Meissner, W. (1981). *Internalization in psychoanalysis.* New York: International Universities Press.

Mellonie, B. & Ingpen, R. (1983). *Lifetimes.* New York: Bantam Books.

Meltzer, H. & O'Kayli, G. (1995). Reduction of suicidality during Clozaphine treatment of neuroleptic-resistant schizophrenia: Impact on benefit assessment. *American Journal of Psychiatry, 152,* 183–190.

Menninger, K. (1938). *Man against himself.* New York: Harcourt, Brace & Co.

Merikangas, K., Foeldenyi, M. & Angst, J. (1993). The Zurich study. *European Archives of Psychiatry, 243,* 23–32.

Michel, K. (1988). Suicide in young people is different. *Crisis, 9,* 135–145.

Michel, K. & Valach, L. (1997). Suicide as goal-directed action. *Archives of Suicide Research, 3,* 213–221.

Michel, K., Maltsberger, J., Jobes, D., Leenaars, A., Orbach, I., Stadler, K., Dey, P., Young, R. & Valach, L. (2002). Discovering the truth in attempted suicide. *American Journal of Psychotherapy, 56,* 424–437.

Mill, J. (1984). *Systems of logic.* London: George Routledge. (Original work published 1892.)

Miller, A. (1981). *Das drama des begabten kindes.* In R. Ward (Trans.), *The drama of the gifted child.* New York: Basic Books.

Miller, A. (1986). *Thou shalt not be aware.* New York: Meridian Books.

Minois, G. (1999). *History of suicide: Voluntary death in western culture.* Baltimore: The Johns Hopkins University Press.

Möller, H.-J. (2001). Pharmacological treatment of underlying psychiatric disorders in suicidal patients. In D. Wasserman (Ed.), *Suicide and unnecessary death* (pp. 173–178). London: Martin Dunitz.

Montgomery, S. (1997). Suicide and antidepressants. *Annals of New York Academy of Sciences, 836*, 329–338.

Morgan, H., Pocock, H. & Pottle, S. (1975). The urban distribution of non-fatal deliberate self-harm. *British Journal of Psychiatry, 126*, 319–328.

Motto, J. (1985). Preliminary field testing of a risk estimator for suicide. *Suicide and Life-Threatening Behavior, 15*, 139–150.

Motto, J. & Reus, V. (1991). Biological correlates of suicide across the life span. In A. Leenaars (Ed.), *Life span perspectives of suicide* (pp. 171–186). New York: Plenum.

Muller, M. (1887). *The science of thought*, 2 Vols. New York.

Muller-Oerlinghausen, B. (2001). Antisuicidal effects of lithium. In O. Grad (Ed.), *Suicide risk and protective factors in the new millennium* (pp. 85–90). Ljubljana: Cantarjeudom.

Murray, H. (1938). *Explorations in personality*. New York: Oxford University Press.

Murray, H. (1943). *Thematic Apperception Test* (Manual). Cambridge, MA: Harvard University Press.

Murray, H. (1967). Death to the world: The passions of Herman Melville. In E. Shneidman (Ed.), *Essays in self-destruction* (pp. 3–29). New York: Science House.

Murphy, G. (1992). *Suicide in alcoholism*. New York: Oxford University Press.

Murphy, G. & Robins, E. (1967). Social factors in suicide. *The Journal of the American Medical Association, 199*, 303–308.

Nagy, M. (1948). The child's view of death. *Journal of Genetic Psychology, 73*, 3–27.

National Police Agency (1986). *National Police Agency's 1985 annual report*. Tokyo: Printing Section of Ministry of Finance.

National Police Agency (1997). *National Police Agency's 1996 annual report*. Tokyo: Printing Section of Ministry of Finance.

Neihardt, J. (1932). *Black Elk speaks*. London: University of Nebraska Press.

Neugarten, B., Moore, J. & Lowe, J. (1965). Age norms, age constraints, and adult socialization. *American Journal of Sociology, 70*, 710–717.

Neuringer, C. (1962). Methodological problems in suicide research. *Journal of Consulting Psychology, 26*, 273–278.

Nietzsche, F. (1966). *Thus spoke Zarathustra* (W. Kaufmann, Trans.). New York: Viking Press.

Noreik, K. (1975). Attempted suicide and suicide in functional psychosis. *Acta Psychiatrica Scandinavica, 52*, 81–106.

NRC Handelsblad (1998, July). *Conformist Nonchalance*, 31.

O'Carroll, P. (1989). A consideration of the validity and reliability of suicide mortality data. *Suicide and Life-Threatening Behavior, 19*, 1–16.

O'Connor, R. & Leenaars, A. (2003). Suicide notes from Northern Ireland and the United States. *Current Psychology*. In press.

O'Connor, R., Sheeby, N. & O'Connor, D. (1999). A thematic analysis of suicide notes. *Crisis, 20*, 106–114.

Ogilvie, D., Stone, P. & Shneidman, E. (1969). Some characteristics of genuine versus simulated suicide notes. *Bulletin of Suicidology*, March: 19–26.

Ogloff, J. & Cronshaw, S. (2001). Expert psychological testimony: Assisting or misleading the trier of fact? *Canadian Psychology, 42*, 87–91.

Oliver, R. & Hetzel, B. (1972). Rise and fall of suicide rates in Australia: Relation to sedative availability. *The Medical Journal of Australia, 2*, 919–923.

Orbach, I. (1988). *Children who don't want to live*. San Francisco: Jossey-Bass.

Orbach, I. (2003). Suicide and the suicidal body. *Suicide and Life-Threatening Behaviour, 33*, 1–8.

Paciocco, D. (1999). Coping with expert evidence about human behaviour. *Queen's Law Journal, 25*, 305–346.

Palmer, B. & Bostwick, J. (2002, Sept.). *Suicide risk in schizophrenia: A meta-analysis*. Paper presented at the 9th European Symposium on suicide and suicidal behavior, University of Warwick, England.

Parad, H. (Ed.) (1965). *Crisis intervention*. New York: Family Service Association of America.

Pavese, C. (1961). *The burning brand: Diary 1935–1950* (A. Murch, Trans.). New York: Walker.

Peck, D. (1983). The last moments of life: Learning to cope. *Deviant Behavior, 4*, 313–332.

Peck. R. (1956). Psychological developments in the second half of life. In J. Anderson (Ed.), *Psychological aspects of aging*. Washington, DC: American Psychological Association.

Pfeffer, C. (1981a). Suicidal behavior in children: A review with implication for research and practice. *American Journal of Psychiatry, 138*, 154–160.

Pfeffer, C. (1981b). The family system of suicidal children. *American Journal of Psychotherapy, 35*, 330–341.

Pfeffer, C. (1986). *The suicidal child*. New York: Guilford.

Pfeffer, C. (1993). Suicidal children. In A. Leenaars (Ed.), *Suicidology: Essays in honor of Edwin Shneidman* (pp. 173–185). New York: Jason Aronson.

Philips, D. (1974). The influence of suggestion on suicide: Substantive and theoretical implications of the Werther effect. *American Sociological Review, 39*, 240–253.

Philips, D. (1986, April). *Effects of the media*. Paper presented at the American Association of Suicidology Conference, Atlanta, GA.

Phillips, M. & Liu, H. (1996, July). *Suicide in China*. Paper presented at the Befriender Conference, Kuala Lumpur, Malaysia.

Piaget, J. (1970). *Structuralism* (C. Maschler, Trans.). New York: Harper & Row.

Piaget, J. (1972). Language and thought from the genetic point of view. In P. Adams (Ed.), *Language in thinking* (pp. 170–179). Middlesex, England: Penguin.

Piaget, J. & Inhelder, B. (1969). *The psychology of the child*. New York: Harper Torchbooks.

Plath, S. (1975). *Letters home* (A. Plath, Ed.). New York: Harper & Row.

Plath, S. (1981). *The collected poems of S. Plath* (T. Hughes, Ed.). New York: Harper & Row.

Pokorny, A. (1983). Prediction of suicide in psychiatric patients. *Archives of General Psychiatry, 40*, 249–257.

Posner, J., Lahaye, A. & Cheifetz, P. (1989). Suicide notes in adolescence. *Canadian Journal of Psychiatry, 34*, 171–176.

Pritchard, C. (1996). Suicide in the People's Republic of China categorized by age and gender: Evidence of the influence of culture on suicide. *Acta Psychiatrica Scandinavica, 93*, 362–367.

R. vs *Beland* [1987] 2 SCR 398.

R. vs *D.D.* [1998] MJ No. 322.

R. vs *D.D.* [2000] SCC 43.

R. vs *Hawkins* [2001] NSWC 420.

R. vs *Mohan* [1994] 2 SCR 9.

Ramson, S., Bancroft, J. & Skumshire, A. (1975). Attitudes towards self-poisoning among physicians and nurses in a general hospital. *British Journal of Psychiatry, 127*, 257–264.

Reimer, C. & Arantewicz, G. (1986). Physician's attitudes towards suicide and their influence on suicide prevention. *Crisis, 7*, 80–83.

Reisman, J. (1973). *Principles of psychotherapy with children*. New York: John Wiley & Sons.

Resnick, P. (1969). Child murder by parents. *American Journal of Psychiatry, 126*, 325–334.

Richman, J. (1986). *Family therapy for suicidal people*. New York: Springer.

Richman, J. (1991). Suicide and the elderly. In A. Leenaars (Ed.), *Life span perspectives of suicide* (pp. 153–167). New York: Plenum.

Richman, J. (1993). *Preventing elderly suicide*. New York: Springer.

Rickgarn, R. (1994). *Perspectives in college student suicide*. Amityville, NY: Baywood.

Rifai, A., Reynolds, C. & Mann, J. (1992). Biology of elderly suicide. In A. Leenaars, R. Maris, J. McIntosh & J. Richman (Eds), *Suicide and the older adult* (pp. 48–61). New York: Guilford.

Robertson, J. (1988). *Psychiatric malpractice*. New York: John Wiley & Sons.

Robinson, E. (1953). Richard Cory. In L. Thompson (Ed.), *Tilbury Town: Selected poems of Edwin Arlington Robinson*. New York: Macmillan.

Rosen, A. (1954). Detection of suicidal patients: An example of some limitations in the prediction of infrequent events. *Journal of Consulting Psychology, 18*, 397–403.

Rosenblatt, P. (1983). *Bitter, bitter tears*. Minneapolis: University of Minnesota Press.

Rosenberg, M., Davidson, L., Smith, J., Berman, A., Ganter, G., Gay, G., Moore-Lewis, B., Mills, D., Murray, D., O'Carroll, P. & Jobes, D. (1988). Operational criteria for the determination of suicide. *Journal of Forensic Sciences, 32*, 1445–1455.

Roskill, M. (Ed.) (2000). *The letters of Vincent van Gogh*. London: Flamingo.

Rourke, R. & Fisk, J. (1981). Socio-emotional disturbances of learning disabled children: The role of central processing deficits. *Bulletin of the Orthopsychiatry Society*, *31*, 77–78.

Rourke, R., Young, G. & Leenaars, A. (1989). A childhood learning disability that predisposes those affected to adolescent and adult depression and suicide risk. *Journal of Learning Disabilities*, *22*, 169–175.

Rudestam, K. (1992). Research contributions to understanding the suicide survivor. *Crisis*, *13*, 41–46.

Runyan, W. (1982a). In defense of the case study method. *American Journal of Orthopsychiatry*, *52*, 440–446.

Runyan, W. (1982b). *Life histories and psychobiology*. New York: Oxford University Press.

Runyan, W. (1983). Idiographic goals and methods in the study of lives. *Journal of Personality*, *51*, 413–432.

Rutz, W., von Knorring, L. & Willinder, J. (1992). Long term effects of an educational program for general practitioners given by the Swedish Committee for the Prevention and Treatment of Depression. *Acta Psychiatrica Scandinavica*, *85*, 83–88.

SAS Institute, Inc. (1985). *SAS users guide. Statistics* (5th edn). Gary, N.C.: Author.

SAS Institute, Inc. (1995). *SAS users guide. Statistics*. Gary, N.C.: Author.

Sainsbury, P. & Barraclough, B. (1968). Differences between suicide rates. *Nature*, *220*, 1252.

Satcher, D. (1998). Bringing the public health approach to the problem of suicide. *Suicide and Life-Threatening Behavior*, *28*, 325–327.

Saunders, J. (2001). Experts in court: A view from the bench. *Canadian Psychology*, *42*, 109–118.

Schlebusch, L. & Bosch, B. (2000, April). *The Durban parasuicide study*. Paper presented at the South African Conference on Suicidology, Durban, South Africa.

Schmidtke, A. (1997). Perspectives: Suicide in Europe. In A. Leenaars, R. Maris & Y. Takahashi (Eds), *Suicide: Individual, cultural, international perspectives* (pp. 127–136). New York: Guilford.

Schwilbe, M. & Rader, K. (1982). Content analytic studies of emotionality in suicide letters and other texts written near death. *Zeitschrift für klinische Psychologie Forschung und Praxis*, *11*, 280–291.

Sederer, L. (1994). Managing suicidal inpatients. In A. Leenaars, J. Maltsberger & R. Neimeyer (Eds), *Treatment of suicidal people* (pp. 167–176). Washington, DC: Taylor & Francis.

Seiden, R. (1984). The youthful suicide epidemic. *Public Affair Report*. Los Angeles: Regents of the University of California.

Seuss, Dr (1954). *Horton hears a who!* New York: Random House.

Shakespeare, W. (1952). *Hamlet*. Chicago: William Benton.

Shneidman, E. (1949). Some comparison among Four Picture Test, Thematic Apperception Test, and Make a Picture Test. *Rorschach Research Exchange and Journal of Projective Techniques*, *13*, 150–154.

Shneidman, E. (1951). *Thematic Tests Analysis*. New York: Grune & Stratton.

Shneidman, E. (1963). Orientations toward suicide. In R. White (Ed.), *The study of lives*. New York: Atherton.

Shneidman, E. (1967). Sleep and self-destruction: A phenomenological approach. In E. Shneidman (Ed.), *Essays in self-destruction* (pp. 510–539). New York: Science House.

Shneidman, E. (1971). Suicide among the gifted. *Suicide and Life-threatening Behavior*, *1*, 23–45.

Shneidman, E. (1972). Foreword. In A. Cain (Ed.), *Survivors of suicide* (pp. ix–xi). Springfield, IL: Charles C. Thomas.

Shneidman, E. (1973). Suicide. In *Encyclopedia Britannica*, Vol. 21, 383–385. Chicago: Williams Benton.

Shneidman, E. (1975). Postvention: Care of the bereaved. In R. Pasnau (Ed.), *Consultation-liaison psychiatry* (pp. 245–256). New York: Grune & Stratton.

Shneidman, E. (1977). The psychological autopsy. In G. Gattschalh et al. (Eds), *Guide to the investigating and reporting of drug-abuse deaths* (pp. 42–56). Washington, DC: US PHEW, US Government Printing Office.

Shneidman, E. (1980). *Voices of death*. New York: Harper & Row.

Shneidman, E. (1981a). *Suicide thoughts and reflections: 1960–1980*. New York: Human Science Press.

Shneidman, E. (1981b). Logical content analysis. In E. Shneidman, *Suicide Thoughts and Reflections, 1960–1980*. New York: Human Science Press.

Shneidman, E. (1981c). Psychotherapy with suicidal patients. *Suicide and Life-threatening Behavior, 11*, 341–348.

Shneidman, E. (1982a). On "Therefore I must kill myself". *Suicide and Life-threatening Behavior, 12*, 52–55.

Shneidman, E. (1982b). The suicidal logic of Cesare Pavese. *Journal of the American Academy of Psychoanalysis, 10*, 547–563.

Shneidman, E. (1984). Aphorisms of suicide and some implications for psychotherapy. *American Journal of Psychotherapy, 38*, 319–28.

Shneidman, E. (1985). *Definition of suicide*. New York: John Wiley & Sons.

Shneidman, E. (1988). Foreword. In A. Leenaars, *Suicide notes* (pp. 9–10). New York: Human Sciences Press.

Shneidman, E. (1991). The commonalities of suicide across the life span. In A. Leenaars (Ed.), *Life span perspectives of suicide* (pp. 39–52). New York: Plenum.

Shneidman, E. (1992). Letter to the Editor: Rational suicide and psychiatric disorders. *New England Journal of Medicine, 326*, 889.

Shneidman, E. (1993). *Suicide as psychache*. Northvale, NJ: Aronson.

Shneidman, E. (1994a). Clues to suicide reconsidered. *Suicide and Life-threatening Behavior, 24*, 395–397.

Shneidman, E. (1994b). The Inman diary: Some reflections. In A. Leenaars, J. Maltsberger & R. Neimeyer (Eds), *Treatment of suicidal people* (pp. 3–15). Washington, DC: Taylor & Francis.

Shneidman, E. (1996). *The suicidal mind*. New York: Oxford University Press.

Shneidman, E. (1999a). An example of an equivocal death classified in a court of law. In A. Leenaars (Ed.), *Lives and deaths: Selections from the works of Edwin S. Shneidman* (pp. 415–443). Philadelphia: Brunner/Mazel.

Shneidman, E. (1999b). Psychotherapy with suicidal patients. In A. Leenaars (Ed.), *Lives and deaths: Selections from the works of Edwin S. Shneidman* (pp. 363–371). Philadelphia: Brunner/Mazel.

Shneidman, E. (1999c). Aphorisms of suicide and some implications for therapy. In A. Leenaars (Ed.), *Lives and deaths: Selections from the works of Edwin S. Shneidman* (pp. 372–382). Philadelphia: Brunner/Mazel.

Shneidman, E. (2001). Anodyne therapy: Relieving the suicidal patient's psychache. In H. Rosenthal (Ed.), *Favorite counseling and therapy homework assignments* (pp. 180–183). Philadelphia: Taylor & Francis.

Shneidman, E. & Farberow, N. (Eds) (1957a). *Clues to suicide*. New York: Harper & Row.

Shneidman, E. & Farberow, N. (1957b). The logic of suicide. In E. Shneidman & N. Farberow (Eds), *Clues to suicide* (pp. 31–40). New York: McGraw-Hill.

Shneidman, E. & Farberow, N. (1961). Statistical comparisons between attempted and committed suicides. In N. Farberow & E. Shneidman (Eds), *The cry for help* (pp. 19–47). New York: McGraw-Hill.

Shneidman, E. & Farberow, N. (1999). The Los Angeles Suicide Prevention Centre: A demonstration of public health feasibilities. In A. Leenaars (Ed.), *Lives and deaths: Selections from the works of Edwin S. Shneidman* (pp. 313–320). Philadelphia, PA: Brunner/Mazel.

Shneidman, E. & Mandelkorn, P. (1967). *How to prevent suicide*. Public Affairs Pamphlet. New York: Public Affairs Pamphlets, No. 406.

Siegel, S. (1956). *Nonparametric statistics*. New York: McGraw-Hill.

Silverman, E., Range, L. & Olverholser, J. (1994–95). Bereavement from suicide as compared to other forms of bereavement. *Omega, 30*, 41–51.

Skutsch, G. (1981a). Manic depression. *Medical Hypotheses, 7*, 737–746.

Skutsch, G. (1981b). Sex differences in seasonal variations in suicide rate. *British Journal of Psychiatry, 139*, 80–81.

Slaby, A. (1992). Creativity, depression and suicide. *Suicide and Life-threatening Behavior, 22*, 157–166.

Slaby, A. (1994). Psychopharmacotherapy of suicide. In A. Leenaars, J. Maltsberger & R. Neimeyer (Eds), *Treatment of suicidal people* (pp. 141–151). London: Taylor & Francis.

Slaby, A. (1995). Suicide as an indica of biologically based brain disease. *Archives of Suicide Research, 1,* 59–73

Smith, K. (1990). Therapeutic care of the suicidal student. In A. Leenaars & S. Wenckstern (Eds), *Suicide prevention in schools* (pp. 135–146). Washington, DC: Hemisphere.

Smith, K. & Maris, R. (1986). Suggested recommendations for the study of suicide and other life-threatening behaviors. *Suicide and Life-threatening Behavior, 16,* 67–69.

Smith, K., Conroy, M. & Ehler, P. (1984). Lethality of suicide attempt rating scale. *Suicide and Life-threatening Behavior, 14,* 215–242.

Sonneck, G., Etzersdorfer, E. & Nagel-Kuess, S. (1994). Imitative suicide in Viennese subway. *Social Science and Medicine, 38,* 453–457.

Soubrier, J. (1993). Definitions of suicide. In A. Leenaars (Ed.), *Suicidology: Essays in honor of Edwin Shneidman* (pp. 35–41). Northvale, NJ: Jason Aronson.

Speijer, N. & Diekstra, R. (1980). *Assisted suicide: A study of the problems related to self-chosen death.* Peventer: van Loghun Slaterur.

Spiegel, D. & Neuringer, C. (1963). Role of dread in suicidal behavior. *Journal of Abnormal and Social Psychology, 66,* 507–511.

Spirito, A. (2001, Nov.). *Psychotherapeutic interventions–short and long term.* Paper presented at "No Suicide" International Congress, Geneva, Switzerland.

Stack, S. (1991). Social correlates of suicide by age: Media impacts. In A. Leenaars (Ed.), *Life-span perspectives of suicide* (pp. 187–214). New York: Plenum.

Stahl, S. (2000). *Essential psychopharmacology.* Cambridge: Cambridge University Press.

Steer, R. & Beck, A. (1988). Use of the Beck Depression Inventory, Hopelessness Scale, Scale for Suicide Ideation and Suicide Intent Scale with adolescents. *Advanced Adolescent Mental Health, 3,* 219–231.

Stengel, E. (1964). *Suicide and attempted suicide.* Baltimore, MD: Penguin.

Stenger, E. & Stenger, E. (2000). Physical illness and suicidal behaviour. In K. Hawton & C. van Heeringen (Eds), *The international handbook of suicide and attempted suicide* (pp. 405–420). London: John Wiley & Sons.

Stoff, D. & Mann, J. (Eds) (1997). *The neurobiology of suicide: From the bench to the clinic.* New York: New York Academy of Sciences.

Stoller, R. (1973). *Splitting.* New York: Quadrangle Books.

Stone, A. & Shein, H. (1968). Psychotherapy of the hospitalized suicidal patient. *American Journal of Psychotherapy, 22,* 15–25.

Styron, W. (1990). *Darkness visible.* New York: Random House.

Sullivan, H. (1962). Schizophrenia as a human process, In H. Perry, N. Gorvell & M. Gibbens (Eds), *The collected works of Harry Stack Sullivan,* Vol. II. New York: W.W. Norton.

Sullivan, H. (1964). The fusion of psychiatry and social sciences. In H. Perry, N. Gorvell & M. Gibbens (Eds), *The collected works of Harry Stack Sullivan.* New York: W.W. Norton.

Sutton, L., Hawton, K., Haw, C., Sinclair, J. & Deeks, J. (2002, Sept.). *Risk factors for suicide in schizophrenia: A systematic review.* Paper presented at the 9th European Symposium on Suicide and Suicidal Behaviour, University of Warwick, England.

Takahashi, Y. (1992). *Clinical evaluation of suicide risk and crisis intervention.* Tokyo: Kongo-Shuppan.

Takahashi, Y. (1993). Suicide prevention in Japan. In A. Leenaars (Ed.), *Suicidology: Essays in honor of Edwin S. Shneidman* (pp. 324–334). Northvale, NJ: Jason Aronson.

Takahashi, Y. (1997). *Psychology of suicide.* Tokyo: Kodansha.

Takahashi, Y., Hirasawa, H. & Koyama, K. (1998). Restriction of suicide methods: A Japanese perspective. *Archives of Suicide Research, 4,* 101–107.

Tanyo, S. (2001, Nov.). *Psychopharmacotherapeutical synthesis of suicidal adolescents.* Paper presented at "No Suicide" International Congress, Geneva, Switzerland.

Tarachow, S. (1963). *An introduction to psychotherapy.* New York: International Universities Press, Inc.

Targum, S., Caputo, K. & Ball, S. (1991). Menstrual cycle phase and psychiatric admissions. *Journal of Affective Disorders, 22,* 49–53.

Task Force on Empirically Supported Therapy Relationships (2001). *Empirically sup-ported therapy relationships: Conclusions and recommendations of the Division 29 task force.* http://academic.uofs.edu/faculty/NORCROSS/empir.htm

Thakur, U. (1963). *History of suicide in India.* Munshi: Ram Manohar Lal.

The Medical Council of Ireland (1994). *Guide to Ethical Conduct.* Cork: Author.

Thomas, C. (1980). First suicide note? *British Medical Journal, 281,* 284–285.

Thorson, J. & Öberg, P.-A. (2003). Was there a suicide epidemic after Goethe's Werther? *Archives of Suicide Research, 7,* 69–72.

Tobin vs *Smith Kline Beecham* [2000], Wyoming Federal District Court.

Tomlinson-Keasey, C., Warren, L. & Elliot, J. (1986). Suicide among gifted women. *Journal of Abnormal Psychology, 95,* 123–130.

Toolan, J. (1981). Depression and suicide in children: An overview. *American Journal of Psychotherapy, 35,* 311–322.

Toynbee, A. (1968). *Man's concern with death.* New York: McGraw-Hill. Quoted in E. Shneidman (Ed.) *Death: Current perspectives.* Palo Alto: Mayfield Publishing Co.

Trad, P. (1990). *Treating suicide like behavior in a preschooler.* Madison, CN: International Universities Press.

Treolar, A. & Pinfold, T. (1993). Deliberate self-harm: An assessment of patients' attitudes to the care they receive. *Crisis, 14,* 83–89.

Tripodes, P. (1976). Reasoning patterns in suicide notes. In E. Shneidman (Ed.), *Suicidology: Contemporary developments* (pp. 203–228). New York: Grune & Stratton.

Tuckman, J. & Ziegler, R. (1968). A comparison of single and multiple note writers among suicides. *Journal of Clinical Psychology, 24,* 179–180.

Tuckman, J., Kleiner, R. & Lavell, M. (1959). Emotional content of suicide notes. *American Journal of Psychiatry, 116,* 1104–1106.

United Nations (1991). *Human rights and scientific and technological developments.* Report of the working group on the principles for the protection of persons with mental illness and for the improvement of mental health care. Resolution 98B. New York: Author.

US Department of Health and Human Services (1989). *Report of the secretary's task force on youth suicide.* Washington, DC: US Government Printing Office.

US Department of Health and Human Services, Indian Health Service (1996). *Trends in Indian Health—1996.* Rockville, MD: Office of Planning, Evaluation and Legislation Division of Program Statistics.

US Secretary Task Force on Youth Suicide (1980). *Report of the Secretary's Task Force on Youth Suicide,* Vols 1–4. Washington, DC: US Dept of Health & Human Services.

Van den Berg, J. & Grealish, E. (1996). Individualized services and supports through the wraparound process: Philosophy and procedures. *Journal of Child and Family Studies, 5,* 7–21.

Van der Maas, P., Van Delden, J. & Pijnenborg, L. (1992). *Euthanasia and other medical decisions concerning end of life.* Amsterdam: Elsevier Science.

Van der Wal, J. (1989–90). The aftermath of suicide: A review of the empirical evidence. *Omega, 20,* 149–171.

Van Heeringen, K. (2000). Multidisciplinary approaches to the management of suicidal behavior. In K. Hawton & K. van Heeringen (Eds), *The international handbook of suicide and attempted suicide* (pp. 571–581). New York: John Wiley & Sons.

Van Heeringen, K. & Apter, A. (2002, Sept.). *The Novartis workshop on schizophrenia.* Workshop presented at the 9th European Symposium on Suicide and Suicidal Behaviour, University of Warwick, England.

Van Hooff, A. (1990). *From autothanasia to suicide: Self-killing in classical antiquity.* London: Routledge.

Van Praag, H. (1997). Some biological and psychological aspects of suicidal behavior: An attempt to bridge the gap. In A. Botsis, C. Soldatos & C. Stefanis (Eds), *Suicide: Biopsychosocial approaches* (pp. 73–92). Amsterdam: Elsevier.

Varah, C. (Ed.) (1978). *Answers to suicide.* London: Constable.

Varah, C. (Ed.) (1985). *The Samaritans: Befriending the suicidal.* London: Constable.

Vergara, Y., Gonzales, I. & Rodriguez, Y. (1998). *Euthanasia*. Unpublished manuscript.

Verkes, R. & Cowen, P. (2000). Pharmacotherapy of suicidal ideation and behaviour. In K. Hawton & K. van Heeringen (Eds), *The international handbook of suicide and attempted suicide* (pp. 487–502). London: John Wiley & Sons.

Vessey, M., McPherson, K., Lawless, M. & Yeates, D. (1985). Oral contraception and serious psychiatric illness. *British Journal of Psychiatry, 146*, 45–49.

Victoroff, V. (1983). *The suicidal patient*. Oradell, NJ: Medical Economics Books.

Von Bertalanffy, L. (1967). *Robots, men and minds*. New York: George Braziller.

Vygotsky, L. (1962). *Thought and language* (E. Hanfmann & G. Vakar, Eds & Trans). Cambridge: The MIT Press.

Wagner, F. (1960). Suicide notes. *Danish Medical Journal, 7*, 62–64.

Wang H. (1989). Euthanasia in China. *Chinese Social Medicine, 6*, 11.

Wasserman, D. (Ed.) (2001). *Suicide—An unnecessary death*. London: Martin Dunitz.

Wasserman, D. (2001, Nov.). *The prevention of repeated suicide attempts*. Paper presented at "No Suicide" International Congress, Geneva, Switzerland.

Watzlawick, P., Beavin, J. & Jackson, D. (1967). *Pragmatics of human communication*. New York: Norton.

Wenckstern, S., Weizman, F. & Leenaars, A. (1984). Temperament and tempo of play in eight month old infants. *Child Development, 55*, 1195–1199.

West, L. (1993). Reflection on the right to die. In A. Leenaars (Ed.), *Suicidology: Essays in honor of Edwin Shneidman* (pp. 359–376). Northvale, NJ: Aronson.

White, R., Gribble, R., Corr, M. & Large, M. (1995). Jumping from a general hospital. *General Hospital Psychiatry, 17*, 208–215.

Wilkins, J. (1967). Suicidal behavior. *American Sociological Review, 32*, 286–298.

Wilson vs State (1961) 14 App. Div. 2d 976, 221 N.Y.S. 2d 354.

Windelband, W. (1904). *Geschichte und Naturwissenschaft* (3rd edn). Strassburg: Hertz.

Wislar, J., Grossman, J., Kruesi, J., Fendrich, M., Franke, C. & Ignatowicz, N. (1998). Youth suicide-related visits in an emergency department serving rural counties: Implications for means restriction. *Archives of Suicide Research, 4*, 75–87.

Wolff, H. (1931). Suicide notes. *American Mercury, 24*, 264–272.

World Health Organization (1992). *Statistics annual*. Geneva, Switzerland: Author.

World Health Organization (annual). Mortality data. *http://www.who.int*.

Wotton, K. (1985). Labrador mortality. In R. Fontaine (Ed.), *Circumpolar Health* (pp. 139–142). Seattle: University of Washington Press.

Zilboorg, G. (1936). Suicide among civilized and primitive races. *American Journal of Psychiatry, 92*, 1347–1369.

Zilboorg, G. (1937). Considerations on suicide, with particular reference to that of the young. *American Journal of Orthopsychiatry, 7*, 15–31.

Zubin, J. (1974). Observations on nosological issues in the classification of suicidal behavior. In A. Beck, H. Resnik & D. Lettieri (Eds), *The prediction of suicide* (pp. 3–25). Bowie, MA: Charles Press.

Index

depression (*cont.*)
  suicidal children 241–2, 248–9
  suicide relation 18, 19, 24–5, 46, 362–5
deprivation 18
Descartes, René 9, 22
desipramine 364
despair 349–51
  see also integrity vs despair
detoxification of environment 371–2, 374
development, elliptical 357
developmental perspective 55, 244–5,
    346–8, 368
Dexedrine 364
Dharmashastras (ancient Indian codes of
    living) 397–8
diagnosis
  DSM 91, 94, 98
  failure to diagnose 409–10
Diagnostic and Statistical Manual (DSM) 91,
    94, 98
diaries 127–8
Diekstra, René 36, 399
Diggory, James 85
Dillman vs Hellman 410
discharge from hospital 371
disorders in adjustment 382, 386
dissembling
  Dan 298
  Joe case 352
  Rick case 67, 148
  Shneidman 137, 150
  Susan case 294
  see also masking
dissociation 296–7
distortions 73–4
DNA 360–1
dominance need 47, 328
Don Schell case 363, 364, 366
Dora 74, 77
Dostoevsky, Fyodor 419–20
drawings, Justin's 233–5, 236, 237, 240–2
drug abuse 284–5, 329, 339, 368
DSM *see Diagnostic and Statistical Manual*
Durkheim, Émile 11, 33–4
duty 33–4
dynamic unconscious 73

education
  drug use 284–5
  means restriction 374, 415
  prevention 311
Effexor 364
ego
  adolescent suicide 55
  identifications 74
  Joe case 350

  Peter case 321
  positive egression 329
  Rick case 146
  Scott Dell case 157
  suicidal children 249
  suicide risk 99–100
  Susan case 295, 302, 315
  template 46–7
  therapists' responses 221
  Vincent Foster case 103
  Werther 64
  young adults 51
egression 20
  alcoholics 336
  attachment 129
  having sex 338
  Jennifer case 286–7
  Peter 324–5
  positive 329
  see also identification–egression
Elavil 360
elderly people
  hospitalization 368
  life-span developmental perspective
    355
  reasons for suicide 31
  suicide notes 356
  suicide rates 6
Eliot, T.S. 49
elliptical development 357
emotional clues 29
empirical research 50–61
empirical uniformities 385
environmental control 367, 369, 371–5
  see also means restriction
environmental factors 19
environmental precipitating events 25–6
Epicurus 8
epidemiology of suicide 5–6
Epstein, S. 67
Erikson, Erik
  age stages 50–1
  age-specific processes 55
  crisis 320
  developmental perspective 54, 244–5
  integrity vs despair 311, 320, 346–8, 356
  intimacy 299, 319
  late adulthood 346–8
  middle adulthood 319–20
  old people and death 356
  trust vs mistrust 330, 339
  young adulthood 319
ethical and legal issues 394–417
euthanasia 35–7, 399–404
excommunication 397
exhibition need 47

therapists, transference and
    countertransference 101–2, 205–6,
    308
therapists responses
    cognitive constriction 216–18
    ego 221
    identification–egression 226
    inability to adjust 219–21
    indirect expressions 218–19
    interpersonal relations 221–3
    rejection–aggression 224–5
    relationship implications 212–13
    unbearable psychological pain
        213–16
therapy relationships 211–12
Thioridazine 366
Thomas, C. 62
thought
    errors of 18
    suicidal 349
time-lines 31–2, 138, 346
Tomlinson-Keasey, C. 56
toxic substances 372, 374, 413
Toynbee, Arnold 310
transference
    and countertransference 101–4, 205–6,
        220, 280, 308–9
    healthy 313–14
    Joe case 353
    Peter case 333
trazadone 365
treatment
    of children 255–7
    termination 200, 204–5, 289–90, 306–7,
        314–15
Treolar, A. 369
triad of motives 75
trunk of suicide 31, 39–40, 98, 379
trust vs mistrust 330, 333, 339,
    341–2
Turtle Island 6, 394–5, 397, 398
    attitudes to suicide 32
    euthanasia 404
    responsibility of care 407–8
unbearable psychological pain
    adolescent suicide 55
    concept 20, 45, 98
    Jennifer case 290
    Plath 132
    Rick case 144
    Scott Dell case 156
    suicidal children 246–7
    TGSP-2 381–2, 385–6
    therapists' responses 213–16
    Vincent Foster 102
    Werther 63

unbearable suffering 400–1
unconscious
    attachment 74–6
    concept 16, 20, 66–7
    indirect expression 218–19
    Justin case 231, 252–5
    Natalie case 76–82
    Peter case 334–6, 339
    speculations 73–6
    suicide notes study 69–73
    Susan case 303–4
understanding 1
understanding need 48
unforgivable, forgiveness of the 342
United Nations Working Group on the
    Principles for the Protection of Persons
    with Mental Illness... 408–9
United States (US) 398
    euthanasia 403
    failure in care 410, 411
    legal issues 396
    means restriction 414
    negligence 412
    reasonable and prudent care standards
        404–6
    Task Force on Youth Suicide 35
    see also Turtle Island
unity thema 88, 131–2
USSR see Soviet Union

validation of TGSP 384–5
validity 86
Valium 360
van Gogh, Vincent 92, 267, 420–4
Varclus procedure 381
vengefulness–aggression 18, 79, 283, 383–4,
    386–7
Venlafaxine 364
verbal statements and behavioural clues
    28
verifiability of protocol sentences 20–1
Vienna 373
Vincent Foster Jr case see Foster
voices see introjects
voir dire (Scott Dell case) 189–93
Vorstellung (permanent existing idea) 385
Vygotsky, L. 84

Wasserman, D. 212
Weist, K. 33
Wenckstern, Susanne xiii
Werther 10, 62–5, 373
what have I learned 379–93
what have we learned 269–70, 290, 315,
    345, 357–8
WHO see World Health Organization

Compiled by Indexing Specialists (UK) Ltd.

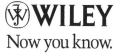

Printed and bound by CPI Group (UK) Ltd, Croydon, CR0 4YY

10/06/2025

14686745-0001